PSYCHIATRY

THE STATE OF THE ART

Volume 1
Clinical Psychopathology
Nomenclature and Classification

PSYCHIATRY
THE STATE OF THE ART

PSYCHIATRY

THE STATE OF THE ART

Volume 1
Clinical Psychopathology
Nomenclature and Classification

Edited by

P. PICHOT
Académie de Paris
Université René Descartes
Paris, France

and

P. BERNER, R. WOLF, and K. THAU
University of Vienna
Vienna, Austria

SPRINGER SCIENCE+BUSINESS MEDIA, LLC

Library of Congress Cataloging in Publication Data

World Congress of Psychiatry (7th: 1983: Vienna, Austria)
  Clinical psychopathology.

  (Psychiatry, the state of the art; v. 1)
  "Proceedings of the VII World Congress of Psychiatry, held July 11–16, 1983, in Vienna, Austria"—T.p. verso.
  Chiefly in English, with several papers in French and German.
  Includes bibliographies and indexes.
  1. Psychiatry—Congresses. 2. Psychiatry—Research—Congresses. 3. Psychology, Pathological—Nomenclature—Congresses. 4. Psychology, Pathological—Classification—Congresses. I. Pichot, Pierre. II. Title. III. Series. [DNLM: 1. Mental Disorders—classification—congresses. 2. Mental Disorders—congresses. 3. Psychiatry—congresses. W3 W05385 7th 1983c/WM 15 W9265 1983c]
  RC327.W63 1983a   616.89′0012   85-6314
  ISBN 978-1-4899-5051-2   ISBN 978-1-4899-5049-9 (eBook)
  DOI 10.1007/978-1-4899-5049-9

Proceedings of the VII World Congress of Psychiatry,
held July 11–16, 1983, in Vienna, Austria

© Springer Science+Business Media New York 1985
Originally published by Plenum Press, New York in 1985
Softcover reprint of the hardcover 1st edition 1985

PREFACE

The purpose of the World Psychiatric Association is to coordinate the activities of its Member Societies on a world-wide scale and to advance enquiry into the etiology, pathology, and treatment of mental illness. To further this purpose, the Association organizes mono- or multithematic Regional Symposia in different parts of the world twice a year, and World Congresses dealing with all individual fields of psychiatry once every five or six years. Between these meetings the continuation of the Association's scientific work is assured through the activities of its specialty sections, each covering an important field of psychiatry.

The programs of the World Congresses reflect on the one hand the intention to present the coordinating functions of the Association and on the other to open a broad platform for a free exchange of views. Thus, the VII World Congress of Psychiatry, held in Vienna from July 11 to 16, 1983, was composed of two types of scientific events - those structured by the Association and those left to the initiative of the participants. The first type comprised Plenary Sessions, planned by the Scientific Program Committee, and Section Symposia, organized by the WPA sections; the second embraced Free Symposia, free papers, video sessions, and poster presentations prepared by the participants. Altogether, 10 Plenary Sessions, 52 Section Symposia, and 105 Free Symposia took place, and 78 free papers and poster sessions and 10 video sessions were held.

The editors of the Proceedings of the VII World Congress of Psychiatry were immediately faced with two major problems, namely how to deal with such a great number of presentations and how to present them to the reader. The only way to solve the first difficulty was to restrict the Proceedings to Plenary Sessions and Symposia. The second obstacle was surmounted by grouping the Plenary Sessions and Symposia according to their scientific content, which meant waiving the chronological order of the Congress. In order to achieve reasonable uniformity in the lengths of the volumes, it was not possible to devote each of the eight books comprising the Proceedings to a single theme. Nevertheless, we hope that the final arrangement will enable colleagues interested in only certain subjects to restrict their purchases to the

particular volume or volumes of their choice. The Proceedings in
their entirety, however, represent a complete and comprehensive
spectrum of the current areas of concern in psychiatry - the state
of the art.

We are greatly indebted to our colleagues Rainer Wolf and
Kenneth Thau. Their untiring efforts made the publication of these
Proceedings possible.

Peter Berner

Secretary General, WPA
  at the time of the VII
  World Congress of Psychiatry
President, Organizing Committee
  VII World Congress of
  Psychiatry
Chief Editor, Congress Proceedings

ACKNOWLEDGMENTS

First and foremost, we should like to express our sincere appreciation to all colleagues whose scientific contributions comprise the content of these Proceedings.

We should also like to thank the immediate administrators of the VII World Congress of Psychiatry (Congress Team International), as well as the staff of the Vienna Secretariat of the World Psychiatric Association, for their collaboration in the compilation of this publication.

We should finally like to explain that, for technical reasons connected with the actual printing process, it has not been possible in every instance to eliminate minor typing errors.

Various reasons also prevented the compilation of all chapters in exact conformity with the presentations as contained in Plenary and Symposium Sessions.

Despite these problems, we hope that our aim to structure the content of the individual volumes as clearly as possible has met with an adequate measure of success.

INTRODUCTORY REMARKS

The World Psychiatric Association was born out of the Organizing Committee of the World Congress of Psychiatry. The first World Congress, held in Paris in 1950, was an event of the utmost importance. For the first time, psychiatrists of the whole world met to exchange their ideas and experiences and to promote the progress of our specialty. It later became obvious that such large congresses, convening every five or six years, needed to be complemented by a more permanent organization and by more frequent meetings smaller in scope and of a more specialized nature. The national psychiatric societies decided on the creation of a World Association which could assume all the responsibilities connected with such a complex task. I had the honor to be elected President of this Association at the VI World Congress in Honolulu and to hold this responsibility for six years until the advent of the Vienna Congress.

Whatever the importance of the various functions of the WPA, the organization of these World Congresses has remained its major task. It has become fashionable to criticize World Congresses because they attract too many participants, because the scientific presentations are not always of the highest quality, and because the multiplicity of the subjects discussed in simultaneous sessions obliges the participants to limit attendance to only part of the entire program. Some of the criticisms may be justified, but the fact remains that such congresses fulfill an important function. The majority of the psychiatrists of the world are not highly specialized research workers but practitioners. Many of them live in countries where they are relatively isolated and where there is little opportunity for scientific interchange. The World Congresses, by presenting not only the latest technical discoveries but also general surveys through leading specialists in the different fields of psychiatry, allow every participant to keep abreast of the state of the art. There is no better opportunity to become acquainted with developing trends, and personal experience of this type cannot be replaced by the reading of scientific journals. Of course, the value of such Congresses depends on the care with which the program is prepared. The readers of these Proceedings will have the opportunity to convince themselves that the Austrian Organizing Committee, under the chairmanship of Prof. Peter Berner,

Secretary General of the WPA at the time of the Congress, has attained this goal, and that the scientific quality of the papers presented and now printed is worthy of the tradition of our World Congresses of Psychiatry.

Pierre Pichot

President, WPA
  at the time of the VII
  World Congress of Psychiatry
President, Scientific Committee

CONTENTS

COMPREHENSIVE PSYCHOPATHOLOGICAL SCALES AND SYSTEMS

TRANSLATIONS OF THE AMDP SYSTEM

METHODOLOGICAL PROBLEMS IN THERAPEUTIC RESEARCH

EVALUATION OF TREATMENT METHODS

SYSTEMATIC AND SYSTEMIC PSYCHOPATHOLOGY

PLUS AND MINUS SYMPTOMATOLOGY IN SCHIZOPHRENIA

NEWER CONCEPTS OF BASIC DISORDERS AND BASIC SYMPTOMS IN ENDOGENOUS PSYCHOSES

ACTUAL PROBLEMS IN PARANOID PSYCHOSES

AETIOLOGY OF DEPRESSION IN SCHIZOPHRENIA

CONCEPTS IN NEUROTIC AND PERSONALITY DISTURBANCES

PANIC AND OTHER ANXIETY DISORDERS:
DIAGNOSIS AND TREATMENT

THE DELUSIONAL MISIDENTIFICATION SYNDROMES

PSYCHOPATHOLOGY OF SELF-DESTRUCTIVE BEHAVIOUR

RESEARCH IN SUICIDOLOGY

PSYCHOPATHOLOGY OF EXPRESSION

PSYCHOPATHOLOGY IN CRISIS?
3. GERMAN-JAPANESE-AUSTRIAN CONFERENCE

DIE PSYCHIATRIE IM PANORAMAWANDEL

DES 20. JAHRHUNDERTS

Heinrich Schipperges
Institut f. Geschichte der Medizin
Im Neuenheimer Feld 305
D-6900 Heidelberg 1

Vor wenigen Tagen erst haben wir - die Universitäten zu Basel und Heidelberg - ihn gefeiert, den 100. Geburtstag von Karl Jaspers, Arzt, Philosoph, Politiker, Weltbürger und, seiner Herkunft nach, Psychiater -: Jaspers, den einen ein Meilenstein in der Entwicklung der Psychiatrie, den anderen ein Memento für Stagnation und Resignation, alles in allem zweifellos ein Paradigma psychopathologischer Problematik. "Was in den letzten vierzig Jahren wissenschaftlich geschah", schreibt Jaspers (1942) in seiner "Psychopathologie", das sei nicht so ohne weiteres in eine einheitliche Ordnung zu bringen.

Um 1900 habe die Psychoanalyse zu wirken begonnen; Bleuler sei ihren Auswirkungen begegnet und habe damals "den haltbaren Bestand der Freudschen Lehren in das Gesamtbewußtsein der wissenschaftlichen Psychiatrie" hinübergerettet. Die großen biologischen Forschungsbewegungen, die Endokrinologie, die Vererbungslehre, die experimentelle Psychologie, sie alle hätten den Horizont der Psychiater wesentlich erweitert; seit Kretschmer (1921) sei zudem eine "Umprägung der Auffassung des Menschen als Konstitution" erfolgt.

Es sind freilich nicht die großen Männer, welche hier Geschichte machen oder gar das Schicksal der Psychiatrie im 20. Jahrhundert gestaltet haben, es sind - wie ich meinen möchte - letztlich die Phänomene, immer noch lebendig aus der weiterwirkenden Kraft älterer Traditionen, für die allerdings der Name "Psych-iatrie" am wenigsten zu bürgen in der Lage sein dürfte, geht es doch hier weder um die Selle noch um den Geist noch gar um das Gehirn -: hier geht es um das Ganze! Und damit sind wir am Thema!

Ich bin gebeten worden, in kurzen Zügen, in straffen Strichen die so markante Entwicklung der neueren Psychiatrie nachzuzeichnen, wobei ich

1

mich - als Historiker wie als Psychiater - zunächst einmal an dem offensichtlich vor sich gehenden Panoramawandel der Medizin im 20. Jahrhundert orientieren möchte. Das Wort "Panorama" will dabei ganz wörtlich genommen werden: als Überblick über eine weitgegliederte Landschaft von einem möglichst hohen Standpunkt aus, der dennoch Einblicke erlaubt in die Einzelheiten, eine prismatische Perspektive also, noch einmal dramaturgisch gesteigert durch die zeitlichen Veränderungen, die strukturellen Entwicklungen und Verkümmerungen, durch ein Geschehen, wie es nirgendwo in der modernen Medizin abenteuerlicher vor sich geht als auf den Gebieten der Psychiatrie.

Vor einer notwendigen Wandlung, und mehr noch Wendung, hatte Viktor von Weizsäcker bereits (1928) die Medizin seiner Zeit gesehen, als er schrieb: "Eine Situation ist gegeben, eine Tendenz kommt auf, eine Spannung steigt an, eine Krise spitzt sich zu ..... und mit ihr, nach ihr ist die Entscheidung da; eine neue Situation ist geschaffen und kommt zu einer Ruhe, Gewinne und Verluste sind jetzt zu übersehen. Das Ganze ist wie eine historische Einheit: Wendung, kritische Unterbrechung, Wandlung".

Mit dieser geradezu klassischen Beschreibung eines Paradigmawechsels ließe sich nun auch der Panoramawandel in der Psychiatrie genauer fassen, wobei das Psychische und alle Psychosen ein Rätsel sind und bleiben. "Daß es das gibt" - schreibt Jaspers in seiner "Psychopathologie" (1913) -, "daß Welt und Mensch derart ist, daß dieses möglich und notwendig ist, läßt uns nicht nur staunen, sondern auch schaudern".

Lassen Sie mich gleichwohl versuchen, in dieser festlichen Runde, in einer knappen halben Stunde, drei Problemkreise herauszugreifen: 1. und zuoberst die so dynamisch aufflutenden Strömungen des 20. Jahrhunders, die wir kaum schon zu fassen vermögen und die uns in jene Krise geführt haben, die ich 2. als die Psychiatrie im Dilemma bezeichnen möchte, eine drohende und bedrohliche Aporie, eine Ausweglosikeit, aus der wir 3. und abschließend die sich heute schon abzeichnenden Wege für eine Psychiatrie von morgen wenigstens andeuten sollten.

1. Die Strömungen des 20. Jahrhunderts

Die Psychiatrie ist in der Tat im Verlaufe des 20. Jahrhunderts in eine stürmische Bewegung geraten, wobei es weniger die seelischen Störungen waren, kaum auch die Geistes-Krankheiten, was hier als Motor gewirkt hat, sondern eher die Begenung der Psychiatrie mit dem ganzen Menschen. Psychiatrie ist auf dem Wege - so vor 150 Jahren schon J. M. Leupoldt (1833) - "im Ganzen mehr und mehr wahrhaftig anthropolgische" zu werden. Vor diesem Hintergrund erst werden wir in der Lage sein, die Strömungen und ihre Richtungen, alle Markierungen und Verknotungen deutlicher zu gewahren.

Geschichte der Psychiatrie, das wäre immer auch die Psychiatrie selbst! Der

2

Historiker der Medizin, der die Entwicklungen der letzten drei Jahrhunderte einigermaßen zu überblicken in der Lage ist, findet freilich nirgendwo ein Fach oder auch nur ein Phänomen vor wie "die Psychiatrie". Wie jung ist dieses Fach! Um 1870 erst wurde im deutschsprachigen Raum ein klinisch-psychiatrischer Unterricht als notwendig empfunden. Um 1880 begann man Universitätskliniken zu errichten. Seit dem Jahre 1901 erst ist die Psychiatrie bei uns ein Prüfungsfach im Staatsexamen.

Dabei hatte es die "Allgemeine Zeitschrift für Psychiatrie", 1844 gegründen von Damerow, Flemming und Roller, bereits um die Mitte des vorigen Jahrhunderts vestanden, die verschiedensten konstituierenden Elemente dieser Psychiatrie "wie die Stimmen einer Fuge" nacheinander hervortreten zu lassen: die naturwissenschaftliche Forschung wie die klinische Psychopathologie und synoptisch über beiden eine anthropologische Gesamtschau (Bodamer, 1953). Für das 20. Jahrhundert sucht man im wuchernden Zeitschriftenwald vergebens nach einem gleichrangigen repräsentativen Organ, das die modernen Entwicklungen adäquat zu spiegeln in der Lage wäre.

Darf ich dennoch erinnern an das, was wir alle erlebt haben: Um 1900 erst konnten die hirnanatomischen Forschungen (von Wernicke zu Kleist) in Blüte kommen. Um 1910 stand die Klinische Forschung ganz und gar unter der Kontrolle der Pathologischen Anatomie. Der organischen Raumpsychiatrie begegneten gleichzeitig die tiefen-psychologischen Bewegungen. Mit den 20er Jahren erlebten wir die Konstitutionspsychiatrie, mit den 30er Jahren den Aufbau einer Sozielpsychiatrie, gesteigert durch den Einbruch der Antipsychiatrie. Seit dem Jahre 1952 wurden systematisch Psychopharmaka in Form von Neuroleptika und Thymoleptika zum Einsatz gebracht und zu strategischen Verfahren entwickelt, mit biologischen und psychischen Nebenwirkungen, aber auch einem uns alle frappierenden Wandel der klinischen Atmosphäre. In den letzen zwanzig Jahren kam es zu weiteren stürmischen Entwicklungen in allen Lagern: der Neurophysiologie und Neuropsychiatrie ebenso wie der Vererbungslehre, der Verhaltenspsychologie, der Familienforschung, der Gruppentherapie, der Personalen Psychiatrie.

Wer uns freilich zumutet, so Gaupp schon 1903, darauf zu warten, bis uns der Zusammenhang der psychischen mit den materiellen Vorgängen im Gehirn bekannt ist, "der vertröstet uns auf eine Zunkunft, die wohl niemals Wirklichkeit wird". Wollen wir warten, bis wir alle die klinischen Bilder aus ihren anatomischen Grundlagen begreifen, "so können wir bis an der Welt Ende warten". Bis dahin aber bliebe die Psychiatrie nicht viel mehr als die "idiotische Schwester der anderen medizinischen Disziplinen".

Thomas S. Kuhn (1962) unterscheidet denn auch zwei Typen der wissenschaftlichen Entwicklung: den normalen, ständig wachsenden, sich stetig perfektionierenden Duktus und den revolutionären, nichtkumulativen Umbruch, wo Gedankenfragmente sich immer wieder neu zusammensetzen und Denkmuster offenbar werden, wie sie zuvor nicht sichtbar waren. Aus vielen Aspekten erst ergibt das Ganze einen Sinn, der aus den isolierten

Teilen nicht ersichtlich war. Es genügt sicherlich nicht, die Strömungen in ihre Elemente zu zerlegen; revolutionäre Verhältnisse haben eine ganzheitliche Struktur, liefern ein System von Generalisierungen, als deren Prüfstein uns z. B. die Sprache erscheint. Hier zeigt sich der janusköpfige Charakter jeder wissenschaftlichen Sprache, mit der sich unabdingbar verbunden auch unser Wissen über die Natur verändert, wobei man sich davor hüten sollte, die "Veränderung des Jargons" schon als "Fortschritt der Erkenntnis" gelten zu lassen (Jaspers, 1913).

Wir erkennen heute, am Ausgang des 20. Jahrhunderts, daß diese "Psychiatrie in Bewegung" nicht zu begreifen sein wird ohne die Motivationen und Tendenzen jenes 19. Jahrhunderts, das in allem eher Vorfeld ist als Geschichte, gleichwohl die "dunkelste aller Epochen", wie Heidegger sie genannt hat, zumal keines der tragenden Probleme dieses Zeitalters der Naturwissenschaft bis zum Tage eine gültige und glaubwürdige Lösung hat finden können.

Den somatischen Generalansatz Griesingers glaubte Meynert (1835 - 1892), Schüler von Hyrth und Rokitansky in Wien, vor mehr als 100 Jahren schon so weit gesichert, daß er alle bisherige Psychiatrie als "Wolkenwelt" (1876) verlästern konnte, um dann seinerseit im Urwald des Hirnfaserdickichts auf nebulöse psychische Beute zu gehen. Am konsequentesten wohl hat Wernicke (1848 - 1905) die Struktur der Seele mit der Struktur des Gehirns in eine verbindliche Kongruenz gebracht. Damals wurde das grundgelegt , was sich ein Jahrhundert lang hat halten können, was ich selber noch aus dem Munde von Oskar und Cecile Vogt - vor genau 30 Jahren (1953) bei einem Besuch in Neustadt - erfahren durfte "daß somatische Hirnveränderungen die letzte Grundlage der pathologischhen Phänomene bilden".

Organisches Leitbild psychischer Krankheit blieb nicht von ungefähr und für lange Zeit jene Progressive Paralyse, die - wieder hier in Wien - Wagner v. Jauregg zum diagnostischen Prototyp, zur "Krankheitseinheit", zum therapeutischen Leitbild gestalten konnte. Hier in Wien erscheinen auch Meynerts "Vorlesungen über Psychiatrie auf wissenschaftlichen Grundlagen" (1890). Das primär somatopathologische Erscheinungsbild, es war jedesmal nur Ausdruck eines abnormen Spiels des Hirnmechanismus, wobei es zu einer höchst charakteristischen Phasenverschiebung vom physikalischen Modell zum dynamischeren Biochemismus gekommen ist.

Gegenüber dieser Strömung bildete sich mit dem neuen Jahrhundert bald schon eine Gegenbewegung, die mit dem Namen Sigmund Freuds verbunden ist und bleibt. Die geschichtliche Rolle der Psychoanalyse war sicherlich von weittragender Bedeutung, aber diese Rolle scheint ausgespielt. Ihre Entwicklung und Entfaltung erscheint uns heute voller Brüche, Umbrüche und Absprünge, ohne daß daraus eine Richtung oder gar eine Psychiatrie in Bewegung geworden wäre.

Wir haben heute genug Distanz von Freud, um konstatieren zu können, daß etwa die Hälfte aller Literatur des 20. Jahrhunderts ohne Freud nicht das

Licht der Welt erblickt hätte. Wir haben aber auch genug Kritik an der Hand, um differenzieren und urteilen zu können, daß die Psychoanalyse weder die einzige, noch die beste oder gar die ideale Methode wäre (vgl. Kretschmer, 1982). Wer anfangs geglaubt hatte, mit einer Analyse den "Gang zu den Müttern" angetreten zu haben, der fand sich bitter enttäuscht.

Freud, so möchte man meinen, ist ein Versprechen gewesen, das wohl nie gehalten werden kann. Immerhin gewann die Psychoanalyse einen Zugang zu jener Theorie der Therapeutik, wie sie bisher weder von der Physiologie noch von der Pathologie konzipiert werden konnte; sie gewann ein neues System der Semiotik, wobei die Anamnese aus der Verdrängung, die Diagnose mit der Analytik, die Prognose im Individuationsprozeß jeweils semantisch interpretiert werden. Die Medizin als Naturkunde, sie gewinnt Kontakt zu Geschichte und Gesellschaft. Der Mensch als der Architekt seines Leibes, er wird wieder - wie Schopenhauer ihn kannte und nannte - der Dramaturg seines eigenen Schicksals.

Eine spätere Generation vielleicht schon wird eher die Abfall-Bewegungen verfolgen, die dieses ganze Jahrhundert durchzittern, am entschiedensten vollzogen von Carl Gustav Jung (1875 - 1961), der sich energisch von der dogmatischen Lehre gelöst hat, die er (1930) entartet fand "zu einem krankhaften Kellergewächs". Mit den Wandlungsgesetzen der "Seele als eines subjektiven Kosmos" versuchte Jung die Bedeutungtiefe des Daseins psychologisch zu erschließen. Das gilt noch einmal gesteigert für Viktor E. Frankl, der mit seiner "Logotherapie" im Gespräch mit dem Patienten die jeweils erreichbaren Sinnbereiche zu erarbeiten suchte und darin zu einer Art "ärztlicher Seelsorge" kam, zu einer Logotherapie wahrhaftig "in spiritu Apollinis".

Lassen Sie mich den ersten Aspekt ganz kurz zusammenfassen! Am Ausgang des 20. Jahrhunderts imponiert uns die Psychiatrie als ein Erbe der Biologie, die als Psychopharmakologie über die Naturprozesse des Gehirns verfügen lernte, als Erbe der Psychologie, wobei die physikalische Programmatik bald schon aufgegeben wurde zugunsten einer seelischen Trieblehre, nicht zuletzt auch als Erbe der Philosophie, deren Hermeneutik einer phänomeologischen Psychopathologie die Leitlinien gab, um damit aber auch die Bezugssysteme zu jener Gesellschaft offenzulegen, die unsere Realität am konkretesten widerspiegelt.

Die Psychiatrie hat ganz bewußt und sehr energisch den Anschluß an die naturwissenschaftliche Medizin gesucht und - über die Hirnforschung - auch gefunden. Aber sie ist nie wirklich in die Medizin integriert worden. Die Neurologie hat sich längst emanzipiert; die Psychoanalyse geht ihren eigenen, eigensinnigen Weg. "Psychotherapie" als eigenes Fach aber wäre ein Nonsens zu einer Zeit, wo man einsieht, daß Leib und Seele keine Sonderheiten sind, sondern Aspekte des Ganzen. "Meine Seele" - schreibt Kant in "Träume eines Geistersehers" -, sie "ist ganz im ganzen Körper und ganz in jedem seiner Teile".

2. Psychiatrie im Dilemma

Damit aber sind wir schon mitten in unserem zweiten, empfindlichsten Fragenfeld, einer Psychiatrie im Dilemma, im Zwiespalt, einer Zwickmühle und Zwangslage, vielleicht einer Ausweglosigkeit, der Aporie.

Vor hundert Jahren schon glaubte die moderne Medizin, ihren wissenschaftlichen Standard erreicht zu haben und im Reigen der Naturwissenschaften parmanenten Fortschritt spielen zu können. Sie hatte "tabula rasa" gemacht mit aller Tratidion, um mit bewährten physikalischen und chemische Methoden jener umfassenden Heiltechnik den Weg zu bahnen, die zu immer weiteren Erfolgen prädestiniert schien und die unerschöpflichen Segen zum Wohle der Menschheit zu produzieren versprach. In diese Entwicklung der neuen Medizin eingeschlossen wurde - zwar verspätet, aber dann doch auffallend systematisch - auch die moderne Psychiatrie, obschon gerade sie immer zwielichtig bleib als Naturwissenschaft, wie sie auch in kein seriöses Verhältnis kam zu den Geisteswissenschaften, von den Gesellschaftswissenschaften gar nicht zu reden.

Dieses wissenschaftliche Fundament der Medizin ist in den letzten Jahrzehnten, wie Sie alle wissen und spüren, erschüttert worden. Die Medizin als eine angewandte Naturwissenschaft, zunehmend begleitet von sozialen Kompetenzverlagerungen und systemimmanenten Gleichgewichtsverlusten, wurde überholt und untergraben oder kompensiert durch eine gegenstrebige Medizin in Bewegung -: und sie wird heute insgesamt und als System attackiert.

Die Medizin gilt - wenn man den kritischen Stimmen glauben will - längst nicht mehr als die Wohltäterin der Menschheit; sie dient eher der Profitmaximierung einer bürgerlichen Leistungsgesellschaft. Der Arzt wird folglich definiert und diffamiert als der "Kesselflicker des Kapitals", insonderheit der Psychiater, der seine Gehirnwäsche betreibt, um aus wachen und unruhigen Kranken brave und gesunde Marionetten zu machen, wo es doch seine Aufgabe sein sollte, psychisches Leiden transparent zu halten, um es zu transformieren auf politische Aktion. Soweit die Schalgworte!

Mit Freud hat - so scheint es - eine gewaltige dionysische Gegenbewegung eingesetzt gegen die Grundpositionen jener Medizin, die seit jeher auf das Apollinische eingeschworen war: auf Apollon, den Arzt, den Heilgott. Auf keinem Gebiete unserer Wissenschaft hat sich denn auch die Theorie von den "zwei Kulturen" unheilvoller auswirken können als in den psychiatrischen Disziplinen. Alexander Mitscherlich hat mit Recht von "den beiden Medizinern der Gegenwart" gesprochen, die in ihrer Intoleranz nirgendwo offenkundiger wird als in der Psychiatrie.

Hervorgegangen aus einem humanisierenden Engagement (von Paracelsus bis zu Pinel) kam es auch in der Psychiatrie zu einer charakteristischen

Konversion zur naturwissenschaftlichen Methodik (über Griesinger zu Kraepelin), ehe sie wieder aufgebrochen wurde in die personalen Dimensionen (bei Freud, bei Weizsäcker u.a.). Während zur reinen Philantropie sich die strenge Naturwissenschaft gesellt, wird diese hinwiederum zu kompensieren versucht durch die Hermeneutik. Die moderne Psychiatrie ist daher ebenso das Erbe der Naturwissenschaft wie auch der Seelenwissenschaft oder der Geisteswissenschaft. Neben solchen methodologischen Grundfragen werden in Zukunft zweifellos auch konkretere Realitäten dominieren: das massenhafte Auftreten akuter exogener Zustandsbilder, etwa der Suchten, die erschreckende Zunahme der Defekt- und Abbausyndrome, etwa bei Alterspsychosen, die mißlungenen Anpassungssyndrome einer unter- wie auch überentwickelten Massengesellschaft und damit ein eklatanter Wandel der psychiatrischen Klientel. Es sind längst nicht mehr die Ordnungprinzipien von Klöstern, Kasernen und Kliniken, welche die Unterbringung und Versorgung von psychisch Kranken garantieren.

Unter dem Stichwort der "Anti-Psychiatrie", dieser blauen Blume einer rosaroten Romantik, läßt sich denn auch die mit den 70er Jahren aufkommende elementare Unsicherheit auf allen Gebieten der Psychietrie am ehesten verstehen als eine fundamentale Verunsicherung dieser unserer für Idologien so anfälligen Disziplin. Die Antipsychiatrie sollte daher auch als eine Antwort auf die Krise der Schulpsychiatrie und der Asylpsychiatrie gewertet werden. Sie ist nicht von ungefähr zum Kampfbegriff der "kritischen" Psychiatrie geworden, ohne damit schon "Polit-Psychiatrie" zu sein. Sie ist augenscheinlich aber auch jenen uralten utopischen Vorstellungen erlegen, die besagen, die Psychiatrie könne und müsse der Vorläufer einer Kulturrevolution werden, sollte "gegen alles ankämpfen, was die Solidarität zwischen den Menschen untereinander und die Solidarität zwischen dem Menschen und seiner Umwelt bedroht", Psychiatrie müsse - mit einem Wort -zu einem "authentischen Menschsein" führen (so Jean Foundraine, 1976).

Vor dem Hintergrund der letzten hundert Jahre jedenfalls spricht nichts für jene "dritte Revolution in der Psychiatrie", die man postuliert hat als eine neue, die dynamische und soziale Psychiatrie (Basaglia), wobei als "erste Revolution" die legendäre Befreiung der Irren von ihren Ketten angesehen wird uns als "zweite Revolution" jene psychoanalytische Bewegung, die eher zu einem Mythos verbrämt wurde als daß sie dem Logos gedient hat. Wir können es uns einfach nicht leisten, einer anti-wissenschaftlichen Spekulation oder aber rein politischen Protesten das Wort zu reden, wie wir auch niemals huldigen sollten dem ehemals in Wien so drastisch demonstrierten und auch heute wieder so modisch gewordenen therapeutischen Nihilismus.

Auf keinem Felde der modernen Medizin hat sich die Kluft zwischen Theorie und Praxis verhängnisvoller ausgewirkt: hier die vornehmere Installation einer letztlich im akademischen Raume doch nicht anerkannten Universitäts-Psychiatrie, dort die Asyle, die Heilanstalten einer blassen Versorgungs-Psychiatrie, während doch Forschung und Lehre, Behandlung und Versorgung zugleich nur möglich erscheinen in einem hochkomplexen integrativen Verbundsystem.

Von den "drei Hügeln" im Panorama der Psychiatrie hatte - um die Mitte des 20. Jahrhunderts noch - Kurt Schneider gesprochen: einer mittleren gewaltigen Hügelkette, repräsentiert durch die psychopathologische Forschung, einer weiteren Bergkette, welche "die Wissenschaft von den körperlichen Grundlagen der Psychosen" symbolosiere und jener Hügellandschaft der psychogenen Störungen schließlich, "bei denen die Psychotherapie unbestritten im Recht war ". Das gilt auch heute noch, wo man meinen könnte, der mittlere Hügel sei völlig abgetragen, das "Bergwerk der Psychopathologie" (wie Schneider das nannte) erschöpft und die "klinische Psychiatrie" am Ende (Schneider, 1952). Und damit sind wir abermals auf den empfindlichsten Punkt, das "punctum saliens", gestoßen: das klinische Interesse an Grundphänomenen um Natur und Geist, Leib und Seele, Person und Welt, die ohne philosophische Prinzipien und Kriterien kaum zu klären und ohne klinischen Einsatz der ganzen Person nicht zu behandeln sind.

Der Mensch als Ganzes freilich, er wird nie - so Jaspers - "Gegenstand der Erkenntnis. Es gibt kein System des Menschseins ..... Alle Erkenntnnis geschieht in partikularen Aspekten, zeigt jedesmal eine Wirklichkeit, aber nicht die Wirklichkeit des Menschen, ist schwebend, nicht endgültig. Der Mensch ist immer mehr, als er von sich weiß und wissen kann und als irgendein anderer von ihm weiß". Aus dieser Einsicht des Philosophen Jaspers das Bekenntnis des Klinikers: "Wir möchten das Bewußtsein der Unerschöpflichkeit und Rätselhaftigkeit jedes einzelnen geisteskranken Menschen auch den scheinbar alltäglichsten Fällen gegenüber nicht verlieren".

Hier im Alltag erst beginnt die Sache ernst zu werden, ruft nach Normen und einem verbindlichen Bezugssystem. Ethische Grundfragen dieser Art begleiten und belasten das gesamte Indikations-Spektrum der Psychiatrie, angefangen vom immer bedenklichen Eingriff und einer Motivation zum Eingreifen über die ganze Kette intervenierender Maßnahmen, der Prävention und Kuration ebenso wie der Rehabilitation und Resozialisierung, bis hin zur immer von neuem notwendigen Legitimation eines Eingriffs, der immer auch verbunden bleibt mit Mißgriff, Fehlgriff, Übergriffen. Versuchsplanung und Qualitätssicherung, sie sind neuerdings, und in Zukunft vermehrt, zum Thema sog. "Ethikkommissionen" geworden, wie sie in Europa allerorts von Ärztegremien, Medizinischen Fakultäten und Standesorganisationen eingerichtet werden und bald auch im Raum der Psychiatrie.

Mit seinem therapeutischen Optimismus hat vor allem Adolf Meyer in den USA einer Psychiatrie die Bahn gebrochen, in welcher der klinische Aspekt - und nicht die Therapie der Menschheit - im Mittelpunkt steht. Bei allen Kreisbewegungen - in die Öffentlichkeit, über die Laienbewegung, mit den Methoden der "re-education" - erwartet auch Erwin Straus von der Psychiatrie, daß sie wieder zurückfinden werde zur klinischen Betrachtungsweise (Straus, 1950).

"Das Zeitalter der Krankheiten ist vorüber. Die Ära des kranken Menschen hat unleugbar begonnen". So schrieb mir Eugen Kahn am 3. Februar 1966, und weiter. "Wird der Kranke sich selber kurieren können oder mit den bisher verfehlten Behandlungsmethoden nur seinen Hinschied beschleunigen? Lassen Sie uns versuchen, optimistisch zu sein" -, ein prinzipieller Rat meines väterlichen Freundes Eugen Kahn, den ich dankbar weitergeben darf.

3. Neue Wege der Psychiatrie

Mit diesem therapeutischen Optimismus sind wir nun im dritten und letzten Aspekt auf die neuen Wege der Psychiatrie gestoßen, uralte Pfade im Grunde genommen, Wege in die Welt von morgen, die ich wenigstens andeuten sollte. Als Kern aller Psychiatrie bleibt - wie ich meinen möchte - der ärztliche Auftrag, fachkundige Hilfe zu leisten in seelischer Not, um die Not zu wenden, zu lindern, zu helfen, zu heilen. Aus dem reißenden Strudel begrifflicher Relativierung rettet uns letzten Endes immer wieder und immer nur die klinische Erfahrung, das, was einem Arzte an Erscheinungen begegnet mit jedem einzelnen Kranken. Der klinische Aspekt bildet nun einmal das Zentrum: als der Blick auf den einzelnen Menschen, der gestört ist und gekränkt wurde und nun als krank erscheint, als hilfebedürftig.

Erinnern darf ich an dieser Stelle an das eindrucksvolle Memento meines verehrten Lehrers Manfred Bleuler, der kürzlich (1975) davor gewarnt hat, daß der Arzt sich von der Seite des Kranken entferne und der Kranke immer einsamer werde. "Je mehr wir uns vom Kranken weglocken lassen und unsere Aufgabe als Ärzte und sogar als psychiatrische Fachärzte in anderen Bereichen als am Kranken sehen, desto mehr zerfällt die Medizin und die Psychiatrie als medizinisches Fach, desto weniger verdienen wir, Arzt genannt zu werden. Verdienen wir es nicht mehr und treten andere an unsere Stelle, so werden humanitäre Werte von größter gesellschaftlicher Bedeutung, die bisher uns Ärzten zufielen, in andere Hände gelegt - oder sie gehen verloren".

Mit diesem Memento kommen wir abschließend noch kurz auf die Konzepte der "patientenorientierten", einer sog. Anthropologischen Psychiatrie zu sprechen, auf ihre Möglichkeiten - und mehr noch Grenzen. Aus drohender Erstarrung befreit wurde die Kraepelin'sche Psychiatrie in erster Linie - wie ich glaube - durch die Phänomenologische Psychiatrie mit vier universalen Repräsentanten: dem Franzosen Minkowski, dem Amerikaner Strauss, dem Schweizer Binswanger oder auch dem deutschen Freiherrn v. Gebsattel. Im Vorfeld dieser klinisch zentrierten, antrhopologisch fundierten Psychiatrie haben wir nicht nur die tiefenpsychologischen Schulen zu suchen und zu verarbeiten, sondern auch die moderne Lebensphilosophie (mit Nietzsche und Dilthey), die Existenzphilosophie (mit Husserl und Heidegger), nicht zuletzt die Philosophische Anthropologie (mit Scheler und Plessner, mit Martin Buber vor allem).

Wenn hier von einer "Anthropologische Psychiatrie" die Rede sein soll, dann ist nichts weniger gemeint als ein "Paradigma": Paradigma für die Begegnung einer medizinischen Disziplin mit den Geistes- und Sozialwissenschaften, Paradigma aber auch für die wechselseitige Befruchtung biologischer, psychologischer und soziologischer Partialwissenschaften, Paradigma nicht zuletzt für ein neues, integratives Plateau der modernen Psychiatrie in Bewegung, das uns mit der Umstrukturierung der Anstalten, einer Rehumanisierung der Pflege- und Behandlungsformen, der Optimierung der Rehabilitation nicht zuletzt auch die Bedeutng der Primären Prävention wieder vor Augen stellt: eine Resozialisierungskette in jener "Therapeutischen Gemeinschaft", die letzten Endes eine Kultur-Bewegung in Gang bringt, wie dies von allen Wellen einer modernen Psychohygiene-Bewegung nicht geleistet werden konnte.

Als neues Paradigma imponiert uns nunmehr der Leib, weitaus mehr als Körperlichkeit oder intraphysische Realität. Subjekt und Objekt, sie begegnen als leibhaftige Einheit einer Welt, zu der sie komplementär angelegt sind. Ausgebrochen aus dem monadischen Menschenbild, ist in diesem Konzept von einem "logos" des "anthropopos" Rede, der sich auf das Wesen jenes gesunden und kranken Menschen bezieht, der mehr ist als das "Seelische" oder auch "Geistiges", der vielmehr "Leib" ist und damit Mensch ganz und gar: in seiner Umwelt, mit seiner Mitwelt, in seinen Erlebniswelten. Und genau das ist das Phänomen! Wir sind einfach nicht mehr wir selber -heißt es bei Shakespeare im "King Lear" -: "Wir sind nicht wir selbst, wenn die Natur im Druck die Seele zwingt zu leiden mit dem Körper" (King Lear, Act 2, Scene IV: "we are not ourselves when nature, being oppressed, commands the mind to suffer with the body").

Von diesem Konzept der Leiblichkeit her lassen sich neue Strategien einer umfassenden Hygiene in allen Lebensbereichen erwarten, eine primäre Grundversorgung mit Methoden und Modellen jener präventiven Medizin, die im Umgang mit Kranksein und einer Partizipation an der pathischen Situation versucht, eine Prophylaxe großen Stils auf weltweitem Niveau zur Vermeidung seelischer Leiden in die Wege zu leiten und die dann auch in der Lage wäre, den Lebensprozeß selbst umzuformen zu einem Lebensstil.

Nicht von ungefähr tauchen in solchen Modellen eines Lebenssils die Schlüsselbegriffe antiker Heilkunst auf: eine "diaita" als die Ordnung humaner Lebensführung, und die "paideia" mit den Prinzipien jener Bildung, die nicht zu verstehen wären ohne "eukrasia", die Harmonie, "mesotes", die Mitte, beide aber im Verbund mit "nomos" und "kosmos", einer Ordnung im All, die einfach nicht zu denken wäre ohne den "oikos", einem geregelten "Haushalt" und die "oikonomia" das Muster zivilisierter Lebensführung.

Bei allen naturwissenschaftlichen Kriterien, geistesgeschitlichen Impulsen, soziokulturellen Verknüpfungen bleibt uns letzten Endes nur ein pluralistisches Konzept der Psychiatrie, einer der unsichersten und zweideutigsten Disziplinen der Heilkunst, aber auch eine der interessantesten und aufregendsten. Kurz vor seinem frühen Tod hatte Ernst Freiherr von Feuchtersleben (1806 - 1849) darauf hingewiesen, daß gerade die Psychiatrie die verschiedensten Richtungen der Medizin, diese "beständig ordnend, begrenzend, verbindend, berichtigend", systematisch zu begleiten habe, um sie alle hinwiederum zu versöhnen in der "Idee einer höheren Einheit". Daß alle Richtungen von einer Gesamtschau getragen sein sollten, das in erster Linie war das Programm seiner "Fünf Vorlesungen über Anthropologie", die 1849 in Wien veröffentlicht wurde, ein großangelegter Entwurf jener umfassenden "Psycho-Physiologie der Menschennatur", welche der Bonner Kliniker Christian Friedrich Nasse (1823) mit dem Namen "Anthropologie" bezeichnet hat und welche umfaßt hat: 1. die genetische Matris, 2. die frühkindlichen Stadien und darauf sich entwickelnd das gesamte biographische Szenarium, 3. das psychosoziale Fluidum -, und damit "das Verhältnis des Menschen zum Menschen, und das des Menschen zu allem anderen, womit er das Erdendasein teilt", ein sehr spezifisches Verhältnis also zu Habitus und Sexus, Alter und Temperament, Gestik und Mimik, zur Sprache vor allem, kurzum: jene ganze "Naturgeschichte des Menschen" in Umwelt, Mitwelt, Erlebniswelt, die Nasse genannt hat "die eigentliche Anthropologie". Und dann wäre auch die ganze Historie nichts anderes als "angewandte Anthropologie" (Novalis).

Gegenwärtiges freilich lasse sich historisch kaum überblicken, hat Karl Jaspers einmal skeptisch gemeint, um dann umso energischer fortzufahren: "Aber spüren läßt sich die Tiefe des Umbruchs, der langsam in den letzten Jahren erfolgt ist", erfolgt ist und in diesen unseren Tagen so dramatisch vor sich geht -: keine einlineare Sequenz von wissenschaftlichen Errungenschaften, sondern eher die Ausfaltung eines ethischen Auftrags, ein mühsames Ringen um die verschiedensten Alternativen aller nur möglichen neuen und älteren Betrachtungsweisen. "Es gibt kein Vergangenes", so Goethe, "das man zurücksehen dürfte, es gibt nur ein ewig Neues, das sich aus den erweiterten Elementen des Vergangenen gestaltet" - heute gestaltet, und für morgen!

CHANGES IN PSYCHIATRY: AN ASPECT OF THE PANORAMA

OF THE XXth CENTURY

H. Schipperges
Institut f. Geschichte der Medizin
Im Neuenheimer Feld 305
D-6900 Heidelberg 1

Only a few days ago the universities of Basle and Heidelberg celebrated the 100th birthday of Karl Jaspers, physician, philosopher, politician, cosmopolite and initially a psychiatrist -: for some, Jaspers was a milestone in the development of psychiatry, for others, a reminder of stagnation and resignation, all in all doubtlessly a paradigm of the problems of psychopathology. He wrote in his "Psychopathology" (1942) that, "what happened in science during the last forty years", could not be unified so easily without any further ado.

Approximately in the year 1900 psychiatry began to be effective: Bleuler had met with its results and was, at that time, able to save "the tenable inventory of Freud's teaching into the overall consciousness of scientific psychiatry". The great biological research movements, endocrinology, experimental psychology, all of them had greatly expanded the psychiatrist's horizon; since Kretschmer's time (1921) a "re-development" of the view of the human being as a constitution " had taken place.

But it was not the great men who made history or indeed characterized the fate of psychiatry during the 20th century. In my opinion there were the phenomena, still alive as the continuing force of older traditions, for which the designation of " Psych - iatry " could scarce guarantee as the focus of our concern can neither be the psyche, nor the mind nor yet the brain -: we need be concerned with the whole and this brings us to the theme at large!

I was asked to sketch rather haphazardly, in tout strokes, the most salient developments of the century's psychiatry, orientating myself - as a historian as well as a psychiatrist -initially with the obviously ongoing transformation of the medical panorama during the 20th century. The concept of "panorama" is to be taken literally:as a review taken of a far-flung landscape from the highest possible vantage point, permitting nevertheless insights into the details, a prismatic perspective therefore, further dramatically heightened by the changes in time, the structural developments and atrophies, events that were never more venturesome than in the aspects of psychiatry.

Already in 1928 Victor von Weizsäcker had seen the medicine of his time in need of transformation, and even more of change, when he wrote: "A situation exists, a tendency develops, tension rises .... and with it, after it, a decision comes about; a new situation has been created, a period of rest ensues, earnings and losses can be assessed. The whole is like a historic entity: transformation, critical interruption, metamorphosis ".
Such a really classical description of paradigmatic change permits a closer examination of the panoramic change in psychiatry, while the psychic and all the psychoses remain an enigma. Jaspers wrote in his "Psychopathology" (1913), "that this might be, that the world and man should be that way, that this is possible and necessary, is not only astonishing, but makes us shudder".

Let me try nevertheless, in a short half hour in this festive round, to address three problem areas: 1st and foremost, the most dynamically arising currents of the 2oth century, which we can scarcely assess yet, and which have brought us to this crisis, that I would secondly refer to as "Psychiatry in the Dilemma", a threatening and menacing aporia, a cul - de -sac, from which thirdly, we should try to trace the possibilities already being outlined for a psychiatry of tomorrow.

I. The Trends of the 20th Century

During this century psychiatry has indeed been subject to stormy movements, although it wasn't the mental disturbances nor the psychopathies that triggered these events, but rather psychiatry's confrontation with man as an entity. As Leupold already thought 150 years ago (1833), psychiatry is about "to become more and more truly anthropological". Only against this background can we become more clearly conscious of its currents and tendencies, of all the pointers and knottings.
History of psychiatry-this must always also be also psychiatry itself! The medical historian, if he is fairly able to review the developments of the last three centuries in some detail, will nowhere find a subject or even merely a phenomenon such as "psychiatry proper". As a subject, think how young it is! It was only around 1870 that in the German language area a need was felt for clinical -psychiatric teaching. University clinics began to be set up in the Eighties. Only since 1901 has psychiatry become an examination subject in the large exams in Germany.

But about the middle of the last century the "Allgemeine Zeitschrift für Psychiatrie" (General Journal of Psychiatry), founded in 1844 by Damerow, Flemming and Roller, had already been able to present the most salient constitutive factors of such a psychiatry, one after the other "like voices in a fugue": scientific research as well as clinical psychopathology, and synoptically across the two, an anthropological overview (Bodamer, 1953). In the flourishing jungle of journals of the 20th century you would seek in vain for an equally representative journal of high standing, able to reflect modern developments adequately.

May I, nevertheless, remind you of what we have all experienced: cerebroanatomical research only began to florish around the turn of the century (from Wernicke to Kleist). Approx. in 1910, clinical research was totally under the control of pathological anatomy. At the same time, organic spatial psychiatry was meeting with the depth-psychological movements. During the Twenties we experienced Constitutional Psychiatry, during the Thirties the development of a Social Psychiatry, heightened still by the break-in of Anti-Psychiatry. From 1952 on psychopharmaceuticals, such as neuroleptics and thymoleptics, went into systematical use and were used for strategic procedures, with their biological and psychic sequelae, but also with a change of clinical atmosphere striking for us all. The last two decades saw further stormy developments in all camps: Neurophysiology and Neuropsychiatry, as well as Genetics, in Behavioral Psychology, in Family Research, Group Therapy and Personal Therapy.

Those, who - like Gaupp already in 1903 - demand that we wait until the inter-relationship between the psychic and material processes in the brain are known, are "holding out promises for a future, never likely to materiaslize ". If we were to wait until we understand all clinical syndromes from their anatomical bases, we might as well " wait for the Last Trump ". Up to such a time psychiatry would stay a little more than the " idiot sister of the other medical disciplines ".

Thomas S. Kuhn (1962) therefore distinguishes between two types of scientific development: the normal, continuoulsy growing, continuously perfectioning ductus and the revolutionary, non-cumulative upheaval, where fragmented thoughts always recompose anew and patterns of thought become visible, that were not revealed before. The whole receives a meaning from many aspects, which was not discernible from the isolated parts. It is surely insufficient to dissect the tendencies as to their parts; revolutionary conditions possess a holistic structure, supply a system of generalisations, of which, e.g. language seems to be a touchstone to us. It demonstrates the janus - headed character of any scientific jargon, linked to which unalterably our knowledge of nature is change, but there is need to be careful not to take " changes is the jargon " as a " progress in cognition " (Jaspers, 1913).

Today, going towards the end of the 20th century, we can see that this "psychiatry in motion" will be inconceivable without the motivations and tendencies of that 19th century, which all in all was more forefield than history amd at the same time "the darkest of all epochs", as Heidegger called it, since none of the burdening problems of this age of science has to this very day found any valid believable solution.

Meynert (1833 - 1892), the pupil of Hyrth and Rokitansky in Vienna, held Griesinger's general somatic approach to be so far assured, that he slandered all previous psychiatry "cloud - cuckoo land" (1876), about to enter the jungle of cerebral fibre thickets in search of nebulous psychic prey. Wernicke (1848 - 1905) developed the most congruent structure of the psyche with the structure of the brain. This formed the basis for a belief spanning a century, that I myself still hear 30 years ago (1953) from the mouths of Oskar and Cecile Vogt, during a visit to Neustadt: "somatic cerebral changes were the final basis of pathological phenomena".

For a long time and not by chance the organic ideal of psychic disease was held to be that Progressive Paralysis, which - again here in Vienna - Wagner v. Jauregg designated as the diagnostic prototype, the "unit of sichness", as a therapeutic model. Also here in Vienna Meynerth published his "Lectures on Psychiatry on A Scientific Basis" (1890). In each case the primary somato -pathological syndrome, was only an expression of the abnormal play of cerebral mechanisms, resulting in a most characteristic phase shift from the physical model to the more dynamic biochemism.

Faced with this tendency, the new century soon created a counter - movement, that became linked with the name of Freud and has remained so. Historically psychoanalysis was surely far - reaching and important, but this role seems to be over. Today to us this development seems full of cracks, transformations and reflexions, without its having become a lead or indeed a psychiatry in movement.

We are sufficiently removed from Freud, to be able to state, that without Freud half the literature of the 20th century would have remained unwritten. But we are also possessed of sufficient criticism to allow us to differentiate and to judge that Psychoanalysis was neither the only, not the best nor indeed the ideal method (cf. Kretschmer, 1982). Those, who initially believed that analysis would show them "the way to the Mothers", were bitterly disappointed.

I prefer to believe, that Freud was a promise that could never be kept. Psychoanalysis, however, opened a way to that theory of therepeutics, that could hitherto be conceived neither by physiology nor by pathology; it attained a new system of semiotics, wherein anamnesis is interpreted semantically from suppression, diagnmosis with analytics and prognosis in the process of individuation. Medicine as a natural science makes contact with history and society. Man as the architect of his body becomes again -as he was known to and named by Schopenhauer - the dramatic producer of his own fate.

A later generation will probably rather study the movements of secession, that took place tentatively all through this century, most decisively realized by Carl Gustav Jung (1875 - 1961), who most energetically rejected the dogmatic teaching, which - in 1930 - he found to have degenerated to a "pathological subterranean growth". With the laws of the transformation of

the "Psyche as a Subjective Cosmos " Jung endeavoured to pathologically
open up the depth significance of existence. This was done on an even higher
level by Victor E. Frankl, who, with his "Logotherapy" tried to work up the
areas of meaning attainable in talks with the patient and thus achieved a
kind of "medico - religious pastoral care", a logotherapy indeed "in spiritu
Apollinis".
Now let me review the first aspect as a whole!

At the turn of the 20th century psychiatry impresses us as the inheritrix of
biology, which as psycho - pharmacology has learnt to control the natural
processes of the brain, as the inheritrix of psychology, wherein physical
programmatics were soon left in favour of a motivational science, last but
not least as the inherity of philosophy, whose hermeneutics supplied guide
lines to a phenomenological psychopathology, also revealing frames of
reference to that society, which reflects our reality most concretely.
Psychiatry has sought the link - up with scientific medicine very consciously
and energetically and found it - by way of brain research. But it has never
really become integrated into medicine. Neurology has long become
emancipated; psychoanalysis is going its own, willful way. At a point of
time, when we have realized that body and soul are nothing special, but only
aspects of the whole, it would be stupid to claim "Psychotherapy" as a
separate subject. As Kant wrote in his "Dreams of a Ghost -Seer": "My soul
is in the whole body and whole in each of its parts".

2. Psychiatry's Dilemma

This brings us right to the centre of our second, most sensitive area, dealing
with psychiatry in dilemma, is discord, in a quandary and in exigencies,
maybe - aporia.

Already a hundred years ago modern medicine believed it had attained its
scientific standard and would be able to play at permanent progress within
the round of natural sciences, with regard to all tradition it had declared
"tabula rasa", so as to be able to open up the way with proven physical and
chemical methods to that all- inclusive therapeutical methodology, that
seemed predestined for ever further successes and promised to produce
inexhaustible blessings for mankind. Modern psychiatry was also included in
this development of a newer medicine - though delayed, yet with remarkable
systematicity - always remaining somewhat ambiguous as a science, never
being able to attain any serious relationship with the arts, not to speak of
the social sciences.

As you all know and have felt, during the last few decades this scientific
foundation of medicine has been severely shaken. Medicine as an applied
science, ever more accompanied by social shifts of competency and systems
-immanent loss of balance, has been overtaken and undermined or
compensated by a counter - determined medicine in movement -: and it is
today being attacked in toto and as a system. If you believe the critical
voices, medicine is no longer held to be the benefactress of mandkind; it is

said to serve profit maximisation of a bourgeois productive society. Therefore the physician is defined and defamed as the "Tinker of Capital", in particular the psychiatrist, who is said to brainwash his patients to turn wake and agitated people into wellbehaved and healthy marionettes, when it should be his task to keep psychic suffering transparent, to transform it into political action. So much for catchwords!

An enormous Dyonisian conter - movement began with Freud - it would seem - against those basic positions of that medicine, which was ever sworn to the Apollinic: to Apollon, the Physician, the God of Healing. In no field of science has the theory of the "two cultures" had a more baneful effect than in the disciplines of psychiatry. Alexander Mitscherlich spoke justifiably of the " two medical sciences of the present", something that is nowhere more intolerant than in psychiatry.

Emerging from a humanizing engagement (from Paracelsus till Pinel), psychiatry also experienced that characteristic conversion to scientific methodology (via Griesinger up to Kraepelin), before it was again forced to open into personal dimensions (with Freud, with Weizsäcker, amongst others). While stringent science is joined with pure phialntropy, an attempt is made once more to compensate this by hermeneutics. Modern psychiatry is therefore as much the heir of science, as of psychology or of the arts. Apart from such basic methodological questions, in future doubtlessly more concrete realities will perdominate: the massiv appearance of acute exogenous syndromes, e. g. the addictions, the horrifying increase of defect - and deterioration syndromes, e.g. with senile psychoses, the failed adaption syndromes of an under-, as well as over- developed mass society and thereby a striking transformation of the psychiatric patient group. There are no longer the ranking principles of monasteries, army barracks and clinics, that guarantee the accomodation and maintainance of psychic patients. The insecurity developing in all fields of psychiatry will best be explained with the catchword of " Anti - Psychiatry ", this blue blossom of rose - colored romanticism, as a fundamental loss of security in our discipline, which is so susceptible for ideologies.

Anti-Psychiatry should therefore be assessed as an answer to the crisis of school psychiatry and asylum psychiatry. Not by chance has it become the fighting concept of "critical" psychiatry, without already being "polit-psychiatry". It has obviously fallen prey to those age- old utopian ideas, which say: psychiatry might and should be the precursor of a cultural revolution, should "fight against everything threatening solidarity between human beings and the solidarity between man and his environment", psychiatry having to lead - with one word - to an "authentic human existence" (cf. Jean Foudraine, 1976).

Looked at against the background of the last hundred years, in any case, nothing speaks in favour of that "third revolution in psychiatry", which was postualted as a new, dynamic and truly social psychiatry (Basaglia), the legendary liberation of the lunatics from their chains being regarded as the " first revolution" and that psychoanalytical movement, which was more trended towards mythos than to serve logos, as the " second revolution ". We simply cannot afford to speak for an anti - scientific speculation or in favour of purely political protests, just as we must never pander to that therapeutic nihilism, which was once so drastically demonstrated in Vienna and has become such a fashion again.

In no field of modern medicine has the gap between theory and practice been more disastrous: on the one hand the more noble installation of an academic psychiatry, which has not yet been finally accepted within the groves of academe, on the other the asylums, the medical establishments of a sickly treatment psychiatry, at a time when research and teaching, tratment and maintainance only seem possible at one and the same time within a highly complex integrative compound system.

Around the middle of the 20th century Kurt Schneider still spoke of "the three hills" in the psychiatric panorama: a central mighty chain of hills, representing psychopathological research, a further chain of mountains, symbolizing " the science of the physiological bases of the psychoses" and finally that hilly landscape of psychogenic disturbances, "in which psychotherapy was undoubtedly justified". This is still valid today, when we could think that that central hill had been totally eroded, the "mine of psychopathology" (as Schneider called it) exhausted and " clinical psychiatry" at an end (Schneider, 1952). Herewith we have once again arrived at the most sensitive point, the " punctum saliens": the clinical interest in the basic phenomena of nature and psyche, body and mens, persona and the world, which can scarcely be explained without philosophical principles and criteria and cannot be treated without the clinical inclusion of the whole person.

Man as an entity, however, can never be - so Jsapers - "the object of knowledge. There is no system of being human...... All knowledge takes place in particular aspects, demonstrates a reality in each case, but not the reality of man, is in suspense, not final. Man is always more than he knows of himself and can know and is more than others may know of him."

From this insight of Jaspers, the philosopher to the creed of the clinician: "We would not want to lose the knowledge of the inexhaustibility and the enigma of every individual mentally ill person, even in the face of the seemingly most trite veryday cases".

Here, in everyday life, things begin to get serious, requiring standards and an obligatory system of relationships. Basic ethical questions of this kind accompany and charge the whole spectrum of psychiatric indications, starting from the always doubtful intervention and a motivation to intervene, via the whole chain of intervening measures, of prevention and curation, as well as rehabilitaion and re- socialsation, all the way to the ever again needful legitimation of intervention, which will always remain linked up with blunder, mistake and excesses. Test planning and quality assurance, these are newly and in future increasingly become the themes of socalled " ethical commissions", which are being set up all over Europe by medical institutions, medical faculties and professional organizations and soon also will exist within the framework of psychiatry.

With this psychiatric optimism, Adolf Meyer, most of all, opened up the way for psychiatry in the United States, where the clinical aspect - and not the therapy of mankind - is at the center of endeavour. In all circular movements, among the public, through the lay of movements, with the methods of "re-education", Erwin Strauss also expects of psychiatry, that it will find back to a clinical mode of observations (Strauss, 195o).

On the 3rd of February 1966 Eugen Kahn wrote to me:"The age of disease is over. The era of man as an ill person has indubitably begun" and further: " will the patient be able to cure himself or will he only speed his demise by means of the hitherto unsuccessful treatment methods? Let us try to remain optimistic" - a basic counsel of my fatherly friend Eugen Kahn, which I gladly pass on to you.

3. New Ways of Psychiatry

With this therapeutic optimism, we have now hit on the third and last aspect of the new ways of psychiatry, basically age-old paths, ways towards the world of tomorrow, which I would at least like to sketch. I would think, that at the core of all psychiatry there remains the medical mission, the need to grant expert aid in a mental emergency, to prevent exigencies, to vitiate, to help and heal. Only clinical experience can save us ever and again from the torrential vortex of conceptual relativation, those phenomena, that the physician meets with in every individual patient. The clinical aspect must ever be the centre: the examination of an individual, who is disturbed and has been hurt and now appears to be ill and in need of help.

At this point I would like to remind you of the impressive recollection of my revered teacher, Manfred Bleuler, who warned us lately (1975) that the physician and that the patient was becoming ever more lonely. "The more we permit ourselves to be enticed away from the patient and to see our tasks as physicians and even psychiatric experts in other fields than with the patient, the more will medicine disintegrate and psychiatry as well as a medical subject, the less will we deserve to be called physicians. If we no longer deserve it and if others will supplant us, humanitarian values of the greatest social importance, that had hither been in our hands, will be laid into the hands of others - or they will be lost".

With this reminder we come - in closing - shortly to the concept of a "patient oriented", socalled Anthropological Psychiatry, to its possibilities - and even more its fronties. Kraepeline's psychiatry was liberated primarily from threatening rigidification - as I believe - through Phenomenological Psychiatry with its four universal representatives: Minkowski, the Frenchman, Straus, the American, Binswanger, the Swiss and last not least Freiherr v. Gebsattel, the German. In the forefield of this clinically centered, anthropologically founded psychiatry, we must not only seek the depth - psychological schools and to process their teaching, but also modern Life Style Philosophy (with Nietzsche and Dilthey), Existential Philosophy (with Husserl and Heidegger), and last but not least Philosophical Anthropology (with Scheler and Plessner and Martin Buber, chief of all).

If here we are to speak of an "Anthropological Psychiatry", we are speaking of nothing less than a "paradigm": a paradigm for the encounter of a medical discipline with the arts and social sciences, but also a paradigm for the interactive fertilization of biological, psychological and sociological part sciences, a paradigm last but not least for a new integrative level of modern psychiatry in motion, which again requires us to deal with a reconstruction of institutions, a rehumanisation of the forms of care and treatment, the optimation of rehabilitation and last but not least the importance of Primary Prevention: a chain of resocialisation in that "Therapeutic Community", which will finally set in motion a cultural movement, that could not be achieved by the waves of a modern psycho - hygienic movement.

As a new paradigm we are now impressed by the body, which is much more than mere corporality or intraphysical reality. Subject and object we meet as the incarnate entity of a world, to which they apply in a complementary manner. Breaking away from the mondiac image of man, this concept speaks about a " logos" of the "anthropopos", which relates to the essence of that healthy or sick individual and which is more than the "psychic" or also the " spiritual", which is rather the " corporality " and thus altogether human: man in this environment, with his contemporary world, in the world of his experience. We are simply no longer ourselves - that is exactly the phenomenon - as is said in Shakespeare's "King Lear", Act 2, Scene IV:
"We are not ourselves when nature, being oppressed, commands the mind to suffer with the body".
From this concept of corporality, we may expect to gain new strategies of an all-inclusive hygiene for all areas of life, a primary basic maintainance with methods and models of that preventive medicine, which attempts participation in an intercourse with sickness from the pathic situation, to introduce a grand style prophylaxis on a worldwide level to avoid mental suffering and which would then also be able to reform the life process itself into a life style.

The key concepts of healing arts from antiquity do not by chance reappear in such life style models: a "diaita" as an order of humane life conduct and the "paideia" with the principles of that education, that cannot be understood without "eukrasia", harmony, "mesotes" the center, both however linked with "nomos" and "kosmos", an orderly system in space, which could simply not be envisaged without "oikos", an orderly "household" and without "oikonomia", the pattern of civilized life conduct.

With all scientific criteria, impulses from the arts, socio-cultural links, finally there remains for us only a pluralistic concept of psychiatry, one of the most insecure and ambiguous disciplines among the medical sciences, but also one of the most interesting and exciting ones. Shortly before his untimely death, Ernst Freiherr von Feuchtersleben (1806 - 1849) had pointed out, that psychiatry had in particular to accompany the most differenciated sections of medicine systematically; "continuously arranging, limiting, linking, rectifying", so as to reconcile all these again in an " idea of higher entity". That all theses sections should be included in an overview, this was primarily the program of his " Five Lectures of Anthropology", published in Vienna in 1949, a major outline of that all- inclusive "Psycho -Physiology of Human Nature", which the Bonn clinician, Christian Friedrich Nasse (1823) designated as "Anthropology" to include: 1. the genetic matrix, 2. the stages of early childhood and developing therefrom the complete biographic scenarium, 3. the psycho-social fluidum - and thereby the " relationship from man to man and that of man with all the others, with whom he shares his earthly existence", therefore a very specific relationship to habitus and sexus, age and temperament, gestics and mimics, with language most of all, in short: that whole "natural history of man" in his environment, contemporary world, experienced world, which Nasse designated " Anthropology per se ". And thereby all of history would be nothing but "applied anthropology" (Novalis).

Jaspers said sceptically at one time, that the present can scarce be reviewed historically, but then continued all the more forcefully: "but we can feel the depth of the transformation, which has slowly been taking place during the last few years", this has happened and is dramatically taking place in our days-: not a single linear sequence of scientific achievement, but rather the unfolding of an ethical mandate, a laborious struggle for the most differenciated alternatives to all the least possible older and newer visions. To speak with Goethe:"There is nothing past, that should be wished to return, there is only the eternally New, which has been designed from the enlarged elements of the past" - has been designed for today and for tomorrow!

THE PROGRAMMES OF THE WORLD HEALTH ORGANIZATION DIRECTED TO THE

IMPROVEMENT OF NOMENCLATURE AND CLASSIFICATION IN MENTAL HEALTH

Norman Sartorius

Director, Division of Mental Health
World Health Organization
Geneva, Switzerland

Mr Chairman, Ladies and Gentlemen:

Before starting I wish to thank the organizers for their invitation to present to you the work of the World Health Organization
on Psychiatric Diagnosis, Nomenclatures and Classification.

Constraints of time will only allow me to touch upon the various
activities undertaken in this area. I, therefore, wish to apologize
to all those among you and to the many others all of whose many
contributions and efforts make WHO's programme but can only be
mentioned rather than described in detail which their quality would
so amply deserve.

The standardization of diagnostic procedures and the establishment and revision of international classifications of diseases are
constitutional functions of the World Health Organization.

To fulfil them the World Health Organization has undertaken
a long-term programme on diagnosis and classification, which has
over the last two decades, involved a large number of experts and
institutions from most countries of the world. The products of
WHO's efforts in this field have been the classifications of mental
and neurological disorders in the successive revisions of the
International Classification of Diseases, classifications of impairments and disabilities due to mental disorder, international
glossaries of psychiatric diagnostic terms; techniques for the
exploration of the diagnostic process; and a series of transculturally
applicable methods for the assessment of patients and for the recording
and presentation of data about mentally and neurologically ill people.

In recent years this work has acquired even greater prominence because of a series of developments, among which the following eight stand out particularly clearly :

(1)   In many countries mental health programmes are in ferment and in a process of revision.   These reformulations are due to several factors including the recognition that mental health problems are serious public health concerns, that the resources for their resolution are insufficient, and that the present organization of mental health services is inadequate to deal with these problems.   The availability of new methods of treatment in psychiatry with a shift towards the incorporation of mental health into general health care, further strengthen the need for radically new strategies of mental health care which involve major changes of all components of health information systems, thus also of classificatory and diagnostic systems.

(2)   Over the past few years a mixture of trends inimical to agreement on a diagnostic system and a classification have occurred. These trends include the re-emergence of national, and even sub-national diagnostic schemes without any attempts to provide a translation of these schemes into a reference classification.   Decisions to limit or eliminate person- and diagnosis-linked information systems have sharply reduced the interest in all matters concerning diagnosis and its recording in a number of countries.   The reluctance of practitioners to follow a classificatory system (often because of its complexity), also seems to be on the increase.   Teaching on systematic psychopathology and diagnosis shows a decline in many parts of the world.   The growth of emphasis on the use of national languages in the teaching of medical students (and in clinical work) laudable as it may be in many respects, decreased the liklihood of agreement on classifications.

(3)   A number of culture-bound epistemological constraints to agreement on diagnostic and classificatory systems have gained importance in recent years.   Most of these are well known and do not need enumeration.   Some, however, are less obvious and therefore more difficult to tackle.   These include, for example, the manner in which knowledge is organized in different cultures.   Approaching information by classifying it is not the preferred way of all cultures for dealing with masses of data.   Tolerance for unresolved conflict and contradiction varies among cultures.   Those who prefer to maintain indeterminancy for a large part of the data pool may be reluctant to operate with classifications requiring immediate final assignment to classes on the basis of more or less incomplete information.

The mind-body dichotomy inherent in many of the classificatory systems which emerged in the 19th century's industrializing Europe is discontinuous with the underlying philosophies of other cultures and makes agreement on classifications difficult. The concepts of time and of its use in the description of phenomena vary between cultures and affect understanding of classificatory schemes.

(4) After a period of high hopes, there is a feeling of profound disappointment with the fact that research, so far, has failed to help us create either disease concepts or disease entities. In psychiatry, syndromes (such as schizophrenia) which have a lower epidemiological rank than a disease entity are still widely used. Classifications which have to accommodate heterogenous groupings of syndromes, disease concepts and disease entities appearing alongside one another are becoming less and less popular.

(5) The need to have different classifications and diagnoses for different purposes has become more obvious and more frequently demanded. General health care personnel now deal with mentally ill people and demand a classification for their use. Increasing sophistication of research in psychiatry brings demand for research classifications. The fact that in developed countries some 40 per cent. of all disability can be ascribed to mental and neurological disorders helped to bring about the development of classifications used by insurance and invalidity schemes. These and other classifications are being produced without any special efforts to ensure their translation into a reference classification. As a result the same conditions change labels as patients pass through health care, research and social welfare facilities and communication in pooling of information from different systems becomes an expensive utopia.

(6) The needs of developing countries have emerged as a powerful factor in determining acceptability of classifications. The problems which are occurring in developing countries are probably to a large extent similar to those that occur elsewhere: the needs of service and the differences that have been observed in the prognosis and outcome of mental disorders in these countries, however, impose new ways of classifying problems and cause profound dissatisfaction with currently existing schemes.

(7) The controversy about ways to handle reporting and classification of medical aspects of behaviour related disorders - such as drug and alcohol related problems - has gained new strength and importance in recent years from the increase of prevalence and severity of these problems and from the growing vigour of inter-professional territorial struggle in this area of health care.

(8) The significant technological advances in recent years make prospects for advances of classification less gloomy. These include

revolutionary achievements in the technology of computer assisted clinical, radiological and radio-isotope examinations and the use of computers in the organization and analysis of findings of patient assessments. New knowledge stemming from experience with polydiagnostic and multiaxial classification schemes has become available. There are important advances in psychometrics. The operationalization of diagnostic criteria and - in some countries - the significant mobilization of interest in classification are further assets and steps forward.

These and other developments of recent years are among determinants of a classification proposed for international use. They will have to be considered together with constraints inherent in any international classification.

Such a classification - if it is to be useful and used - must be based on points of agreement among mental health professionals and between them and other users of the classification. It must at all times be a servant rather than a master of communication. It must not aim to oust or replace regional or local classifications which have often valuable functions and are likely to be well adjusted to the situation in which they have come into existence. It must be sufficiently well liked as a tool of information exchange to generate translations of national or special-purpose classifications into the reference classification. It must be rather conservative and theoretically unenterprising to remain attractive or at least acceptable to a wide variety of people of different orientations and knowledge. Changes can only be introduced when sufficient scientific data has become available to support the change and facilitate its acceptance. It must take into account languages into or from which the classification will be translated. A certain amount of continuity must be preserved between successive revisions, for economical and scientific reasons.

The multitude of factors which influence revisions of classifications and the many people and agencies that are consulted in this process make it difficult or impossible to predict changes in content of international classification in any detail. It is, however, possible to foresee tasks that will have to be done in preparation for the new revision. So, for example, it is likely that concerted research will be necessary to obtain data required to improve classifications, and that mechanisms which will facilitate its conduct have to be strengthened. Participation of many nations and many disciplines as well as continuing interest and the support of all national authorities to both national and international efforts in this area are of essential importance. More energetic attention will have to be given to training on classification and diagnosis. Ways to monitor how well the

classification is used will have to be found. An intensive effort
will have to be directed to the adjustment of the classification
to the real situation in the countries of the Third World.

It is also possible to speculate about directions in which
research may have to go. Functional psychoses, for example, until
now received the lion's share of attention of most researchers;
perhaps this is because of their great public health importance.
Some 40 million people in the world suffer from such conditions.
Perhaps this is because of their puzzling and dramatic appearance
or because institutions in which many of to-day's psychiatrists
were taught and worked, still contain so many patients with these
syndromes. These are good reasons for the fascination researchers
have for these conditions: yet there is no doubt that research will
have to shift its emphasis to include diagnosis and classification
of childhood mental disorders, organic brain disorders and mental
retardation, all of which are conditions of tremendous public
health importance, particularly in developing countries. Similarly,
the problems of diagnosis (and classification) in instances of the
co-appearance of conditions such as dementia in a retarded individual,
neurosis in a person with a frontal lobe syndrome, require significant
attention as well as iatrogenies ranging from drug dependence in
infants to tardive dyskinesia, alcohol and drug dependence and somatic
and non-specific complaints.

In many of these areas inadequacy of classification and diagnosis
rest on total inadequacy of our knowledge. This is particularly true
for non-specific multiple complaints - an array of conditions which
are often on the borderline between disease and misery, psychological
distress and inadequate communication about unhappiness and malaise.
Research, particularly in these conditions which even in developing
countries occupy at least one quarter of all health service potentials,
will have to proceed into ways of handling those conditions rather
than to be restricted on ways of classifying them better.

New approaches to classification will also have to be developed.
Among these is the need to use and assess the value of new paradigms
of classification based on other types of logic, on other modes of
approaching the field. Cultural psychiatry and psychiatry from
developing countries may help to enlarge the pool of inspiration.
Other branches of medicine as well as systems of traditional medicine
may have to be re-examined in the search for different classificatory
systems. Broad multidisciplinary consultation may yield new hints
and open new avenues of search.

Some of the issues I have described were raised recently in a
conference on diagnosis and classification of mental disorder,
alcohol and drug-related problems which took place in April 1982 in

Copenhagen. This conference, perhaps the most significant ever held, brought together 150 participants from 47 countries from all continents. It was organized as one of the activities in the framework of a project on diagnosis and classification undertaken by the World Health Organization in collaboration with the Alcohol, Drug Abuse and Mental Health Administration of the USA.

The aims of this joint endeavour were to review the present state of diagnosis and classification, identify gaps in knowledge and define priority objectives for future research. The project has had the benefit of guidance of an international advisory group with some 30 mental health experts representing all WHO Regions and all the major schools and traditions of world psychiatry. Prior to the Conference, a series of scientific meetings was organized to examine different parts of the field involving experts from some 60 countries. The conference reviewed current issues and major traditions in psychiatric diagnosis and classification, proceeded to examine strategies for generating and validating nosological classes and then critically assessed the contributions to the development of classification stemming from a variety of disciplines.

Several themes emerged forcefully. There was an impression that there is a revival of interest in the issue of psychiatric diagnosis and classification among scientists parallel to a rather apathetic acceptance or rejection of classification by the practitioners. There was a wide-spread discontent with the state of theory underlying the classification of mental disorders. The question of psychiatric practice and research in the Third World received major attention. The conference marked areas which need intensive work including the development of assessment instruments, glossaries and research on nonpsychotic disorders, personality types and personality disorders, alcohol and drug-related problems, and psychiatric problems in primary care. The multidisciplinary approach to problems of classification and diagnosis received general approbation.

The further development and maintenance of the international classification was seen as one of the major tasks and prerequisites of international collaboration.

As a result of these efforts, a series of specific recommendations and suggestions about future research was produced, and a comprehensive and compelling agenda for research in the 80's emerged, complementing results of consultations with Member States and non-governmental organizations about immediate needs and opportunities for action.

To respond to the challenge which these demands represent, WHO will have to continue working closely together with all those who can make a positive contribution to knowledge and to international understanding and collaboration in an intensive and extensive way. Such joint work with many countries, institutions and individuals, without any doubt, remains the only way to achieve progress in this field which is of such essential importance for the improvement of care for the mentally ill, their families and their communities.

IMPROVING THE QUALITY OF DIAGNOSTIC SYSTEMS: MULTIAXIALITY AND
THE POLYDIAGNOSTIC APPROACH

P.Berner and H.Katschnig

Psychiatric University Clinic
Vienna
Austria

Multiaxial classification has become one of the major methodological issues in psychiatric research. At the 6th World Congress
of Psychiatry, Mezzich (1) reported on patterns and issues of multi-
axial psychiatric diagnosis. The statements of his excellent analysis
in essence still hold today and it is not intended to rediscuss them
here. The purpose of the following reflections is to discuss the
different uses of multiaxial classification.

USES OF MULTIAXIAL CLASSIFICATIONS

The original idea of multiaxial classifications was that assessment of a psychiatric patient should be carried out in different
areas, such as symptomatology, course, putative aetiological factors,
etc., independently, and that the different information gathered
should not be prematurely combined into diagnostic entities. Multi-
axial classification is only possible if data collection itself has
been multiaxial. It is perhaps best to start with the topic of
'multiaxial data collection', because this brings us down to earth
and away from mere theoretical reflections, and then proceed to the
two main uses of multiaxial classification: psychiatric diagnosis and
the validation of psychiatric diagnosis through research.

1. Multiaxial Data Collection

For research workers it is common sense to collect information
in one area after the other, usually by means of separate collecting
instruments, and, when possible, employing different interviewers.
This principle is not generally followed in clinical practice, where
the clinician gathers information more or less unsystematically and
then synthesizes it to a judgement. The type of data gathered in

31

different areas, usually called axes, is very different in respect to the levels of measurement employed: Some data correspond to categorical yes/no information, some are rank-ordered, some are real continuous measures of a dimensional nature. Only for the latter is the term 'axis' justified (2).

There is no agreement about the number of areas into which psychiatrically relevant information should be distributed, and it is partly a question of terminology whether large areas such as 'social adjustment' should include several subareas, or whether the latter should be conceived as independent areas. In a symposium of the 7th World Congress of Psychiatry the problem as to the adequate number of axes is raised; a questionnaire sent out for the preparation of this symposium contained 21 different proposed axes.

The information contained in one axis may serve different purposes: Genetic data or illness course may for instance be regarded in one research design as elements necessary for diagnostic assignment, in others as appropriate tools for its validation. Therefore, axes should not be conceived and labelled with regard to a possible interpretation (for instance, 'aetiology', 'precipitating factors') but rather with regard to the area of information they cover (for instance, 'abnormal psychiatric or somatic conditions', duration or course of symptoms', 'proceeding life events', etc.). The interpretation of the data contained in the different axes should be left to alogrithms formulated for precise purposes, such as attaining diagnoses, validating hypothetical diagnostic assignments, searching for aetiological or pathogenetic influences, etc.

Special attention has to be given to the 'time axis', which up to now has been widely neglected or restricted to the time aspects of symptomatology (such as age of onset, duration of episode, etc.). In addition it must be stressed that for some purposes, such as for aetiological models and for prognostic studies, recording the chronological relationship between symptomatology and other variables as well, is crucial. Finally, depending on the use of the data collected in a multiaxial way, it may be of utmost importance to document the time relationship between variables of the nonsymptomatological axes. The practical solution to this problem is not easy, as the only correct one would be to add a time axis to most of the areas included in the system.

Multiaxial classification can best be used if information is first recorded as raw data and not put immediately into categories. Thus, if age of onset is documented, the factual age should be recorded instead of using several predetermined categories (e.g. 0-20, 21-40, 41-60, 60+). Equally, psychopathological information should be recorded on a symptom and not on a syndrome level.

2. Multiaxial Classification and Psychiatric Diagnosis

Diagnostic criteria used in practical work and in research are composed of elements extracted from at least the symptomatological area and from other areas which cover possible etiological factors. Apart from 'syndrome classes' which do not claim to be identical with a diagnosis, such as the CATEGO classes (3), even the most parsimonious definitions of diagnosis incorporate both psychopathological symptoms and etiological information, if only in the assumption of the absence of a plausible organic etiology. However, many diagnostic criteria additionally contain characteristics belonging to other areas.

In any case, the choice of elements, regardless of whether they are used as inclusion or exclusion criteria, is determined by reasons which vary from one set of criteria to the other. These reasons may be of theoretical or empirical nature, as can best be exemplified with regard to the diagnosis of schizophrenia.

The main theories taken into account in diagnostic formulations for this disorder are:

a) The hypothesis (derived from Moebius (4), and Kraepelin (5) that schizophrenia is an endogenous psychosis following a chronic course to a state of deficiency.

b) The hypothesis derived from Bleuler (6) that the basic disturbances of schizophrenia disorders are dissociation (to be grasped mainly in formal thought disorders) and affective blunting.

c) The assumption (derived from Janazarik's concept of 'structural dynamic coherency', (7)) that first and second rank symptoms may occur in states of psychotic turmoil stemming from various origins and thus are nosologically unspecific.

d) The stipulation (derived from Japsers' hierachical principle, (8)) that schizophrenic symptoms determine the diagnosis when occurring simultaneously with or consecutively to manic depressive features.

Empirical reasons for the choice of elements for diagnostic algorithms are generally based on experiences of follow-up or validation studies. Thus the observation that patients who have once exhibited affective and certain 'schizophrenic' features (for instance first rank symptoms) and later become clear cut manic-depressive has led some researchers to use affective symptoms as excluding criteria (which is tantamount to a reversal of Jaspers' principles). Many such empirical elements are prognosis indicators: they are only empirical in so far as their relation to good or bad prognosis is not derived from a theory. The underlying identification of bad prognosis with the diagnosis of schizophrenia is clearly theoretical.

Kurt Schneider (9) with regard to his first rank symptoms claims to use a purely pragmatical approach without any explicit reference to an underlying theory. It must, however, be assumed that his selection of symptoms is based at least on his clinical experience and is thus to a certain degree empirical. Furthermore it is evident that he adheres to Jaspers' hierarchical principle.

Diagnostic formulations and their elements may be described as to whether and to what extent they are theoretical or empirical and according to the kind and number of areas of information they use. Most of the diagnostic criteria on hand are mixed, containing a combination of theoretical and empirical elements (for instance the St. Louis Criteria for Schizophrenia, (10)).

In analysing and comparing different diagnostic systems in this way, a 'comparative nosology' could emerge which would make the whole diagnostic field more transparent and understandable. An overview of the most important diagnostic systems and formulations for the schizophrenic and affective psychoses is available in a book published for the WPA on the occasion of this world congress (11).

On the basis of such comparative analysis of several diagnostic systems one can work out a multiarea data gathering instrument which will cover all the information necessary for making a diagnosis according to the different systems. Thus a so-called 'polydiagnostic approach' (2) which implies the simultaneous application of several diagnostic formulations for one and the same nosological concept such as schizophrenia becomes feasible. This means that the patients included in a study can be grouped differently according to the various diagnostic criteria used.

In this way, comparisons with all past and future studies dealing with the same topic, such as genetic influences in schizophrenia or life events in depression, and using only one specific diagnostic formulation will become possible. Thus, one of the major barriers to building up a coherent body of knowledge in psychiatry, the lack of diagnostic comparability, would gradually fade away if more and more projects are carried out using a polydiagnostic approach.

The polydiagnostic approach has been shown to be feasible with little extra effort. At the Psychiatric Clinic of the University of Vienna it is currently applied in two comprehensive follow-up studies, one on depression and the other on the major psychoses. In order to collect all relevant information, the Present State Examination (3) was expanded by those symptoms which were required by the diagnostic algorithms used but were not contained in the PSE. Together with information from other areas, including course, personality, genetic loading, etc., a number of diagnostic formulations for depression and schizophrenia can be simulated by a computer programme especially developed for this purpose.

3. Multiaxial Classification and Validation of Diagnosis

Diagnostic formulations can at present best be regarded as
hypotheses concerning the homogeneity of groups of psychiatric
patients in relation to criteria regarded as relevant. Such hypothetical classes still have to be validated and one purpose of the
polydiagnostic approach is to determine which of the diagnostic
formulations is best correlated with external criteria, such as
putative etiological factors, outcome, age of onset, etc. The more
elements from different axes are used for a diagnostic algorithm
the less will remain for its validation. Therefore, we would suggest
sampling psychiatric patients for studies basically on psychopathological grounds, i.e. on syndrome groups, and using all the other
axes including therapeutic response, as validating criteria for the
syndromes.

4. Conclusion

Using a multiaxial approach for the collection of data, for
classification, and for validation means establishing an 'open
methodology' in psychiatric research. Whenever necessary, supplementary axes or items may be easily incorporated into the basic
areas of data collection. This proceudre has considerable advantages
over the usual 'compromise classification' systems and meets Adolf
Meyer's common-sense and to some extent provocative statement formulated as early as 1906 (12): 'An order presentation of the facts
alone is a real diagnosis'.

REFERENCES

1. J. E. Mezzich, Patterns and Issues in Multiaxial Pscyhiatric
    Diagnosis. Psychological Medicine 9: 125-137, 1979.
2. P. Berner and H. Katschnig, Principles of 'Multiaxial'
    Classification in Psychiatry as a Basis of Modern Methodology.
    In: Helgason, T. (Ed.) Methods in Evluation of Psychiatric
    Treatment. Cambridge University Press, Cambridge 1983.
3. J. K. Wing, J. E. Cooper and N. Sartorius, Measurement and
    Classification of Psychiatric Symptoms. Cambridge University
    Press, Cambridge 1974.
4. P. J. Moebius, Abriß der Lehre von den Nervenkrankheiten.
    Leipzig 1889
5. E. Kraepelin, Psychiatrie. Barth, Leipzig (6 Aufl.) 1899. Tran-
    slated by Barclay, R. M. from the 8th edition of Psychiatrie.
    Livingstone, Edinburgh 1919.
6. E. Bleuler, Die Prognose der Dementia Praecox (Schizophrenie-
    gruppe). Allg. Z. Psychiat. 65: 536-464, 1908.
7. W. Janzarik, Dynamische Grundkonstellationen in Endogenen
    Psychosen, Springer, Berlin-Göttingen-Heidelberg 1959
8. K. Jaspers, Allgemeine Pscyhopathologie. Springer, Berlin 1913.
    English translation by Hoenig, J. and M. W. Hamilton:
    General Psychopathology. Manchester University Press 1962.

9. K. Schneider, Klinische Psychopathologie. 12., Gegenüber der 8. Univeränderten Aufl. Thieme, Suttgart 1980. English edition: Clincial Psychopathology, translated from 3rd ed. by Hamilton M. W. and Anderson, E. W., Grune and Stratton, New York 1959.

10. J. P. Feighner, E. Robins, S. R. Guze, R. A. Woodruff, G. Winokur and R. Munoz, Diagnostic Criteria for Use in Psychiatric Research. Arch. Gen. Psychiat. 26: 57-63, 1972.

11. P. Berner, E. Gabriel, H. Katschnig, W. Kieffer, K. Koehler, G Lenz and Ch. Simhandl, Diagnostic Criteria for Schizophrenic and Affective Psychoses. American Psychiatric Press, Washington D.C. 1983.

12. A. Meyer, Principles in Grouping Facts in Psychiatry. Report of the Pathological Institute, 1904-1905, p.8, State of New York 1906.

PROBLEMS OF TERMINOLOGY AND CLASSIFICATION

IN FORENSIC PSYCHIATRY

Helmut E. Ehrhardt

Professor of Legal and Social Psychiatry
University of Marburg
Ortenbergstrasse 8,   D-3550 Marburg, F.R.G.

Within the overlapping areas of psychiatry and law, physicians
and jurists have always found it difficult to reach a true understanding. In addition to the barrier of professional language the
main obstacle of a common consensus is represented by the contrast
existing between psychiatry as natural science and psychology, as
opposed to the normative and evaluative discipline of jurisprudence.
Psychiatric concepts and terminology emanate only partly from
biology. To a large extent they are determined by questions of
meaning and motivation, by psychodynamic problems. Misunderstandings
might thus result from a transitory lack of biologically based
knowledge, but could also represent a fundamental issue. Although
psychology and psychopathology are empirical sciences, they are not
only and not purely biochemistry or biophysics. The ambivalence inherent in psychiatry, represents a heavy obstacle to the jurist's
access to a science which views behaviour and activities of human
beings from a different perspective to the one he is familiar with.

Apparently well defined notions like normality or abnormality,
sickness or health, have become increasingly controversial and today,
we lack a universally recognized health or disease concept. What is
"health"? - In the preamble to their Constitution, WHO has coined
one of the familiar, but also one of the most misleading definitions,
according to which the health concept denotes not merely the absence
of disease, infirmity or disability, but appears as a state of complete physical, mental and social well-being. This concept encompasses a strong political aspect and the most recent WHO slogan of
"Health for All by the Year 2000", goes conform with that dimension.
This slogan necessarily promotes the absurd notion that all forms
of sickness or disability could be done away with, within the next
two decades. As in the concept of "complete well-being" however,

the slogan merely describes a norm-ideal, the approach of which should be the ultimate aim of all concrete endeavours, under the existing circumstances and in this world full of insufficiencies and conflicting oppositional forces.

The incorporation of the political dimension into the general health concept, might be considered justified or even practical, but in that case it would be advisable, as a consequence, to closely examine and analyze a diminution or possibly even exclusion of a common denominator for ultimate realization of that concept within the area of tension existing between the individual and society.

A universally applicable rating scale for a health concept in the sense of mental and social well-being, does not exist. Socialists and communists, liberals and conservatives, obviously cater to different notions of a citizen's mental and social well-being and, naturally, envisage different ways and means to obtain such a state; in addition to which, the significance of historical and cultural backgrounds for divergent social structures, remains subject to misinterpretation and underestimation. In this connection, it is necessary to stress the fundamental differences between the individualistic concept of basic rights in the western democracies and the traditional, group- and family oriented value-system, still predominant in most of the developing countries. The collectivistic understanding of basic rights within socialistic and communistic ideologies is a third value system, likewise not to compare and not to combine with the two others. – The ubiquitous and plausible acclaim of a "complete well-being", of a certain life quality as the basic requisite for a worthwhile existence resulted, unfortunately, in an ambiguous formula which lends itself to the glossing-over of a very real and concrete dissent in reference to the subject matter.

The discussions about the "right to employment" have proved, that the attempt to postulate a "right to health" as a basic social prerequisite, will not constitute a problem solution. Social rights of that kind cannot be constitutionalized, because their realization depends on the available conditions. The "right to health" slogan therefore will merely serve to foster unrealistic expectations and demands which detract from the individual's own contribution to the maintenance of his health and will thus promote the diminishment of his liability share and deteriorate his value as an adult citizen.

In its dependency upon the results of scientific research and attainment of further knowledge, the "medical-illness-concept" is subject to constant change. Because the diagnostic, pathogenetic and nosological deliberations of the physician mostly constitute juridically irrelevant aspects, the jurist is obliged to extract from the varied and shifting notions of the physician as to the nature of an illness, a legally operationable illness concept. Juridically, it is necessary to determine whether the pertinent disorder repre-

sents a deviation from the norm and especially on whether that deviation has assumed a proportion which is of juridical consequence.
In determination of criminal responsibility for instance, it is of
relevance whether an illness or disorder gravely impedes or exclu-
des the capacity for understanding and/or the capacity to act
according to such understanding. Depending upon the extent of a de-
bilitating illness, civil law for example, contains different
protective mechanisms for the benefit of the patient, whereas
the application of social legislation hinges upon the measure in
which a disease or handicap diminishes an individual's ability to
meet the demands of his occupation. The juridical illness concept
is therefore, of necessity, a quantitatively accentuated one. The
allegorical figure Justitia with her scales, may thus be understood
as a symbolization of this concept.

In forensic psychiatry, the general problematic connected with
the illness concept is further aggravated by the fact that legislative texts contain neither medically nor juridically clear termini
technici in regard to mental diorders and defects, because their
formulations stem from non-scientific, popular diction. The highly
differentiating and - owing to the progress resulting from ongoing
research - continually changing denominations utilized in psychiatric
diagnosis, are not part of popular language. For the jurist it remains difficult therefore, to relate the possibly disabling effect
of organic disease or psychogenic disorder, of psychopathy (personality disorder) or of behavioural aberration with neurotic or
psychosocial background, to a person's accountability in regard to
penal or civil law. It should additionally be considered, that the
diagnostic demarcations in psychopathology - characterized by the
peculiarities of psychological conceptualization - tend to be of an
accentuative nature, in contrast to the determinative one they would
assume in natural science.

Psychiatrists and politicians engaged alike upon the field of
public health, must be held responsible for the present confusion,
which became even more evident in the recent arguments concerning:
informed consent, right to demand or refuse treatment, confidentiality and data protection. The trend, noticeable within the anglo-
american sphere of influence, within the WHO and UN bodies, to
abolish the concept of mental illness or disease in favour of the
foggy term "mental disorder", must be considered as a characteristic
example in justification of this accusation.

The International Commission of Jurists (ICJ) and the International Association of Penal Law (IAPL) for instance, presented 1981,
to the UN Human Rights Commission and the Council of Europe, a
"Draft Body of Principles for the Protection of Persons suffering
from Mental Disorder", the amended version of which subsequently
figured under the title of "Draft Guidelines·.....", - although
the text of both documents, conceptualized mainly by jurists, com-

pletely lacked an adequate denomination for the state of "mental disease". Since however, the concept of "mental disorder" is utilized in reference to grave brain lesions , as well as for psychosocial disorders of behaviour, it becomes inapplicable in the juridical sense. During the course of his lifetime, almost every individual's behaviour may be adversely affected over shorter or longer periods of time by psychoneurotic or psychosocial disturbances, so that it appears impossible to postulate, in regard to such cases, the identical legislative stipulations applied to psychotic patients whose disease has impaired their mental capacities and their sense of liability toward society.

During recent years, WHO has contributed to the promotion of questionable perceptions and initiatives, by the issue of statements to the effect that - in the latter half of this century - the policy of individual countries has concentrated on the improvement of mental health, rather than on the cure of mental illness. If that were indeed the case, WHO should make an effort to impress on politicians engaged upon the public health issue, that they should primarily concern themselves with the improvement of care- and treatment facilities, since the promotion of "mental health" - under any denomination, and certainly in the sense of primary prevention - should preferably remain the responsibility of social and educational policy.

By accentuating the marginal zones and borderline aspects of mental illness, WHO professes to attempt a re-orientation of public opinion in reference to the mental health issue. However, several years ago, it was asserted that approximately 40 million individuals of the world's entire population, suffer from the effects of severe mental illness, such as for instance: psychoses, organic brain syndromes and oligophrenias. Up to the year 2000, the expected increase of such diseases and defects has been estimated with about 20% within the industrialized-, and approximately 72% in developing countries. A 23% resp. 87% rise is expected in regard to the schizophrenias, whereas senile dementia patients are expected to increase by 54% to 123% respectively. Regarding the less serious to slight mental disorders, the numbers-as far as they have become at all available - are appreciably higher, whereby attention should be drawn to the fact that a diagnostic scale, which encompasses organic brain defects as well as psychosocial behaviour aberrations, represents a diminutive record, additionally diluted by subjectively based evaluations, thus resulting in a further softening of data.

The increasing tendency of the "hard data" is nothing less than frightening. It is therefore difficult to understand why, in the face of such a situation, WHO promotes a re-orientation of thought and a shift of public policy away from the issue of mental disease, toward the concept of "mental health". This gives rise to the question as to who will then care for the rapidly increasing number of seriously mentally ill patients and who, moreover, is going to provide the financial wherewithal, if the politicians concerned are further encouraged to deploy the revenues derived from tax- and social security payments, upon the undefined and limitless area of "soft data"?

Examples for the terminological confusion and perceptual complexity, and the noteworthy consequences in the care for psychiatric patients, may be found in all areas of legislation. In this paper, it is impossible to provide more than just a few brief references: only recently , the United States have witnessed a resurgence of public debate concerning the prerequisites determining a delinquent's criminal responsibility. Immediate cause for the debate was John R. Hinckley's attempted assassination of President Reagan. Hinckley has been diagnosed as mentally sick, pronounced irresponsible and was admitted for treatment into a psychiatric hospital. Under German law, this case would not represent a problem, as long as the delinquent suffers indeed from schizophrenia, which in some of its characteristic forms results in the inability to understand and/or to act according to such understanding.

In this particular case however, it seems that psychiatrists failed to come to an agreement as to the delinquent's mental state. The deliberations of American jurists who, at present, advocate a revision of the entire concept in regard to insanity defense, in the USA until today exercised with differing accentuations, add to the general confusion. Jurists are of course aware of the fact that out of the vast conglomerate of mental disorders, only a very small percentage justifies the acceptance of criminal irresponsibility. To the legal mind, it must be a matter of considerable irritation, when psychiatrists discuss neuroses and psychoses upon the same level as abnormal social reaction patterns. If psychiatrists were in a position to improve upon the objectivation and concretization of their diagnostic statements, jurists would much more readily accept their recommendations.

Civil law confronts us with similar problems: legal incapacitation, guardianship, civil committment etc. - represent protection and aid mechanisms which are similarly incorporated into legislation and judicature of many countries. Legal incapacitation or the appointment of guardianship are based on certain prerequisites determined by the psychiatrist. The pertinent and very similar stipulations of German-, Austrian- and Swiss law, utilize the terms "mental illness" and "mental debility", although these denominations do not entirely conform with psychiatric terminology, and their juridical interpretation in the three countries is not identical. These terms, moreover, do not represent a psychiatric diagnosis, but rather a juridical concept, the content of which necessitates - by detour, so to speak - precise interpretation and concretization through the psychiatrist. The pertinent legislative stipulations were formulated, in the German-speaking countries, around the turn of the century.

In the course of time, their practical application has been adjusted to changing circumstances. Meanwhile however - and in consideration of the preceptions gained by today's psychiatry - it has become obvious that detailed revisions should urgently be undertaken but should not of course remain limited to the terminological aspect.

The legislative amendations planned - or already effected - in other countries, could be utilized in many ways as patterns or guidelines: in France, the stipulations governing appointment of guardianship have been basically reformed by the law of Jan.3,1968, and several of the newly formulated solutions can be considered to have model character. Mention should here be made of the fact that the entire procedure has become largely independent of psychiatric diagnosis and terminology and has been accomodated mainly to individual care requirements. - Another example is to be found in Great Britain's recently formulated "Mental Health (Amendment) Act 1982", which replaces the first version (1959) from Sept.30,1983 onward. Within these revisions may also be found several juridical solutions upon which the legislator of other European countries might orient himself; whereas other stipulations, regarding the extension of mechanisms for additional legal protection of patients, the concept of a patient's representative for instance, should be viewed sceptically and with due reservation.

Social law encompasses numerous vague formulations and confused notions,and many juridical concepts received their subsequent - but not always convincing - interpretation by court decisions over a lengthy period of time. The"handicap"-concept e.g., represents a typical example: in German law, the extent of handicap is evaluated in regard to the percentage of one's occupational or professional disability. Whenever a 50% diminishment can be diagnosed, the person in question meets the stipulations determining "severe handicap" and becomes the beneficiary of numerous social as well as financial privileges. By simple addition of several trivial and practically insignificant complaints such as e.g.: mild forms of diabetes, hypotonia, myopia, rheumatism , etc. - it is comparatively easy to reach the desired 50% incapacity. Thanks to the legislative stipulations governing the state of "severe handicap" - initially considered a social innovation of considerable merit - the FRG numbers to date approximately 4,5 mio citizens of that category and the country is well on the way to developing into a nation of "severely handicapped" people, whereby the possibilities inherent in the concept of mentally or psychosocially based handicaps, has not as yet been thoroughly explored. Handicaps caused by the aging process, represent an additional and practically unsolvable problem. The attempt, initiated by WHO, to distinguish between impairment, disability and handicap, is an interesting proposition, but remains inadequate for the solution of practical problems. For that reason, this triple sub-classification has not been incorporated into the ICD.

If in closing, we attempt to explore the means by which a diminishment of the conceptual misunderstandings between the two disciplines may be effected, the intensivation of the dialogue between psychiatrists and jurists appears as the prime requisite. An attitude of resignation on the part of either profession, would defeat all efforts at an improvement and would negatively affect the situation of the patients entrusted to us. In the USA, recent discussions regarding the patient's right to demand – or reversely to refuse – treatment, have proved that subject oriented, unbiased debate can produce positive results. Not every psychiatrist however, represents a suitable partner in dialogue with the jurist. It would be advisable to delegate for such discussions, psychiatrists with broad clinical and forensic experiences, who have supplemented their medicinal knowledge by juridical and legislative studies.

Recently established methods for improved concretization and classification of psychiatric symptoms, represent an additional instrument for attainment of the desired goal. Mention should be made in this connection, of the PSE-system of Wing, Cooper et al. and of the AMDP-system developed by several psychiatrists in German speaking countries. These, and similar systems, aim at homogenization and objectivation of diagnostic criteria in psychopathology, and by such means, a terminology similarly acceptable and adequate to the demands posed by both disciplines, might be developed. However, it remains the forensic psychiatrist's foremost competency to elucidate, to the pertinent court, the implication of his medical diagnosis in reference to: accountability in confrontation with demands of criminal or civil law or, in confrontation upon the sector of social legislation, the extent of one's capacity to earn one's own livelihood.

References

AMDP, Hrsg.,"Das AMDP-System, Manual zur Dokumentation psychiatrischer Befunde", 4.Aufl., Springer, Berlin (1981).
Ehrhardt, H., Psychiatrie, in: "Handwörterbuch der Kriminologie", R. Sieverts,Hrsg., 2.Aufl. Bd.II, de Gruyter, Berlin (1971).
Gross, R., Gesundheit und Krankheit in ihren verschiedenen Aspekten, Dtsch. Ärztebl. 77:1397 (1980).
Häfner, H., Allgemeine und spezielle Krankheitsbegriffe in der Psychiatrie, Nervenarzt 54:231 (1983).
Helgason, T., ed., "Methods in Evaluation of Psychiatric Treatment", University Press, Cambridge (1983).
Spitzer,R.L.,Williams,J.B.W.,Skodol,A.E.,eds., "International Perspectives on DSM III", Am.Psychiat.Press,Washington,DC (1983).
Wing,J.K.,Cooper,J.E.,Sartorius,N., "Measurement and Classification of Psychiatric Symptoms", Univ. Press, Cambridge (1974).
World Psychiatric Association, ed., "Diagnostic Criteria for Schizophrenic and Affective Psychoses", American Psychiatric Press, Washington, D.C. (1983).

PSYCHIATRIC CLASSIFICATION – A VIEW FROM THE THIRD WORLD

Narendra N. Wig

Prof. & Head, Department of Psychiatry
All India Institute of Medical Sciences
New Delhi, India

INTRODUCTION

More than three-fourths of the world's mentally ill live in
the countries of Asia, Africa and Latin America – the so-called
third world. Yet, the current systems of psychiatric diagnosis
and classification have hardly taken into account the different
patterns of psychiatric symptomatology present in these countries,
or the special needs of these regions as regards psychiatric classification.

The mental health professionals of the third world countries
thus face a special problem in the field of psychiatric diagnosis
and classification. Most of them have been trained in the psychiatric centres of Europe or U.S.A. and have learnt their psychiatry
by seeing Western patients and reading the text books written by
European and American authors. In contrast, their own upbringing
has often been considerably different. They have picked up, in
their own respective cultures, many ideas of mental processes in
health and disease which are at variance with the teachings of
psychiatric text books but which are nonetheless shared by many of
the patients in their own countries.

SOME CONCEPTUAL DIFFERENCES BETWEEN EUROPEAN AND OTHER CULTURES IN
PSYCHIATRIC DIAGNOSIS AND CLASSIFICATION

Psychiatric classification is not simply a convenient list of
disease categories: it is, indirectly a way of looking at the whole
concept of mental ill health. It is often not realized that current
psychiatric classification has many conceptual biases that have

their origins in 19th century European philosophical & psychiatric thinking. Some of these conceptual differences as seen from the point of view of the Third World are discussed below.

a)   One striking difference between European psychiatry and ancient systems of medicine is the concept of psychogenesis i.e. intrapsychic forces being the underlying causes of mental illness. Insanity as a grossly disturbed behaviour with loss of insight seems to be well recognised in most of the ancient medical texts. However, such a diagnosis was based predominantly on observation of external behaviour. Intra-psychic processes, as such, were neither given prominence in the understanding of symptoms, nor used as the basis of diagnosis or classification. For example, in Indian Ayurvedic texts there is no clear recognition of separate affective or mood disorders nor is there any clear description of insanity resembling paranoid psychosis, while states of excitement, severe withdrawl and socially inappropriate behaviour are well described.

b)   The European mind has a habit of thinking in terms of duality i.e., either/or principles like Good and Evil. As a result of this tendency there are many intellectual themes which have become major controversies for the European mind while they have never been so important for people of other cultures. In the field of medical sciences, endless time has been spent during the last hundred years to sort out the nature of the body versus mind, importance of genetic versus environmental factors, endogenous versus reactive illness, organic versus functional symptoms, and so on. It is perhaps difficult for the European mind to accept and understand that for many other cultures in the world these either-or controversies are really not so important, and life is often seen more in terms of continuity rather than in terms of such sharp division between two poles.

Perhaps the same European influence has resulted in the current dichotomy between Schizophrenia and Affective Psychosis in the classification of Psychosis. In nineteenth century European psychology, it was popular to divide mental functions into thinking and feeling, as two distinct faculties. As a logical extension of that thought there has evolved an "Insanity of thinking" and an "Insanity of feeling" leading on to the present day Schizophrenia and Affective psychosis. As a result of this thinking, even if there are clear delusions present in mania or depression, these are always explained on "underlying" affective disturbances, just as depression or elation present in schizophrenia is always supposed to be "secondary".

c)   The concept of Neurosis is also essentially a product of European thought. While the role of life events and strong emotions in health and disease has been accepted by all cultures, the concept of somatic symptoms being produced by "Underlying" psychological factors or "Subconcious" conflicts is the contribution of European medicine. In the indigenous systems of medicine of India, China or other Afro-Asian countries, there is no such separation of bodily symptoms due to bodily causes, and bodily symptoms due to mental causes, a distinction which is at the root of modern psychiatry.

This concept of neurotic symptoms being essentially psychogenic has probably created more problems than it has solved. On the positive side it has perhaps given birth to modern psychotherapy as a method of treatment, though with congroversial results. In the bargain it has produced serious problems in medical diagnosis and classification, and in many ways has slowed down the process of our understanding of these compoex human reactions. Grouping together of such diverse conditions as acute panic reactions, hysteria, obsessions, hypochondriasis and compensation neurosis does not appear to be very logical. The common thread in all such diverse conditions is presumed to be the underlying "anxiety", or some mysterious psychological tension. Many of the people in the third world countries including the health staff find it very difficult to understand how diverse bodily symptoms can be produced by "hidden" psychological causes. Those who are practicing medicine in a developing country would appreciate how frustating it can be to explain to the relatives of a young girl with hysterical paralysis or aphonia, brought in an emergency, that these symptoms are really not physical but are all in the mind. It immediately downgrades the patient as a malingerer or as psychologically inferior. No wonder most such patients prefer to go to indigenous healers rather than to modern doctors.

d) Many cultures all over the world have recognized the harmful effect of excessive emotions. Modern European psychiatry has however arbitrarily selected two of the emotions viz: anxiety and depression as abnormal, and projected them as serious psychiatric diseases. Anxiety and depression have become the two commonest diagnoses in general practice. It is difficult to understand that if excess of fear or sadness is bad, why are excess of anger, jealousy, hate, greed or eroticism not abnormal? The only group which seems to have benefitted by such frequent diagnoses of anxiety and depression is, perhaps the pharmaceutical industry. As soon as the psychiatrists have labelled anxiety and depression as diseases, the drug companies have come out with "anti-anxiety" and "anti-depressant" drugs.

IMPORTANT VARIATIONS IN PSYCHIATRIC SYMPTOMATOLOGY BETWEEN EUROPE & THIRD WORLD COUNTRIES

How are the mental health professionals in Third World countries using psychiatric terminology and what are their impressions of the usefulness of psychiatric classification in their day-to-day work ? Unfortunately psychiatric research is still in its infancy in the Third World and research publications are scanty. Inspite of these limitations many observers from the developing countries have repeatedly recorded considerable variations between the psychiatric phenomenon as seen in these countries and those described in Western countries. Interestingly, there is a close similarity between these reports from different parts of the developing world. These differences can be summed up in the following way. Firstly, the gross psychiatric symptoms, particularly psychotic reactions in developing countries, tend to be acute and short-lived. Secondly, the psychiatric symptoms appear (at least to the western-trained observer) more dramatic and exaggerated. Thirdly, the psychological expression of symptoms is often global, mixed, or amorphous, as a result of which differentiation between various psychiatric categories and even between psychosis and nourosis becomes very difficult. Fourthly, somatic complaints are quite frequently present along with the classical psychological syndromes. Fifthly, the primitive reactions of fear and panic are quite common.

USE OF PSYCHIATRIC CLASSIFICATION IN THE THIRD WORLD

In the most of the developing countries modern medicine and psychiatry has evolved through the European influence. Consequently, the medical education and training in these countries has heavilly modelled itself on the parent European country. For example, in the countries of the erstwhile British Empire, the British system of medical education still dominates, while the French influence in medical education is still supreme in the countries of the former French Empire. This is to a degree inevitable because the language of science in developing countries is often a modern European language like English, French, German etc.

As a result of this, psychiatric nomenclature in each developing country has borrowed heavily from the original European source. While the English-speaking countries have adopted the English views of psychiatric diagnosis and classification, the French-speaking countries of Asia and Africa have stuck to the traditional French systems of psychiatric nosology. As a result, while certain concepts and diagnostic terms (like Boufees Delirantes) are common in French psychiatry, they are virtually unknown to an English-speaking psychiatrist in the third world.

Since the emergence of WHO International Classification of Disease (ICD), many developing countries have tried to adopt this for national medical records. However, in the psychiatric education and research, the influence of earlier dominant European thought remains. In the English-speaking countries a very powerful influence in recent years has been that of the American Psychiatric Association's Diagnostic and Statistical Manual (D.S.M.). Its third edition with its new emphasis on criteria and use of different axes, has made a strong impact on modern psychiatry. However, one would have to wait for sometime to assess its long-term influence.

CERTAIN SPECIAL NEEDS OF PSYCHIATRIC CLASSIFICATION FOR THE
DEVELOPING COUNTRIES

One of the major difficulties in the developing countries at
present, is the limited availability of trained manpower for the
health services. For example, the psychiatrist-to-population ratio
is roughly one to a million in most of the countries of the third
world (WHO T.R.S., 1975). Obviously, there can never be enough
specialists in these countries in the foreseeable future to provide
mental health care to all the people. The bulk of the mental health
services would have to be undertaken by primary care physicians and
health workers. It is doubtful if the current psychiatric classification, with all its controversies, would be able to meet this
need. It is thus necessary that a parallel, management-oriented,
simple psychiatric classification for use at the primary level be
prepared.

An initial effort at such a classification should be at an
international level, the resulting classification being then adapted
to local conditions and to the various levels of health workers
wherever necessary. It is hoped, as indicated earlier, that the
more elaborate classification for use by specialists may eventually
be built on such a simpler classification.

CONCLUSIONS

a)   The mental health professionals in the third world countries
find themselves in a difficult position in the matter of psychiatric
diagnosis and classification. The psychological concepts and psychiatric nomenclature prevalent in the old indigenous systems of medicine, though still popular with the lay public and many health
professionals, are insufficient to accommodate the growing knowledge
in psychiatry or the complex health needs of the modern health
services. On the other hand, a total switch to an European or
American classification proves equally frustrating.

b)   Psychiatrists in the third world are impressed by many psychiatric phenomena that cannot be satisfactorily classified in the current classification. Perhaps there are still undescribed psychiatric diseases and syndromes present among the vast populations of
third world countries, or may be there are only different presentations of the essentially common human psychopathology. On both
counts, there is urgent need for recognizing such different psychiatric presentations for the growth and future of world psychiatry.

c)   Much of what today forms the modern psychiatric classification was largely developed in the nineteenth century European mental hospitals. For some time now, psychiatry has moved out into the general hospitals and the community. General hospital psychiatry has already thrown new challenges to diagnosis and classification, especially in the developing countries. It is, thus, imperative that a fresh look be taken at the classification in the light of general hospital and community psychiatry. It is necessary that a parallel, simple, management-oriented classification be prepared for use at the primary health care level.

AN INTERNATIONAL CONSULTATION ON MULTIAXIAL DIAGNOSIS

Juan E. Mezzich, Horacio Fabrega, Jr.,
and Ada C. Mezzich

Western Psychiatric Institute and Clinic
University of Pittsburgh
3811 O'Hara Street, Pittsburgh, Pennsylvania 15213

INTRODUCTION

Essen-Möller and Wohlfahrt[1] in Sweden in 1947 and Leme Lopes[2] in Brazil in 1954 inaugurated a new approach to diagnostic formulation in psychiatry. This approach, currently known as the multiaxial model, attempts to articulate in an explicit and formal manner the key elements of the patient's condition. These elements, termed axes, are evaluated separately from each other and basically include clinical syndromes and etiological or associated factors. During the past decade at least 13 other multiaxial systems, originating from ten different countries, have been published.[3] A variety of axes have been included in these systems, with the common intentions of providing a more comprehensive representation of the clinically pertinent factors of a psychiatric condition and of making the formulation more useful for the various basic diagnostic purposes (i.e., clinical description, treatment, prognosis, and etiological and theoretical research).

Correspondingly, the multiaxial approach is attracting considerable interest for the development of standard diagnostic systems, such as the next revision of the International Classification of Diseases. However, little systematic information has been available at the international level about actual experience with multiaxial systems and on the most appropriate number and most promising types of axes to include. These questions were addressed by the present study, sponsored by the World Psychiatric Association (WPA), through a consultation by mail with a broad international panel of diagnostic experts.

METHOD

The first phase of the study involved the development of the panel of experts. To this end, with the help of the secretariat of the WPA and its Section on Nomenclature and Classification, presidents of national psychiatric societies, contacted during the first half of 1982, were asked to furnish names of distinguished colleagues with recognized expertise in psychiatric diagnosis and nosology, and, if possible, familiarity with multiaxial systems. Out of 60 national societies, 55 responded positively, one negatively, and five did not respond. Also contacted were officers of the World Health Organization (WHO) and some of its regional offices, as well as key contributors to the international literature on multiaxial systems, most of which responded positively. Through this procedure, the names and addresses of 250 experts from 55 countries spanning the six WHO world regions were obtained.

Also during this preparatory phase, a questionnaire was devised to explore: the professional characteristics of the prospective participants; their experience with standard diagnostic systems and special diagnostic procedures; their use and perceived usefulness of and problems with multiaxial systems; their views on the value of 21 potential axes (extracted from previously proposed multiaxial systems); and their suggestions for refining the conceptualization and assessment of proposed axes and for developing additional ones.

Mostly during the first half of 1983, the 250 identified experts were contacted and non-respondents received two follow-up letters. At final count, 175 experts (70%) completed the study questionnaire, 9 (4%) declined participation, and 66 (26%) did not respond (wrong addresses being a contributing factor). The 175 participants, representing 52 countries, are listed in the Appendix and were distributed as follows: 39 from the Americas, 59 from Europe, 15 from Africa, 13 from the Eastern Mediterranean, 38 from Southeast Asia, and 11 from the Western Pacific.

The mean profile of proffered theoretical orientation of the participants was as follows: 39% biological, 23% psychodynamic, 21% social/community, 10% behavioristic, and 7% "other." Their mean profile of professional activities included: 26% outpatient practice, 22% research, 20% teaching, 19% inpatient practice, 12% administration, and 10% "other." The average distribution of their patients' age-developmental status was 8% children, 17% adolescents, 63% adults, and 12% elderly. Regarding participation in future empirical studies on multiaxial systems using actual case material, 63% reported high interest, 28% moderate interest, and 9% no interest.

RESULTS

In the first substantive section of the study respondents were asked about their experiences with standard diagnostic systems. Table 1 presents the use and perceived usefulness of ICD-8,[4] ICD-9,[5] and

DSM-III[6] by WHO regions. The system most frequently used was ICD-9 (77%), followed closely by DSM-III (72%) (this order being inverted only among the Eastern Mediterranean and Western Pacific experts). High usefulness was most frequently reported for DSM-III (46%) and next for ICD-9 (29%) (except in Africa where this order was inverted).

Additionally, 40% of the participants reported using 64 diagnostic systems other than those listed above (although many of them entailed slight modifications of these). Special diagnostic procedures reported as "used frequently" included structured interviews (51%), psychological tests (30%), checklists of clinical manifestations (29%), and biological tests (23%).

The most frequent recommendations offered for the improvement of psychiatric diagnostic systems included: the furtherance of the use and refinement of multiaxial diagnosis (21%), advances in the procedures for patient evaluation (19%), the development of internationally useful diagnostic systems (15%), better descriptions of diagnostic categories (13%), and the empirical evaluation of diagnostic systems (10%).

Table 1

Use and Perceived Usefulness of ICD-8, ICD-9, and DSM-III
As Reported by the ICMD Participants by W.H.O. Regions

Use and Usefulness of Diagnostic Systems	Americas (n=39) %	Europe (n=59) %	Africa (n=15) %	E. Mediterranean (n=13) %	S.E. Asia (n=38) %	Western Pacific (n=11) %	TOTAL PANEL (n=175) %
ICD-8							
Users	45	68	53	45	65	45	58
Usefulness:							
Low	47	31	37	60	29	60	37
Medium	24	36	50	20	54	40	39
High	29	33	13	20	17	0	24
ICD-9							
Users	76	72	73	67	89	82	77
Usefulness:							
Low	14	24	27	12	18	33	20
Medium	48	45	45	50	59	56	51
High	38	31	28	38	23	11	29
DSM-III							
Users	76	70	47	83	70	91	72
Usefulness:							
Low	14	28	14	30	19	10	21
Medium	27	23	72	10	46	50	33
High	59	49	14	60	35	40	46

The second section of the study investigated the participants' experiences with multiaxial diagnosis. Table 2 displays the use and perceived usefulness of multiaxial systems by WHO regions. Eighty-three percent of the participants had used a multiaxial approach and 67% of these considered its usefulness high. Interestingly, in Africa, where the lowest percentage of multiaxial users (69%) was found, the greatest percentage of high usefulness was accorded to this approach (89%).

The most frequently used specific multiaxial systems by far were DSM-III and close derivatives (56%), followed by the system developed by Rutter et al[7] for child psychiatry (11%).

The principal ways in which multiaxial systems were found useful were by: providing a comprehensive evaluative formulation (25%), facilitating treatment planning and management (18%), allowing greater comparability of diagnoses (9%), teasing out key clinical/diagnostic elements (7%), enhancing the usefulness of diagnosis for different purposes (7%), elucidating areas of consensus and divergence (5%), and facilitating teaching (5%).

The main difficulties reported in the use of multiaxial systems were unclear or problematic definitions (24%) and cumbersome or time-consuming usage (16%).

The number of axes considered feasible or manageable to use in regular clinical work was two by 2% of the respondents, three by 25%, four by 21%, five by 30%, and six or more by 21%.

The third substantive section of the study elicited the views of the experts on the value of individual potential axes regarding four

Table 2

Use and Usefulness of Multiaxial Systems
as Reported by ICMD Participants by W.H.O. Regions

Use and Usefulness of Multiaxial Systems	Americas (n=39) %	Europe (n=59) %	Africa (n=15) %	E. Mediterranean (n=13) %	S.E. Asia (n=38) %	Western Pacific (n=11) %	TOTAL PANEL (n=175) %
Users	90	83	69	83	78	100	83
Usefulness:							
None	0	2	0	0	4	0	1
Medium	32	25	11	40	35	60	32
High	68	73	89	60	61	40	67

diagnostic purposes (clinical description, treatment decisions, prediction of illness outcome, and theory development), and on whether they are essential for an efficient multiaxial system. This information is summarized in Table 3, which shows that the best rated axes, in decreasing order of importance, were psychiatric syndromes, physical disorders , course of illness, personality disorders, specific psychosocial stressors, psychoticism, adaptive functioning, etiology specified by clinician, specific developmental delays, and intelligence level/mental retardation. Ranking order varied noticeably according to diagnostic purpose. On the other hand, there was almost no variation in overall mean ratings across world regions.

The most frequently suggested axial additions, in decreasing order, were an axis on family structure and functioning; the combin-

Table 3

Potential Axes, Their Mean Ratings for Various Diagnostic Purposes, and Percent Checked as Essential by ICMD Participants

Potential Axes	Ratings for Various Diagnostic Purposes*					Percent Checked As Essential
	Description $\bar{X}$	Treatment $\bar{X}$	Prediction $\bar{X}$	Theory $\bar{X}$	Overall $\bar{X}$	%
1. Psychiatric Syndromes	3.0	2.8	2.5	2.3	2.6	85
2. Personality Disorders	2.4	2.3	2.4	2.1	2.3	68
3. Specific Developmental Delays	2.2	2.1	2.1	1.9	2.1	25
4. Intelligence Level/M.R.	2.2	2.1	2.1	1.6	2.0	40
5. Severity of Symptomatology	2.3	2.4	1.9	1.5	2.0	26
6. Psychoticism	2.4	2.4	2.1	1.8	2.2	20
7. Age at Onset of Illness	2.1	1.9	2.2	1.9	2.0	21
8. Speed of Illness Onset	2.2	2.1	2.3	1.8	2.1	22
9. Duration of Illness	2.3	2.3	2.6	1.8	2.3	29
10. Course of Illness	2.4	2.5	2.6	2.0	2.4	41
11. Highest Level of Adaptive Functioning in Past Year	1.9	2.2	2.4	1.8	2.1	37
12. Current Level of Adaptive Functioning	2.2	2.3	2.3	1.7	2.1	36
13. Physical Disorders with Brain Dysfunction	2.7	2.7	2.5	2.2	2.5	64
14. Physical Disorders without Brain Dysfunction	2.1	2.1	1.9	1.6	1.9	30
15. Neurobehavioral Functioning	2.1	2.0	1.9	2.0	2.0	19
16. Psychodynamic Factors	2.0	2.1	2.0	2.1	2.1	30
17. Specific Psychosocial Stressors	2.2	2.3	2.3	2.3	2.2	41
18. Overall Psychosocial Stressor Severity	1.9	2.1	2.1	1.9	2.0	30
19. Support Systems	1.6	2.3	2.2	1.8	2.0	25
20. Etiology Specified by Clinician	2.0	2.2	2.1	2.3	2.1	35
21. Conceptualization of Illness by Patient/Family	1.5	1.9	1.9	1.5	1.7	13

* 1 = Not Important; 2 = Somewhat Important; 3 = Very Important

ation of course, duration, speed of onset, and age at onset of illness; and the combination of personality, developmental delays, and I.Q.

COMMENT

The findings of this study documented the considerable usefulness accorded to the multiaxial approach by diagnostic experts around the world. The prominence of DSM-III was striking among all multiaxial systems, as was the tendency to consider it as more useful than the current International Classification. The differential ratings obtained for individual axes may be helpful when selecting and organizing those to be involved in future diagnostic systems.

Further appraisals of multiaxial systems should consider their reliability, perceived usefulness among clinicians, impact on treatment decisions, and ability to predict illness outcome.

REFERENCES

1. E Essen-Möller, S Wohlfahrt, Suggestions for the amendment of the official Swedish classification of mental disorders. Acta Psychia. Scan. Supp., 47:551 (1947).
2. J Leme Lopes, As dimensões do diagnóstico psiquiátrico: Rio de Janeiro, Agir (1954).
3. JE Mezzich, Multiaxial diagnostic systems in psychiatry. In: Comprehensive Textbook of Psychiatry, 4th Ed.. HI Kaplan & BJ Sadock, Eds. Baltimore, Williams & Wilkins, in press.
4. W.H.O., Manual of the International Classification of Diseases, Injuries and Causes of Death, 8th Rev. (ICD-8), WHO, Geneva (1967).
5. W.H.O., Manual of the International Classification of Diseases, Injuries and Causes of Death, 9th Rev. (ICD-9), WHO, Geneva (1978).
6. American Psychiatric Association, Diagnostic and Statistical Manual of Mental Disorders, 3rd Ed. (DSM-III). Washington, D.C., APA (1980).
7. M Rutter, D Shaffer, M Shepherd, A Multiaxial Classification of Child Psychiatric Disorders. Geneva, W.H.O. (1975).

APPENDIX - International Consultation on Multiaxial Diagnosis Participants

Argentina: C Hernández, J Herrera, G Vidal. Australia: R Adler, PJV Beaumont, H Brodaty, AS Henderson, B Klug, G Parker, J Price. Austria: H Katschnig, G Lenz, W Schony. Belgium: J Janssen, E Suy. Brazil: J Caruso Madalena, E Busnello, J Leme Lopes, G Loreto. Bulgaria: I Ignev, Z Ivanov, K Milenkov, V Milew. Canada: P Barker, S Hirsch, W Junek, KI Pearce. Chile: E Covarrubias, R Florenzano, H Montenegro, R Ruiz, M Trucco, O Dörr Zegers. China: S Yucun. Colombia: CA León. Costa Rica: J Rodríguez, A Gallegos-Chacón. Cuba: JA Bustamante Oleary. Denmark: T Isager, M Mellergaard, N Reisby. Egypt: M Abdel Gawad, MK Ismail, A Okasha, TY Rakahwy, O Shaheen. Finland: B Furman, MD Huttunen, J Lonnqvist. France: P Marchais, E Zarifian. Germany (East): GE Kuehne. Germany (West): H Dilling, S Haas, H Helmchen, A Pietzcker, D von Zerssen. Greece: E Frangos, A Liakos, G Lyketsos, YG Papakostas. Iceland: H Hannesdottir. India: VN Bagadia, SB Chatterjee, DD Doongaji, RS Master, S Menon, V Ramchandran, AV Rao, G Singh, VN Vahia, VK Varma, N Wig. Iran: N Ameri, M Behfar-Rad, H Darabi, H Davidian, A Mohit. Israel: A Apter, H Dasberg, Y Ginath, Y Levav. Italy: G Cassano, D Kemali. Japan: T Fukuda, Y Kasahara, A Mori, R Takahashi, S Takahashi, N Yamaguchi. Lebanon: F Antun, C Baddoura. Luxembourg: GE Muller, C Pull. Malaysia: MP Deva, M Subramaniam. Mexico: C Campillo-Serrano, J Sepúlveda-Amor. Morocco: F Benchekroun, J Ktiouet, D Moussaoui, M Paes. The Netherlands: CJAJ Slooff, AL van Bemmel, K van Groos, P Chr. Mussert, Fr. van Ree, W van Tilburg. New Zealand: TLU Fernando, B James, J Werry. Nigeria: A Binitie, RO Jegede, R Makanjuola. Norway: AA Dahl. Pakistan: SH Ahmed, KZ Hasan, HAG Kazi, MH Mubbashar, M Shafique. Panama: J Arroyo Sucre, OA DeLeón, J Kravcio. Papua-New Guinea: TL Sawa. Peru: R Llanos, J Mariátegui, H Rotondo Grimaldi. The Philippines: L Ladrido-Ignacio, JP Lopez. Poland: A Bilikiewicz, J Bomba. Singapore: TW Foo, TS Hock, PW Ngui. South Africa: MB Feldman, G Hart. Spain: DC Ballus Pascual, J Giner Ubago, J Guimón Ugartechea, JJ López-Ibor Aliño, DJ Rodríguez Sacristán. Sweden: H Agren, E Essen-Möller, J-O Ottosson, C Perris, B-E Roos. Switzerland: J Angst, MT Gastpar. Taiwan: C-H Chan, H-G Hwu, H-N Lin, W-T Soong, J-K Wen. Thailand: S Dejatawongse, S Suvanashiep, S Suwanlert. Turkey: O Köknel, G Koptagel-Ilal. United Kingdom: I Brockington, J Cooper, J Copeland, RE Kendell, M Rutter, M Shepherd. United States: D Cantwell, P Clayton, J Gunderson, L Judd, D Shaffer, R Spitzer, JS Strauss. Venezuela: A Hernández Carstens, L Meléndez de Nucette, A Pacheco Hernández. Zambia: A Haworth.

A LOGICAL BASIS FOR THE STRUCTURE OF MULTI-AXIAL DESCRIPTIONS OF

PSYCHIATRIC PATIENTS

John E. Cooper

University of Nottingham
Department of Psychiatry
United Kingdom

The first section of this paper is a critical discussion of
the nature and purposes of what is nowadays usually called "multi-
axial classification".   The characteristics of so-called "axes"
are discussed, in order to examine the relationships between them.
Suggestions are then made as to how the information in published
multi-axial systems can be viewed in relation to the complete set
of clinical and social information that comprises the conventional
clinical formulation.   A simple basic division into unchanging
and changing categories is suggested.   Finally, a particular
hierarchical system of classification is suggested as suitable for
classifying some physical, personal and social aspects of the
patient.

The interest being shown in "multi-axial classification " in
psychiatric research is well illustrated by the review of Mezzich
(1979) and by his presentation today.   In the review, he
discussed and compared nine systems that had appeared in the
psychiatric literature between 1970 and 1978.   The most recent
of these (and the most complicated) is the DSM-111, (Diagnostic
and Statistical Manual, Third Edition, of the American Psychiatric
Association), which many psychiatrists in the United States are
now obliged to use whether they like it or not.   With regard to
the future, it is already widely supposed that the Mental Disorder
Section (Chapter V of the 10th revision of the International
Classification of Diseases sponsored by the World Health
Organisation will be "multi-axial".   In other words, multi-axial
classification in psychiatry seems to be here to stay, and
deserves attention.

As the review of Mezzich shows, even a cursory glance at the

many multi-axial systems now in existence indicates that they
differ in purpose, content and organisation. This could be
admirable and useful if the variations were systematic and if
the systems were planned in relation to one another, but this
is not so. As with many other simpler forms of classification
used in psychiatry, the elementary rules of classification are
often not followed by those who put together multi-axial systems,
and there is little discussion which justifies the number, form
and content of the axes. The usefulness of the term "axis"
itself has been questioned, and a more general term such as
"aspects" is preferred by many. The Oxford English Dictionary
defines axis as "a straight line about which a thing revolves or
is symmetrically arranged". These properties are not possessed
by the sections of most systems. In addition, some 'axes' are
categorical and some are dimensional, and some hardly specified
at all. I shall therefore use the word "aspect" as a more
general term.

It is clear that psychiatrists and social scientists in a
number of countries are now looking for ways of systematically
classifying and recording several things about their patients at
the same time, in a way which other research workers can understand
and duplicate.

This interest in systematic, reliable and communicable
systems of description stem from the fairly recent realisation
that it is now possible to use information with the above
properties in psychiatric research. In other words, as a profession
we are accepting that some form of measurement is both possible
and necessary in many types of psychiatric activity. I suggest
that this is the fundamental change that has come about and which
is now manifest in the developments that we are discussing. The
last ten years or so has seen the first stage of this move towards
scientific respectability in the form of the production and
widespread use of standardised rating systems for mental state
and behaviour. (At first even these were thought to be impractical
and not applicable to the subtle fields of psychiatry). However,
having satisfied the psychiatrist's traditional preoccupation with
presenting symptoms, syndromes and diagnoses, we are now approaching the next stage, which is to bring the even more difficult
field of psychosocial data under some form of control.

What is being classified?

In the currently available systems the following are found:-

1.   The patient's premorbid characteristics.
2.   The illness or illnesses, both physical and psychiatric,

and statements about severity and course over time of
the illness.
3. The causes of his illness.
4. The psycho-social environment of the patient.
5. The social functioning of the patient as a result of
the illness.

Strictly speaking, most of the published multi-aspect systems
are incorrectly named, since they almost all refer to "psychiatric"
or "mental" disorders or diagnosis in their titles. In fact,
some are multi-aspect classifications of psychiatric disorders,
some are multi-aspect classification of patients and their disorders, and some include also psycho-social aspects of the
patient's environment. In Mezzich's review, all except two of
the systems he described are far more than classifications of
mental disorders or diagnosis. It seems therefore to be preferable to talk of developing a "classificatory profile" for whatever collection of concepts is required.

The above list of five aspects is by no means exhaustive.
For instance, an interesting example of requests for the
inclusion of yet more types of information came to light in the
meeting of Scientific Working Group No. 8. (Psychosocial Aspects
of General Health and Primary Health Care), conducted as part of
the recent WHO-ADAMHA International Collaborative Research Project.
Primary care physicians noted their interest in recording the
reason for consultation, and also the actions taken by the primary
care workers as part of a method of "classification of the
encounter".

Quite reasonable pleas are sometimes also made for inclusion
of "conventional" data such as age, sex and occupation in these
new descriptive systems. These data describe the patient before
the onset of the illness which brings him to psychiatric attention;
they serve a different purpose and are of a very different nature
to the information about the illness itself, or about its
consequences.

To sum up at this stage, we have concluded that :-

1. Most of the existing systems are misnamed, in that much
more than the psychiatric diagnosis is being classified.

2. The choice of aspects is no doubt reasonable, but there
has been little or no debate about the nature of the
aspects, the relationships between them, and the type
of information they contain.

I have already suggested that so-called "multi-axial
classification" is really nothing more than a necessary attempt

to put essential clinical information into a systematic standardised and reliable form; the novelty is in the attempt to be systematic and standardised rather than in the nature of the information. Existing systems are brave beginnings in a complicated process, but they can all be viewed as partial versions of a more comprehensive system that encompasses all the information relevant to clinical assessment and research.

In other words, multi-aspect systems are simply trying to deal with our old and familiar friend - the clinical formulation - in which all the most important information about the patient, his pre-morbid state, his illness and its causes and consequences, are brought together in a set of brief but comprehensive statements. The modern change that is now accepted is that each statement must be referable to a stated and defined list or system of classification, so that other workers can understand what the terms mean.

We are therefore likely to arrive at a satisfactory multi-aspect system if we recognise this from the start, and examine the implications of trying to systematise and standardise a collection of items of information of very different types and purposes. The suggestions that follow are based upon the simple, logical and practical sequence that forms the basis of ordinary clinical assessment. It is first necessary to describe the patient's pre-morbid characteristics and state, then various aspects of his illness, and finally the consequences of his illness.

To organise a sequence of events a reference point is needed, so the whole process will be viewed from the mental and psycho-social state of the patient just before the onset of his illness (or at the key service contact for patients with chronic disorders). The first of these three basic types of information noted above is unchanging, the second is concerned very much with change from pre-morbid to morbid and the reasons for the changes, and the third type describes the consequences.

These basic requirements have been listed in Figure 1. The completeness of any "multi-axial" systems can be assessed by referral to this comprehensive outline. Sections 1 and 2 of Figure 1 give the framework of the sequence, but section 3 is of a different nature. Many of the items in Figure 1 have other properties which also need to be recorded, such as severity, speed of onset and course over time, and whether they were the reason for consultation or a basis for action. A schema (or rating sheet) which gave space for the rating of all such possible properties of all items alongside the item itself would be very large indeed. For the purposes of this discussion, a few of the

1. <u>Unchanging data base</u>

    1.1.   Age, Sex, Marital Status, Occupation etc

    1.2.   Physical State.

    1.3.   Pre-morbid psycho-social function.

        1.31   Intellect and perception.

        1.32   Individual personality
                                  features

        1.33   Dyadic function

        1.34   Group function.

2. <u>New data base (date of change)</u>

    2.1   Classification of <u>changes</u> associated
                             <u>with illness</u>.

        2.11.   Symptoms

        2.12   Inferred syndromes or diagnoses

    2.2   Classification of <u>causes</u> of change in

        2.21   Physical state

        2.22   Pre-morbid psycho-social function

            2.221   Intellect and Perception

            2.222   Individual personality
                                      features

            2.223   Dyadic functions

            2.224   Group function.

    2.3   Classification of <u>effects</u> of change upon

        2.31   Physical state

        2.32   Pre-morbid psycho-social function

            2.321   Intellect and Perception

            2.322   Individual Personality
                                      features

            2.323   Dyadic function

            2.324   Group functions.

3. <u>Other properties</u> of items in Section 2 above.

    3.1.   Rapidity of onset   ) each

    3.2   Severity   ) requires

    3.3   Course over time   ) a classif-

    3.4   Reason for consultation) ication.

    3.5   Basis for action   )

FIGURE 1:   A COMPREHENSIVE CLASSIFICATION PROFILE FOR PSYCHIATRIC
PATIENTS

most commonly specified extra properties are listed in Section 3 of Figure 1, and in practice this is probably the easiest way of arranging a schedule based upon this model.

There is nothing particularly new or unfamiliar about the arrangement of information in Figure 1, but it emphasizes the different nature and uses of the various types of information that must be put into any systematic multi-aspect description of a patient. Section 2 of Figure 1 covers most parts of the majority of published "multi-axial" systems, but some popular items are to be found in Section 1, and some in Section 3. To see a comprehensive and systematic layout of potentially usable information, as in Figure 1, emphasizes the partial nature of most of the published multi-axial systems. In practice, of course, multi-aspect classifications will never cover all the items in Figure 1, and will quite legitimately use only selected sections, depending upon the purposes for which they are being designed and used. The over-all scheme contained in Figure 1 can be called a "Comprehensive Classificatory Profile", to distinguish it from the multi-aspect classifications which may be derived from it.

One particular group of items recurs three times in Sections 1 and 2 of Figure 1, i.e. those which cover the functioning of the patient at several levels, ranging from physical to groups (items in 1.3, 2.2, and 2.3).

There is clearly a need for a comprehensive classification of the physical and social functioning (or lack of functioning) of the patient in relation to his psycho-social environment. No such comprehensive system has yet been developed into a form in which it has appeared as a useable rating schedule, but an outline scheme upon which schedules can be based has been produced in the form of a "taxonomic hierarchy of social functioning", described in outline at a meeting of the W.P.A. Section on Epidemiology and Community Psychiatry in Aarhus in 1980 (Cooper, 1980). Since this part of the system deals with the all-important psycho-social functioning of the patient, I will go into this in more detail, so as to remind you of the basic characteristics of this hierarchical classification.

Using the principles of hierarchical classification, a set of ranks or levels can be devised which are conceptually related to each other according to stated principles. Each rank contains a number of 'taxons' or groups of social functions, each of which needs to be defined within the confines of the concepts of that rank.

Figure 2 shows the outline structure of this hierarchy, giving emphasis to the four middle ranks, i.e. 6 - groups, 5 -

Rank 1   ANATOMY: The Body

Intact organ.   Intact CNS   Intact joints and
                                                     limbs

Rank 2   HOMEOSTASIS: Physiological Homeostasis and simple
                        movements.

Physiological Systems   CNS   Simple Movements.

Cardiovascular, renal   Reflex responses Simple individual
Respiratory   Reflex learning   muscle and
Hormonal, blood etc.   joint
                                             movements.

Rank 3   AWARENESS: Psychological function and behaviour sequence

Alimentary   Arousal   Affect & sensorium

Mechanisms for   Orientation,   Normal affect &
   drinking   concentration   perception.
   eating   attention.   Special Senses
   excretion.   Memory, learning   functions
                      Conditioned learning. (speech, vision,
                                                hearing etc).

Movement Sequence

Walk, jump, run
Push, grip, Lift.

Rank 4   CONTROL: Individual response to and control of immediate
                   environment.

Personal Comfort	Intellect & Information	Emotional learning	Physical Activity.
Social procedures for eating. excreting washing dressing handling money	Read, write, draw. Make decisions cope with change. Operant learning.	Control of affective responses Fight, flight & sex response.	Use of tools to manipulate environment. Work activity sequences.

FIGURE 2

Rank 5   DIADIC : Relationships and roles.

Personal	Social Skills	Social Status
Marital	Verbal	Hierarchical position
Parental	Non-verbal	behaviour
Sibling	Dyadic manners	
Sexual	Coping with change	
Mimetic learning	in relationships	

Supportive

Provider
Career

Rank 6   GROUPS: Small group roles.

Family	Domestic	Social	Group skills
Father	Breadwinner	Leisure groups	Group manners
Mother	Housekeeper.	Neighbourhood	Travel and causal
Son, daughter.		groups.	groups.

Work

Task group roles
Work/Social roles.

Rank 7   AFFILIATION : Profession, union, minor religious groups

Rank 8   ORIGINS: Race, nation, tribe, cultural groups.

FIGURE 2 (Continued)

dyadic, 4 - control and 3 - awareness.

The appendix to the written version of this paper contains
an account of how hierarchies can be constructed, using a
simple non-medical model of football behaviour as an example.
For the purposes of the present discussion it is necessary to
summarise only the principles by which each level differs
conceptually from the next. These are:-

1. The constituent elements (or taxons) of each level are
    homogenous according to a few stated criteria - such
    as those required to define the essential aspects of
    social functions between two persons in rank 5 - DYADIC.

2. The Behaviour defined in one level is necessary for
    achieving the behaviours defined in the next level above
    but it is not explicitly repeated in the defining
    features of the rank above. For instance, it is
    necessary to have one's eating and drinking mechanisms
    correctly functioning (Rank 3) to carry out the correct
    social procedures of eating a meal (Rank 4).

3. The concepts and characteristics that define a rank will
    be of a different nature to those identifying all other
    ranks, and the farther apart the ranks, the more
    different their identifying features will be. For
    instance, the defining concepts of "small group roles"
    - rank 6, can hardly be confused with those of rank 4
    - "control of and response to immediate environment",
    but yet are not all that different from those that
    define larger group roles found in rank 7 - "Affiliation
    to professions, unions, etc".

The principle of these ranks can be used to define two at
the bottom of this particular hierarchy, which cover what might
crudely be called physiological functions and anatomical
integrity - i.e. rank 2 - homeostasis and rank 1 - Anatomy.
When developed a little more, these can be included in the
structure of Sections 1 & 2, of the system just described, as a
means of recording organic aetiology and consequences of the
illness, just as the three ranks of "groups" (6), "Diadic" (5)
and "control" (4) in Figure 2 can be used to deal with different
levels of social functioning.

These three social and two physical ranks offer a
conceptual basis for the development of rating schedules for
social functioning and dysfunctioning that have known relationships between them and which could be developed not only into

useful lists of items, but into properly organised systems of classification. There are also obvious advantages in using the same set of ideas for statements in Section 1, about the premorbid functioning of the patient, as in Section 2 when dealing with both causes and effects of the illness.

To conclude, it needs to be said once more that I have been describing a conceptual framework or "Comprehensive classificatory profile" that is nothing more than a systematic and potentially standardisable model that encompasses inform- ation very familiar to any clinician. Put at its simplest, this system is merely a systematised clinical formulation, organised with a view to finishing up with coded information that is easy to store, retrieve, and manipulate. Any one investigation is likely to use only a part or parts of the whole system, but if this system, or something like it, is used, then it will be easier to see clearly what type of information is being used, and how it is related to other types.

REFERENCES

Cooper, J.E. (1980) The description and classification of social disability by means of a taxonomic hierarchy. Acta Psychiatrica Scandinavica, Supplement 285. Vol 62.
Mezzich, J.E., (1979). Pattern and Issues in multi-axial Psychiatric Diagnosis. Psychological Medicine 9 125-137.

APPENDIX:

The structure of a taxonomic hierarchy illustrated by a simple non-medical example

Before approaching directly the complicated problem of a general classification of social behaviour, it is worthwhile constructing a taxonomic hierarchy for a simple model of one limited type of behaviour so as to identify as many points and principles as possible about the construction of schemes of classification of this type. The game of football (soccer) will be used as a comparatively simple non-medical model.

If a classification of behaviour relevant to playing football was required, it would need to contain at one level a set of ideas such as "attacking movement on the right wing" or "defence positioning for a corner kick". At other levels in the classification there would need to be a place for less complicated but essential behaviour such as "flexion and extension of the right knee". Somewhere between these two would be behaviour describing different ways of passing the ball from one player to another. An outline of part of such a system might be as follows, using common-sense and thinking briefly about the training programme of footballers:-

Rank 1   Movement of limbs such as flexion, extension and rotation of joints of arms and legs.

Rank 2   Sequences of purposeful movements: such as jumping, running, walking (which need the elements in Level 1 but have additional qualities and relationships, such as change of position of the whole body, and the idea of speed of movement).

Rank 3   Methods of contact with the football such as kicking, dribbling and heading (which need the sequences in 2 but have additional ideas about relationships between the ball and the body and movements of one player).

Rank 4   Types of pass from one player to another such as cross-field, forward, backwards, along the ground, in the air (which need the elements in level 3 but bring in ideas of patterns of play and spatial relationships between ball and several players).

Rank 5   Types of attacking and defending movements involving groups of players, some with and some without the ball (which need the elements in 4 but involve concepts of attack, defence and territory).

All of these "levels" are football behaviour of some sort, and players practice them as such independently. The general relationships between the levels have three main qualities. The first is that the elements of one level of classification are homogenous according to a few stated criteria (e.g. level 1 - simple limb movements; level 2 - purposeful sequences of movements changing the position of the whole body). The second is that behaviour in one level is necessary for the achievement of the next level about it (e.g. kicking and dribbling in level 3 cannot be done without the limb movements in level 2). The third is that additional concepts and relationships are present in a level which are not present in the level below, and in turn are also necessary for the performance of behaviours in the next level above.

Thus each unit of behaviour in a particular level of the scheme is not identifiable as such in subsequent levels, but is necessarily implied in the progressively more complicated and summarised levels that are developed. (For instance, it is necessary to bend the left knee in order to take part in an attacking move down the left wing, but knee movements are not described as such in level 5 in the example above).

The number of levels chosen for a system of classification is presumably variable and arbitrary, and will depend upon the purposes of the classification. The above 5 levels of football behaviour could be sub-divided or condensed without going against the principles just noted, or more levels could be added, for instance, extension of the scheme to include 6 types of football (rugby, soccer, Australian, Gaelic) 7 all team ball-games, 8 all team games, 9 all games, and so on.

PERSONALITY AS AN AXIS IN A MULTIAXIAL PSYCHIATRIC

CLASSIFICATION SYSTEM

Andreas Baumgartner and Hanfried Helmchen

Psychiatrische Klinik und Poliklinik
Freie Universität Berlin
Eschenallee 3 - D-1000 Berlin 19 - FRG

Every psychiatrist has experienced how important the "personality" of the patient is for the origin, appearance, and course of the psychic illness through all the diagnoses and thus for his diagnostic and therapeutic action. In striking opposition is the fact that this subject has to date been absolutely inadequately investigated scientifically and has led to almost no practically useful results: Most of the investigations lack clearly falsifiable hypotheses, precise theoretical reasoning, operationalization of the constructs used, empirical control of influential factors, e.g. sociodemographical background variables; and practical instruments for the standardized recording of the personality for the use in psychiatric routine are missing too.

In this situation it seems sensible(1) to name some arguments in favor of a more intensive occupation with the subject of "personality" in psychiatry; (2) to point out the numerous theoretical, methodological, and practical difficulties facing this investigation; and (3) to make some suggestions for further research, whereby above all the importance of multiaxial classification will be emphasized.

To the first point:

a) The importance of specific personality characteristics for the origin and development, and thus also for the diagnosis and prognosis, particularly with affective and schizophrenic psychoses, has been repeatedly pointed out. Frequently investigated examples are the "typus melancholicus" in unipolar depressions (H.TELLENBACH 1961, SHIMODA, s.SHINFUKU und IHDA 1969, v.ZERSSEN 1977) and, less clearly, the "schizoid character" in schizophrenics (BRÄUTIGAM 1974, FRITSCH 1976). For the descriptively diagnostic validity of the connection between premorbid personality and psychosis one can point out that diagnostically unclear first episodes of psychotic illnesses could be more than coincidentally correctly nosologically diagnosed based just on knowledge of anamnestic personality characteristics (R.TELLENBACH 1975). Against the assumption of too high a specificity among such originally only descriptive correlations one can mention that, for example, the tendency to schizoidism was found not only with schizophrenics, but was also found significantly more frequently premorbidly with neurotics in comparison to healthy control persons (v.ZERSSEN 1977,1979,1980). Even less is known about the mechanism of connection between such personality disposition and psychic illness, such as, for instance, how this can be a precondition for illness manifestation. Examples for a specific kind of connection between premorbid personaliy structure and psychic illness are the delusion of sensitive reference described by KRETSCHMER, which develops in sensitive personalities after a specific offending "key" experience, or the hypothesis from TELLENBACH about the manifestation of endogenous depression if the typus melancholicus, characterized by a narrowness of existence (Inkludenz) as a result of orderliness and conscientiousness, remains for some reason behind the high requirements he has set for himself (Remanenz). Better knowledge of such perhaps even specific vulnerability, the ability to recognize it, and the measurability of its extent with the help of particular indicators could contribute to prevention for instance in risk families that have a history of schizophrenia or to relaps prophylaxis with depressions.

b) Similar arguments are valid for the interpretation of the connection between premorbid personality and the development and course of the illness. Thus BLEULER (1972) and HUBER (1973) proved on the basis of longitudinal investigations covering decades the unfavorable influence of an asthenic schizoid character on the degree of remission and the further development of schizophrenic illness. However, it is not clear to what extent this connection is specific to the diagnosis, if one considers that the development is influenced by a number of factors, such as how the patient, with his personality, experiences the beginning of the illness, what processing and coping strategies he has at his disposal, and what attitude he can find toward the limitations imposed by the illness. These reactions, determined by the personality, can be expressed especially clearly in problems of compliance as well as with the chronification of psychic illness.Thus the development of a practicable personality theory within the framework of a psychiatric psycho- and sociotherapy could improve and stabilize its successes, and, besides this, could be a step toward reining in the various psychotherapeutic procedures that are becoming more and more numerous and uncontrollable on the far side of psychiatry.

c) Finally, personality can also determine the appearance of a psychic disturbance. We speak of personality disturbance as its own diagnostic category when the personality tends to leave the norm of human experience and behavior (K.SCHNEIDER:"the extent of human existance"). This deviation from the norm can be more closely determined, when ubiquitous personality characteristics are too strong or too weak and are disproportionally pronounced (disturbances of patterns and traits), when this deviation shows itself again and again in sterotyped ways with fluctuating intensity, and when it leads to a breakdown of the individual or to a disturbance in his sur- roundings (and thus takes on the quality of an illness). This defini- tion contains problems that have hardly been solved to date.

The quantitative character of this norm deviation determines that it moves in a dimensional continuum from normal or healthy to abnor- mal or disturbed or ill. We have not yet been successful in estab- lishing a generally acceptable and practicable out-off point between normal and abnormal (TYRER and ALEXANDER 1979, SHEPHERD and SARTORIUS 1974, WALTON and PRESLEY 1973, MANN et al.1981, HELMCHEN 1980, STRAUSS und HELMCHEN 1982). Considering the changability of norms and their very wide and indistinct boundaries, especially today, it is probably not possible to establish a cut-off point. Rather than going by norms that one cannot grasp, it would probably be more sensible to define pragmatically the border to a disturbance and, for example, to vali- date this prospectively toward the need to psychitric care. A series of studies points out that the category of personality disturbance is especially important in out-patient treatment.for instance in the treatment of addicts, patients with psychosomatic illnesses, and those with persistent and deep sexual disturbances.

A further area of problems is as follows: The above-mentioned defini- tion of personality disturbance is only valid if other psychic ill- nesses can be excluded. This can be established generally by corres- ponding, qualitatively abnormal, psychopathological or relevant so- matic findings or on the basis of a clearly progressive or regressive development of the disturbance (departure from the individual norm). However, it is difficult or impossible, for example, with personality disturbances after minimal perinatal ("pseudopsychopathy", adult MBD) or traumatic (postraumatic personality change) brain damage or with gradual "personality sharpening" as a result of a beginning dementa. In the case of so-called cognitive basis distrubances, it is not yet clear whether they are "advance post symptoms" (HUBER) of a slowly developing schizophrenia or else the expression of a preschizophrenic personality disturbance (JANZARIK: "preceding defect"). Finally, the border to neurotic illness is completely unclear (MOMBOUR). This be- comes especially obvious if the personality disturbance is explained psychodynamically and then called character neurosis.

The question of therapy possibilities and prognosis of personality disturbances is just as open. Although WATSON's opinion from 1928 that "a zebra will lose its stripes before an adult his personality" has been confirmed in some investigations (PARNAS et al.1982, SUND 1973), other studies come to the opposite conclusion (TÖLLE 1968), so that further longitudinal investigations are necessary.

To the second point:

The most important conceptual and methodological problems are as follows:

a) There is no unified and generally acceptable personality con- struct. A compromise between the theoretically necessary number of description dimensions to grasp the personality in a way that says something and their clinical practicability has also not yet been found. This is the reason why the clinically customary categories of personality typology, to be sure evident and practicable but very unclear around the edges and thus unreliable, have been so long-lived.

b) Personality and personality disturbances could up to now not be separated quantitatively from each other. Also personality disturbances in a narrower sense could be separated from certain other psychiatric illnesses only with difficulty or not at all.

c) The reliability of the diagnosis personality disturbance is inadequate. Most authors agree that it is difficult or impossible to judge the personality of a patient during a single hospital stay, especially during an active psychosis. A personality diagnosis should rather be a longitudinal diagnosis and include outside anamnestic data, both of which often present considerable problems in practice.

In the face of all these problems it is obvious that a satisfactory classification of personality 'cannot be developed around a table and not in the near future either, but will grow step for step out of the framework of progress in many areas of personality research.

To the third point:

What specific steps are now necessary in order to move foreward in psychiatric personality research, and what meaning does a multi-axial classification system have for this?

a) Relationship analyses that provide a basis for hypotheses are epidemiologically or at least partly epidemiologically only feasible, e.g., on complete and non selected hospital populations. The precondition for this is the routine and practicable compilation of defined personality characteristics independent of other data. It is important for this start to refer to a multiaxial classification that has as its goal the explicit, systematic, and individually independent compilation of data for different aspects of the patient (HELMCHEN 1983). If in such a multiaxial system an axis exists to record the personality, then the relationship of data from this axis and data from other axes such as organic illness or life events or course characteristics can be investigated. A condition analysis of these relationships is, however, no longer possible on the basis of clinical routine data and retrospectively, but rather only with the help of special research designs and prospectively (SPITZER and ENDIKOTT 1980).

b) The area "personality" is represented in most multiaxial systems, either as an aspect of the axis symptomatology or also etiology or more frequently as its own axis. There are differences especially as to whether the personality should be comprehended for itself (ESSEN-MÖLLER 1961, HELMCHEN 1975), or only the personality disturbance should be compiled (WING 1970, DSM-III) or both (OTTOSSON and PERRIS 1973). As mentioned above, we consider the complete understanding of the personality to be a condition of improved therapy and feel therefore that the personality should be classified as such, regardless of whether a disturbance as illness is assumed or not. Considering the unclear relationships among personality characteristics and psychiatric illnesses, the former should be compiled on their own axis.

c) A basic disadvantage of all research to data in this area lies in the lack of comparability of the studies because of differing diagnostic assumptions. Because the usual classification systems (e.g. DSM-III and ICD-9) are scarcely usable due to their poor reliability, each research group uses its own classification. One hears over and over again in this respect that the reliability in compiling personality dimensions is greater than in the category compilation of personality types. Thus the next step would be to develop an inventory of standardized instruments for the quantitative compilation of personality dimensions as a basis for the elaboration, clinical testing, and unification over a larger geographical area of a new diagnostic system of personality comprehension.

The difficulties that would arise in a clinical personality diagnosis in the framework of a dimensional classification system would pay off in the long run. It might be helpful to consider that the extent and especially the success of every standard therapy, e.g. pharmacotherapy, are put in question wherever the indicidual characteristics of the patient's personality are not taken into account. A multiaxial system, in which the personality has its own axis, can meet this danger for didactic reasons, not to mention its scientific importance.

Acknowledgement: the authors thank for help in translation are due to Mrs. Jane HELMCHEN, M.A.

References

1) BLEULER,M.,1972, Die schizophrenen Geistesstörungen im Lichte langjähriger Kranken- und Familiengeschichten, Thieme, Stuttgart
2) BRÄUTIGAM,W.,1974, Untersuchungen zur Persönlichkeitsentwicklung im Vorfeld der Schizophrenie, Nervenarzt 45: 298-304
3) ESSEN-MÖLLER,E.,1961, On classification of mental disorders. Acta psychiat.scand. 37: 119-126
4) FRITSCH,W.,1976, Die prämorbide Persönlichkeit der Schizophrenen in der Literatur der letzten hundert Jahre. Fortschr.Neurol.Psychiat. 44: 323-372
5) HELMCHEN,H.,1975, Schizophrenia: Diagnostic concepts in the ICD-8. in: Studies in Schizophrenia, M.H.LADER,ed. Brit.J.Psychiat., Spec.Publ.Nr.10, 10-18
6) HELMCHEN,H.,1980, Multiaxial systems of classification. Acta psychiat. scand. 61: 43-55
7) HELMCHEN,H.,1983, Multiaxial Classification in Psychiatry. Compreh.Psychiat. 24: 20-24
8) HUBER,G.,G.GROSS,R.SCHÜTTLER,1979, Schizophrenie, eine Verlaufs- und sozialpsychiatrische Langzeitstudie. Springer, Berlin-Heidelberg-New York

9) MANN,A.H.,R.JENKINS,E.BELSEY, 1981, The twelve-month outcome of patients with neurotic illness in general practice. Psychological Medicine 11: 535-550

10) MOMBOUR,W.,1975, Klassifikation, Patientenstatistik, Register, in: KISKER,K.P.,J.E.MEYER, C.MÜLLER, E.STRÖMGREN, Hrsg., Psychiatrie der Gegenwart,3, Springer, Berlin-Heidelberg-New York, 87-118

11) OTTOSSON,J.O., C.PERRIS,1973, Multidimensional classification of mental disorders. Psychological Medicine 3:238-243

12) PARNAS,J.,T.W.TEASDALE, H.SCHULSINGER,1982, Continuity of character neurosis from childhood to adulthood.

13) SHEPHERD,M., N.SARTORIUS,1974, Personality Disorder and the International Classification of Diseases. Psychological Medicine 4: 141-146

14) SHIMODA,S.N.,SHINFUKU, S.IDA, 1969, Über den prämorbiden Charakter der endogenen Depression. Fortschr.Neurol.Psychiat. 37: 545-556

15) SPITZER,R.L., J.ENDIKOTT, 1980, Classification of Mental Disorders and DSM-III, in: Comprehensive Textbook of Psychiatry III, KAPLAN,FREEDMAN,SADOCK, eds., Williams & Wilkins, Baltimore-London

16) STRAUSS,J., H.HELMCHEN, 1982, Working Paper on Multiaxial Diagnosis, WHO/ADMHA: International conference on classification and diagnosis of mental disorders and alcohol- and drug-related problems. Copenhagen, 13-17 April 1982

17) SUND, A., 1973, The Prognosis of Psychiatric Disorders in Young Norwegian Men. Brit.J.Psychiat. 122: 125-139

18) TELLENBACH, H., 1976, Melancholie. Springer,Berlin-Heidelberg-New York

19) TELLENBACH, R., 1975, Typologische Untersuchungen zur praemorbiden Persönlichkeit von Psychotikern unter besonderer Berücksichtigung Manisch-Depressiver. Confin.Psychiatr.18:1-15

20) TÖLLE, R., 1968, The Mastery of Life by Psychopathic Personalities, Psychiat.clin. 1: 1-14

21) TYRER,P.,J.ALEXANDER, 1979, Classification of Personality Disorders.Brit.J.Psychiat. 135: 163-167

22) WATSON,J.B., 1928, The Ways of Behaviorism, New York

23) WALTON,H.J., A.S.PRESLEY, 1973b, Dimensions of Abnormal Personality. Brit.J.Psychiat. 122: 269-276

24) WING,L., 1970, Observations on the psychiatric section of the International Classification of Diseases and the British Glossary of Mental Disorders.Psychological Medicine 1:79-85

25) ZERSSEN,D.v.,1977, Premorbid personality and affective psychoses. in: Handbook of studies on depression, BURROWS,G.D.,ed., Excerpta Medica, Amsterdam-London-New York, p.79-83

26) ZERSSEN,D.v., 1980, Konstitution, in: Psychiatrie der Gegenwart I/2, Springer,Berlin-Heidelberg-New York, S.619-705

CHOICE OF THE AXES IN MULTI-AXIAL CLASSIFICATIONS OF MENTAL DISORDERS

Carlo Perris

Department of Psychiatry
Umeå University
S- 901 85 UMEÅ   SWEDEN

The categorical classification of mental disorders, that with a few modifications we still use, was born early in this century and was based on naturalistic principles comprised of both theoretical assumptions and empirical observations made in that historical epoch. In the course of time that has elapsed since most of the classical concepts were first introduced, the inadequacy of the theoretical foundations on which our previous knowledge on their origins, manifestations, and outcome was based has become manifest, and unsatisfaction with current classifications more and more evident.

There is a general agreement that classifications in medicine have a number of aims. The principal of them are summarized in the following:

1. To gather information on morbidity: e.g. in epidemiological studies, in cross-cultural comparisons, in the detection of changes in morbidity over time;
2. As a basis for structuring information: e.g. both to be able to communicate within as well as outside the medical profession, and for teaching purposes;
3. As a basis for research work: e.g. for the collection of homogeneous series of patients and for the description of the patients in a study;
4. As a basis for planning appropriate psychiatric services;
5. To make predictions: e.g. in relation to different treatment procedures and to forecast outcome and thus, future needs;
6. To discover new fields of research and thus to increase knowledge.

Unsatisfaction with current classification systems has been expressed with reference to almost all the above mentioned purposes.

During the last decades there has been a marked progress in most fields of psychiatric research, mainly due to the consistent application of a developing scientific technology. However, no sophisticated technical methodology can ever compensate for inconsistencies in the identification of the patients on which such technology is applied and for unsolved issues in the theoretical formulations which underly the taxonomic concepts which are used. Although it is very difficult to make any correct estimate of the extent to which inconsistently applied diagnostic principles have lead to obtain non-replicable research results, it is tempting to assume that classification problems have represented at least one major source of error, thus contributing to an enormous waste of time and money.

More recently, an improvement in the use of current diagnostic concepts has been obtained by the introduction of a glossary to complement the 9th edition of the ICD and by the development and introduction of explicit diagnostic criteria in the DSM-III. However, although these additions have undoubtely contributed to enhance the diagnostic reliability of both systems, it is not yet full established to what extent they have contributed in enhancing, also the validity of the taxonomic concepts to which the criteria are applied. In particular, we do not know yet whether an improved diagnosis enhances, also the prognostic usefulness and the clinical meaningfulness of the typal constructs. In fact, according to Kendell (1) all daignostic concepts stand or fall by the strength of the prognostic and therapeutic implications they embody.

An important issue to be dealt with when planning classificatory work is to decide whether to start with the specification of a theoretical model, for example about the aetiology of the disorders to classify, or to accept to stay at an early stage of development (2), that is that of a descriptive approach based on empirical observations. In the last decades there have been several proposals of classifications in psychiatry based on either of the two above mentioned perspectives. Some of these proposals have taken into account the specification of a theoretical model to be used to predict the criterion (3,4), while others have been based upon the use of clustering techniques (5,6). Unfortunately, research work based on such approaches has been limited in its coverage and has not lead to any radical revision of psychiatric classification.

A further approach at the descriptive level has consisted of attempts to make explicitily the characterization of the psychiatric patients more detailed. It is in this context that proposals of multi-axial models have to be considered.

I will not indulge at this juncture on a discussion about the use of the term "multi-axial". It is quite clear that the majority of the models proposed so far are not comprised of "axes" in the correct meaning of the term but more properly of descriptive "elements" or "aspects" of the condition observed in the patient. However, although we have preferred the use of the term "multi-aspects" in our system (7,8) we are aware that the term multi-axial has already become deeply rooted in the psychiatric literature, and we suspect that it will probably survive despite its uncorrectness.

Multi-aspects models are composite structures which are basically pragmatic, atheoretical, and of heuristic value. They are based on the general assumption that we still badly need descriptive research at various levels before being able to formulate well worked-out theories from which to proceed to a taxonomic classification. Since multi-aspects models are relatively free from binding theoretical formulations, they are expected to have a very high degree of generalizability and coverage and thus can be applied to every condition in all cultural settings.

Recent reviews of the principal multi-axial models proposed so far have been published by Mezzich (9), Spitzer and Williams (10), and Helmchen (11). It is unclear, however, to what extent they are consistently used in clinical work. Our own MACM has been consistently used to classify in-patients at our Department since January 1975 and to classify out-patients since 1981. In addition it has been used by the Board of Social Welfare in a nationwide census of the in-patient population in mental hospitals.

In considering multi-axial models one has to take into account the number and content of the axes and the fact whether they are cathegorical or dimensional. Table 1 shows the content of the axes that has been taken into account in the different models. There are no established rules to decide which axes should be comprised in a multi-axial model. However, there are some limitations which have to be taken into account if the system has to be feasible.

Ideally, a thorough knowledge of a disorder, that would enable us to use it in a taxonomic system would imply that we have a correct information about its aetiopathogenesis, its clinical manifestations, its course, and its outcome both in a natural setting and when influenced by therapeutic interventions. Since for most of the mental disorders currently classified under specific diagnostic labels we still lack valid information at one or more of the above mentioned levels it can be maintained that one principal rationale in the choice of the elements to be comprised in a multi-axial model is that of covering as many as possible of the variables about which information is needed in order to find out how they correlate with each other. One major limitation in this respect is imposed by a principle of persimony dictated both by the objective or preventing to overload the

Table 1. Content of the axes most often taken into account

PHENOMENOLOGY	Symptoms, syndromes, personality characteristics;
SEVERITY	Psychotic, non-psychotic, occasionally psychotic - severe, moderate, mild;
TIME ASPECTS	Microcourse (within the episode, e.g. onset, fluctuations, sensitivity to environmental changes), macrocourse;
AETIOLOGICAL AND ASSOCIATED FACTORS	Somatic illnesses, brain organic conditions, situational stresses, developmental defects, cryptogenesis;
SOCIAL FUNCTIONING	Work, personal relations, adaptive functioning;

clinician who has to conceptualize the patient's disorder and by the objective of obtaining a system that is both clinically meaningful and easy to handle statistically.

A look at the multi-axial models which have been proposed so far shows that the choice of elements to be included has been fairly limited. In fact, the modal number of axes in the nine multi-axial systems reviewed by Mezzich (9) is five. In addition, there is also a high degree of consistency in the choice of the content of the axes among the different proponents of multi-axial models.

An element that occurs consistently in all the multi-axial models deals with psychopathology registered either as syndrome or as symptoms. There are several reasons why just this variable is regarded as one of the most important. Abnormal behaviour manifestations are one of the most immediate and characteristic features of persons with a particular disorder, which are relatively easy to identify and to communicate to others. The assessment of symptomatology is the basis of all clinical work and there are several instruments which allow to do that with a high degree of accuracy, consistency and reliability. Furthermore, most of the treatments currently used are symptomatic, or at their best syndromatic and not yet directed against the possible cause of the disorders. Thus, a correct definition of present psychopathology might be a first important step in the identification of variables which could allow the prediction of treatment outcome.

Table 2 shows the aspects taken into account in the MACM. While most of the multi-axial systems take into account sydromes, the MACM has been successively changed to focus more on symptoms. The rationale for doing so has been to try to avoid the use of comprehensive labels for the denomination of syndromes, as in the proposal by Ottosson and Perris (12) and to try to detect new combinations of symptoms which occurred consistently together and which did not corres-

Table 2. Aspects covered by the "Multi-aspects classification model" MACM, developed at Umeå

PSYCHOPATHOLOGY	The three most prominent symptoms which allow to characterize the patient clinically (according to a code list);
SEVERITY	Not ill, non-psychotic, psychotic, occasionally psychotic (according to given definitions;
COURSE	Episodic, recurrent of the same or of different type, chronic progressive, chronic stable (habitual) (according to given definitions);
AETIOLOGICAL AND ASSOCIATED FACTORS	Somatogenic factors (histogenic, chemogenic, hereditary), sociogenic (stressful environmental factors), characterogenic (more habitual disorder of personality development): any association of the above cryptogenic;

---

pond to stereotypical concepts. For example, in the original edition of the MACM were comprised "schizophrenic" and "schizo-phreniform" symptoms. We felt that this approach was not longer merely descriptive but implied, also some theoretical formulation of what had to be regarded as proper schizophrenic and what had to be regarded as schizophreniform. In the MACM we have not any longer comprised personality disturbances as a detailed subgroup under the heading symptomatology since we believe that these should be separetely assessed and separately coded as for example in the German system (11).

The second element in the MACM refers to the severity of the clinical picture presented by the patient. The rationale behind an explicit indication of severity has been the unsatisfaction with the current use of diagnostic labels as for example manic-depressive psychosis, also when the patient is not actually psychotic. We feel that a correct indication of severity is of great importance both as a variable which could help in predicting outcome, and even more for the planning of appropriate psychiatric services. Since we have defined "psychotic" with regard to impaired reality testing, it could be maintained that information about a patient being "psychotic" is redundant when for example the presence of clear cut delusions or hallucinations is listed among the symptoms. However, we felt that it would perhaps have been more difficult to give a generally acceptable definition of terms such severe, moderate or mild as used in other systems. To be coherent in avoiding controversial terms, the term "neurosis" comprised in the Ottosson and Perris's original proposal has been substituted by that of "non-psychotic". In addition two additional terms have been introduced to be able to classify subjects not mentally ill who occasionally consulted the department and patients who were not constantly psychotic during their morbid episode.

The element referring to course is, in our opinion one of the most important both from an epidemiological point of view to easily detect for example new patients (episodic), and for research purposes (for example a separation of unipolar from bipolar depressed patients or the identification of patients with a recurrent course). Information about course and duration, implicit under the heading of chronicity is important, also to make predictions and for the planning of appropriate services to meet the needs of the chronic patient population. It must be observed that the coding of the course in the MACM refers to what has in fact occurred up to the time when the coding is made without any preconceived assumption about what will occur in the future.

The last element, common to all multi-axial systems refers to aetiological and associated conditions and does reflect the hope to be able to link causative factors with clinical manifestations and course variables. Very likely, this element is the weakest in all the multi-axial models since it is unsure to what extent its coding will reflect the idiosyncratic theoretical orientation of the judge. However, in our experience now lasting for more than seven years it seems that the fact that the doctors have to code also this variable implies a more comprehensive evaluation of all the circumstancies which might have contributed to the fact that someone has become mentally ill and consequently the application of a broader range of therapeutic interventions.

REFERENCES

1. R.E. Kendell, "The role of diagnosis in psychiatry", Blackwell Sci. Publ., Oxford (1975).
2. C.G. Hempel, "Aspects of scientific explanation", The Free Press, New York (1965).
3. P.E. Meehl, Amer. Psychol. 17:827 (1962).
4. L.S. Benjamin, Psychol. Review, 81:392 (1974).
5. M. Lorr, "Explorations in typing psychotics", Pergamon Press, Oxford (1966).
6. J.E. Overall, L.E. Hollister, M. Johnson, and V. Pennington, J.A.M.A. 195:946 (1966).
7. L. Jacobsson, L. von Knorring, and C. Perris, Nord. Psykiatr. Tidskr. 31:435 (1977).
8. L. von Knorring, C. Perris, L. Jacobsson, and B. Rosenberg, Neuropsychobiology 6:101 (1980).
9. J.E. Mezzich, Psychol. Med. 9:125 (1979).
10. R.L. Spitzer, and J.B.W. Williams, in: "Comprehensive Textbook of Psychiatry", A.M. Freedman et al., eds. Chapter 14, Williams and Wilkins, Baltimore (1980).
11. H. Helmchen, Acta Psychiatr. Scand. 61:43 (1980).
12. J.-O. Ottosson, and C. Perris, Psychol. Med. 3:238 (1973).

CONCEPTUAL ISSUES IN COMPARING RESULTS FROM THE NIMH DIS WITH

CLASSIFICATION SYSTEMS USED INTERNATIONALLY

Jack D. Burke, Jr. and Darrel A. Regier

Division of Biometry and Epidemiology, NIMH
Room 18C-26, 5600 Fishers Lane
Rockville, MD 20857, U.S.A

Probably the most difficult question in psychiatric epidemiology has been: What is a Case? (1) Dealing with that problem almost invariably creates a second one: How does that method of case-identification compare to those used in other studies conducted around the world?

In addressing these two problems, this abstract will outline the operational approach to psychiatric diagnosis that has been developed in the United States, with an emphasis on its application in a multi-site epidemiologic survey, the NIMH Epidemiologic Catchment Area (ECA) program. (2) The ECA is a longitudinal study being conducted at five sites, each of which is performing a total community survey, with at least 3500 household and institutional respondents at each site. Case assessments are produced by the Diagnostic Interview Schedule (DIS), which uses fully specified questions, elaborate probes, and a computer algorithm to make diagnostic assignments according to DSM-III criteria. (3)

OPERATIONAL STAGE OF CLASSIFICATION:

This ambitious effort to use a fully structured interview to produce diagnoses of specific mental disorders was made possible by the recent move to an operational stage of psychiatric classification. In 1965, discussing the relationship between nosology and epidemiology, Ernest Gruenberg distinguished two approaches to diagnosis, which he called ostensive and operational. An "ostensive" system is one that attempts to express the concept of a disorder. In this approach, a category is defined by illustrative examples. Consider, Gruenberg said, "a group of cases, each of whom describes a thought or idea which he says keeps troubling him in a meaningless way; we can say we mean by 'obsession' the disorder which all of these people have." Such an approach conveys a concept of the illness, but does not produce homogeneous or logically separate categories; it has also been hard to use in epidemiologic surveys. By contrast, an operational approach emphasizes the importance of measurement according to specified criteria; in the natural sciences, for example, rather than defining a concept like "force", physicists establish criteria for a unit of force and indicate how that unit, called a dyne, can be measured in a standardized way. This combination of explicit criteria and a method of assessing them produces an operational approach. (4)

DSM-III provides half the operational approach by providing a set of explicit criteria. Also important, though, is a procedure for assessing subjects to determine if the criteria have been met. In the ECA program, that has been done by use of the DIS. In discussing the possible uses of early data from the ECA, we will review two questions that arise from this operational approach: (a) Is a DSM-III diagnosis produced by one assessment instrument the same as produced by another instrument?", and (b) How does a DSM-III diagnosis produced by the DIS compare to ICD-9 diagnoses produced in other studies?

COMPARISONS BASED ON DSM-III

Relevant to the first question, of potential differences in DSM-III diagnoses produced by different instruments, is a paper by Gerald Klerman and colleagues, which outlined six different criteria that could be derived from the description of Neurotic Depression in DSM-II. With data from the SADS interview, they demonstrated that these different criteria produced different meanings for the category and identified somewhat different types of patients. (5) Although DSM-III has reduced ambiguity considerably, there may be a limit on the precision and clarity of any classification system that is intended for routine clinical use. If we assume that DSM-III is reasonably clear, our question now is not about ambiguity itself, but about potential differences in the way assessment instruments apply DSM-III criteria. If there are differences, that fact has major implications for the capacity to make straightforward comparisons between DSM-III diagnoses as assessed by different instruments. This potential problem would be especially important for the future. The DIS used in the ECA was the first interview available to make DSM-III diagnoses, but many others are under development. In fact, at the American Psychiatric Association meeting in May, 1983, at least five new interviews to

82

make DSM-III diagnoses were presented. The extent to which comparisons can be made between ECA data and findings based on any of these interviews is not yet clear.

Three examples can be discussed to illustrate possible differences. The first problem is differing interpretations of individual symptoms. Even a simple symptom, like insomnia, can be considered only as difficulty falling asleep; or as early morning waking; or as difficulty staying asleep as well. In fact, each of these approaches is represented in at least one of the various standardized instruments being developed for DSM-III assessments.

There are also potential differences in the way that the required clustering of symptoms within a specified time period is assessed for various DSM-III disorders. Panic disorder, for example, requires that the characteristic panic attacks must occur together, with at least three attacks within a three-week period. An instrument that assesses lifetime occurrence for a subject, as the DIS does, may inquire whether the three panic attacks have ever occurred together within a three-week time period; if so, a current diagnosis for the past month can be assigned if the subject reports that the illness has continued as shown by at least one panic attack within the past month. However, an instrument that concentrates on the subject's current experience may ask only whether there have been three attacks within the past month. If only one or two panic attacks have occurred in the past month, the subject would be found negative regardless of whether the required clustering has occurred earlier than that. With these two different approaches, the two instruments will yield different rates of current disorder. In fact, just such an approach has been taken in one instrument that has been used as a reference measure for the DIS, and not surprisingly, the two interviews produced quite different results. These differences have little to do with whether the clinical phenomena associated with panic attacks are present but depend only on the different timeframe used for assessing the subject's disorder.

A related source of variation derives from the time period used for determining rates of "current" illness. Two methods for dating a current disorder are provided on the DIS. The "standard" approach identifies illnesses which continue to have some symptomatic activity within the time period of interest, for example, the one month prior to interview. In this method, a subject who has a history of Major Depression is asked, for example, when he last experienced the mood disturbance and some of the other symptoms that contribute to the disorder. If he answers in the past one month, then he is identified as having a current illness. Note that the minimum requirement of having at least four associated symptoms, such as sleep or appetite disturbances, is not used to assess current activity. So an episode that started several months earlier but has had partial recovery will still be counted as present.

In an alternative approach, the DIS recency probes are used. That is, after each positive symptom, the subject is asked when he most recently had the symptom. With this information, the requirement for a mood disturbance and at least four associated symptoms can be assessed directly. Michael von Korff and colleagues have reported that this method produces smaller rates for current Major Depression than the standard approach that assesses recent activity of illness. In the first 51 cases from the Baltimore community survey who had current Major Depression in the month prior to interview by the standard approach, only 32 had met the full DSM-III criteria with at least four associated symptoms in that month. (6)

How important are these differences between assessment instruments? This question can be asked in the ECA because three of the sites have used some other assessment instruments for DSM-III to compare to the DSM-III diagnoses produced by the DIS. The simplest way to evaluate those comparisons is to calculate standard measures of agreement. Such an approach has been used in clinical studies of patient populations, but that approach is not easily transferred to an epidemiologic survey of the general population because the standard measures of agreement are severely affected when the baseline rates of disorders are low.

In a review of kappa as a measure of agreement, Grove and colleagues demonstrated that for samples with rare disorders, the maximum value of kappa is considerably reduced in cases of less than perfect agreement. (7) For this reason, Grove recommended that kappa not be used when the prevalence rate is below 5%.

Similarly, Shrout and Fleiss (8) have demonstrated that positive predictive value is attenuated with low prevalence rates, even when the instrument's characteristics are constant. David Goldberg has also demonstrated this effect in studying the characteristics of screening questionnaires. (9)

With rare disorders, the apparent values for sensitivity and specificity are also affected when the reference measure is less than perfect. Since that is always the case in psychiatry, it becomes difficult to make simple comparisons between two instruments and calculate the apparent sensitivity and specificity of one of them. Of course, with the dilemmas described earlier about different interpretations of the fundamental criteria for a diagnosis, simple comparisons are not likely to be useful anyway. (10)

COMPARISONS WITH OTHER STUDIES

To facilitate international comparisons, it is important to be able to compare DIS results with ICD-9 diagnoses from studies using the PSE-CATEGO or DiaSiKa-AMDP. Two approaches have been tried to make "ICD-9" equivalent diagnoses from the DIS. The first is to combine similar categories into groupings, e.g., of Depressive disorders, and to compare rates of these broad categories. Since the individual categories in ICD do not always correspond with DSM-III, the grouping permits only rough comparisons to be made with the community surveys in Camberwell, U.K., and Canberra, Australia, based on the PSE and equivalent ICD-9 categories, and the differences in rates are difficult to interpret.

Another attempt to produce ICD-9 information from the DIS was even less successful. With John Helzer from St. Louis, we attempted to rewrite the ICD-9 glossary into the "explicit" format used by DSM-III. Since the glossary was meant to provide a concept of the disorder, rather than explicit criteria to serve as the basis for standardized assessments, this translation effort was not immediately helpful for that purpose. (11) However, it did help clarify the differences between ICD-9 and DSM-III disorders, and pointed to the kind of gaps in information that would have to be supplied if the ICD were to support the "operational" level of DSM-III.

CONCLUSION:

One conclusion from the ECA results is that there is no pure DSM-III diagnosis; a principle inherent in the operational approach is that both the set of explicit criteria and the assessment technique used are important in determining the basis of a diagnostic assignment for a given subject. With the diversity of approaches to assessment even within the framework of DSM-III, it seems clear that simple comparisons of instruments will not be possible even if convenient statistical measures can be found. Comparability on a broad scale internationally will likely require instruments designed to be comprehensive in their coverage of clinical phenomena and to be linked directly to various classification systems. For that reason, the WHO-ADAMHA Collaborative Project on Diagnosis and Classification has sponsored a Task Force on Psychiatric Assessment Instruments to produce assessment schedules for use in epidemiologic and clinical studies. Under the chairmanship of John Wing, the Task Force has produced a Composite International Diagnostic Interview (CIDI) that merges the DIS and the PSE. That combined interview may provide a true basis for international comparability with studies that use either the PSE or DIS for epidemiologic investigations.

References

1. J. K. Wing, P. Bebbington, and L. N. Robins, eds.: "What is a Case?", Grant McIntyre, London (1981).
2. D. A. Regier, J. K. Myers, M. Kramer, et al: The NIMH Epidemiologic Catchment Area (ECA) Program: Historical Context, Major Objectives, and Study Population Characteristics, Arch Gen Psychiatry (in press, 1984)
3. L. N. Robins, J. E. Helzer, J. Croughan, et al: NIMH Diagnostic Interview Schedule, Arch Gen Psychiatry, 38:381 (1981).
4. E. M. Gruenberg: Epidemiology and Medical Statistics, in "The Role and Methodology of Classification in Psychiatry and Psychopathology", M. M. Katz, J. O. Cole, and W. E Barton, eds., Government Printing Office, Washington, DC (1967).
5. G. L. Klerman, J. Endicott, R. Spitzer, et al: Neurotic Depressions: A Systematic Analysis of Multiple Criteria and Meanings, Am J Psychiatry 136:57 (1979).
6. M. R. von Korff and J. C. Anthony: The NIMH Diagnostic Interview Schedule Modified to Record Current Mental Status, J Affective Disorders, 4:365 (1982).
7. W. M. Grove, N. C. Andreasen, P. McDonald-Scott, et al: Reliability Studies of Psychiatric Diagnosis, Arch Gen Psychiatry, 38:408 (1981).
8. P. E. Shrout and J. L. Fleiss: Reliability and case detection, in "What is a Case?", J. K. Wing, P. Bebbington, L. N. Robins, eds., Grant McIntyre, London (1981).
9. D. Goldberg, "Manual of The General Health Questionnaire", NFER Publishing Co., Windsor, Berks, U.K. (1978).
10. L. A. Thibodeau: Evaluating Diagnostic Tests, Biometrics, 37:801 (1981).
11. J. C. Helzer, and J. D. Burke: Reformatting ICD-9 Diagnostic Criteria. Working paper, prepared for The International Conference on Diagnosis and Classification of Alcohol, Drug Abuse, and Mental Disorders, Copenhagen (1982).

COMPARING FRENCH AND INTERNATIONAL CLASSIFICATION SCHEMES :

I. SCHIZOPHRENIA

C.B. Pull, M.C. Pull, and P. Pichot

Centre Hospitalier, 1210 Luxembourg and
Clinique des Maladies Mentales et de l'Encéphale
75014 Paris

INTRODUCTION

It is generally considered that French psychiatry adopts
an original attitude in several major areas of psychiatric nosology. In particular, French opinions on non-affective psychoses are viewed to depart to a large extent from other
classification systems. Owing to historical reasons, which
have been discussed in detail elsewhere [1] , French psychiatry
divides the non-affective psychoses into three major groups of
disorders which are considered to be nosologically independent : the chronic schizophrenias, the transitory delusional
states and the chronic delusional states.

In the present report, attention will focus on schizophrenia and two specific French diagnostic categories which
retain a considerable influence on French diagnostic practices.
The first, bouffée délirante, relates to acute, transitory delusional states, the second, chronic hallucinatory psychosis,
concerns a chronic delusional state. Results from recent empirical investigations have permitted to elicit operational diagnostic criteria for each of the three categories under discussion. As a consequence, it became possible, for the first
time, to proceed to direct comparisons between the French
classification of mental diseases and conditions described in
the latest edition of the World Health Organization's International Classification of Diseases (ICD-9) [2] as well as disorders defined in the third edition of the American Psychiatric
Association's Diagnostic and Statistical Manual of Mental Disorders (DSM III) [3] .

METHOD

In 1981, a survey [4] was carried out in a sample group representative of French psychiatrists. The group consisted of 87 qualified psychiatrists who had previously collaborated in similar studies. The participants were invited to provide several cases of psychotic conditions, excluding the purely affective psychoses. No criteria were imposed to make a diagnosis. The only requests were that the clinicians should (1) be reasonably positive about their diagnoses and (2) that they should document their diagnoses using a set of internationally understandable criteria.

The instrument used in the investigation was a List of Integrated Criteria for the Evaluation of Taxonomy in the field of non-affective psychoses (LICET-S) [5] which presents a total of 70 criteria for schizophrenia and schizophrenia-related categories. LICET-S assembles all specific criteria for schizophrenia [6] proposed by several prominent authors in the past (KRAEPELIN, BLEULER, SCHNEIDER, LANGFELDT) or more recently by different North-American authors (FEIGHNER, TAYLOR, ASTRACHAN). It also includes the "discriminant" symptoms for schizophrenia emerging from the International Pilot Study of Schizophrenia, as well as all DSM-III inclusion and exclusion criteria for schizophrenic disorder, paranoïd disorder and psychotic disorders not elsewhere classified.

In what concerns the three categories under discussion, the description of cases provided through LICET-S was of a quite remarquable homogeneity. The results were highly consistent in what concerned age of onset, duration, symptom pattern, and exclusions. Moreover, the data relevant to a definition of the concepts consisted of objective observable behaviours and reported feelings for which there is no need for inference. As a consequence, the major elements required to operationalize diagnostic concepts could be elucidated, which in turn permitted to construct the corresponding diagnostic algorithms.

LICET-S also permits to formulate diagnostic decisions based on the specific criteria and algorythmes defining a number of categories included in the classification systems that have been integrated in the list. In particular, the data from our study could be analyzed on the basis of DSM III criteria. A cross-tabulation of French clinical diagnoses and DSM III diagnoses is presented in the following.

SCHIZOPHRENIA

1. French empirical diagnostic criteria

    A. Age of onset : before age 40

    B. Onset : acute (a first acute episode would be given a
       diagnosis of bouffée délirante) or progressive

    C. Chronicity : active phases are followed by a residual
       phase characterized by at least some signs of the
       illness.

    D. Characteristic symptoms : 2 at least of the following

        1. Marked illogicality : patently unrealistic, bizarre
           or magical thinking
        2. Inappropriate affect : blunted and/or
           discordant affect and/or ambivalence
        3. Major formal thought disorder : loosening of
           associations, inefficient thinking, incoherence
        4. Unsystematized delusional ideas having no apparent
           relation to depression or elation

    E. Not due to any organic mental disorder

2. Comparison with ICD-9

    ICD-9 requires the presence, at some time during the
illness, of characteristic disturbance of thought, perception,
mood, conduct, or personality-preferably in at least two of
these areas. This symptom definition seems broader than the
French one. There is, moreover, no threshold for age at onset
in ICD-9 nor is chronicity postulated. As a consequence, the
French concept appears to be narrower.

3. Comparison with DSM III

    DSM III requires the presence of at least one of 6
symptom criteria. The French symptom definition is restricted
to the last DSM III symptom criterion. The DSM III upper limit
for age at onset is higher than the French one. In contrast
to the French definition, chronicity is not a requirement in
DSM III, allthough full recovery is considered exceptional.
Owing to the preceeding differences, the French concept would
be narrower. There is, however, an additional exclusion criterion in DSM III, not to be found in the French definition,
concerning a history of full depression or manic syndrome.
Moreover, some cases of schizotypal personality disorder might
probably be diagnosed as schizophrenias in France.

BOUFFEE DELIRANTE

1. French empirical diagnostic criteria

    A. Age at onset : between 20-40

    B. Onset : acute, without any prior psychiatric history
       (other than identical episodes)*

    C. Duration : active phases fade away completely in
       several weeks or months, possibly recurring under the
       same form, but with the patient remaining devoid of any
       psychopathology in the interval

    D. Characteristic symptoms : all of the following :

        1. Delusions and/or hallucinations of any form
        2. Depersonalization/derealization and/or confusion
        3. Depression and/or elation
        4. Symptoms vary from day to day, even from hour to
           hour

    E. Not due to any organic mental disorder

    F. Bouffée délirante without other specification (or
       "genuine" bouffée délirante) occurs in the absence of
       any identifiable psychosocial stressor. Bouffée déliran-
       te occuring in temporal relation with stress is termed
       "reactive".

2. Comparison with ICD-9
   The definition of acute schizophrenic episode provided in
   the ICD-9 glossary is quite similar to the French definition
   of "genuine" bouffée délirante. The ICD-9 definition of
   acute paranoid reaction obviously corresponds to reactive
   bouffée délirante, and not, as stated in the ICD glossary,
   to "bouffée délirante" without specification.

3. Comparison with DSM III
   DSM III lists at least two categories which would be covered
   by bouffée délirante : (1) schizophreniform disorder
   corresponds to "genuine" bouffée délirante, but is less
   specific in what concerns onset and characteristic symptoms, and (2) brief reactive psychosis corresponds to
   reactive bouffée délirante. In addition, a number of patients with a DSM III diagnosis of Atypical psychosis or
   Acute paranoid disorder would probably be given a diagnosis
   of bouffée délirante in France.

---

*For a minority of clinicians, a history of full manic or
 depressive syndrome does not preclude the diagnosis.

CHRONIC HALLUCINATORY PSYCHOSIS

Diagnostic criteria presented elsewhere [7] link chronic hallucinatory psychosis to paraphrenia (ICD-9 297.2) and late-onset schizophrenic disorder which would be classified as atypical psychosis (DSM III 298.90).

FRENCH TRADITION AND THE NEW AMERICAN CONCEPT OF SCHIZOPHRENIA

The hallmark of traditional French psychiatric nosology consists in restricting the diagnosis of schizophrenia by (1) separating a number of non-schizophrenic delusional states, acute or chronic and (2) insisting on the chronicity of the disorder. Up to recently, North American nosology has used much broader criteria for the concept. As shown in a comparison [8] of French and American diagnostic practices (based on DSM II), American clinicians diagnosed schizophrenia approximately three times more often than French psychiatrists. In the same comparison, chronic hallucinatory psychosis and "bouffée délirante" could be identified as the primary basis for more frequent use of the diagnosis of schizophrenia by American psychiatrists, allthough they did not account for all the differences.

From the comparisons established in the present report, it would appear that DSM III has taken a significant step towards traditional French nosology in this field. Owing to criterion D for schizophrenic disorder (no history of full manic or depressive syndrome), the new American concept of schizophrenia might even have become more restrictive than the French one. First empirical evidence supporting this assumption is reported in table 2 which presents a cross-tabulation of French clinical diagnoses by DSM III criteria.

Table 1. Cross-tabulation of French clinical
diagnoses by DSM III criteria

		DSM III CRITERIA				
		SCHIZO-PHRENIA	SCHIZOPHRENI-FORM +	ATYPICAL PSYCHOSIS	AFFECTIVE DISORDER	OTHER	TOTAL
FRENCH	SCHIZOPHRENIA	164			15	12	191
	CHRONIC HALLUCINATORY PSYCHOSIS	21		14	5	1	41
	ACUTE DELUSIONAL STATES*	12	25	1	8	4	50

* includes "genuine" bouffée délirante, reactive bouffée délirante and acute delusional state presumed to be a prodromal episode of schizophrenia. + includes brief reactive psychosis.

Although further investigation is needed to establish the correspondance between traditional French and new American positions on schizophrenia, the following schematic diagram may serve as a preliminary illustration to understand the similarities and differences between the two concepts.

Table 2. Preliminary diagram comparing traditional French and new American positions on schizophrenia

FRENCH	BOUFFEE DELIRANTE	SCHIZOPHRENIA	CHRONIC HALLUCINATORY PSYCHOSIS

DSM III	SCHIZOPHRENI-FORM DISORDER	AFFECTIVE DISORDER	SCHIZO-TYPAL	SCHIZOPHRENIC DISORDER	ATYPICAL PSYCHOSIS

REFERENCES

1. P. Pichot, The diagnosis and classification of mental disorders in French-speaking countries : background, current views and comparison with other nomenclatures, Psychol. Med., 12, 475 (1982)
2. World Health Organization, Mental Disorders, Glossary and Guide to Their Classification in Accordance with the Ninth Revision of the International Classification of Diseases, W.H.O., Geneva (1978)
3. American Psychiatric Association, Diagnostic and Statistical Manual of Mental Disorders (3rd edn., DSM III), A.P.A., Washington D.C. (1980)
4. C. B. Pull, M. C. Pull, P. Pichot, Etude Nationale sur les Critères de Diagnostic des Psychiatres Français dans les Psychoses Non-Affectives : Premiers Résultats, Comptes-rendus du Congrès des Psychiatres et Neurologues de langue Française, P. Sizaret, ed, Masson, Paris (1981)
5. C. B. Pull, M. C. Pull, P. Pichot, LICET-S : Une Liste Intégrée de Critères d'Evaluation Taxinomiques pour les Psychoses Non-Affectives, J. Psych. Biol. Thérapeut., 1, 33 (1981)
6. C. B. Pull, M. C. Pull, Des Critères pour le diagnostic de schizophrénie, in P. Pichot, ed, Actualité de la Schizophrénie, Masson, Paris (1981)
7. C. B. Pull, M. C. Pull, P. Pichot, Comparing French and International classification systems. III Paranoid disorders Pr.VII World Congr. Psychiat.(1982)
8. C. B. Pull, P. Pichot, J. E. Overall, Comparison of French and American diagnostic practices for schizophrenia, Psychopharmacol. Bull. 16, 43 (1980)

UNCHANGED DISCREPANCY IN INTERNATIONAL DIAGNOSTIC PRACTICE AFTER 1970
CONFIRMING THE PRESERVING FACTOR OF CONVENTION - PERSISTENT
RELUCTANCE TO ACCEPT INTERNATIONAL CLASSIFICATION

L.Saugstad & Ø.Ødegård

National Case Register of Serious Mental Disorder
Gaustad Hospital
Box 16,Oslo 3,Norway

INTRODUCTION

The psychiatric chapter in the International Classification of
Diseases(ICD) was internationally accepted around 1970.The main reason for this reluctance among the psychiatrists to accept international standard,was the significant national discrepancies in diagnostic
practice.In Norway and Denmark,where the Kraepelinian nosology was
accepted early,a need was felt for a third category of functional
psychosis in addition to schizophrenia and manic-depressive psychosis.
An intermediate category,named "constitutional","psychogenic" or "reactive" psychosis was introduced (Wimmer,1916,Ødegård,1968).In Norway
this category was much used,and more than 42 % of first admissions
to psychiatric hospitals 1965 were given this diagnosis,and 19 % only were diagnosed schizophrenics.Similarly in Denmark 1965-6,39% were
classified as "psychogenic" psychoses,as against five percent schizophrenics (Table 1).In France,intermediate categories of functional psychoses (the transitory delusional state(bouffée delirante)
and chronic delusional state) were introduced in the end of last cen-
tury.The present French psychiatric classification INSERM includes
criteria restricting the diagnosis of schizophrenia and increasing
the number of non-schizophrenic delusional states(Pichot,1982).The
transitory delusional state has also been used in Canada(Allodi,1982).
In countries such as Sweden,U.S.A.,U.S.S.R. and the United Kingdom,
the psychiatrists felt no need for an "intermediate " category.In
these countries,we observe either an extremely wide concept of schizophrenia such as is the case in U.S.A. and U.S.S.R.,where nearly
50 % of first admissions are given this diagnosis.Or a similarly wide
concept of manic-depressive(affective) disorder,such as is observed
in England & Wales.In Sweden,the"intermediate" psychoses are probably included in the non-psychotic admissions which comprised more

Table 1. Proportion of First Admissions by Diagnosis(both sexes).

Diagnosis	Denmark (1965-6)	Sweden (1962-4)	Poland (1969)	Norway (1965)	U.S.A. (1969)
295	5.4	13.9	16.7	19.0	46.1
296	15.2*	15.1	5.6**	10.4	8.5
297,298,299	39.3	9.6	37.3	42.2	10.7***
300,306-8	40.1	61.4	40.4	28.4	34.7
Total Adm.	4179	15870	35185	4272	194543

*Incl.306-8. **Incl.290-4 and 298.0. ***26.3 % diagnosis 300.4.

than 60% of first admissions 1962-4 (Table 1).

The WHO decided to reserve the three digit category 298 for the "intermediate"(Other psychosis) in ICD8.It also decided to introduce three new subgroups of schizophrenia,which by definition had a favorable outcome(295.4,-.5 & -.7).The WHO thereby invited to a change in diagnostic practice.This fundamental alteration was probably an important reason why ICD8 was internationall accepted.It is of particular interest to examine whether there is in fact greater uniformity in diagnostic practice following ICD8.It was therefore decided to investigate the diagnostic distribution of first admissions to psychiatric hospitals in countries where official statistics were published.

MATERIAL AND METHODS

Information was available from seven countries:Denmark,Norway,England & Wales,France,Poland,Australia(VIctoria) and U.S.A.The following diagnoses were left out of the analysis:organic & symptomatic psychoses(290-4),personality disorder,alcoholism and drug addiction (301,303-4).These categories do not present international diagnostic problems of similar importance.The functional psychoses were divided in :schizophrenia(295),manic-depressive disorder(296),and"intermediate" psychoses(297,298,299).Non-psychotic admissions(300,306-8) were also investigated.

RESULTS

The proportion of "intermediate" psychoses ranges from 8.3% in Australia,11.8% in U.S.A. and 36.8% in Denmark.Admissions labelled schizophrenia range from 7.4% in Denmark,11.5% in England & Wales to 46.6% in U.S.A.Manic-depressive disorder is used in only 6.4% in Norway as against 37.1 % in U.S.A. where 298.0 and 300.4 are included in this category.The 42.5% of affective disorder in England &

Table 2.Proportion of First Admissions by Diagnosis since 1970

Diagnosis	Denmark (1974-5)	England[1] (1976)	Norway (1972-4)	France[2] (1974)	Poland[3] (1976)	Austr.[4] (1972-5)	U.S.A[5] (1975)
295	7.4	11.5	12.8	14.5	18.0	29.7	46.6
296	25.5	42.5	6.4	17.0	12.2	15.7	37.1
297,298,299	36.8	13.4	28.1	23.3	29.7	8.3	11.8
300,306-8	30.3	32.6	52.7	45.2	41.1	46.3	4.5
Total Adm.	4173	56080	5274	77700	44849	11350	53217

[1]295 incl.297,296 incl.311. [2]298 incl.300.4. [3]297,298,299 incl.292-4. [4]The information is from Victoria. [5]The information is from a sample survey conducted by National Institute of Mental Health.

Wales includes "depressions not elsewhere classified(311)". Non-psychotic admissions range from less than five to more than 50%. A comparison between Tables 1 & 2,shows a decrease in "intermediate" psychoses in Denmark and Poland,accompanied by a rise in schizophrenia and affective disorder.The decrease in "intermediate" psychoses in Norway is concomitant with a reduction in schizophrenia and affective disorder,and non-psychotic admissions now predominate. The diagnostic distribution in U.S.A. is unchanged from 1969 to 1975. No directly comparable information was available from England & Wales before 1970. The proportion of affective disorder and "depressions not elsewhere classified" remained unchanged around 42% 1970-77,as compared with 37% before 1970 (Saugstad & Ødegård,1983).There was no increase in schizophrenia or "intermediate" psychoses.

DISCUSSION

The discrepancy in diagnostic distribution is more or less unchanged from before 1970. The new category 298 (Other psychosis) has had no success in countries with a wide concept of schizophrenia nor in those with a wide concept of affective disorder.In countries with a previous predominance of "intermediate" psychoses,a slight reduction is observed in Denmark,Norway and Poland.This is however accompanied by a further decline in schizophrenia and affective disorder in Norway,where in 1978 only 10 % of first admissions were given these diagnoses (Saugstad & Ødegård,1979,1980).The three new subgroups of schizophrenia were only used in 1.2%.

The veritable flight from the two Kraepelinian disease entities in Norway is also a flight from the term psychosis,as nearly 60% of first admissions 1978 were labelled non-psychotic(300,306-8).This predominance could result from our inability to eliminate the social stigma attached to the term psychosis.The psychiatrists prefer a diagnosis which traditionally implies a favorable outcome.Non-psychotic depressions (300.4) is the preferred diagnosis in 20%.The preference for depressions as the least stigmatizing of the mental disorder,is also characteristic of England & Wales.Here nearly two-thirds are labelled 300.4 or 311(depressions not elsewhere classified).This trend goes back to Aubrey Lewis highly influential paper(1934) where he establihed a concept of affective disorder which included depressive psychoses labelled "intermediate" in Denmark and Norway.That this category also includes cases which in U.S.A. would have been labelled schizophrenia,is evident from Kantor & Glassman's(1977) re-examination of Sir Aubrey Lewis 61 original case reports (1934,1936).According to their judgement,as many as 30 cases would have been diagnosed as schizo-affective psychosis or schizophrenia in U.S.A.

The persistent predominance of schizophrenia in U.S.A. is striking.The social stigma attached to the term psychosis,and more particularly to schizophrenia is of less importance in this country.The DSM-III has replaced ICD as the national classification in 1980.The DSM-III has a considerably narrower concept of schizophrenia(Skodol & Spitzer,1982).It remains to be seen,whether this will result in fewer admissions with this diagnosis.

Most psychiatric cases can be classified in more than one way. Preferences depend upon the purpose,the diagnostic system as well as local diagnostic practice(Rawnsley,1968).The fundamental national differences in diagnostic distribution,must result primarily from differences in diagnostic practice.More information about the ICD would probably lead to significant reduction in certain categories. Zigmond & Sims(1983) have already shown,how the unspecific diagnosis 311 could be reduced to only one percent through issuing the clinical psychiatrists with the WHO glossary and instructing them in its use. In Norway,where more than 30% of functional psychoses 1977-8 were classified as "unspecific"(fourth digit 9),more information would probably reduce this category considerably.

There is a general reluctance to accept internation standard.A reluctance which was barely overcome with the international acceptance of ICD8 around 1970,but which is evident in the persistent national differences in diagnostic practice.The replacement in U.S.A. of ICD by a national classification,such as happened in 1980,could aggrevate this reluctance.More particularly,since during the last ten years or so,we have seen the development of a multitude of such national classificatory systems.In addition to the DSM-III,the RDC and SADS are among the most well-known American,and the PSE,ID and CATEGO are the most well-known British systems (Wing et al.1974). Several of these systems were constructed primarily to serve as guides for less experienced psychiatrists to arrive at a reliable diagnosis.Specific operational criteria have been introduced,as well as multi-axial systems.Fundamentals of psychopathology are frequently disregarded,and there is dissolution of classical disease entities and syndromes (Berner & Küfferle,1982).Because of this non-theoretical approach,the underlying concepts differ.This is evident from the alarming lack of consensus in diagnosis between the British and American systems as verified by Dean et al.(1983).In only 16.7% of cases of anxiety and in 56% of depressions,there was agreement about diagnostic labelling.More importantly,depending upon the particular diagnostic "system" chosen,the proportion of schizophrenics was found to vary from 3% to 38% within the same sample according to Brockington and co-workers(1978).The various operational diagnostic criteria have actually dereased international diagnostic agreement.According to Kendell (1982),the average K-value of the concordance between each pair of 9 operational definitions of schizophrenia varied from "0.41 to as little as 0.14,values lower than the corresponding figures for the reliability of psychiatric diagnoses in the 1960's,before operational definitions were introduced".

When the psychiatric classification in ICD8 became accepted by most WHO member countries around 1970,it was hoped that its wide acceptance would result in official use.Information on first admission by ICD diagnosis,was however available only from seven WHO member countries.Of these,only two (Denmark & Norway) strictly adhere to the ICD categories.The fact that ICD was in official use only in a small number of WHO member countries,does not reduce the importance of preserving the ICD as the official international classification in psychoatry.More information is obviously needed about its concepts as well as its actual practical usage.Further,the use of ICD does not interfere with the introduction of local more detailed systems of classification for research or other special purposes.However,without an internationally accepted psychiatric classification,we are back to the conditions described by dr.Renaudin,director of the asylumn at Meurthe in France in 1856:

" It is therefore essential that we shall agree about the signifi- "
" cance of the words we employ,about the elements of rational clas-"
" sification.In other words,about the evaluation of the signs we   "
" record in our observations.It is evident that no such mutual un- "
" derstanding exists today,and it is to be feared that we shall not"
" reach it in the foreseeable future.After having fought victori-   "
" ously against administrative and judical prejudices,and after ha-"
" ving seen veritable triumphs in the field of medico-legal exper-"
" tise,we now see anarchy in the field of classification threatening
" to split our ranks and robbing us of the victories or our pre-   "
" decessors.

REFERENCES

Allodi,F.(1982) Acute Parnoid Reaction(Bouffée Delirante) in Canada.Can.J.Psychiatry,27:366-373.
Berner,P.& K.Küfferle(1982)British Phenomenological and Psychopathological Concepts:A comparative review:Brit.J.Psych.558-65.
Brockington,I.F.,Kendell,R.E.& Leff,J.P.(1978)Definitions of Schizophrenia:concordance and prediction of outcome.Psychological Medicine,8:387-398.

Dean,C,P.G.Surtee & S.P.Sashidharan(1983) Comparison of Research
    Diagnostic Systems in an Edinburgh Community Sample.Brit.J.of
    Psychiatry:142:247-256.
Kantor,S.J.& A.H.Glassman(1977) Delusional Depressions:Natural
    History and Response to Treatment:Brit.J.Psych.131:351-360.
Kendell,R.E.(1982) The Choice of Diagnostic Criteria for biologi-
    cal Research.Arch.Gen.Psychiatry,39:1334-1339.
Lewis,A,J,(1934) Melancholia:clinical survey of depressed states.
    Journ.Mental Science.80:277-378.
Lewis,A.J.(1936) Melancholia:prognostic study and case material.
    Journ.Mental Science.82:488-558.
Rawnsley,K.(1968) An International Diagnostic Exercise.Proc.IVth
    World Congress of Psychiatry.Vol.4.Amsterdam.
Renaudin,P.(1856) Recherche statistiques relative a l'alienation men-
    tale.Annales Mi dico-Psychologiques.p.339-360.
Pichot,P.(1982) The Diagnosis and Classification of Mental Disorder
    in French-speaking Countries:background,current views and com-
    parison with other nomenclatures.Psychological Medicine,475-92.
Saugstad,L.& Ø.Ødegård (1979) Mortality in Psychiatric Hospitals in
    Norway 1950-74,Acta Psychiat.Scand.59:431-447.
Saugstad,L.& Ø.Ødegård (1980) Ingen International Tilnærming etter
    10 år med den internasjonal diagnoseliste ICD8.Nord.Psyk.Tid-
    skr.34:455-464.In Norwegian.
Saugstad,L.& Ø.Ødegård (1983) Persistent Discrepancy in Internatio-
    nal Diagnostic Practice since 1970.Acta Psychiat.Scand.in Press
Wimmer,A.(1916) Psykogene Sindssygdomsformer.In St.Hans Hospital
    1816 - 1916,Copenhagen,in Danish.
Wing,J.K.,Cooper,J.E.& N.Sartorius(1974) Measurement and Classifica-
    tion of Psychiatric Symptoms.London,Cambridge Univ.Press.
Zigmond,A.S. & A.C.P.Sims (1983).The effect of the Use of the Inter-
    national G assification of Diseases 9th Revision:Upon Hospital
    In-Patient Diagnosis.Brit.J.Psychiatry.142:409-413.
Ødegård,Ø.(1968) Reactive Psychoses.Acta Psychiat.Scand.Suppl.203.

ABSTRACT

    National admission statistics by ICD diagnosis since 1970 were
available from seven WHO member countries.The discrepancy in diagnostic distribution was more or less unchanged from before 1970.
These persistent national differences in diagnostic practice reflect a persistent reluctance to accept international standard.A
reluctance which was barely overcome with the acceptanc of ICD8
around 1970.

    The replacement in U.S.A. of the ICD by a local classification
(DSM-III) in 1980,is a serious move.It is likely to accelerate this
reluctance. We need to preserve the ICD as the official international classification in psychiatry. The use of the ICD does not interfere with the development of local more detailed systems of
classification for research and other special purposes.These local
systems in England and U.S.A.,are however not without problems,
as there is a disturbing lack of consensus in diagnosis between them.

THE POLYDIAGNOSTIC APPROACH

Ian Brockington

Professor of Psychiatry
The University of Birmingham
Birmingham B15 2TH

Psychiatrists have tried to solve their nosological problems
by arbitrary definition of entities like 'schizophrenia'. Scientists
investigating the cause and treatment of mental illness have seized
on these definitions in the hope that their patients will be comparable
with those of other groups using the same definitions, wherever they
may be. Unfortunately a large number of rival diagnostic systems
have been introduced, each with its limited zone of influence. The
'polydiagnostic approach' is a possible remedy for this confusion.
It consists of applying several different diagnostic systems to the
same series of patients, enabling the relationship between clinical
concepts to be examined directly and empirically.

The technique was introduced independently by Carpenter &
Strauss (1974) and Kendell (Brockington, Kendell & Leff, 1978). Both
groups sought to choose between rival definitions of schizophrenia,

Table 1. Netherne study of 6 definitions of schizophrenia

Definition	N	Concordance with final diagnosis	Social Status score
RDC	44	.60	44.7
Catego	56	.59	43.1
Langfeldt	37	.56	44.9
Carpenter (5)	48	.52	45.4
Schneider	38	.39	41.7
Astrachan	48	.36	42.2
All patients	129	-	38.5

by examining their prediction of outcome. These studies had some interesting results. Table 1 shows a comparison of 6 definitions of schizophrenia, all applied to the 'Netherne series' of 129 patients who were followed for about 6 years. Two criteria of outcome are shown in the table – agreement with the 'final diagnosis' made by 2 raters reviewing the whole course of the disease, and the 'social status' score derived from employment record and social involvement (a high score implying a poor outcome). Four definitions (RDC, Catego, Langfeldt's and Carpenter's) had the best concordance with the final diagnosis and selected patients with a relatively poor outcome, while two (Schneider's and Astrachan's) appeared less valid when tested in this way.

A further analysis, using more sensitive outcome measures, demonstrated differences between Catego, RDC and the newly introduced DSM III definitions of schizophrenia. Table 2 shows a comparison of Catego and RDC. When 52 patients meeting Catego criteria for schizophrenia were divided into 24 who met RDC and 28 who did not, it was found that those Meeting RDC had more delusions, passivity and other schizophrenic symptoms during the follow-up period, and were almost always given a final diagnosis of schizophrenia; those not meeting RDC had an excess of affective symptoms during the follow-up period, and were often given a final diagnosis of affective disorder. Thus RDC appears a stricter definition which selects a group of patients with a relatively poor prognosis. DSM III, however, is even more strict (Table 3). RDC schizophrenics meeting DSMIII criteria have more defect symptoms, a poorer social outcome and spend much longer in hospital than those who do not meet DSM III criteria, who often have manic symptoms during the follow-up period. The poly-diagnostic approach allows these differences to be plainly seen.

The technique is commended to biological researchers, because it increases the chances that their results can be compared with those of other laboratories. It is not, however, a panacea. Given the contemporary obsession with structured interviews, there is a danger that laboratory scientists will collect clinical data entirely in the form of interview ratings using a 'respectable' 'instrument',

Table 2. Outcome of catego schizophrenia in Netherne Series (N = 125)

	RDC+	RDC-	p
Number meeting R.D.C.	24	28	
Delusions of control	8	1	.01
Passivity scale	20.7	5.3	.02
Delusions scale	37.2	22.1	.03
Psychopathology score	− 0.16	+ 0.68	.02
Final diagnosis schizophrenia	21	16	.04
Final diagnosis affective	1	9	.03

and apply computer programmes in order to generate a large number of diagnoses. This is a poor man's clinical technique. Apart from the limitations of the data base and ratings, there is a danger that symptoms defined by one system will not correspond to those used in another. Applying the diagnostic methods used by each school requires an intimate knowledge of its concepts. For example, the concept of thought disorder used by the New Haven school (eg. 'bizarre thinking', 'autism or grossly unrealistic private thoughts') was opaque to British psychiatrists, and it was almost impossible to apply Astrachan's definition of schizophrenia. Equally the clinical ideas of Scandinavians like Perris and Langfeldt are unfamiliar to Anglo-American psychiatrists. Some progress can be made by swapping itemized definitions, preferably applied to data based on multiple information sources and multiple raters (Brockington & Meltzer, 1982), but the use of expert diagnosis is probably a superior method. It was used in the Netherne series for the study of 'cycloid psychosis', the diagnoses being made by Perris. The clinical data were scarcely adequate for the task, but it was possible to show that cycloid psychosis had an unusually good prognosis.

These outcome studies are an early and primitive attempt to evaluate clinical concepts. They were based on the inferior method of the 'follow up' study, in which patients are carefully studied during one index admission and are traced and interviewed some years later. There are at present no data using the 'follow-through' method in which patients are identified at their first admission and followed through several episodes. The evaluation of clinical concepts must, however, also include the use of genetic and biological criteria, and treatment response. There are, to my knowledge, no polydiagnostic studies using genetic criteria. Since the clinical techniques are difficult and expensive, it would be wise to apply them only to the best available genetic data. Large twin or adoption series, such as the Danish adoption study or the National Academy of Sciences Twin Panel would be appropriate, as would also be the Danish series of patients born to 2 psychotic parents. The use of the criterion of treatment response also deserves to be done with excellent data, eg. those obtained in large multicentre (double-blind, randomized, controlled) drug trials, such as the 9 hospitals collaborative study of neuroleptics in acute schizophrenic patients. The use of biological criteria is of great interest, and the polydiagnostic technique could be applied to series of patients subjected to hormonal challenge tests, or lumbar puncture and the analysis of CSF neurotransmitter metabolites. In this way the construct validity of definitions of schizophrenia will eventually be elucidated.

The polydiagnostic approach will enable the relationship of diagnostic conepts to be clarified, and may lead to a more widely accepted, more highly differentiated international diagnostic system .

Table 3. Outcome of RDC schizophrenia in Netherne series
(N = 125)

	DSMIII+	DSMIII-	p
Number meeting DSMIII criteria	18	10	
Manic scale	3.6	13.2	.05
Defect symptoms	23.6	10.3	.20
Time in hospital	48.1%	10.8%	.003
Social status	53.1	33.0	.009

References

Brockington I F, Kendell R E, Leff J P (1978)
Definitions of schizophrenia: concordance and prediction of outcome
Psychological Medicine 8, 387-398

Brockington I F, Meltzer H Y (1982)
Documenting an episode of psychiatric illness: need for multiple
    information sources, multiple raters, and narrative
Schizophrenia Bulletin Vol 8, No 3, pp485-492

Strauss J S, Carpenter W T Jnr (1974)
Characteristic symptoms and outcome in schizophrenia
Archives of General Psychiatry 30, 429-434

THE POLYDIAGNOSTIC APPROACH IN PSYCHIATRIC RESEARCH:

SCHIZOAFFECTIVE PSYCHOSES

Gerhard Lenz

Psychiatric Clinic, University of Vienna
Währingergürtel 74-76
A - 1090 Vienna, Austria

INTRODUCTION AND METHODS

The data presented in this paper are part of a larger project on "classification and course of functional psychoses"; in this project a representative sample of 200 patients with an ICD-diagnosis of 295, 296, 297 or 298 at their first admission to either the Psychiatric Clinic, University of Vienna or to the Psychiatric Hospital of the City of Vienna were interviewed during this first admission with an extended version of Present State Examination and each patient was diagnosed by the interviewer according to ICD-9 (1978) and DSM-III (1980) and was rated positive or negative for a series of different diagnostic criteria for functional psychoses:
these included for schizophrenia the criteria of Taylor (1978), RDC Spitzer (1978), Feighner (1972), Berner (1983) and also K. Schneider's FRS (in Berner 1983) and Bleuler's basic symptoms (in Berner 1983),
for schizoaffective disorder RDC Spitzer (1978)
and for affective disorder the criteria for mania and depression of Taylor (1978), Feighner (1972), Spitzer (1978) and the endo-genomorphic cyclothymic axial syndrome (Berner 1983).

RESULTS

Table 1 shows the number of patients assigned to different ICD-diagnoses and also presents the sex-distribution: it is interesting to notice that the sex-distribution in ICD-schizoaffective patients is similar to affective disorder and strikingly different to schizophrenic disorder.

Table 1. ICD - Diagnosis and Sex

	MALE		FEMALE	
295 (without 295.7) n = 64	42	66%	22	34%
295.7 n = 33	11	33%	22	67%
296 n = 69	26	38%	43	62%
297 n = 24	11	46%	13	54%
298 n = 10	4	40%	6	60%
	94	47	106	53%

In looking at the previous outpatients-episodes of patients with a first-admission-diagnosis of ICD 295.7 (table 2) it is interesting to note, that in 24 previous episodes there isn't any previous diagnosis of schizophrenia, only 4 episodes of schizo-affective disorder, but 13 episodes of affective disorder.

Table 3 shows the relationship between different research-criteria and ICD-9 and DSM-III-diagnoses of Schizoaffective Disorder. It is evident from this table that 85 % of the ICD-schizoaffectives have at least one FRS of Schneider and 73 % at least one of Bleuler's basic symptoms. Only very few patients fit into Feighner's or RDC Spitzer's criteria for schizophrenia, mania or depression because of the restrictive exclusion criteria for "schizoaffectives" of these systems. So most of the patients fit into the category of RDC Schizoaffective Disorder.

Table 2. Previous outpatient-episodes of patients with a present diagnosis of ICD 295.7

ICD-Dg	Last epi-sode	Last but one	Last but two
295.7	2	1	1
296	8	4	1
298	1	1	-
30.	3	2	-
NONE	19	25	31

Table 3. Relationship between different research-criteria and
ICD-9 and DSM-III-diagnoses of schizoaffective disorder

N = 200			ICD-9 295.7 n = 33	DSM III 295.70 n = 6
Basic symptoms	FRS SCHNEIDER	n = 121	28	5
	BLEULER	n = 91	24	5
Schizophrenia	TAYLOR	n = 96	13	3
	SPITZER RDC	n = 67	1	1
	FEIGHNER	n = 44	-	-
	BERNER	n = 40	4	3
Schizoaff. Disorder RDC SPITZER				
	Manic type	n = 25	22	1
	Depressive type	n = 16	8	4
Mania	TAYLOR	n = 44	15	1
	SPITZER RDC	n = 31	6	-
	FEIGHNER	n = 27	2	-
Depression	TAYLOR	n = 56	3	1
	FEIGHNER	n = 49	1	-
	SPITZER RDC	n = 47	-	-
Cyclothymic axial-syndrome				
	BERNER	n = 86	29	4

An execption are Taylor's criteria, here used in the version
of 1978: on the one hand they provide a very wide concept of affective disorder but on the other hand, if there is a marked disturbance of affect (like inappropriate affect, which happens quite
often in these schizoaffective patients) these patients are very
quickly moved to the category of schizophrenia: in this study 40 %
of the ICD-9-schizoaffectives fulfil Taylor's criteria for schizophrenia. Berner's Endogenomorphic-Cyclothymic Axial Syndrome
(Berner 1983), which proposes a close relationship to affective
disorder, is fulfilled by 88 % of the ICD-9-schizoaffectives.

The results are similar, if you look at the relationship
between an ICD-diagnosis of 295.7 and DSM-III-diagnoses: it is
quite impressing that the majority of ICD-schizoaffectives belong
to affective disorder in DSM-III (Fig. 1).

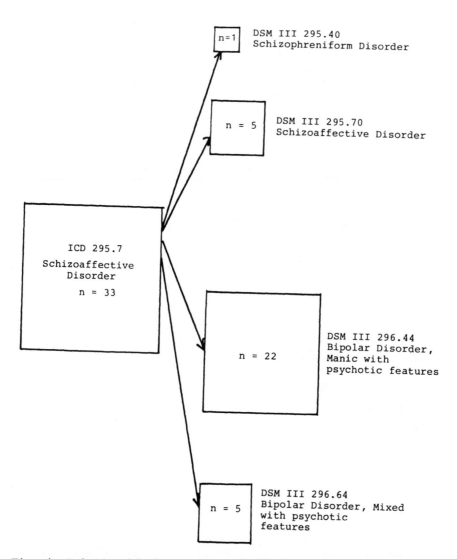

Fig. 1. Relationship between ICD-9 295.7 and DSM-III-diagnoses

In fact 27 of the 33 schizoaffectives had manic features or mixed states and this is in concordance with several studies (Abrams 1976, Brockington et al. 1980 a, Pope et al 1980, Rosenthal et al. 1980) in which the course of schizoaffective mania was found to be very similar to the course of bipolar affective disorder.

This is again shown in Figure 2, where it becomes obvious that a large majority of RDC Spitzer Schizoaffective Disorder. Manic Type belongs to Affective Disorder in DSM-III

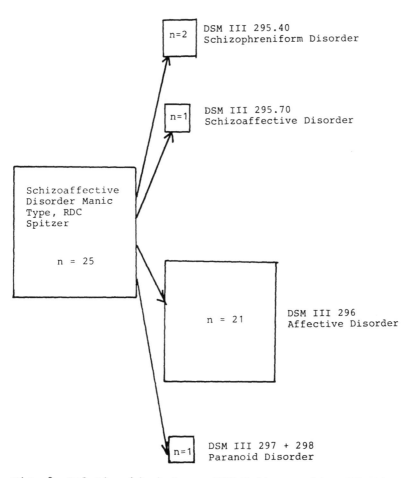

Fig. 2. Relationship between RDC Spitzer schizoaffective
disorder, manic type and DSM III - diagnoses

The situation is quite different for schizoaffective disorder,
depressive type: these patients seem to be more heterogeneous and
in this study the RDC Spitzer Schizoaffective Disorder, Depressive
Type (n = 16) is nearly equally distributed over the DSM-III-
diagnoses of 295 without 295.7 (n = 5), 295.70 (n = 4) and 296
(n = 6). This is in keeping with the study of Brockington et al.
(1980 b), who found their schizoaffective-depressed patients much
more heterogeneous than their schizoaffective manic patients in
past history and clinical features and they also found outcome
inpredictable: some patients followed a typical unipolar depressive
course, others were typically schizophrenic and very few developed
bipolar affective disorder.

CONCLUSION

It seems useful from our study to divide schizoaffective disorder by polarity. This is in concordance with the opinion of Clayton, who - in her review-article on schizoaffective disorders (Clayton 1982) - stressed that much of the data on schizoaffective mania indicate that most cases are very similar in symptomatology, course, family history and response to treatment to bipolar affective disorder patients, whereas the data on the schizoaffective depressed patients are far more confusing and suggest these group of patients to be very heterogeneous.

REFERENCES

Abrams, R. and Taylor, M., 1976, Mania and schizoaffective disorder, manic type: A comparison, Am. J. Psychiatry, 133: 1445-1447.

Berner, P., Gabriel, E., Katschnig, H., Kieffer, W., Koehler, K., Lenz, G. and Simhandl, C., 1983, Diagnostic criteria for Schizophrenic and Affective Psychoses, American Psychiatric Press, Washington D.C.

Brockington, I.F., Wainwright, S. and Kendell, R.E., 1980 a, Manic patients with schizophrenic or paranoid symptoms, Psychol. Med., 10: 73-83.

Brockington, I.F., Kendell, R.E. and Wainwright, S., 1980 b, Depressed patients with schizophrenic or paranoid symptoms, Psychol. Med., 10: 665-675.

Clayton, P.J., 1982, Schizoaffective Disorders, J.Nerv.Ment.Dis. 11: 646-650.

Diagnostic and Statistical Manual of Mental Disorders, 1980, 3rd edition, American Psychiatric Association, Washington D.C.

Feighner, J.P., Robins, E., Guze, S.B., Woodruff, R.A., Winokur, G. and Munoz, R., 1972, Diagnostic criteria for use in psychiatric research, Arch. Gen. Psychiatry, 26: 57-63.

ICD 9 th revision: Mental Disorders, 1978, Glossary and Guide to their Classification in Accordance with the Ninth Revision of the International Classification of Disease, WHO, Geneva.

Pope, H.G., Lipinski, J.F. and Cohen, B.M. et al., 1980, Schizoaffective disorder: An invalid diagnosis; A comparison of schizoaffective disorder, schizophrenia and affective disorder, Am.J. Psychiatry, 137: 921-927.

Rosenthal, N.E., Rosenthal, L.N. and Stallone, F. et al., 1980, Toward the validation of RDC schizoaffective disorder, Arch. Gen. Psychiatry 37: 804-810.

Spitzer, R.L., Endicott, J. and Robins, E., 1978, Research Diagnostic Criteria (RDC) for a Selected Group of Functional Disorders, 3rd edition, New York State Psychiatric Institute, New York.

Taylor, M.A. and Abrams, R., 1978, The prevalence of schizophrenia: A reassessment using modern diagnostic criteria, Am. J. Psychiatry 135:8, 945-948.

THE POLYDIAGNOSTIC APPROACH IN RESEARCH ON DEPRESSION

Heinz Katschnig and Peter Seelig

Psychiatric Clinic, University of Vienna

Währinger Gürtel 74-76, A-1090 Wien, Austria

176 carefully selected depressed patients admitted to the Psychiatric Clinic of the University of Vienna or to a nearby state hospital were included in a study, the main aim of which was the validation of the classical dichotomy of endogenous versus neurotic depression. The validating criteria were life stress preceding the depressive episode, and the course of symptomatology in the two years after discharge.

The definitions of the concepts of "endogenous" and "neurotic" depression, although showing a certain degree of overlap, are very different from diagnostic system to diagnostic system and from author to author.

This is reflected in studies both on the relationship of psychosocial variables, such as life events, and of biological variables, such as the Dexamethason Suppression Text, to these subtypes. Thus, while each of the following studies on the relationship of life events to subtypes of depression is methodologically sound, they are not comparable,because each has used different definitions of these subtypes: Paykel (1971) used a cluster analysis derived grouping, Brown et al.(1979) relied on clinical judgement, and Bebbington et al.(1981) separated their cases in CATEGO classes 'N' (neurotic) and 'R or D' (retarded or psychotic) according to the Present State Examination (PSE)/CATEGO system (Wing et al.,1974) (see table 1).

The results of these studies differ from each other: Paykel (1971) and Brown et al. (1979) did not find a specific relationship between depressive subtypes and life events, whereas Bebbington et al. (1981) demonstrated that a much higher percentage of neurotic than endogenous depressives had suffered from preceding life stress. Apart from the problem that different definitions of diagnostic subtypes were used a second obstacle to comparison are the different life stress indices used in the three studies.

We employed a polydiagnostic approach (Berner and Katschnig, 1983; Katschnig and Berner, 1984), i.e. we used as many definitions of depressive subtypes as were available, in order to be able to compare our results with those of similar studies in which only one specific formulation had been chosen.

Hence, after analyzing a number of definitions of depressive subtypes a data collection instrument, based on the PSE (Wing et al., 1974), was devised containing all elements which were necessary to assign a patient to an "endogenous" or "neurotic" depressive subtype according to the diagnostic formulations included.

The diagnostic formulations used can be divided into three classes:

Table 1: Different definitions of endogenous/neurotic depression:

(1) Psychopathological Definitions

    (a) Research Diagnostic Criteria (Spitzer et al., 1978)
    (b) Viennese Research Diagnostic Criteria (Berner et al., 1983)
    (c) CATEGO - Classes (Wing et al.,1974)
    (d) Cluster Analytic Definition (project)

(2) "Reactivity" diagnosis

    (a) at least one/none life event in week before onset
    (b) at least one/none life event in four weeks before onset
    (c) subjective experience of triggered depression (life events) : yes/no
    (d) subjective experience of triggered depression (chronic social problem) : yes/no
    (e) c or d

(3) Mixed Criteria

    (a) ICD-8 (WHO,]967)
    (b) Newcastle Scale (Carney et al.,1965)
    (c) Depressive Category Type Scale (Sandifer et al.,1966)

A computer program was developed with the special purpose of arriving automatically at a diagnostic assignment for the patients included in our study.

The numbers of patients diagnosed as endogenous varied between 132 (CATEGO classes D or R) and 97 (no subjective experience of depression triggered through either life event or chronic difficulty).

In an analysis of the overlap of these concepts, it could be demonstrated that there was a wide range of different percentages of overlap, reaching from nearly 75% (Research Diagnostic Criteria "endogenous subtype" probable plus definite and CATEGO classes "R or D") to only 42% overlap (Vienna Criteria and no subjectively experienced triggered depression) (see figures 1 and 2).

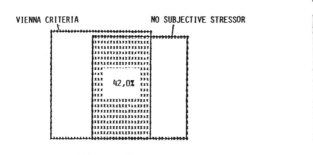

Figure 1

Overlap between different definitions of endogenous depression

Figure 2

Overlap between different definitions of endogenous depression

The reasons for these different overlaps cannot be discussed here but the examples shown can serve as a model of how differences between different diagnostic formulations may be analyzed on empirical grounds. A "comparative" nosology could become one of the uses of the "polydiagnostic approach".

Concerning the relationship between life events and depression we were able to replicate exactly the study design of a similar study by Bebbington et al. (1981), i.e. we were able to use the same stress index (according to the "Life Event and Difficulty Schedule" of Brown (1974)) and the same definition they had used to subdivide depression (CATEGO classes). The results of our study are contrasted with those of Bebbington et al's results in table 2.

Table 2

Percent patients with at least one independent life event with threat 1 or 2 or at least one chronic difficulty with threat 1, 2 or 3 in the 3 months before onset, for CATEGO classes 'N' and 'R or D'

	CATEGO 'N' (neurotic)	CATEGO 'R/D' (retarded/ psychotic)	
Bebbington et al. (1981)	20/36 = 55,6 %	2/13 = 14,4 %	p<0,05
Reanalysis of data from Katschnig et al. (1981)	4/22 = 18,2 %	18/75 = 24,0 %	n.s.

Whereas Bebbington et al. (1981) had found a preponderance of life stress in the neurotic class, we could not reproduce this finding. As the life event methodology is the same in both studies, the reasons for this discrepancy must be sought elsewhere. We can not speculate about these reasons here, but can only name the possibility that the different cultures, the different samples (Bebbington et al. studied community cases and outpatients, whereas we studied inpatients) or other methodological problems may be the reason for this discrepancy (in Bebbington et al.'s study the same interviewer elicited life stress and symptoms, which leaves the possibility open that the correlation between the two are an artifact of the interviewer, whereas we used two different groups of interviewers).

When using the same life event index as Bebbington et al. (1981) and applying it to several other diagnostic formulations, no differences emerged between the depressive subtypes except for ICD-8, where the difference corresponded to the clinical folklore of a "non-endogenous" depression being preceded by more life events (see table 3). This result cannot be discussed here in any detail; it can only be stated that this difference is probably a clinical artifact, as the ICD-8 diagnosis was taken from the clinical records and there are data showing that the doctors on the wards may have been heavily influenced by the mere fact of the existence of life events before the onset in giving an ICD-8 diagnosis.

Table 3

Percent patients with at least one independent life event with threat 1 or 2 or at least one chronic difficulty with threat 1, 2 or 3 in the 3 months before onset for 4 different diagnostic formulation for "non-endogenous" and "endogenous" depression

	"NON-ENDOGENOUS"	"ENDOGENOUS"	
ICD-8	12/32 = 37,5%	10/63 = 15,9%	p<0,05
VIENNA RESEARCH CRITERIA	6/38 = 15,8%	17/64 = 26,6%	N.S.
RDC	4/32 = 12,5%	19/70 = 27,1%	N.S.
CLUSTER ANALYSIS	5/40 = 12,5%	18/62 = 29,0%	N.S.

In a two year follow-up study several outcome variables were used for validating the depressive subclasses. By way of example the results for the outcome variable of "chronicity" (i.e. less than 10% healthy in the two years after discharge) are shown in table 4. No difference was found between the seven diagnostic subtypes selected for this presentation.

Table 4

Diagnostic subclassification: Percent patients with chronic course 2 years after discharge

DIAGNOSTIC CRITERIA	ENDOGENOUS	NON-ENDO-GENOUS	
VIENNESE CRITERIA	26,0%	26,0%	N.S.
CATEGO D/R=END.,N=NON-END.	22,9%	34,5%	N.S.
RDC ("DEFINITE")	27,3%	40,0%	N.S.
CLUSTER ANALYSIS	25,0%	27,3%	N.S.
OBJECTIVE LIFE STRESS(LEDS)	27,5%	22,2%	N.S.
SUBJECTIVE LIFE STRESS	31,4%	19,3%	N.S.
ICD-8	23,5%	30,6%	N.S.
CORE GROUP	29,7%	33,3%	N.S.

In concluding we would like to stress both the heuristic value and the feasibility of the "polydiagnostic approach". On the one hand, comparing different diagnostic formulations may prove to be a valuable activity for finally arriving at the essentials of specific diagnostic formulations, on the other hand, using several diagnostic systems simultaneously will increase the comparability between different studies. We could show that a "polydiagnostic approach" is feasible with surprisingly little extra effort and would like to recommend its use in psychiatric research.

References

Bebbington,P.E., C.Tennant, J.Hurry: Adversity and the nature of psychiatric disorder in the community.1981,J. of Affective Disorders 3:345-366

Berner.P.. E.Gabriel. H.Katschnig et al.: Diagnostic Criteria for Schizophrenic and Affective Psychoses.1983, World Psychiatric Association, American Psychiatric Press, Washington

Berner,P. & H.Katschnig: Principles of "multiaxial" classification in psychiatry as a basis of modern methodology, in "Methods in Evaluation of Psychiatric Treatment", Helgason,T. ed., Cambridge University Press, Cambridge, 1983.

Brown,G.W., M.Nî Bhrolchain, T.O.Harris: Psychotic and neurotic depression: Part 3: Aetiological and background factors.1979, Journal of Affective Disorders 1:195-211

Carney,M.W.P., M.Roth & R.F.Garside: The diagnosis of depressive syndromes and the prediction of ECT response. 1965, British J. of Psychiatry 111:659-674

Katschnig,H. and P.Berner: The Poly-Diagnostic Approach in Psychiatric Research, in World Health Organization: Proceedings of the International Conference on Diagnosis and Classification of Mental Disorders and Alcohol and Drug Related Problems, Copenhagen, April 1982. Geneva: WHO, 1984.

Paykel,E.S.: Classification of depressed patients: A cluster analysis derived grouping. 1971, Brit.J.Psychiatry 118:275-288

Sandifer,M.G., I.C.Wilson, L.Green: The two-type thesis of depressive disorders. 1966,Amer.J.Psychiatry 123: N° 1

Spitzer,R.L., J.Endicott, E.Robins: Research diagnostic criteria: Rational and reliability. 1978,Arch.Gen.Psychiatry 135:772-782

Wing,J.K., J.E.Cooper, N.Sartorius: The Measurement and Classification of Psychiatric Symptoms. Cambridge University Press, London 1974

WHO Manual of the International Statistical Classification of Diseases: ICD 8th Revision, V (1965 revision). Geneva: WHO,1967

THE POLYDIAGNOSTIC APPROACH IN DELUSIONAL SYNDROMES

Hans Schanda, Kenneth Thau, Bernd Küfferle, and
Peter Berner

Psychiatric University Clinic, Vienna, Austria

INTRODUCTION

According to the considerations at the beginning of this symposion we tried to apply the polydiagnostic approach (PDA) (the
simultaneous application of various diagnostic criteria to one and
the same population under study) to a sample of patients with delusional syndromes. The motives for this procedure were: 1. the
concept of axial syndromes has been developed in several cohorts of
delusional patients and 2. the delusional symptomatology itself is
one of the main pitfalls in many of the widely used diagnostic
systems. Productive symptoms have a central position, e.g. in the
FRS, whose validity underwent criticism especially in the last
years (Carpenter et al., 1973), but which on the other hand are
used on a world-wide scale and provide the basis for schizophrenia
diagnosis in several diagnostic systems as for example Taylor et al.
(1978), in part RDC (Spitzer et al., 1978) and ICD-9 (WHO 1978).
The assumption that incongruencies between different diagnostic
systems can be distinctly demonstrated in a sample of delusional
patients, seems to make this diagnostic group especially suitable
for the application of the PDA.

In a follow up study 90 patients with delusional psychoses
were examined and underwent reexamination after intervals of 6 to
9 years. In our descriptive classification we differentiated between theme, structure and constitutent elements of the delusion on
the one hand and the so-called background symptomatology (i.e.
disturbances of mood and drive, thought disorder) on the other.
We subdivided the background symptomatology into three axial
syndromes and assigned our patients to one of them if possible.The
definitions of the axial syndromes are presented in table 1. In

Table 1. Axial Syndromes (AS)

Endogenomorphic-Cyclothymic AS
A) Pronounced alteration of mood
   1. euphoric-expansive 2. depressive 3. dysphoric (hostile)
B) Pronounced alteration of drive
   1. increased (hyperactivity) 2. decreased (hypoactivity)
C) Biorhythmic disturbances
   1. diurnal variations 2. sleep disturbances (interrupted sleep,
      early awakening)
At least one of A plus at least one of B plus at least one of C
are necessary.

Endogenomorphic-Schizophrenic AS
A) Formal thought disorders
   1. blocking 2. derailment 3. pathologically "muddled speech"
B) Deficiency symptoms
   1. affective blunting 2. decrease of vital energy
At least one of A and/or all of B are necessary.

Organomorphic AS
Disturbance of thought and language (slow, viscous, circumstantial,
with or without verbal perseverations) (evidence for organic brain
damage not obligatory)

addition, we diagnosed the patients with Schneider's criteria (1939),
ICD-9 and DSM-III (American Psychiatric Association, 1980).

RESULTS

     Simultaneous application of Berner's AS and Schneider's FRS
at the time of initial examination revealed the following congruen-
cies (table 2). The 7 patients with an endogenomorphic-schizophrenic
AS did have at least one FRS, but 6 of the 16 endogenomorphic-cyclothymic and 6 of the 14 organomorphic patients had at least one as
well. Moreover, 27 patients not classifiable with Berner's criteria
showed FRS.

     A comparison of Berner's criteria with ICD-9 at the time of
initial examination is presented in table 3. Again, the 7 endogenomorphic-schizophrenic patients are included in ICD-9 schizophrenia
(295 excl. 295.7), but also 2 of the organomorphic and 20 of the
non-definable cases. All patients but one with an endogenomorphic-
cyclothymic AS are covered by the ICD-9 concept of schizoaffective
psychosis (295.7). 30 of the 41 paranoid states (297) and psychogenic paranoid psychoses (298.4) are recruited from Berner's non-
definable cases, 10 from the organomorphic ones.

116

Table 2.

Table 3.

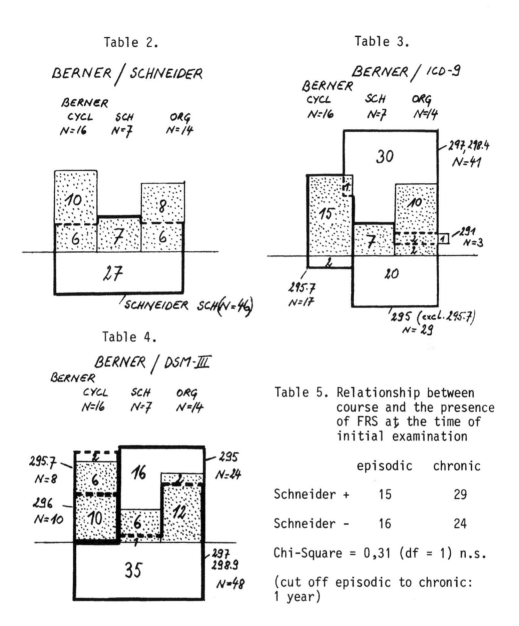

Table 4.

Table 5. Relationship between course and the presence of FRS at the time of initial examination

	episodic	chronic
Schneider +	15	29
Schneider -	16	24

Chi-Square = 0,31 (df = 1) n.s.

(cut off episodic to chronic: 1 year)

The same procedure with Berner's AS and DSM-III is presented in table 4. Of the 16 patients with a cyclothymic AS 10 corresponded to DSM-III affective disorder (296) and 6 to DSM-III schizoaffective disorder (295.7). The distribution of Berner's schizophrenic and organomorphic cases into DSM-III 295, 297 and 298.9 is similar to that in ICD-9.

Aside from genetic findings and treatment response, course and outcome of a disease are supposed to be important factors for establishing homogeneous groups in psychiatric diagnosis. Regarding

Table 6 Relationship between course of the illness and ICD-9
diagnoses at the time of initial examination

ICD-9	episodic	chronic	
295 (incl. 295.7)	18	25	
297	11	27	
298	1	0	Chi-Square = 3,34
291	1	1	(df = 3) n.s.
295 (excl. 295.7)	7	21	
295.7	11	4	
297	11	27	Chi-Square = 13,14
298	1	0	(df = 4)
291	1	1	sign. 5 % level
295.7	11	4	Chi-Square = 10,41
295 (excl. 295.7)			(df = 1)
+ 297 + 298 + 291	20	49	sign. 1 % level

(cut off episodic to chronic = 1 year)

the relationship between course of the illness in the interim between first and follow-up examination and presence of FRS at the
time of initial examination, no statistically significant correlation could be found (table 5). The usual 1:2 distribution of
episodic versus chronic course, as in classically diagnosed schizophrenics is present.

Also, ICD-9 schizophrenics (295) showed no statistically significant difference to the other diagnostic groups (table 6). After
separation of the schizoaffective cases (295.7), however, a relationship significant on the 5 % level developed (middle part of table 6).
Comparing the schizoaffective cases with all other diagnoses, correlation reached significance on the 1 % level in the expected
direction (lower part of table 6).

The main advantage of DSM-III can be seen in table 7. The
removal of the schizoaffective cases from the concept of schizophrenia and the possibility to classify patients with mood incon-
gruent delusions under affective disorder produces from the beginning statistically significant results regarding the course of
the illness.

The same procedure with Berner's AS brought similar results:
the cyclothymic AS group progressed mainly episodic, the schizophrenic and the organomorphic AS group mainly chronic; the non-
definable cases showed the usual 1:2 distribution episodic versus
chronic (table 8). Comparing the cyclothymic cases with all others,

Table 7. Relationship between course of the illness and DSM-III
diagnoses at the time of the initial examination

DSM-III	episodic	chronic	
295	7	16	
295.7	5	2	Chi-Square = 13,82
296	7	2	(df = 4)
297	12	29	sign. 1 % level
298.9	0	4	

(cut off episodic to chronic: 1 year)

Table 8. Relationship between course of the illness and axial
syndromes at the time of initial examination

AS	episodic	chronic	
endogenomorphic-cyclothymic	11	4	
endogenomorphic-schizophrenic	1	6	Chi-Square = 12,02
organomorphic	2	9	(df = 3) sign. 1 % level
atypical	17	34	
endogenomorphic-cyclothymic	11	4	Chi-Square = 8,59
endogenomorphic-schizophrenic,organo-morphic, atypical	20	49	(df = 1) sign.0,5 % level

(cut off episodic to chronic: 1 year)

the statistical significance reached the 0,5 % level. If one takes
the whole course and non only the first cross-section for assignment
to the axial syndromes, the results are significant on the 0,1 %
level.

CONCLUSIONS

1. The delusional symptomatology itself is not able to produce
homogeneous groups, regarding course and outcome. The important
group-establishing factors can be found in the background symptomatology (disturbances of mood and drive, thought disorder, and
affective blunting). According to this, diagnostic systems based
mainly on delusional symptoms for diagnosis of schizophrenia,
produce unsatisfying results. In this regard the FRS are of
differing quality, which could also be shown by Berner (1983) in

the symposion on plus and minus symptomatology in the case of schizoaffective disorder.

2. Regarding the course, ICD-9 schizoaffective disorder showed more affinity to MDI and should therefore be excluded from schizophrenia.

3. The presence of mood-incongruent delusional symptomatology should not be an exclusion criterion for the diagnosis of affective disorder.

REFERENCES

American Psychiatric Association, 1980, Diagnostic and Statistical Manual of Mental Disorders (DSM-III).

Berner, P., Küfferle, B. and Schanda, H., 1983, Are there Plus and Minus Symptoms Specific for Schizophrenia; Proceedings of the 7th World Congress of Psychiatry, Vienna.

Carpenter, J.W.T., Strauss, J.S.S. and Muleh, S., 1973, Are there pathognomonic symptoms in schizophrenia, An empiric investigation of Schneider s first rank symptoms. International pilot study of schizophrenia, Arch.gen.Psychiat. 28: 847.

Schneider, K., 1939, Klinische Psychopathologie, Thieme, Leipzig.

Spitzer, R.L., Endicott, J. and Robins, E., 1978, Research Diagnostic Criteria. Arch.Gen.Psychiat. 35: 773.

Taylor, M.A. and Abrams, R., 1978, The prevalence of schizophrenia: A reassessment using modern diagnostic criteria, Amer.J. Psychiatry 135: 945.

World Health Organisation, 1978, Mental disorders: Glossary and Guide to their classification in accordance with the 9th Revision of the International Classification of Diseases, Geneva.

COMPARING FRENCH AND INTERNATIONAL

CLASSIFICATION SCHEMES : II. DEPRESSION

C. B. Pull, M. C. Pull, A. Stauder, and P. Pichot

Centre Hospitalier, 1210 Luxembourg and
Clinique des Maladies Mentales et de l'Encéphale
75014 Paris

INTRODUCTION

In the French classification of mental diseases [1] , ela-borated by the Institut National de la Santé et de la Recherche Médicale (INSERM), depressive disorder is listed in the three following categories : (1) manic and depressive psychoses (INSERM 01) with basically only two sub-categories, i.e. the melancholic episodes of manic-depressive psychosis and involu-tional melancholia, (2) non-psychotic depressions (INSERM 13) subdivided in neurotic and reactive depressions, and (3) chronic schizophrenia (INSERM 02) which presents a subcategory termed chronic schizophrenia with depression, or atypical de-pression.

The INSERM classification is a simple nomenclature which provides neither glossary like ICD-9 [2] nor diagnostic criteria like DSM III [3] . As a consequence, it would make no sense to proceed to direct comparisons between the French and any other classification system. In the present report, comparison is based on a poly-diagnostic approach, in which clinical diagno-sis is documented by means of a standardized list which inte-grates the diagnostic criteria proposed in a number of recent, mostly North American classification systems.

METHOD

Clinical diagnoses following the INSERM classification were formulated, on the day of discharge, for a total of 50 depressed patients hospitalized at the Centre Hospitalier de Luxembourg. Final diagnosis was reached as a consensus between the chairman and one of the residents. The same resident evaluated each of the patients, after 2 weeks of hospitalization, using a List of Integrated Criteria for the Evaluation of Taxonomy in Depression (LICET-D) [4] .

LICET-D is a diagnostic instrument which integrates, in their exact original formulation, all the diagnostic inclusion and exclusion criteria that are required for all depression categories and sub-categories listed in 7 different classification systems. The composition of LICET-D is presented in the following :

Composition of LICET-D

1. The Saint-Louis criteria for primary and secondary depression [5] .
2. The New-York Research Diagnostic Criteria [6] for the major depressive disorder and minor depressive disorder.
3. The DSM III criteria for major depressive episode (with or without melancholia or psychotic features), cyclothymic disorder and dysthymic disorder.
4. The Vienna criteria defining Berner's [7] endogenomorphic cyclothymic axial syndrome.
5. The Klein [8] criteria for endogenomorphic and non-endogenomorphic depression .
6. The Newcastle [9] criteria for endogenous and neurotic depression.
7. The Winokur [10] criteria for pure depressive disease, sporadic depressive disease and depression spectrum disease.

Diagnostic decisions follow the exact instructions (decision-trees, algorithms, weights) provided by the respective systems. Each set of criteria is used as actually intended.

RESULTS

Cross-tabulations of French clinical diagnoses by DSM III, Saint-Louis and Newcastle criteria are presented in tables 1, 2, and 3.

1. French classification and DSM III

With only 2 exceptions concerning neurotic and reactive depressions, all INSERM diagnoses of depression may be classified into one or another DSM III depression category. All INSERM psychotic depressions, except one, are major depressive episodes according to DSM III. On the other hand, INSERM neurotic and reactive depressions are distributed, in grossly identical proportions, among each of the DSM III depression ca-

tegories. In particular, one fourth of INSERM diagnoses of neurotic and reactive depressions are major depressive episodes
according to DSM III criteria. In addition, the three INSERM
atypical depressions would be major depressive episodes in
DSM III. On the whole, the North American concept of major depressive episode appears to be broader than the French one of
depressive psychosis. All depressive psychoses are major depressive episodes, but not all major depressive episodes are
depressive psychoses.

In the lower part of table 1, major depressive episode is
subdivided according to DSM III criteria for fifth-digit coding
of : with melancholia, with psychotic features, (with both of
the preceeding), and without melancholia. INSERM psychotic depressions are obviously major depressive episodes with melancholia, with or without psychotic features. Our sample size is
too small at the moment to draw any further conclusions.

2. French classification and the Newcastle criteria

As shown in table 2, almost all INSERM neurotic or reactive
depressions are also neurotic depressions according to the
Newcastle criteria. On the other hand, only about two thirds
of the French depressive psychoses would be considered endogenous depressions using the Newcastle criteria. As a consequence,
the Newcastle criteria defining endogenous depression appear
to be more restrictive than the French ones for depressive psychosis.

3. French classification and the Saint-Louis criteria

About one fifth of our patients (listed as "other" in table 3) had to be discarded because duration of illness was less
than one month. As a rule, INSERM neurotic or reactive as well
as "atypical depressions" are secondary depressions. The same
applies, however, to half of the French psychotic depressions
as well. The concept of primary depression, developed for use
in psychiatric research, is obviously based on very narrow criteria and cannot be related to any concept in the French
classification.

4. French classification and other criteria

Proportion of INSERM Psychotic depressions that meet criteria for endogenous major depressive disorder (New York RDC),
endogenomorphic cyclothymic axial syndrome (VIENNA) and endogenomorphic depression (KLEIN) are included in table 4. Additional information will be published at a later time.

Table 1. Cross-tabulation of French clinical diagnoses by DSM III criteria

010 = melancholia
013 = involutional
010+013 = psychotic
130 = neurotic
131 = reactive
024 = atypical

		FRENCH CLINICAL									
		010		013		130 131		024		TOTAL	
		N	%	N	%	N	%	N	%	N	%
DSM III	MAJ. DEPR. EPISODE	15	94	10		5	24	3		33	66
	CYCLOTHYMIC	1	6			6	28			7	14
	DYSTHYMIC					3	14			3	6
	ADJUSTMENT					5	24			5	10
	OTHER					2	10			2	4
	TOTAL	16		10		21		3		50	
MAJOR D. EPIS.	WITHOUT MELANCHOLIA	1				2		2		5	10
	WITH MELANCHOLIA	14		10		3		1		28	56
	WITH PSYCH. FEATURES	3		3		1		2		9	18
	MEL. + PSYCH.	3		3				1		7	14

Table 2. Cross-tabulation of French clinical diagnoses by Newcastle criteria

		FRENCH CLINICAL									
		010		013		130 131		024		TOTAL	
		N	%	N	%	N	%	N	%	N	%
NEWCASTLE	ENDOGENOUS	10	62	7	70	2	10			19	38
	NEUROTIC	6	38	3	30	19	90	3		31	62
	TOTAL	16		10	21			3		50	

Table 3. Cross-tabulation of French clinical diagnoses by Saint-Louis criteria

		\multicolumn{10}{c}{FRENCH CLINICAL}
		010		013		130 131		024		TOTAL	
		N	%	N	%	N	%	N	%	N	%
ST. LOUIS	PRIMARY	6	38	5	50	3	15			14	28
	SECONDARY	8	50	5	50	11	52	3		27	54
	OTHER	2	12			7	33			9	18
	TOTAL	16		10		21		3		50	

Table 4. Proportion of INSERM psychotic depressions meeting criteria for other diagnostic concepts

SYSTEM	DIAGNOSTIC CONCEPT	N	%
DSM III	MAJOR DEPR. EPISODE WITH MELANCHOLIA	24	92
NEW YORK	ENDOGENOUS MAJOR DEPRESSIVE DISORDER	24	92
VIENNA	ENDOGENOMORPHIC CYCLO-THYMIC A. S.	19	73
NEWCASTLE	ENDOGENOUS DEPRESSION	17	65
KLEIN	ENDOGENOMORPHIC DEPRESSION	16	61
ST. LOUIS	PRIMARY DEPRESSION	11	42
\multicolumn{2}{c}{A "CONCORDANT" GROUP OF DEPRESSIONS}	7	27

CONCLUSION : A "CONCORDANT" GROUP OF DEPRESSIONS

Table 4 lists pourcentage of INSERM psychotic depressions meeting criteria for specific concepts defined in 6 different classification systems. INSERM psychotic depressions are major depressive episodes with melancholia (DSM III) or endogenous major depressive disorders (New York RDC). Three out of four INSERM psychotic depressions are endogenomorphic cyclo-thymic axial syndromes (Vienna), two out of three are endogenous depressions (Newcastle) or endogenomorphic depressions (Klein) and less than half are primary depressions. Only one out of four INSERM psychotic depressions would meet the criteria for all of the six other concepts.

This very narrowly defined group of "primary-psychotic-melancholic-endogenous-endogenomorphic" depressions, we propose to call "a concordant group of depressions". It might be interesting to study this group more closely, in particular in what concerns therapeutic response, course of illness, family history and biological characteristics.

REFERENCES

1. Institut National de la Santé et de la Recherche Médicale, ed, Classification française des troubles mentaux, Bull. de l'INSERM, 24, Suppl. to N° 2 (1969)
2. World Health Organization, Mental Disorders, Glossary and Guide to Their Classification in Accordance with the Ninth Revision of the International Classification of Diseases, W.H.O., Geneva (1978)
3. American Psychiatric Association, Diagnostic and Statistical Manual of Mental Disorders (3rd edn, DSM III), A.P.A., Washington D.C. (1980)
4. C. B. Pull, M. C. Pull, P. Pichot, LICET-D : Une Liste Intégrée de Critères d'Evaluation Taxinomiques pour les dépressions, Psychologie Médicale (in press)
5. J. P. Feighner, E. Robins, S. B. Guze, R. A. Woodruff, G. Winokur, R. Munoz, Diagnostic criteria for use in psychiatric research, Arch. Gen. Psychiat., 26, 57 (1972)
6. R. L. Spitzer, J. Endicott, E. Robins, Research Diagnostic Criteria (RDC) for a selected group of functional disorders, 3rd edn, New York State Psychiatric Institute, Biometrics Research (1977)
7. P. Berner, H. Katschnig, Principles of "multiaxial" classification in psychiatry as a basis of modern methodology, in "Methodology in evaluation of psychiatric treatment, T. Helgason, ed. (in press)
8. D. F. Klein, Endogenomorphic depression : A conceptual and terminological revision, Arch. Gen. Psychiat., 34, 447 (1974)
9. M. W. Carney, M. Roth, R. F. Garside, The diagnosis of depressive syndromes and the prediction of E.C.T. response, Brit. J. Psychiat., 111, 659 (1965)
10. G. Winokur, The devision of depressive illness into depression spectrum disease and pure depressive disease, Int. Pharmaco-psychiat., 9, 5, (1974)

RELIABILITY OF PSYCHIATRIC DIAGNOSIS BASED ON CHECKLIST CRITERIA

John E. Overall

University of Texas Medical School at Houston
Department of Psychiatry and Behavioral Sciences
P.O. Box 20708
Houston, Texas 77025

The purpose of my talk today is to consider parameters of the polydiagnostic model that contribute to greater reliability and validity of diagnostic decisions. In so doing, I will mention briefly the particular data that we have used to examine these issues empirically; however, it is not the empirical results that I plan to discuss. The point that I would emphasize, instead, is that psychometric test theory has implications for reliability and validity issues related to psychiatric diagnosis. Ultimately, empirical studies can be used to corroborate conclusions drawn from test theory.

As every psychiatrist is aware, several different sets of characteristics have been proposed by different authors as meaningful criteria for confirming a diagnosis of depression or schizophrenia. Some diagnostic criteria concentrate on phenomenological characteristics, others emphasize psychological states, others emphasize physiological or biological parameters. History and background items have been considered by a few. Quite a long list would result if one were to incorporate into a polydiagnostic model all of the characteristics that have been proposed to distinguish depressive disorders or schizophrenia from other psychiatric conditions. In my talk today, I will use criteria for diagnosis of depressive disorder as an example, but the concerns that I express relate to criteria for diagnosis of other conditions as well.

It is appropriate to consider that a list of diagnostic criteria is a kind of true-false test, like those used in the classroom. An item is true if it represents a symptom or behavior present in the patient. By considering a set of diagnostic criteria to be analogous to a true-false test, certain conclusions can be derived from psychometric test theory.

Operational definitions of depressive disorder which can be conceived as a checklist permit some latitude regarding which particular symptoms and how many of them must be present to establish a diagnosis of depression. The diagnosis is confirmed if a specified number of symptoms from a longer list is recorded as present. I will here use the diagnosis of Major Depressive Episode from the American Psychiatric Association DSM III as an example. As noted earlier, several other sets of diagnostic criteria might be used as alternative examples, and this discussion would apply equally well to them. To qualify for a diagnosis of Major Depressive Episode according to DSM III, a patient must have dysphoric mood or pervasive loss of interest or pleasure, plus at least four of the following eight associated symptoms: poor appetite or weight loss, insomnia or hypersomnia, agitation or retardation, loss of interest or pleasure, loss of energy (fatigue), feelings of worthlessness or guilt, diminished ability to think or concentrate, and recurrent thoughts of death or suicide. It is the list of associated symptoms that I would liken to a true-false test.

A. Dysphoric mood or pervasive loss of interest or pleasure
B. At least four of the following:

_____ 1. Poor appetite or significant weight loss

_____ 2. Insomnia or hypersomnia

_____ 3. Psychomotor agitation or retardation

_____ 4. Loss of interest or pleasure

_____ 5. Loss of energy

_____ 6. Feelings of worthlessness, self-reproach, guilt

_____ 7. Diminished ability to think or concentrate

_____ 8. Recurrent thought of death or suicide

Fig. 1. DSM-III Major Depressive Episode

In recognizing the similarity between checklist criteria for diagnosis and true-false tests, we must also recognize that each item (or symptom) is recorded with some probability of error. The point that I want to make about the DSM III criteria, and about most other checklist criteria, is that a list of only eight items constitutes a rather short true-false test, as we are familiar with them from our classrooms. When the list of symptoms is very short, a mistake in judging the presence or absence of a single symptom can have profound consequences for the accuracy of the diagnostic decision. On the other hand, if the list of symptoms is reasonably long and the presence of several symptoms is required, then a mistake in judging the presence or absence of a single symptom has less effect on the diagnostic conclusion.

Even though the greater importance of accuracy of each item in a very short test is intuitively obvious, psychometric test theory provides a precise mathematical statement concerning the effect of length of a test on its reliability. The well-known relationship is explicit in what is commonly called the Spearman-Brown prophesy formula (also known as Kuder-Richardson formula #21). This formula says that, if the reliability of a test consisting of N items is r_{11}, the reliability of the test can be increased to r_{22} by doubling the length of the test.

$$r_{22} = \frac{2r_{11}}{1 + r_{11}}.$$

Explicit in this formula is the fact that r_{22} must be greater than r_{11}. The implication of this for reliability of psychiatric diagnoses based on checklist criteria is clear. Reliability of diagnoses can be increased by considering larger numbers of relevant patient characteristics. One of the most striking deficiencies in previous attempts to define objective criteria for diagnosis in psychiatry has been the failure to consider much of the relevant information.

This raises the question of what additional information one might consider relevant, as well as how to weight more and less relevant information. I would offer two comments on these issues. The first is that demographic and epidemiologic data have generally been given too little attention in previous attempts to specify objective criteria for psychiatric diagnosis. Depression, in particular, has different relative frequencies of occurrence in different age groups, different sex groups, different ethnic groups, and in different social classes. Marital status and marital history are also important diagnostic clues. These kinds of data can be treated in the same checklist fashion as are signs and symptoms in more abbreviated diagnostic checklists.

As one seeks to extend the list of items that are to be considered in reaching a diagnostic decision, the question of relevance for the decision process is obviously important. The Spearman-Brown formula, which was the starting point for this discussion, implicitly assumes comparable relevance for all items in the extended list. That is actually unlikely, but the general principle holds so long as all items have a reasonable degree of relevance. Appropriate weighting can be used to ensure that an extended list will result in increased reliability and/or validity. This is true, even if the additional items are less discriminating than the original shorter list of diagnostic criteria. Currently used checklist criteria tend to give equal weight to items of unequal importance. For example, "loss of energy" which may result from a variety of causes is given the same weight as "persistent thoughts of suicide".

A related issue concerns the failure of most current diagnostic criteria to consider adequately symptom severity. Most current checklist criteria simply note whether a symptom is present or absent. By considering different levels of severity, one is in effect adding differentially weighted items to the diagnostic checklist. This can affect reliability in much the same way as does extending the list of diagnostic criteria with any other types of items.

To conclude my talk, I would like to mention briefly, the instruments that we have used in applying the polydiagnostic approach to diagnosis of depressive disorders. A composite Diagnostic Checklist for Depression (CDC-Dep) was developed to include the criteria proposed by several different authors, as well as items to delineate DSM III major depressive disorder and its sub-categories. Specifically, the CDC-Dep contains criteria for diagnosis of primary depressive disorder (Feighner, et al, 1972), major depressive disorder (Spitzer, Endicott and Robins, 1975), DSM III major depressive episode, unipolar vs bipolar, with psychotic features or melancholia (American Psychiatric Association, 1980), depressive spectrum disorder (Winokur, 1972), plus demographic and history items identified in our own actuarial studies. This Composite Diagnostic Checklist (CDC-Dep) is reproduced in Figure 2. In recognition of the fact that description of the scoring of the various diagnostic criteria included in this composite checklist has been published elsewhere, that detail need not be repeated here (Overall, 1982; Zisook, Click and Overall, 1980; Overall, Cobb and Click, 1982). The purpose here is simply to present the data form as a research tool which has incorporated the work of several groups in the United States. In a sense, the CDC-Dep is a composite of characteristics that American psychiatrists and psychologists have considered to be most relevant for diagnosis of depression.

Composite Diagnostic Checklist for Depression

Name of Subject _____   Date _____

Name of Interviewer _____

Check all items that are present

A. Dysphoric mood
   ☐ Moderately severe
   ☐ Severe
   ☐ Distinct quality-
     different from grief
   ☐ Worse in morning
   ☐ Unresponsive to
     environmental changes

B. Associated symptoms
   ☐ Looks sad, tearful, or
     depressed
   ☐ Decreased appetite or
     weight loss
   ☐ Increased appetite or
     weight gain
   ☐ Difficulty falling asleep
   ☐ Early awakening or
     middle insomnia
   ☐ Hypersomnia
   ☐ Excessive somatic concern
   ☐ Pessimistic
   ☐ Loss of energy
   ☐ Psychomotor retardation
   ☐ Psychomotor agitation
   ☐ Clinging dependency
   ☐ Anxiety
   ☐ Demandingness
   ☐ Blame projection
   ☐ Self-pity
   ☐ Resentful, irritable,
     angry or complaining
   ☐ Feelings of guilt or
     self-reproach
   ☐ Brooding about
     unpleasant events
   ☐ Loss of interest or
     pleasure
   ☐ Pervasive loss of
     interest
   ☐ Preoccupation with feelings
     of inadequacy
   ☐ Decreased sex drive
   ☐ Increased sex drive
   ☐ Diminished ability to
     concentrate
   ☐ Diminished ability to
     think
   ☐ Thoughts of death or
     suicide
   ☐ Delusions with definite
     depression theme
   ☐ Hallucinations with definite
     depression theme

C. Duration of depressive symptoms
   ☐ Less than two weeks

☐ Two to four weeks
☐ More than four weeks
☐ More than six months

D. Course of illness
   ☐ First episode
   ☐ Chronic state
   ☐ Recurrent unipolar
   ☐ Bipolar (previous manic)
   ☐ Bipolar (previous hypomanic)

E. Depressive Spectrum History
   ☐ Family history of depres-
     sion predominantly
     female relatives
   ☐ Family history of alco-
     holism or sociopathy in
     male relatives
   ☐ Depression about equally
     prevalent in relatives
     of both sexes
   ☐ No significant alcoholism
     in family history
   ☐ No significant socio-
     pathy in family history
   ☐ No significant depression
     in family history
   ☐ Probable schizophrenia
     in family history

F. Demographic characteristics
   ☐ Female
   ☐ Present age 40 or older
   ☐ Onset of first episode
     before ages 40
   ☐ Married or divorces
   ☐ Two or more children
   ☐ Skilled, sales or
     clerical worker, or
     housewife
   ☐ High school graduate
   ☐ College graduate
   ☐ Moderate religious
     attitude
   ☐ Abstain alcohol
   ☐ Frequent or heavy alcohol
     use
   ☐ No previous hospitalization
   ☐ Lower-middle or middle
     S.E.S. class
   ☐ Complaint of marital
     problems
   ☐ Severe discord in child-
     hood home

G. Symptoms suggestive of
   schizophrenia

☐ Thought broadcasting,
  insertion, or withdrawal
☐ Delusions of being controlled
☐ Any recurrent delusion or
  hallucination (except
  typical of depression)
☐ Preoccupation with any non-
  affective delusion or
  hallucination
☐ Auditory hallucination in
  which voice keeps up
  running commentary or two
  voices converse with each
  other
☐ Any non-affective hallucinations throughout the day
  for several days or inter-
  mittantly for a week
☐ Formal though disorder
☐ Period of one month during
  present illness in which
  delusions or hallucinations
  present without prominent
  dysphoric mood

H. Pre-existing psychiatric condition (other than mania or
   depression), such as schizophrenia, alcoholism, drug dependence,
   personality disorder, or
   organic brain syndrome

   ☐ No
   ☐ Probable
   ☐ Definite
   Type

I. Organic etiology
   ☐ No
   ☐ Yes
   Type

J. Precipitating factors
   ☐ None apparent
   ☐ Probable
   ☐ Definite

K. Phenomenological type
   ☐ Anxious depression
   ☐ Agitated depression
   ☐ Retarded depression
   ☐ Hostile depression

L. Endogenous depression
   ☐ No
   ☐ Probable
   ☐ Definite

In summary, psychometric test theory says that reliability can be increased by increasing the length of a test. Objective checklist criteria for diagnosis can be considered to be a type of true-false test in which each item is judged to be either present or absent. The test theory then suggests that the reliability of psychatric disgnoses can be improved by taking into account more of the relevant information. The ploydiagnostic model provides a basis for a more comprehensive approach by incorporating criteria proposed by several different authors. History and demographic data can be included, and symptom severity can be considered. Ultimately, optimal scoring of the combined information may require differential weighting based on empirical determination of differential relevance for diagnostic decisions.

References

American Psychiatric Association, "Diagnostic and Statistical Manual, Third Edition." A.P.A.: Washington, D.C. (1980).

Feighner, J.P., Robins, E., Guze, S.B., Woodruff, R.A., Winokur, G. and Munoz, R., 1972, Diagnostic criteria for use in psychiatric research. Arch. Gen. Psychiat. 26:57-63.

Overall, J.E., 1981, Criteres de diagnostic et de classification des depressions, in: "La Symptomatologie Depressive: Enregistrement et Evaluation," P. Pichot and C. Pull, eds., Geigy-Editions Spire, Paris.

Overall, J.E., Cobb, J.C. and Click, M.A., Jr., 1982, The reliability of psychiatric diagnosis based on alternative research criteria. J. Psychiat. Treat. Eval. 4:209-220.

Spitzer, R.L., Endicott, J., and Robins, E., 1975, Research diagnostic criteria (RDC). Psychopharm Bull. 11:22-24.

Winokur, G., 1972, Types of depressive illness. Brit. J. Psychiat. 120:265-266.

Zisook, S., Click, M.A., Jr. and Overall, J.E., 1980, Research criteria for the diagnosis of depression. Psychiatry Research, 2:13-23.

THE DEVELOPMENT OF THE PRESENT STATE EXAMINATION (P.S.E.)

John E. Cooper

University of Nottingham
Department of Psychiatry
United Kingdom

In this presentation, I shall trace the history and development of the Present State Examination (P.S.E.) from its early beginnings in the 1960's to the present day. The present position is that it is used in many different countries for surveys of both patients and community subjects. It has now been translated into over twenty different languages and obviously fulfills a need which is widley felt. I shall finish by mentioning very briefly the prospects for the next edition of the interview, P.S.E.10.

The P.S.E. originated in work of Professor John Wing and his colleagues in the Social Psychiatry Unit at the Institute of Psychiatry in London. The original purpose was to produce a simple descriptive categorisation of the four leading symptoms of chronic schizophrenia, i.e. flatness of affect, poverty of speech, incoherence of speech, and coherently expressed delusions (Wing 1961). This proved to be successful but indicated a need for more elaborate and extensive schedules. Sections dealing with neurotic symptoms were added during the production of second and third versions, and reliability studies were done during further improvements which formed the fourth and the fifth editions. Work on the fifth edition resulted in the first publication, concerned largely with the reliability of the P.S.E. (Wing, Birley, Cooper, Graham and Isaacs, 1967). By the time the seventh and the eighth editions were produced (these were very similar), it had been adopted for use in the International Pilot Study of Schizophrenia of the World Health Organisation, and in the US/UK Diagnostic Project (between New York and London). The field work for these two large international studies started in 1965 and 1966, and successive versions of the P.S.E. have been used in a variety of studies in many countries since this time.

BASIC PRINCIPLES OF THE PRESENT STATE EXAMINATION

In all its versions, the P.S.E. has been a systematically arranged interview schedule, containing all the conventionally recognised symptoms which are likely to be considered relevant to a present mental state examination. A form of questioning is suggested for each symptom, usually as a major introductory question, followed by a number of optional probing questions. These cover the content of the symptom at which each set of questions is aimed. Set out on the schedule opposite these questions is a rating for the symptom, together with a brief reminder of the main points that define the ratings.

The main principles that guide the conduct of the interview are 1) it is basically clinical and not a questionnaire, 2) the questioning and the rating cover the patient's experience during the last month and state at the time of the interview, and 3) a series of cut-off points are provided at which the interviewer decides whether to proceed with more detailed questions on the same topic, or whether to move on to the next section of the interview.

The principles by which the ratings are made must be learned before the interview can be used properly, by means of a special period of training and experience under the guidance of already experienced interviewers. The interviewer must learn a detailed glossary of terms and definitions so that he can judge whether or not a symptom is present, irrespective of the initial response of the patient to the main question. Each rating is made as the interview proceeds and items are not left to be rated at the end of the interview. However, the ratings are made on the basis of everything that emerges during the interview and at the end of the interview the interviewer checks carefully each item in the schedule in turn, to ensure that it has been rated on the basis of all the information that has become available.

Some further explanation of the meaning of the word 'clinical' is needed here, since this is such an important aspect of this procedure. For every rating, what is required is the interviewer's judgement of whether the symptom is present or not, based upon the whole content of the interview and upon his own observations. For a positive rating, specific examples of the occurrance of the symptom are required and detailed questioning is often needed to elicit these specific examples. In some cases the rating may be 0 even when the patient says 'yes' to initial probes, and equally the rating may be positive even though the patient initially denies its presence. The final rating is decided by the interviewer's judgement and not upon the initial response of the patient. The interviewer must expect to use many conventional and familiar probes and facilitating questions which are not printed in the schedule, such as 'tell me more', 'could you give me an example of that 'when did that last happen'.

The items are rated on the basis of the last month, so in one sense the title 'Present State' is not quite accurate. In practice, this period turns out to be best for achieving the basic purpose of the interview, which is to allow the interviewer to finish up with a reliable and comprehensive set of symptoms upon which to base a clinical diagnosis. When patients are interviewed soon after coming to medical attention or soon after being admitted to hospital, it is often found that the peak of their symptoms was some days or even a week before the occasion of the interview. The interview ratings must therefore go back over a period of time in order to cover this.

These basic principles and properties allow the P.S.E. interview to provide the interviewer with a set of ratings of symptoms upon which a clinical diagnosis can be based. The reliability of the symptom ratings and the syndromes or section scores which may be easily derived from these was well illustrated in the first publication already mentioned, (Wing, et al 1967). The clinical diagnosis based upon this information was also shown to be very reliable in the same study.

STUDIES USING THE P.S.E.

Although the seventh and eighth editions of the P.S.E. contained comprehensive coverage of neurotic symptoms, the main purpose of the development of the interview up till that time had been to allow a thorough description of psychotic symptoms, particularly those of schizophrenia. For this reason the P.S.E. was used in two large international studies that were starting around 1965 and 1966. These were the US/UK Diagnostic Study, done principally between London and New York, and the International Pilot Study of Schizophrenia, of the World Health Organisation. An important and interesting feature of both these studies was the need for extensive training periods in the use of the interview by the field workers in the study. This has remained the case with later editions of the P.S.E. and there is no doubt that to achieve high standards of reliability (and therefore comparability of information between studies), it is necessary to train with already experienced interviewers. The structure of such training courses has been described in some detail (von Cranach and Cooper 1972).

THE CATEGO COMPUTER PROGRAM

Experience gained during the process of the US/UK study, in which the P.S.E. interview was combined with Spitzer's 'Mental Status Schedule', indicated the need to develop a computer program using the P.S.E. items, which would produce a standardised

categorisation of the patient's mental state.   The US/UK study
had found Spitzer's computer program (Spitzer and Endicott, 1968)
to be a most useful tool for making comparisons between patients
in London and New York.   It was clear that a program based on the
P.S.E. items would be of great value in making further progress
with the P.S.E.   In 1967 work was therefore started on the
condensation of the items in the schedule to form symptoms and
syndromes, as a necessary preliminary to the making of diagnostic
statements.   Several members of the US/UK project team worked
with Professor J. Wing on the early stages and Professor Wing
undertook the burden of the later stages of the work, working
closely with several computer programers.   Other programs have
since been added dealing with items of history, and converting the
'categories' used by the computer program into the nearest possible
equivalents in ICD 8 and 9.   The W.H.O. team working on the IPSS
also had access to the first versions of the symptom condensations,
and these were later developed into the 'units of analysis' that
figure in some of the later analyses of the IPSS data.

A comprehensive manual to the P.S.E. was finally published in
1974 (Wing, J.K., Cooper, J.E. and Sartorius, N., 1974).   This
contains an account of the development of the interview, its uses
and its reliability, and lists of how the symptoms, syndromes and
categories of the CATEGO program are derived.   A detailed glossary
of terms is also given, and the interview schedule itself (PSE-9)
is included as an appendix.

THE USE OF THE PSE IN COMMUNITY SURVEYS

By about 1970 it had become clear that the interview was
flexible and useful in a variety of circumstances, and that its
use was by no means restricted to the psychotic patients for whom
it had originally been designed.   George Brown and Tyrill Harris
were at that timedeveloping plans for community surveys of
depressed women and collaborated in the preparation of their studies
with some members of the US/UK Diagnostic Project Team (J. E. Cooper,
J. R. M. Copeland).   Brown and Harris and their colleagues were the
first non-psychiatrists to be taught how to use the neurotic
sections of the P.S.E.   Since then these sections of the P.S.E.
have been used extensively by non-psychiatrists in a variety of
studies of both neurotic patients and community subjects.

Experience in these community studies led to the development
of a further extension of the computer program in the form of the
'Index of Definition' (Wing, J.K., 1980; Wing, J.K., Bebbington, P.,
Hurry, J., and Tennant, C., 1981).   This is an arbitrary but
reasonable set of rules which allows subjects to be given a
grading on an index of 0 - 4 when they do not have sufficient
symptoms to produce a conventional psychiatric syndrome or
category on the CATEGO program.   The higher levels of 5, 6, 7

on the Index of Definition indicate that there is an increasingly high probability of the subject being allotted to specific syndromes and categories on the CATEGO program which will indicate a more conventional diagnosis.

SHORTENING OF THE P.S.E. INTERVIEW PROCEDURES

An experienced P.S.E. interviewer faced with a well subject with no symptoms can complete the interview in around ten to fifteen minutes, in marked contrast to the forty-five to sixty minutes that is often necessary for a patient. However, even ten to fifteen minutes may seem a long time to both the interviewer and interviewee when everything is clearly negative and when there are several other interviewing schedules to be completed during the course of a compound survey interview. In view of these problems, a very short screening procedure taking only two or three minutes was devised by Cooper & Mackenzie (1981) with the aim of predicting those subjects who will not be rated for any symptoms at all on the P.S.E. This is done by asking the subject ten questions without further probes, each question covering a main section of the P.S.E. It has been shown that those subjects who score 0 or 1 on these questions, judged by an experienced P.S.E. interviewer, have an extremely high probability of having no symptoms positive on the complete neurotic sections of the P.S.E.

THE PRESENT POSITION.

The ninth edition of the P.S.E. is in current use in many countries. It has now been translated into more than twenty different languages and in spite of obvious problems of translation (particularly of some items in the neurotic sections), there is no doubt at all that its content can be used in research projects in many different cultures. It is fulfilling its basic purpose as a research instrument which leads to reliable descriptions of symptoms upon which diagnoses can be based. It must also be acting indirectly as an important means of international communication about psychiatric symptoms and concepts, and as a form of education. Its relationships with some of the ratings derived from recently produced standardised interviews in the U.S.A. (such as the D.I.S., Robins, L.N., Helzer, J.E., Croughan, J.L., and Ratcliffe, K., 1981), are now being examined. This work should provide some valuable clues for the production of the next generation of standardised interviewing instruments on both sides of the Atlantic. It is to be hoped that they will emerge with significant similarities.

PROSPECTS FOR P.S.E. 10

The W.H.O. - ADAMHA International Collaborative Study on diagnosis has led, amongst other things, to further collaborative

work between the W.H.O. and N.I.M.H., in the production of a
variety of standardised interviewing schedules. During the
course of this work, Professor J. Wing, is preparing first
drafts of what should become the P.S.E. 10, although it is
impossible at this stage to say when it will be finalised.
However, the basic principles that have been outlined at the
start of this presentation will still be followed, i.e. it will
remain a clinical interview, which is both flexible and thorough.
The same symptoms will form the nucleus of the interview,
because comparisons must be possible with the very extensive
data base now existing from the use of P.S.E. 8 and 9. It is
very likely that more ratings will be contained in the schedule
to deal with the duration and onset of symptoms, so as to allow
comparisons with D.I.S. items and to allow the derivation of
some DSM 111. diagnostic categories. It remains to be seen to
what extent further editions of the interviews from the U.S.A.
and P.S.E. 10 can also generate diagnostic categories that will
be contained in ICD-10 and in DSM ↑V. Obviously a great deal of
work remains to be done but the closer the relationship between
standardised interview schedules and diagnostic classifications,
then the easier it will be to communicate about our research
findings. We must all remember that no one standardised
interviewing or rating procedure can ever claim to be correct or
perfect; they all have their individual purposes and characteristics, and all share the common aims of improving the
reliability of research findings and our ability to communicate
with each other about our results.

REFERENCES

COOPER, J.E., Mackenzie, S. (1981) "The rapid prediction of low
    scores on a standardized psychiatric interview (Present State
    Examination) in What is a Case eds. Wing, Bebbington and
    Robins; Grant McIntyre : London.
Cooper, J.E., Kendell, R.E., Gurland, B.J., Sartorius, N., &
    Farkas, T. (1969). "Cross-National Study of Diagnosis of
    Mental Disorders : Some Results from the first Comparative
    Investigation : American Journal of Psychiatry 125 10
    April 1969 Supplement.
Cooper, J.E., Kendell, R.E., Gurland, B.J., Sharpe, L., Copeland,
    J.R.M., & Skmon, R. (1972) Psychiatric Diagnosis in New
    York and London. Maudsley Monograph no 20. Oxford
    University Press. Oxford.
Cranach, M. von and Cooper, J.E., (1972) Changes in rating
    behaviour during the learning of a standardised psychiatric
    interview. Psychological Medicine 2 373-80.

Robins, L.N., Helzer, J.E., Croughan, J.L., Ratcliffe, K., (1981)
"The NIMH Diagnostic Interview Schedule : its history,
characteristics and validity". in What is a Case eds.
Wing, Bebbington and Robins; Grant McIntyre : London.

Sartorius, N., Shapiro, R., Kimura, M. & Barrett K. (1972)
Preliminary Communication - WHO International Pilot Study
of Schizophrenia. Psychological Medicine, 2 422-425.

Sartorius, N., A. Jablensky, & Shapiro, R., (1977).   Preliminary
Communication.   Two-year follow-up of the patients included
in the WHO International Pilot Study of Schizophrenia.

Spitzer, R.L., and Endicott, J. (1968)   Diagno : a computer
program for psychiatric diagnosis utilising the differential
diagnostic procedure, Archives of General Psychiatry 18
746-56.

Wing, J.K., (1961) "A simple and reliable sub-classification of
chronic schizophrenia".   Journal of Mental Science 107 862.

Wing, J.K. (1980) "The use of the Present State Examination in
General Population Surveys", Acta Psychiatrica Scandinavica
Supplement 285 vol. 62

Wing, J.K., Bebbington, P., Hurry, J. and Tennant, C.   (1981) "The
prevalence in the general population of disorders familiar to
psychiatrists in hospital practice" in What is a Case eds.
Wing, Bebbington & Robins; Grant McIntyre, London.

Wing, J.K., Birley, J.T.L., Cooper, J.E., Graham, P., and Issacs,
A.D. (1967) "A procedure for measuring and classifying Present
Psychiatric State"   British Journal of Psychiatry, 113 499-515

Wing, J.K., Cooper, J.E., Sartorius, N. (1974) The measurement and
classification of psychiatric symptoms.   Cambridge University
Press.

THE AMDP

Hanfried Helmchen

Psychiatrische Klinik und Poliklinik
Freie Universität Berlin
Eschenallee 3 - D-1ooo Berlin 19 - FRG

Background and History

With the introduction of neuroleptic and antidepressant drugs in
the 195o's both neuropsychopharmacology and pharmacopsychiatry
and, in a broader sense, psychiatric therapy research became a fast
growing field of interest. Particularly in psychiatry controlled
clinical trials needed instruments to objectify by standardization
and to quantify the recording of psychopathological findings in
order to improve their comparability. This was especially true with
comparability of findings with those at other times, e.g. in intraindividual comparisons for measurement of change, at other places,
e.g. in multicentred trials for fast collection of large as well
as divergent populations, and with other drugs, e.g. with wellknown
standard drugs for the purpose of finding better drugs.

These needs led to the development of lists of psychopathological
and somatic symptoms by psychiatrists from all 5 Swiss and 5 German
university psychiatric hospitals. In 1965 both groups decided upon
further collaboration, including the Austrian universiy psychiatric
hospital of Vienna. They named their group "Association for Methodology and Documentation in Psychiatry" (AMP-Arbeitsgemeinschaft
für Methodik und Dokumentation in der Psychiatrie). This name reflected the intention of all members of the group not to restrict
themselves to the documentation of drug trials but to deal with all
questions within the scope of psychiatric methodology. The influence of patient, psychiatrist, and their interactional situation
on the different steps of the diagnostic process, on observation,
rating, and coding, was investigated empirically and theoretically.
Especially the reductionistic implications of the common observational
language and the problems of adequacy of algorithms were discussed

intensively and critically. Important consequences of these experiences were to develop a glossary of descriptive definitions of each item, and to implement regular training seminars for users of the AMP system in order to improve reliability. However, it was stated that "agreement coefficients do not prove the instrument as such, but prove the (comparability of) research group working with the documentation system, whose mutuality in the observation language is identified by these coefficients."

From AMP to AMDP: the Revision Process

After the first publication of the system in 1969, and the complete system, including a manual and a glossary, in 1971, a broadly designed and carefully performed revision was undertaken by several small working groups. E.g. the working group "Interrater Reliability" performed a multicenter study, supported by WHO, in 6 different psychiatric hospitals in 2 countries with lo2 psychiatrists as AMP raters of 12 videotaped psychiatric patients. Also, the procedure followed by the working group "Psychic Findings: Glossary" was to delete all non-specific and seldom-found items as well as those with low interrater reliability according to the results of the above mentioned interrater reliability study; some new items were inserted upon request of AMP members. Then the group improved the definition of items with respect to the following objectives: a) more precise formulation of the glossary text; b) more exact distinction among the items; c) better differentiation among items of the so-called experiential and the behavioral levels; d) attempts to operationalize the levels of intensity; e) descriptions of the phenomena without nosological-diagnostic references, as each item was supposed to be considered by itself, independent of diagnoses. The close collaboration of this working group with the very active French-speaking AMP group was very productive. Discussions and mutual translations provided stimulating experiences of recognizing the same psychopathological phenomena from different schools of psychiatric thought and the sometimes different semantics of their wordings. In 1979 the revision was completed and published as a booklet containing the documentation system together with the glossary and manual. Since then it has no longer been called AMP but instead the AMDP system. The reasons for the expansion of the abbreviation were, for one thing, the frequent confusion in the literature with the cyclic AMP and other organizations with the same abbreviation, a problem which had become more significant with the international dissemination of the system. However, this was meant, above all, to indicate that the new version of the documentation system represented the result of an intensive, essential revision over a period of several years and that this clearly differed from the preceding version.

The Documentation System : Data Sheets and Syndrome Scales.

The AMDP system is designed for standardized documentation of data
from the patients' history and findings which are usually recognized
as psychiatrically relevant by a comprehensive psychiatric interview.
Now the AMDP documentation system consists of 5 data-sheets for
1) sociodemographic data, 2) life-events related to the individual
life time schedule, 3) psychiatric history, 4) psychopathological
findings, and 5) somatic findings.
From the 140 symptoms of the last 2 sheets 8 factors were extracted
by several factoranalyses based on symptoms of 2313 patients routinely recorded in 1980 by the university psychiatric hospital in
Berlin and Munich. The factors are stable, reliable, and sample-independent. Because they both are very similar to well-known clinical
syndromes and satisfy statistical test criteria, it is justified to
call them syndrome scales. They can be used for quantitative description of psychopathology in scientific investigations. They show
a close similarity to factor solutions of several previous factor-
analyses of older AMP data. This provides a good comparability between new studies based on AMDP syndrome scales and already published scientific work using the former AMP syndrome scales. The 8
AMDP syndrome scales, with the number of items for each single scale
varying between 13 and 7 are: paranoid-hallucinatory (PARHAL), depressive (DEPRES), psychoorganic (PSYORG), manic (MANI), hostility
(HOST), autonomic (AUTON), apathy (APA), and obsessive-compulsive
(OBSESS) with only 3 items. A further step of data reduction was to
extract second-order factors. Three such stable factors could be
found: a psychotic, a depressive, and a psychoorganic factor. These
factors can be used if a less detailed description of psychopathological findings is sufficient for certain problems.
Decentralized EDP programmes for AMDP data have been developed in
Berlin, Brussels, Liège, Madrid, Munich and Zurich.

Applications

The AMDP system has been applied mainly in a) clinical trials of
psychotropic drugs, b) psychiatric classification, and c) training
in psychopathology, but also in other fields. More than 200 papers
on such AMDP investigations have been published. It has been proven
that the system sensitively and differentiatedly describes psychopathological changes in the course of treatment, especially of endogenous psychoses. The AMP system permits much more differentiated, and for European psychiatrists more familiar, descriptions of
the pertinent psychopathological phenomena and their changes in
the course of illness than the Brief Psychiatric Rating Scale (BPRS)
which is probably the most frequently used psychopathological instrument in the American ECDEU system. This was established by comparisons of the AMP psychopathology data with the BPRS and with the
IMPS. - With respect to rating scales for particular psychopathological phenomena or syndromes such as depressive states, it can be

said that individual AMDP syndrome scales will be used in the same way. But it should be pointed out that the AMDP syndrome scales are based on the full range of psychopathological symptomatology recorded after a comprehensive psychiatric interview. The philosophy of AMDP is to base an evaluation on the whole scope of psychopathology and not on single aspects of it. The need for this becomes evident, e.g., if treatment of schizophrenic symptomatology induces changes of mood and the affective state, or if antidepressive treatment provokes manic or productive psychotic symptoms. Therefore it seems more appropriate clinically to measure treatment-induced changes not by a single and highly specific (and in this regard valid and reliable) syndrome scale but by a set of syndrome scales in order to represent the whole range of changes by syndrome profiles.

Measurement of change can be applied not only to the psychopathological state of patients under therapy but also to psychiatrists as raters of psychopathology in terms of the efficacy of a training seminar. AMDP rating of psychopathological states shown by video tapes followed by a reasoning for the individual ratings and particularly by discussions of discrepancies of the ratings of distinct psychopathological phenomena have a high educational efficacy. Further conclusions from these experiences are that an unexperienced AMDP rater should have supervision for the initial 10 interviews by an experienced AMDP rater, and both raters should use the glossary. The video tape of an AMDP interview together with a standard rating by experienced AMDP raters may serve as an additional training aid. Tapes and ratings should be collected in a "videotheque" and in this way AMDP learners can compare their own ratings with expert ratings.

Further Developments

The AMDP rating is based on a comprehensive and free psychiatric interview. Its free form is the customary mode with which the psychiatrist is acquainted, and it has the advantage that it can be adapted to the state of the patient and the situation. In fact, however, an AMDP directed interview is not a totally free one, insofar as at least its content is predetermined by the items of the psychopathological and somatic findings sheets, each of which must be rated independently from each other as absent or present. But sometimes an unexperienced or an unattentive interviewer fails to explore some items, or others are explored insufficiently for a definite AMDP rating. Therefore we plan to investigate the possibilities of a semi-structured AMDP interview.

Another need for further development comes from the fact that the AMDP sheet for psychic findings is based on the classical German language descriptive psychopathology. Therefore it is most appropriate for the documentation of psychotic symptomatology. But it should provide a more differentiated documentation of neurotic symptomatology. Furthermore, the item list should be extended from the psychopathological symptoms into the normal range of psychic

144

findings in order to comprehend the healthy parts of the personality too, e. g. the abilities and talents of the patient.
Further interest is directed to the use of AMDP data for diagnostic classification. As most of the important criteria for nosological psychiatric diagnoses are included or can be derived from the AMDP anamneses or findings data. We believe that such standardized recorded data of a large number of patients may provide a basis for objectification of the diagnostic process, or algorithm, and perhaps for the improvement of our diagnostic classification, e.g. by methods of cluster analysis.

International Acceptance

In 1976 AMDP implemented an International Secretariat in order to satisfy the increasing international interest in AMDP. The main activities of the AMDP International Secretary, Dr.BOBON, were to stimulate and to foster AMDP working groups in other countries and translations into other languages. Presently there are adaptations of the AMDP system in 11 languages, namely a) an official manual in English, French, and Spanish; b) a recently completed draft in Japanese and Portuguese; c) adaptations at various stages in Croatian, Danish, Dutch, Italian, Greek and Russian. BOBON reports that "the difficult task of securing alltogether the formal comparability on these scales, the identity of the symptoms measured and the specificity of various schools was achieved through numerous video sessions in French at which participated permanent representatives from other languages and through a number of write-in items which allow flexibility without a loss of standardization". And Dr.SARTORIUS, Director of the WHO Division of Mental Health in Geneva, has commented on the value of the AMDP system for its contribution to an urgently needed common language in psychiatry in his foreword to the English edition of the AMDP manual. This booklet (4) as well as the German "mother" edition (1) can be found here in the books-exhibition. Besides these, you will find there the just published authoritative description of the AMDP system including several examples of its application (3), and the AMDP Test Manual including all empirical analyses of the AMDP system itself (2).

References

1. AMDP (Arbeitsgemeinschaft für Methodik und Dokumentation in der Psychiatrie)
   (Hrsgeb.): Das AMDP-System, Manual zur Dokumentation psychiatrischer Befunde. 4. korr. u.erw. Aufl.,
   Springer, Berlin Heidelberg New York, 1981

2. BAUMANN, U., STIEGLITZ, R.-D.: Empirische Studien zur Psychopathologie - Testmanual zum AMDP-System -
   Springer, Berlin Heidelberg New York Tokyo, 1983

3. BOBON, D., BAUMANN, U., ANGST, J., HELMCHEN, H., HIPPIUS, H.
   (Eds.): The AMDP System in Pharmacopsychiatry,
   S. Karger, Basel München Paris London New York Tokyo,
   Sydney, 1983

4. GUY, W., BAN, T.A. (Eds.): The AMDP System
   Springer, Berlin Heidelberg New York, 1982

THE COMPUTERIZED UNIFIED PSYCHIATRIC CLINICAL RECORD (H.C.U.)

Juan J. López-Ibor Jr., Rafael Abad, German Rey,
Javier López-Ibor, and Manuel Rodriguez-Gamazo

Departments of Psychiatry and of Radiotherapy-
Oncology, Centro Ramón y Cajal and Instituto de
Investigaciones Neuropsiquiátricas.
Av. de Nueva Zelanda num.44, Madrid (35), Spain

INTRODUCTION

The Computerized Unified Psychiatric Clinical Record, or more briefly in Spanish "Historia Clínica Unificada" (H.C.U.) aims to solve, with the help of computers, the problem of filing and recalling with speed and reliablility, the most significant and valuable of the clinical records. These are the basic psychopathological documents, they derive from the relational activity between the doctor and the patient and they have a very important value, not always well utilized, in psychiatric and sociological research.

None of the methods of the gathering of computerized clinical and psychopathological data fulfills the functions of a clinical record, since they are additional documents to same. A computerized clinical record has to have the following characteristics:

a) Easy handling to improve administrative functions and unification of data collection to allow statistical analysis.
b) Maintain the philosophy of the traditional clinical records, respecting the intimacy of the medical act, gathering the details of the biography of the patient and his environment, and keeping as a primary function that of helping to make and be the support of decisions related to the patient to which the record refers.
c) The characteristics described in a) should not be achieved to the detriment of b), the method should at the same time, facilitate the daily clinical work.

d) A coding system forming part of the clinical record, not requiring additional manuals or documents.
e) A flexible set of alphabetical and numerical codes and free texts, to permit recovering completely all the information.
f) Simplicity in the analysis of collections of clinical records to help establish systems of vigilance for epidemiological, organizational and research purposes.
g) Possibility of permanently updating the data of each case.
h) Provide the physician directly and immediately with the information of each patient to be used in the daily practice.

With this in mind we have elaborated a SYSTEM OF HEALTH INFORMATION (S.H.I.), made up of a subsystem of gathering of data, a specially designed version of the "Stratos" folder, and an informatics subsystem. This S.H.I. is a dynamic unit. The informationalization of an isolated document does not give rise to the creation of a S.H.I. An essential part of the S.H.I. is that the information circulates constantly, feeding itself retrospectively with the results obtained.

The H.C.U. serves, first for the control of the information of each patient individually, and second for the analysis of collections of clinical records. These last can be applied to clinical and research studies in each unit and in multi-center studies. The S.H.I. even permits that these last ones be carried out partially in different languages.

The concrete data and the **typological** classifications of epidemiological research, are not always useful in every day practice. The clinician, even more the psychiatrist has to consider nuances and peculiarities in every patient, whose pathology he prefers to classify according to **dimensional** systems. Although one must take into account that scientific medicine is constituted from typological categories, the nosological entities, being different from the other sciences that as in psychology, use dimensional classifications. Psychiatry resorts to both and the clinician, even within the excluding categories, likes to be able to distribute his patients dimensionally in accordance with certain criteria, such as for example, that of severity.

But there is more, the clinician acts with immediate interest, conditioned by the patient he has before him; he gathers the information progressively, extracting conclusions, and from them the directions for the taking of decisions.

THE STRATOS FOLDER

The Stratos Folder has as a fundamental characteristic that its pages become progressively longer from the first one on, in such a way that the last centimeter of each page overlaps the last one. This space is designed to write the codes and texts which are to be processed by the computer. In this way it is possible have on sight the data for informatics and even be able to photocopy them. Each one of the pages is designed to one aspect of a clinical record and contains three clearly defined parts.

a) One blank space of a large enough size to be able to write up a text of a conventional clinical record.
b) The codes and coding instructions corresponding to the corresponding section of each page.
c) The last line with the respective spaces for the codes and blank spaces for free texts which permit clarification of the codes or abstracts of the text of the clinical record.

This arrangement allows having together the conventional text of the clinical record, the coding instructions and the information for the computer.

A workshop of members of the Spanish Psychiatric Society chaired by Llavero defined criteria to unify the contents of the psychiatric clinical records. We have included them in the H.C.U. The folder has several sections each one of which, in general occupies a page. The closed folder is shown in figure 1.

THE HANDLING OF THE INFORMATION

The System is operating in BASIC language in a CBM 3032 micro-computer and in UCSD-PASCAL language in a PHILIPS (P-2000) micro-computer.

The input of data is carried out with a program which presents successively on the screen, and in its same shape, the codified lines of the H.C.U., which are visible in the closed folder.

Once the information is introduced into and stored in the computer, it provides by means of a program of text processing an abstract of the clinical record in correct Spanish. This one can be used as a discharge report, which since it is signed by the doctor is a guarantee of the exactness of the information filed. If a unit does not have a computer it can in spite of it, use the system, since it is enough to make a photocopy of the closed folder to have the informational data. Afterwards this photocopy can be sent to the adequate place for its processing.

CHARACTERISTICS OF THE COMPUTERIZED UNIFIED CLINICAL RECORD

It is a customary Clinical Record. The H.C.U. is simply a Clinical Record. It is not a system of documentation, nor a group of scales, nor a systematic protocol of clinical research. The H.C.U. does not gather epidemiological data, only **judgements** of the clinician, which are the result of an evaluation of the facts

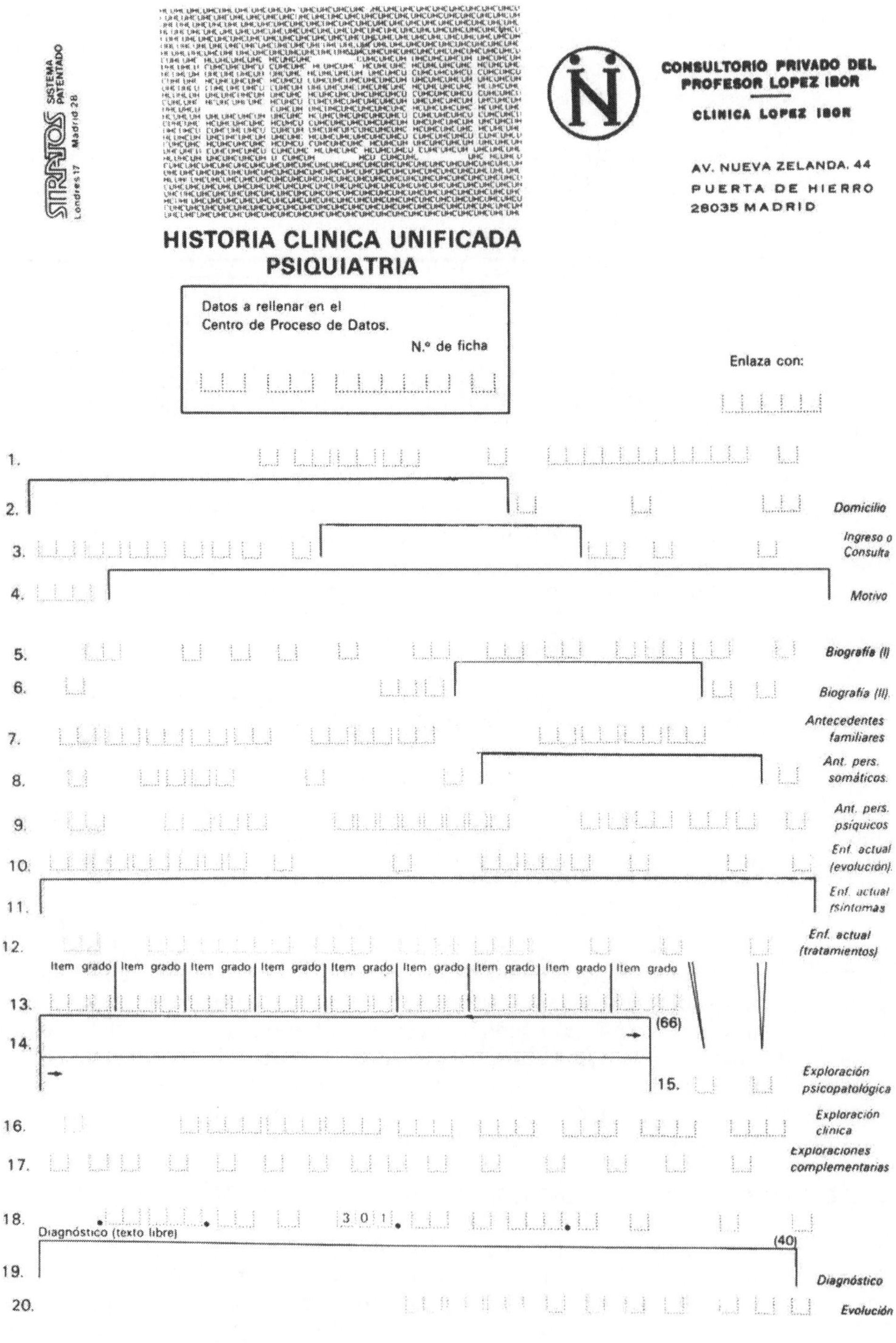

Figure 1: The closed STRATOS folder.

obtained in everyday practice, and so it raises less rejection and interferes less with the doctor-patient relationship than other systems aimed for research purposes.

Unification: The H.C.U. is called unified because it expects that the group of users be numerous, independently of the clinical situation, of the characteristics and of the type of patient and even of the difference in perspectives of the different schools. The numerical codes permit uniformity based on the principle of the "maximum common denominator". The H.C.U. is a single document for diverse applications, writing up the clinical record, coding manual, page of notes for the data that has to be filed and evaluated.

Simplicity: The H.C.U. is simple. It does not require more work than the customary clinical record, in some sense even less.

Flexibility: The blank spaces permit each physician to write according to his training and perspective, adapting to the patient and the clinical situation. The free texts of the last line embody the information which is necessary to write up an individualized abstract. The H.C.U. makes compatible uniform data with others having a greater utility in the treatment of an individual problem.

Reliability: The reliability is based on the codified information noted. A Manual provides definitions, however, and this is one of the characteristics of the system, the reliability is not sought at the expense of flexibility. The system permits an intra-rater reliability as high as he wants it, provided that he always uses the same terms for each concept, on the other hand the inter-rater reliability can be very low. This complementary relationship between reliability and flexibility is very important in two sections: the mental state and the diagnostic. In both there are two types of lines, one for codes (more clearly defined in the diagnosis from the ICD-9 and the DSM-III) and another for free texts, in which the physician will write according to his own terms the most relevant aspects of the psychopathological exploration and a clinical diagnosis more adjusted to the reality confronting him, if the rigidity of the ICD-9 should prove excessive.

Immediate utility for the clinician: Experience shows that the longer the time elapsed between gathering the information and its use, the lesser is its reliability. The interest of the clinicial and his diligence in noting down of the facts decreases if he cannot employ them in a short period of time, if they are not applicable in the specific case which concerns him and above all, if the one who is going to make use of his work is not going to be him but someone else who will extract results in scientific publications or statistical studies.

The H.C.U. has an immediate use for the clinician since it puts at his disposal an abstract of the clinical history, with hardly any effort. Of course, not everything will be included in it, but certainly the most significant facts. The second advantage is the availability of statistical analysis.

Confidentiality: The folder of the H.C.U. does not need to nor should it leave the Unit or the Center. In the cases in which the processing of the information has to be done in another place, the photocopy sent does not have the name of the patient, nor anything that would identify him since the first folded page conceals it.

Ethical aspects: The mechanized writing of a report compels the supplying of all those receving it with complete and uniform information. It is an effort to avoid barriers of communication between the patient and those that live with him. This is another aspect of the **unification** which we forsee is going to be more and more important.

THE H.C.U. IN THE TOXIC OIL SYNDROME DISASTER

The Toxic Oil Syndrome disaster has allowed to test the H.C.U. in a difficult task. None of the users had previous experience with the system and even the majority of them had never had a special interest in the methodology of psychopathological documentation. The Toxic Oil Syndrome was a new pathology of unforseen reach and evolution. The number of users was large (25 psychiatrists) and dispersed throughout various centers (15 hospitals initially to which were added various out-patient units). The psychiatrists contracted did not come from the same school and neither at the moment had the H.C.U. been used and they did not even have available a manuel.

Clinical research in health disasters presents very particular ethical and strategic problems. By their own nature, disasters are something new, unforseen, in which it is not possible to resort to pre-established solutions. The first task of the health personnel in a catastrophe is to care for the individual needs of those affected and only when this is satisfied is when one can begin to think about clinical research. If this is not one hundred percent exact, it is indeed lived through by those affected. For example, a few days ago, the press reported the complaints of the associations of the affected by the Toxic Oil Syndrome who mentioned the scientific advantage of this catastrophe that had been taken by the physicians. The H.C.U. designed to be a conventional clinical record has been a method that has absolutely not interfered with this delicate psychological aspect, since it begins and finishes in the individual patient to whom it refers.

REFERENCE

Lopéz-Ibor Jr., J.J., "Manual de la Historia Clínica Unifica-
    da", Garsi, Madrid, 1982.

152

XXI. BIOMETRICS

CONCLUSIONS

Norman Sartorius

Director, Division of Mental Health
World Health Organization
Geneva, Switzerland

The last two decades have seen a paradoxical development
with regard to comprehensive assessment of psychopathological
states. On the one hand, there is an incomparably better acceptance and a growing sophistication of assessment methods. A number
of them have been developed and there is sufficient evidence of
their validity, reliability and sensitivity. On the other hand,
however, the excitement and enthusiasm have left the field of
assessment. The novelty has worn off and the use of instruments
and standardized methods of assessment has become a boring chore
often applied mechanically.

To an extent this lack of popularity of assessment technique
is linked to the decrease in popularity of epidemiology in
psychiatry. Now that the curiosity about the forms and frequency
of mental disorders in different settings has been satisfied and
that it has been demonstrated that these diseases are ubiquitous
and serious everywhere, attention of the scientific community
appears to have been attached to biological studies and towards
service provision. If this observation is correct, there are two
directions in which scales would have to be developed for the
future.

First scales should be developed that will be applicable
in biological and treatment studies. This means that they have
to be simple in application, valid in repeated applications and
sensitive to relatively minor changes, both in the overall state
of the individual and in changes in functions (e.g. cognitive performance.

Secondly, instruments for the assessment of the state of the mentally ill in relation to services, their changes and their impact should be developed. These are scales which can be used routinely in conditions of service and which will be capable of demonstrating difference as an effect of service interventions.

RECENT DEVELOPMENT OF THE AMDP-SYSTEM

Urs Baumann

Institut für Psychologie der Universität
Akademiestr.22, A-5020 Salzburg
Austria

INTRODUCTION

The official history of the German-language 'Association for
Documentation in Psychiatry' (AMDP) is marked by the year
1969 and the year 1979. In 1969, the AMP-manual was edited
for AMP, and in 1979, the extensive revision was completed by
the edition of the AMDP-revision. The AMP-system has been
evaluated in numerous empirical studies, which were mainly
publicized during the seventies and early eighties. A few
studies concerning the AMDP-system have been conducted to
date. In "Test-Manual für das AMDP-System-Empirische Studien
zur Psychopathologie" (1983) the extensive data have been
presented in a comprehensive manner. The aboundance of results
is not only of importance for AMDP, but represents a significant contribution to the empirical research of psychopathology. The development of the AMDP-system has found a tentative
termination, due to the revised AMDP-system manual (AMDP,
1981), which contains the definitions of symptoms in particular
and the recently published test-manual (Testmanual AMDP,
1983), which presents the empirical findings.

It is prudent to consider the AMP-system's level of evaluation
as satisfactory. The purpose of the present contribution is
to examine, to what degree this holds true for AMDP, which
areas have been evaluated for AMDP to date, and which
areas remain to be evaluated. The standard for the
evaluation of AMDP is the level of evaluation of AMP.

The studies concerning the AMP-system can be subdivided into the following categories: (1) studies on the decision-making-process and on symptom-characteristics. (2) studies for the generation of first and second order syndrome-scales. (3) reliability-studies on the symptom-level and the syndrome-level. (4) validity-studies on the symptom-level and the syndrome-level.

AMP-EVALUATION: STANDARD FOR THE AMDP-EVALUATION

Studies on the Decision-Making Process and on Symptom-Characteristics

In the AMP-system, accessibility and certainty have been documented separately. Our own extensive studies on material in Zurich and Berlin have led us to combine the two categories under the code "not ascestained" (if no quotation is made in the subsequent text: see the comprehensive account in the Test-Manual für das AMDP-System, 1983). Also, Mombour's studies led to the consequence, that the absence of symptoms, not previously documented in AMP, was integrated in AMDP as a category of its own.

Woggon contributed the analyses of the basis of judgement of symptoms, which are of importance for symptom definitions. They differentiate symptoms, which are judged primarily on the basis of subjective information from the patient (i.e. verbal hallucinations), symptoms which are judged on the basis of an assessor's behavioral observation (i.e. tangential thinking), and symptoms, where it can not be distinguished to what degree subjective information and direct behavioral observation mingle (i.e. concentration).
Further studies dealt with the frequency distribution of individual symptoms. Symptoms which are unspecific, rare and insignificant in the course of treatment are of little interest for a documentation system; and were therefore eliminated in the revision.

Such analyses are of importance for the AMDP-System as well, because the previously used characteristics have become questionable due to changed definitions and the addition of new symptoms.

First and Second Order Syndrome-Scales

Five different first order factorial solutions were proposed for the AMP-system. These are the studies by Baumann, Gebhardt et al., Mombour et al., Sulz-Blume et al., and Wegscheider (factorial analyses, which were conducted in more homogenous samples or that deals with special problems, will not be mentioned here). Empirical studies for comparing the different solutions on the basis of scale-values had the following results:
- Sample-independent syndromes: Apathy, hostility, manic syndrome,

psycho-organic syndrome, autonomic syndrome
- <u>Sample-independent syndromes (solutions, in which a few individual syndromes are split into partial syndromes</u>): depressive syndrome (Zurich: somatic depressive syndrome, retarded depressive syndrome, hypochondriasis), paranoid-hallucinatory syndrome (Zurich: hallucinatory syndrome, paranoid syndrome)
- <u>Comparable syndromes (middle correlations in the individual solutions</u>): Catatonic syndrome/stuporous syndrome, obsessive-compulsive syndrome.

Over all, a high degree of concurrence between the five different factorial solutions was evident. Out of the five authors, though, only two, Baumann and Gebhardt et al., carried out test-analyses, in other words, they computed selectivity, consistency and distribution-characteristics.

Baumann, Angst and Woggon, Dittrich suggested second order factors, whereby the last-named authors also developed scales (manic depressive syndrome and schizophrenic syndrome), which are distinguished by invariance in time.

The different first order factorial solutions for the AMP-system did document the eagerness of the German-speaking AMP-researchers - perhaps also a little bit of competition -. But, they were also an annoyence. The comparability of empirical studies, which are based on the syndromes or scales, is limited, despite the concurrence of the different solutions. Therefore, AMDP sought to find a unified, compulsory solution for first and second order scales.

The cooperation of the psychiatric university clinics of Berlin and Munich helped to achieve this goal; some authors are Gebhardt, Pietzcker, Strauss, Stoeckel, Langer, Freudenthal (Gebhardt et al., 1983). In constructing the scales, the authors used the follwing criteria for guidelines: (1) Solution must be replicable within clinic sub-samples, but also between clinics. (2) Solutions developed by factorial analysis must show sufficient results in item-analyses. (3) Solutions should be as similar as possible to the sample-independent syndromes of the AMP-system.

The analyses were based on admission reports of 1654 patients (Munich), and 659 patients (Berlin) respectively. The analyses conducted in accordance with the criteria mentioned before led to the following 8 primary scales: 1) paranoid-hallucinatory syndrome, 2) depressive syndrome, 3) psycho-organic syndrome, 4) manic syndrome, 5) hostility syndrome, 6) autonomic syndrome, 7) apathy syndrome, 8) obsessive-compulsive syndrome.

In addition a neurological syndrome - built on the basis of clinical consideration - was constructed for description of side

effects in the course of psychopharmacological treatments. The
8 primary AMDP-scales are to large degree concurrent with the
sample-independent scales of the AMP-system. In addition to the
8 primary scales, the authors developed 3 second order scales:
(I) paranoid-hallucinatory scale, (II) depressive scale, (III)
psycho-organic scale.

It can be concluded that for AMDP generally obligatory first-
and second order scales could be presented and that they are
test-statistically satisfactory. Therefore, no more
evaluations will be necessary in this respect, except for cross-
validations.

Reliability

Several different studies have been executed concerning the
reliability of the AMP-system. On the symptom-level, we have retest-studies and studies on interrater-reliability. While the
interrater-studies by Gebhardt and Helmchen, as well as those by
Woggon et al. were evaluated in a traditional manner (a.o. percent
and kappa), a special coefficient was used in Renfort et al.'s
multicenter-study, in which video-recordings were rated. They
differentiated concurrence in 'existence' and 'non-existence' of
a symptom. The authors showed, that the absence of symptoms can
usually be judged reliably, whereas proof of existence is often
not possible. Despite their different approaches, in all of the
three studies symptoms could be identified with good and with low
reliability. The interrater-studies were largely evaluated
according to "symptom present/absent". The investigation of degrees
(not present-mild-moderate-severe) on the symptom-level has yet
to occour for AMP.

For first and second order scales, we have retest-studies, we have
results on inner consistency and interrater-coefficients. These
results cannot be discussed in great detail here. Conclusively
one could say that none of the AMP-scales have proved to be
thouroughly unreliable. The coefficients are usually between
$0.6 < r_{tt} < 0.8$, which is satisfactory for ratings, if the number
of items is considered.

Reliability-studies have been conducted for the AMDP-system on the
symptom- and syndrome-levels. In a direct comparison of AMP-rating
and AMDP-rating, Kuny et al. (1983) showed that a mild improvement of interrater-reliability could be achieved for the AMDP-
system. Also, the analyses of Gebhardt et al. (1983), concerning
the inner consistency of the scales showed results, which reached
the previous AMP-scale values or even surpassed them mildly.
Judging from the results thusfar, one can expect the interrater-
results on the AMDP-scale level to be at least as satisfactory as
they are with AMP. The necessary computations need yet to be done.

Validity

Since the publication of AMP, many studies on the symptom- and syndrone-levels contributing to the validation of the system have been executed.
Mainly, the following areas are to be named: (1) group comparisons (symptom-, scale-level), (2) comparison with other assessment methods, (3) drug trials in clinical psychopharmacology, (4) other psychiatric fields (e.g. Diasika), (5) nonpsychiatric studies (e.g. openheart surgery). With the use of the AMP-scales, diagnostical groups could be separated satisfactorily. First studies with the AMDP-scales indicated that the new scales are at least equal to the old ones; partially, they are apt to separate diagnostical groups even better.
Of particular interest are validating studies in which scales are compared to other diagnostical tools (e.g. Hamilton-Depression-scale, BPRS). The results indicate, that, compared to BPRS, Hamilton rating scale for depression, and other rating scales, the AMP scales show a good criterion-related validity. For exact evaluation of the new AMDP-scales vis a vis other methods, respective comparative studies including the most important psychiatric rating procedures will be essential.

The other areas of validity can not be discussed in any detail here. It is to be expected that within a brief period of time, very many validation results can be won for the new scales, largely as a result of psychopharmacological studies.

CONCLUSIONS FOR THE AMDP-EVALUATION

If we reconsider the areas of evaluation that have been mentioned, several areas can be seen as dealt with, whereas other yet remain to be worked upon: (1) The development of primary and secondary order scales is finished. (2) On the symptom and syndrome-levels first reliability-results have been obtained. Additional investigations must be executed and results on interrater-reliability are neccessary. (3) First validity-results have been obtained. Further studies, particularly comparisons with other rating-systems, must be conducted. (4) Analyses of specificity, frequency in the initial status, and during the course of treatment need to be conducted.
Due to the revision, the AMP has clearly been altered, but nevertheless there still exist structurally and in terms of content great similarities between AMP and AMDP. The evaluation-results generated for AMP can therefore be used as general validation-results for the AMDP-System, so that the level of evaluation for AMDP may be considered altogether positive.

Finally, some more points shall be mentioned which have not been solved to satisfaction for AMP or for AMDP, such as: (1) Relia-

bility data for part 1 (demographic data), 2 (life events), 3
(psychiatric history). Respective data can be obtained from inter-
view-research, exact results should be obtained especially for
AMDP, though. (2) The problem of interview structure for the
AMDP-data-obtaining process, particularly for part 4 (psychopathological symptoms) and 5 (somatic signs). (3) The question, whether
parts 1 through 5 should be supplemented by data pertaining to
social adjustment, particularly for long-term studies. (4) The
position of AMDP within the frame-work of diagnosis-formation.
Pilot work has been done at DIASIKA (by von Zerssen).

If one considers AMDP as an attempt to yield relevant data on the
psychic and social areas more precise, than its development has
not come to an end with the 1979 revision. Moreover, it trans-
cends the evaluation of the data documented in parts 1 to 5. The
necessity of paying greater attention to biological parameters
must not lead to the neglect of psychic and social parameters.
Therefore, one can hope that these will continue to receive
attention by researchers.

REFERENCES

AMDP, 1981, Das AMDP-System. Testmanual zur Dokumentation
   psychiatrischer Befunde, Springer, Berlin (4.ed.).
Gebhardt, R., Pietzcker, A., Strauss, A., Stoeckel, M., Langer, C.
   and Freudenthal, K., 1983, Skalenbildung im AMDP-System, Arch.
   Psychiat. Nervenkr., in press.
Kuny, S., Luckner, N. von., Baeninger, R., Baur, P., Eichenberger,
   G. and Woggon, B., 1983, Interrater reliability of AMDP- and
   AMP-symptoms. In: AMDP-system in pharmacopsychiatry, D.Bobon,
   U.Baumann, J.Angst, H.Helmchen and H.Hippius, ed., Karger, Basel.
Testmanual für das AMDP-System - empirische Befunde zur Psycho-
   pathologie (verfaßt von U.Baumann, R.D.Stieglitz), 1983, Springer,
   Berlin.

THE AMDP-SYSTEM : THE FRENCH-SPEAKING GROUP

C.B. Pull

Centre Hospitalier de Luxembourg
4 Rue Barblé
1210 Luxembourg

INTRODUCTION

The first edition of the French AMDP Manual [1] was released in 1978. This edition included only the psychopathological and somatic scales and was intended primarily at elucidating difficulties encountered by French-speaking clinicians in applying German concepts. The second edition [2], which is fully compatible with the latest German revision [3] was published in 1981. It includes all 5 parts that are integrated in the current system : part 1 (Demographic data), part 2 (Life events), part 3 (Psychiatric history), part 4 (Psychopathology) and part 5 (Somatic signs).

A. BACKGROUND [4]

The French-speaking AMDP group was founded on the occasion of the 9 th CINP Congress in Paris, in 1974, by a small group of psychiatrists from Belgium, France, Germany and Switzerland. Shortly after, this group was joined by participants from Algeria, Austria, Canada, Greece, Italy, Luxembourg, Portugal, Spain and Zaire. From the beginning, the group has been coordinated by D.P. BOBON from the University of Liège, who also acts as the International Secretary of the AMDP Committee. In the 9 years since its foundation, the group has held 16 international meetings with a number of different purposes. For obvious reasons, the initial goal was to elucidate, discuss and solve various difficulties encountered in translating the AMDP System into French. The experience accumulated in this field was to prove highly valuable to those participants who later on decided to adapt the system into their own national languages, especially Spanish, Portuguese and Greek. In fact, however, the French-speaking group did not restrict its activities to adaptation problems, but rapidly decided to study the metrological characteristics of the system as well as applicability in various fields such as psychopharmacology, teaching or nosology. Finally, the French group took an active part in the third revision of the original German AMDP version. Results from the principal investigations with the French adaptation are presented in the following.

B. FRENCH ADAPTATION

The AMDP System is a German instrument and as such relies on German concepts, some of which do not have direct correspondants in French psychopathology. As a consequence, a number of terminological misunderstandings and conceptual differences had to be recognized, analysed and eliminated during the process of the French adaptation. The fact that the French group holds several participants who are bilingual and moreover well acquainted with both French and German psychopathology was very helpful in this respect.

Prominent among AMDP concepts for which no direct correspondant could be elucidated in French psychopathology was the German "Antrieb". After many discussions, the French concept "élan vital" was considered to correspond closest to "Antrieb". In a comprehensive analysis of this particular problem, BOBON [5] agrees with the translation proposed by the French group, in spite of certain differences bearing on the scope of symptoms characterizing either concept.

A second major difficulty concerned several important items pertaining to delusions. In this field, both German and French psychopathology attribute a major significance to a number of rigorously defined concepts. Some of these concepts exist only in one of the two traditions, others in both but bearing different meanings. As a consequence, thorough reflexion was needed to find the equivalents of "Wahnstimmung" (pressentiment délirant), "Wahneinfall" (intuition délirante) and "Wahnwahrnehmung" (perception délirante). The concept "Phantastischer Wahn", the meaning of which was significantly different from "fabulation délirante" was finally eliminated from the latest edition.

Other, more trivial misunderstandings could be resolved more easily. For further comments see a recent article by BOBON [6].

C. INTER-RATER RELIABILITY

Over the years, the French group has developed a video methodology for the measurement of inter-rater reliability. Video equipment has been installed in almost all the participants' facilities. A semi-structured interview was designed for videotaped evaluations. A modified obverse factor analysis was chosen as the method of choice for statistical analysis.

The reliability of the psychopathology scale has been tested in several studies [7,8] during video-sessions attended by a majority of the group's members. Probably owing to the fact that the group met frequently from the beginning and regularly trained together, the results proved highly satisfactory. The only major disagreement concerned several specific items, such as agitation, hyperactivity or complaintiveness, for which there was a systematic discrepancy between participants from Northern and Southern countries, and which was interpreted as a culture bias.

The fact that inter-rater reliability is highly satisfactory among the group's members should not, however, be interpreted as evidence of good reliability for the system as such. For new potential users of the system, the French group insists on the necessity of training sessions under the direction of experienced AMDP members. Seminars, including presentation and discussion of the system as well as practice of the system through evaluation of videotaped examinations are held twice a year in Liège.

A major contribution of the French group to improve inter-rater reliability was the development of semi-structured interviews for the psychopathology and somatic scales. A provisional French standardized somatic interview was slightly modified by the German group. This modified version was subsequently adopted by the French group. Both the psychopathology and somatic semi-structured interviews are currently used by the French group at large.

D. FACTOR STRUCTURE [9]

In 1982, ten centers from the French group participated in a study the aim of which was to elucidate the factor structure of the second French version of the AMDP psychopathology scale. Data were obtained on a sample of 388 unselected patients. Principal components analysis followed by varimax rotation yielded the following 10 factors : obsessions-phobias, dramatization, anxiety, depression, retardation, organicity, dissociation, delusions, mania and dysphoria.

The factor structure is similar to the one found in analyses previously reported by the German group, except for the
anxiety which does not appear in the German studies, probably
because the German edition has a smaller number of items for
description of anxiety. This fact needs to be explained.

In the development of successive editions and language
adaptations, a main concern of the international AMDP group
has been to strictly adhere to an identical common core instrument. On the other hand, specific additional write-in "reserve"
items, suggested by one particular language group, were allowed to be integrated in a given adaptation. Clinicians in the
French speaking group unanimously considered that the psychopathology scale did not allow to adequately evaluate the
various anxiety disorders and for this reason decided to include a number of additional items pertaining to this field.
More recently a second analysis has been performed on an expanded sample. The results confirm the factor structure listed
above.

E. SUBSCALES

Subscales constitute one of the few major topics for
which there is considerable disagreement between the French
and the German speaking groups. Although the first AMDP subscale, for mania and depression, has been proposed by the
Zurich center [10], the German group as a whole does not favor
the development of specific subscales. The French group has,
on the contrary, shown considerable interest in this field and
is currently investigating the validity of several specific
subscales.

A first step in this direction was the development of a
syndromic scale [4]. A provisional 12 factor scale, FACT-Lg,
was elaborated in Liège on the basis of factors elucidated in
several German studies. FACT-Lg was incorporated in the French
group's 1982 study mentioned above. The provisional factor
scale proved highly satisfactory for global evaluation of psychopathology. Moreover, individual FACT-Lg factors or "syndromes" had high correlations with the corresponding factors
emerging from the French principal componants analysis. The
final French AMDP syndromic scale concerns 13 syndromes :
(1) obsessions-phobias, (2) hypochondriasis, (3) dramatization,
(4) anxiety, (5) depression, (6) retardation, (7) agitation,
(8) mania, (9) tension, (10) delusions, (11) hallucinations,
(12) dissociation, (13) organicity.

While the Zurich Mania-Depression subscale has not yet
been adopted by the German group at large, it has been accepted without restraint by the French group. The subscale

164

consists of 20 depression and 7 mania items and is a second-order scale derived from several factor analyses. The Zurich group has reported an inter-rater reliability coefficient of .87 and acceptable correlations with the Hamilton Depression Scale, the Brief Psychiatric Rating Scale and the Inpatient Multidimensional Personality Scale. The French 1982 study confirmed the stability of the subscale. According to more recent investigations by the Liège group, the subscale discriminates between depressed and nondepressed individuals, correlates significantly with the Hamilton Depression Scale and with von ZERSSEN's Self-Rating Mood Scale, and is sensitive to antidepressant treatment.

The French group favors the development of other subscales and is currently working on a subscale for schizophrenia.

F. NOSOLOGY AND DIAGNOSIS

Up to now, attention of the French AMDP group has focussed on the psychopathology and somatic scales, i.e. on parts IV and V of the AMDP system. It should be pointed out however, that the group also participated actively in the revision of parts I (demographic data), II (life events) and III (psychiatric history) and that the whole system is currently available in French.

The five integrated parts of the system permit evaluation and documentation of all the data that are required to make a diagnostic formulation. There have been, however, only a few attempts up to now to link the system with the diagnostic process. In the French speaking group, a first step in this direction was recently taken by PIREE and PICHOT [11] . Starting from the German DIASIKA program, the authors developed a sequential computer method which applies empirically derived criteria and rules for the categories of the French classification of Mental Disorders (INSERM) to sign and symptom information provided in the AMDP System. The concordance between computer diagnosis and clinical diagnosis was by and large encouraging, in spite of a number of difficulties that remain to be solved. In particular, the authors were compelled to include additional signs and symptoms not contained in the original system.

Current investigations trying to establish the validity of the AMDP System for diagnostic purposes are based on Lists of Integrated Criteria for the Evaluation of Taxonomy (L.I.C.E.T)[12,13].

REFERENCES

1. D. P. Bobon, ed, Le Manuel AMDP, Presses
   Universitaires, Liège (1978)
2. D. P. Bobon, ed, Le Système AMDP, 2e édition,
   Mardaga, Bruxelles (1981)
3. Arbeitsgemeinschaft für Methodik und Dokumentation
   in der Psychiatrie, ed, Das AMDP-System, 3. Auflage, Springer, Berlin (1979)
4. D. P. Bobon, Foreign adaptations of the AMDP System,
   in : "The AMDP System", D. P. Bobon, ed,
   Karger, Basel (1983)
5. D. P. Bobon, Le concept d'Antrieb dans l'adaptation
   française de l'échelle psychopathologique AMP,
   Ann. Méd.-Psychol. 135 : 478 (1977)
6. D. P. Bobon, Conceptual and semantic problems raised
   by the French translation of the AMP Psychopathology Scale, in : "Neuro-psychopharmacology,
   P. Deniker, ed, Pergamon Press, Oxford (1978)
7. R. v. Frenckell et al., Preliminary Study of the
   Interrater Reliability of the AMDP Psychopathological Scale, in : "Comptes rendus du Congrès de
   Psychiatrie et de Neurologie de Langue Française,
   P. Sizaret, ed, Masson, Paris (1979)
8. J. Mirel et al., Fidélité intercotateurs de l'échelle
   psychopathologique AMDP. II. Distances entre cota-
   teurs et analyse d'items d'une délirante et d'une
   déprimée, in : "Comptes rendus du Congrès de Psychiatrie et de Neurologie de Langue Française",
   P. Sizaret, ed, Masson, Paris (1979)
9. D. P. Bobon et al., Analyse factorielle de la révision française de l'échelle AMDP. Résultats d'une
   étude internationale de 388 cas, Acta psychiat.
   belg. 82 : 371 (1982)
10. B. Woggon, A. Dittrich, Konstruktion übergeordneter
    AMP-Skalen : "manisch-depressives" und "schizo-
    phrenes Syndrom", Int. Pharmacopsychiat 14 :
    325 (1979)
11. P. Pichot, B. Samuel-Lajeunesse, S. Pirée, Un systè-
    me de diagnostic par ordinateur. Version française
    du D.I.A.S.I.K.A. Ann. Méd.-Psychol. (in press)
12. C. B. Pull, M. C. Pull, P. Pichot, L.I.C.E.T.-S :
    Une Liste Intégrée de Critères d'Evaluation Taxi-
    nomiques pour les psychoses non-affectives,
    J. Psychiat. Biol. et Thérapeut. 1 : 33 (1981)
13. C. B. Pull, M. C. Pull, P. Pichot, L.I.C.E.T.-D :
    Une Liste Intégrée de Critères d'Evaluation
    Taxinomiques pour les dépressions, Psychol. Méd.
    (in press)

SPANISH ADAPTATION OF THE SYSTEM OF THE ASSOCIATION FOR METHODOLOGY AND DOCUMENTATION IN PSYCHIATRY (AMDP SYSTEM)

Juan J. López-Ibor Jr., Amadeo Sanchez Blanqué, and
Javier San Sebastian

Centro Ramón y Cajal, Madrid, and Departament of
Psychiatry, University of Zaragoza, and Instituto de
Investigaciones Neuropsiquiátricas, Madrid
Av. Nueva Zelanda, 44, Madrid, Spain

The interest of Spanish speaking psychiatrists in the AMDP System is old. It was initiated through contacts or stays of Spanish or Iberoamerican psychiatrists in German, Belgian or French clinics. Translations of the second version of the AMDP System were made in Mexico (Heinze) and in Madrid and Salamanca (López-Ibor Jr.). In 1974 Heinze and Hinojosa made known the AMDP System in a publication of the Mexican Psychiatric Association and from 1980 there exists a Spanish version of the third edition (López-Ibor Jr.).

Although the AMDP System began to be applied in clinical research, primarily in the field of measuring psychopathological changes induced by treatments especially psychopharmacological ones, little by little other virtues and possibilities of the System have come to be appreciated. At present, the AMDP System tends to be used more and more in teaching and in psychopathological research.

Another reason that makes the System more attractive is that it uses psychopathological and clinical criteria, derived from the psychopathology that today we could call more classic, in which the major part of Spanish psychiatrists have been trained. The definitions in the manual are a summary of concepts of the most ordinary treatises with precise and operative definitions. It is a psychopathological system which gathers the richness of this discipline, and which permits its application to the daily clinic. Other methods come from more epidemiological perspectives which

167

makes them operationalize the definitions more, pinpoint the mode of exploration and they definitely move away from the everyday clinical practice interfering more in a normal doctor-patient relationship.

One of the most suggested applications of the AMDP System is the research on equivalencies of psychopathological concepts among the diverse languages and schools. To start with it is possible to say that the Spanish version has had less difficulties that the French version. Spanish psychiatry relies on a long tradition of model quality care which was interrupted in the middle of the XIX century coinciding with the development of French and German psychopathology. Also, it is traditional in Spanish psychiatry a clear forensic basis, precise and very appropriate in which the regulation of commitments, of incapacities or of responsibility is based on scientific and medical criteria outside the concrete social circumstances. So, when today we read old dispositions they appear to be very "modern". In this context, Spanish psychiatry received very important influences simultaneously from German and French psychopathology which coexisted with others that arrived later. Already in this century the prestige of Ramón y Cajal, histologist, lead to the development of a school of neuropathological orientation, and coinciding with it the influence of Freud arrived early to Spain. It should be remembered that the first translation of Freud's complete works took place into Spanish. Also during this time, which corresponds to the period between the two World Wars, translations of psychopathologists of anthropological orientation were made known in Spain, and therefore those of Zutt, V.v. Weizsaecker, etc. prove to be very early. The so-called school of Heidelberg had a great circulation in Spanish psychiatry. On the other hand, if such different tendencies have been able to blend and coexist together it is because from all of them Spanish psychiatry obtained something that it could compare with and apply to clinical practice.

The AMDP System is evolving in the Spanish speaking countries in several directions:

1) In psychopathological training, using the methodology of pedagogical work-shops with the evaluation of non-structured or structured interviews taped in video (Heinze, Sanchez Blanqué).
2) The use of scales 1, 2 and 3 in clinical and epidemiological studies in areas for which initially the AMDP System had not been forseen and in which the pages of psychopathological and somatic records are not applicable. It's a question of studies of heroin dependencies (López-Ibor Jr. and A. Rodriguez), alcoholism, psychiatric consultation and liaison psychiatry.
3) Use of the AMDP System as a routine instrument in the daily clinic. J. Giner is doing just that in Sevilla (see his

communication to this Congress) in spite of the difficulties entailed in a complex system.

4) Inter-rater reliability studies from interviews taped in video. At present there exist two studies underway (López-Ibor Jr., J. San Sebastian, Sanchez Blanqué).

5) The use of the AMDP System in clinical research. It is very difficult to make here a reference of the studies carried out or that are being carried out, although it must be said that , in general, there are serious studies in which there is no skimping of methodological effort.

6) The conversational version for the use f the AMDP System with a micro-computer. The first one made in the world was ours (López-Ibor Jr.) in the Centro Ramón y Cajal which continues to function just as it was described in 1980 which supposes a considerable saving of time, immediate availability of information and the possibility of applying statistical treatments over same.

7) At present, some Spanish groups are collaborating with the International Secretary of the AMDP System (Bobon) in a study of international inter-rater reliability.

In October of 1980 there took place in Madrid an International Symposium on the AMDP System in research, teaching and the international standardization of psychopathology, which interested many psychiatrists in the System in such a way that there is no lack of communications about it in national congresses of our discipline and the attendance at seminars of evaluation of patients is becoming more and more numerous.

The AMDP System is at the present moment the most complete in existence for documentation and quantification measures in psychiatry (Bobon), which makes it very attractive for its use in teaching and research centers, and thereby, the interest aroused by it in the Spanish speaking countries (Sanchez Blanqué and Giraldez Revuelta, 1981; Sanchez Blanqué, 1982). Certainly, the major part of the research has been centered on the psychometric qualities of the psychopathological scale (AMDP-4) and its use for the quantification of psychiatric symptomatology in therapeutic trials, in its application to automatized diagnoses (DiaSika program of von Zerssen) and in the teaching of psychiatry (Conde López, 1980; Berner, 1982). But the advantage of the AMDP System over other proceedures of psychopathological objectivity and evaluation resides, precisely, in the fact that it has three anamnestic cards (AMDP-1, 2 and 3) and a somatic card (AMDP-5) which permit summarizing in a significant way a great number of clinical and ancillary data facts about the patient (Bobon, 1978).

Of the three anamnesic cards, the first one gathers the most important references on the psychosocial environment of the patient: family structure, habitat, professional situation, economic means, and religious or ideological attitudes.

The second card serves to reflect the life events of the patient through two items: one permits the evaluation of the "possible influences provoking the illness" (item No. 22), and in the other the "alterations of the life situation" are pointed out (or "major events of the existence", such as the death of parents, marriage, divorce, birth and death of children, alterations in the work situation, etc.).

Finally, the third anamnesic card permits recording the psychiatric history: beginning of the illness, previous episodes, early disturbances in the development, family history, therapy to which the patient has been submitted and results obtained, etc.

Our experience concurs with that of Mormont (1982), who has calculated the time spent in administrating each one of these three cards: 17, 15 and 15 minutes respectively, with typical deviations of around 5 minutes each. In total, the performance of the anamnesic cards of the AMDP System takes 45-60 minutes, with the advantage that all the relevant facts have been gathered systematically.

The research into the provoking factors of psychic pathology with the second card of the AMDP System, has shown in a heterogeneous sample of psychiatric patients (Sánchez Blanqué and Giráldez Revuelta, 1981), that the ones most frequently involved in the three months before the beginning of the illness are: unspecific psychic stress (inadaptation, unrest, nervousness, exhaustion, etc., 29.31% of the cases), sexual conflicts (20.69%), family problems (excluding marital conflicts), 17.24% of the cases, loneliness (17.24%) and the problems with inter-personal relations (not sexual) with the spouse or partner (15.52% of the cases).

When one studies the presence of such psychosocial influences with a presumed pathogenic influence in different groups of mental patients with homogeneous diagnoses, significant differences are confirmed among them. Therefore, comparing the frequency with which the provoking of the illness is attributed to unfavorable conditions occurring in the three previous months in 30 patients affected with endogenous depression and 36 diagnosed with neurotic depression ("dysthimic disturbance", DSM-III,1980), we observe that among these it is more frequent to attribute a pathogenic power to the different socio-environmental circumstances and especially to family conflicts, problems relating to sexuality and to loneliness. (Sánchez Blanqué, 1982).

In the same way, the comparison between a sample of 49 schizophrenic patients and a mixed heterogenous group formed by 40 psychic patients with different diagnoses, has shown (Sánchez Blanqué et al., 1983) that the former demonstrate with less frequency the existence of provoking factors of the illness. The most relevant ones were loneliness (in 12.25% of the cases) and sexual problems (10.,20%), but they always showed up less often than among the patients of the mixed group. The most significant differences between both groups refer to a lower frequency, among the schizophrenics, of marital conflicts, family problems, economic difficulties and unspecfic psychic stress.

The AMDP System has shown, then, in Spanish research, its use for the evaluation of stress factors and life events in psychiatry. However, as we have commented in another paper (Sánchez Blanqué and Giráldez Revuelta, 1983), the anamnesic card No. 2 can be improved introducing the following modifications:

a) Quantify the severity of the stress factors (item 22) with a similar system to that of the psychopathological scale, on five levels (0,1,2,3 and 4). Thereby, for example, "family problems" can oscilate in their severity from a discrete lack of understanding to verbal disputes, physical aggression or abandoning the home.

b) Point out with precision the exact moment in which the life events (item 23) have occurred. The compartments to note down the age of the patient when he suffered these psychic traumas are too wide. Therefore, the death of the father of a young man of 14 is noted in the space corresponding to the period between 5 and 15 years, thereby losing much information and it is not possible to evaluate afterwards the real reach and significance of the fact, and therefore, his pathogenic role. It would preferable, then, to indicate the exact age on one continuous line instead of using compartments with a range of ages.

We think that the introduction of these modifications in future editions of the AMDP Manual and of the anamnesic cards N° 2 could improve the quality of the System for the research into the life events in psychiatry from a strictly clinical perspective, and it would furnish a greater amount of information on each concrete case in particular.

In the future versions of the AMDP System we would like to see a configuration of the sheets and a definition of the choices of the items not limited by the structure of optical reading computerized forms. This will add more flexibility and precision to the System.

REFERENCES

Berner, P., 1982, Las funciones del Sistema AMDP en la formación y la investigación en Psiquiatría. Actas Luso-
Españolas Neurol. Psiquiatr., 10, 405-408.
Bobon, D. P., 1978, Comparaison du Système AMDP à d'autres
dossiers Psychiatriques standardisés et échélles

multifactorielles d'évaluation de la psychopathologie Acta Psychiatr. Belg., 78, 559-572.

Conde López, V., 1980, El sistema AMDP en la formación de psiquiatras. Symposium Internacional AMDP, Madrid.

DSM-III, 1980, "Diagnostical and Statistical Manual of Mental Disorders". American Psychiatric Association, Washington,

Heinze, G., 1982, La versión española del Sistema AMDP en la enseñanza e investigación en México, Actas Luso-Esp. Neurol. Psiquiatr.y C.A., 6, 427-429.

López-Ibor Jr., J.J., ed., 1980, "El Sistema AMDP", Grupo para el Progreso de la Psiquiatría, Garsi, Madrid.

López-Ibor Jr., J.J., Rey Portolés, G., Benitez Hita, F. and Rodríguez Gamazo, M., 1982, Versión conversacional directa del Sistema AMDP, Actas Luso-Esp. Neurol. Psiquiatr. y C.A., 10, 429-444.

Mormont, I., 1982, Premières impressions sur l'application multicentrique des fiches anamnestiques de l'AMDP, XIV Symposium Francophone International de l'AMDP, Liège.

Sánchez Blanqué, A., 1982, La notation des événements pathogènes en psychiatrie par le Système AMDP. Différences entre malades déprimés et non déprimés, Acta Psychiatr. Belg.,82,390-397.

Sánchez Blanqué, and Giraldez Revuelta, E., 1981, Utilidad clínica del Sistema AMDP para la evaluación de los acontecimientos biográficos en enfermos psiquiátricos, Comunicación Psiquiátrica, 8, 111-119.

Sánchez-Blanqué, A. and Giraldez Revuelta, E., 1983, La investigación de los acontecimientos vitales en el contexto del Sistema AMDP, Actas Luso-Esp. Neurol. Psiquiatr. y C.A., in press.

Sánchez-Blanqué, A., Giraldez Revuelta, E. and López Plaza, J.J., Les influences psychosociales dans le déclenchement de la schizophrénie. Un étude au moyen du système AMDP, Acta Psychiatr. Belg.,in press.

COMPATABILITY BETWEEN THE AMDP
AND THE BLIPS/BDP DOCUMENTATION SYSTEM*

Luciano Conti

Institue of Clinical Psychiatry – University of Pisa
56100 Pisa – Italy

Giovanni B. Cassano

2nd Chair of Clinical Psychaitry – University of Pisa
Pisa – Italy

Gabriele Massimetti

Institute of Clinical Psychiatry – University of Pisa
Pisa – Italy

Jerome Levine

Pharmacologic and Somatic Treatments Research Branch
NIMH Rockville, Maryland – USA

─────────────
*This study was supported by NIMH Grant No. 1U01 MH33922-03

In the past decade the planning and conduct of clinical trials in psychopharmacology has undergone a continuous process of harmonization which has been founded mainly on a scientific basis and has attained a general consensus and acceptance by clinical investigators as well as by regulatory agencies of various countries. The phases used for establishing efficacy and safety of new psychotherapeutic compounds are well known as are the assessment criteria and methods. Moreover some assessment instruments are widely used for the evaluation of symptom change in clinical trials. Nevertheless, to date we are far from attaining general agreement on the method of documenting, analyzing, and presenting the large amounts of data arising from clinical investigations. Though for each trial a special set of analyses may be required, a routine documentation procedure should be available systematically providing the fundamental information. As previously stated currently we are far from attaining general agreement on a methodology of analyzing, documenting, and presenting data arising from clinical investigations.

Agreement would allow easier accomplishment of multicenter international trials, utilization of the same data by regulatory agencies of different countries, and easier communication and comparison of results derived from different populations of patients evaluated by investigators of different cultures. Even though the process of documenting clinical trials needs to be uniform and unified, the different cultural and clincial backgrounds of individual investigators of different countries may result in different attitudes toward the assessment criteria and toward the choice of rating instruments for measuring psychopathology. Therfore a comprehensive and standard system for clinical psychopharmacological documentation should enable use of both those rating instruments which are widely used internationally and those which are an expression of the scientific and cultural traditions of each country.

The major objective of the Center for Clinical Psychopharmacology Data Documentation (CCPDD), jointly established by the U.S. National Institute of Mental Health (NIMH) and the University of Pisa, at the Institute of Clinical Psychiatry of Pisa University, is to improve the quality of clincial trials of psychopharmacologic agents performed internationally. This is attempted by utilizing and disseminating computer based data documentation techniques which allow more understandable, comprehensive and standardized data analysis and data presentation and which require better planning of clinical trials. This results in clinical reports which are more useable and acceptable internationally.

The basic flexibility of the Biometric Laboratory Information Processing System (BLIPS) and the Banca dei Dati Psicofarmacologici (BDP) systems have been unified with a substantial enhancement of the power of the resulting BLIPS/BDP documentation system now available at the CCPDD in Pisa.

The flexibility and the compatibility of the BLIPS/BDP is demonstrated by its successful incorporation and utilization of other selected rating instruments. Sociologically oriented clinical investigators may require a deeper and more detailed documentation of the psychosocial profile of subjects responding or not to certain type of treatment and in order to do that the Social Adjustment Scale-SAS II (SCHOOLER, HOGARTY, WEISSMAN, 1979) was added to the BLIPS standard forms and supplemented by detailed analyses and displays.

An Italian self-rating scale for depression (Self Assessment Depression Scale - SADS - by CASSANO & CASTROGIOVANNI) has become part of the standard set of forms, analyses and displays of the system.

A further step in international harmonization of clincal psychopharmacology data documentation has been attained with the integration of the Psychopathology Assessment Scale (PAS) of the AMDP system with the BLIPS/BDP system.The last version of the AMDP's PAS has been utilized following the French and Italian translations in which the last 15 optional items are substituted with fixed ones. The PAS's items explore all areas of psychopathology following a systematic traditional approach to the evaluation of mental status. The format of the PAS has been modified by adding the identification block variables of the BLIPS system. The first 19 columns identify the center, the study, the patient, the form, the assessment period, the rater and the group to which the patient is assigned (Fig. 1). A special control file has been created which allows automatic insertion of the PAS in the routine BLIPS/BDP data processing. According to the standard BLIPS/BDP procedure all the item scores of the PAS are edited to achieve quality control. The program (PREPROC), a preprocessing procedure, allows identification of missing data as well as out of range scores. After quality control a Master Data File is created on which the routine BLIPS analyses can be performed through the DATRAN program.

A special program can, at this point, provide for the storage of the corrected raw data into the BLIPS/BDP Data Bank. From this bank the stored data may be retrieved by means of the MMSEL, a very sophisticated selection program, and utilized for other standard and/or non-standard analyses within the same study or in a pool of studies.

The BLIPS/BDP program of data analysis of the PAS provides:

1. tabulation of the raw scoress for each subject and for each evaluation (fig. 2);

2. the item scores are combined in two different types of composite scores, the psychopathological areas in which the PAS is divided (Fig. 3) and the factor scores derived from the factor analysis performed by BOBON & COWORKERS (in press) (Fig. 4). For each subject and for each assessment period the composite scores are tabulated (Fig. 5 & 6) and the mean and the standard deviation is calculated (Fig. 7 & 8);

3. cross-tabulation analysis between two different assessment periods is performed for each factor (Fig. 9);

4. a bar-graph display for the same time intervals used in the cross-tabulation is provided for the mean scores of the factors (Fig. 10);

5. variance and/or covariance analysis is performed on the two types of composite scores (psychopathological areas and factor scores) to verify if it is likely changes in symptomatology are due to chance (Fig. 11 & 12);

6. additional non standard statistical analyses may be easily performed and the results may became part of the standard BLIPS/BDP output.

Similar in documentation philosophy, BLIPS differs primarily from the AMDP in its generality since it was designed to process all types of clinical assessment data. The AMDP system was designed specifically for the AMDP forms. Therefore the PAS could be successfully integrated into the BLIPS/BDP demonstrating the possibility of utilizing the BLIPS/BDP procedures of data analysis and documentation for the AMDP.

The PAS now can be processed automatically resulting in a wide variety of analyses offered rountinely by the BLIPS/BDP system creating uniform data displays and analyses which are easily readable and interpretable. Due to the structural characteristics of BLIPS/BDP once data analysis and display procedures for the PAS are set up in one center they can easily be transferred and become operative in other centers using the BLIPS/BDP system.

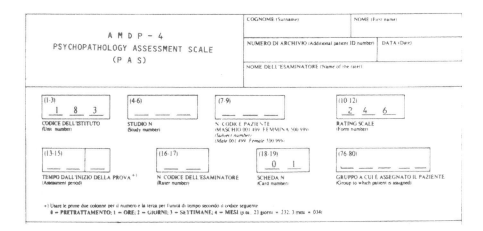

Figure 1

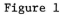

Figure 2

```
                    AMDP - 4   ABBREVIATION LEGEND
                    -------------------------------


          AREAS                    ITEMS      ---ABBREVIATIONS---

    DISORDERS OF CONSCIOUSNESS       01-04          CONS

    DISORDERS OF ORIENTATION         05-08          ORNT

    DISTURBANCES OF ATTENTION & MEM. 09-14          ATTN

    FORMAL DISORDERS OF THOUGHT      15-26          THGT

    PHOBIAS AND COMPULSIONS          27-32          PHOB

    DELUSIONS                        33-46          DELU

    DISORDERS OF PERCEPTION          47-52          PRCP

    DISORDERS OF EGO                 53-58          EGOO

    DISTURBANCES OF AFFECT           59-79          AFCT

    DISORDERS OF DRIVE & MOTILITY    80-88          MOTL

    CIRCADIAN DISTURBANCES           89-91          CIRC

    OTHER DISTURBANCES               92-100         OTHD

    OTHER SYMPTOMS                   101-115        OTHS
```

Figure 3

PSYCHOPATHOLOGICAL   SYMPTOMS   AMDP - 4   (FORM 246)   FACTOR LISTING

ORGANIC DISTURBANCES (ORGO)

```
  7  ORNT/SITUATION
  6  ORNT/PLACE
  5  ORNT/TIME
  9  ATTN/APPERCEPTION
  2  CONS/CLOUDED
 19  THGT/PERSEVERATION
 12  ATTN/RETENTION
  8  ORNT/SELF
100  OTHD/LACK SELF CARE
 11  ATTN/MEMORIZATION
  1  CONS/LOWERED
  3  CONS/NARROWED
 13  ATTN/CONFABULATION
 18  THGT/RESTRICTED THINKING
 10  ATTN/CONCENTRATION
 23  THGT/TANGENTIAL THINKING
```

DEPRESSION (DEPR)

```
 64  AFCT/HOPELESSNESS
102  OTHS/LOSS OF DESIRE TO LIVE
 60  AFCT/LOSS OF FEELINGS
 63  AFCT/DEPRESSED MOOD
 92  OTHD/SOC.WITHDRAWL
 71  AFCT/INADEQUACY
 95  OTHD/SUICIDE
 61  AFCT/BLUNTED EFFECT
 16  THGT/RETARDED  THINKING
 81  MOTL/INHIB.DRIVE
 62  AFCT/LOSS VITALITY
 80  MOTL/LACK DRIVE
 74  AFCT/FEEL. IMPOVERISH.
 73  AFCT/FEELING OF GUILT
 15  THGT/INHIB. THINKING
103  OTHS/ASTHENIA
 89  CIRC/WORSE AM
 20  THGT/RUMINATION
110  OTHS/REDUCED SEXUAL INTEREST
 87  EGOD/MUTISM
```


MANIA (MANI)

```
104  OTHS/ACCELERATED THINKING
 82  MOTL/INC. DRIVE
 22  THGT/FLIGHT OF IDEAS
 66  AFCT/EUPHORIA
 88  MOTL/LOGORRHEA
 93  OTHD/EXC. SOC. CONTACT
 83  MOTL/MOTR. RESTLESS
 72  AFCT/EXAG. SELF-ESTEEM
111  OTHS/INCREASED SEXUAL INTEREST
 97  OTHD/LACK. FEEL. ILL
```

DELUSION (DELU)

```
 40  DELU/DEL. PERSECUTION
 38  DELU/DEL.DYNAMICS
 35  DELU/SUDDEN DEL. IDEA
 34  DELU/DEL. PERCEPTION
 39  DELU/DEL. REFERENCE
 37  DELU/SYSTEMATIC DEL.
 36  DELU/DELUSIONAL IDEAS
 44  DELU/HYPOCHON. DEL.
 48  PRCP/VERBAL HALLUC.
 57  EGOD/INSERTION
 58  EGOD/OTHER SYMPTOMS
 45  DELU/DEL. GRANDEUR
 55  EGOD/BROADCASTING
 98  OTHD/LACK INSIGHT
 42  DELU/DEL. GUILT
 14  ATTN/PARAMNESIAS
```


DYSPHORIA (DYSP)

```
 76  AFCT/PARATHYMIA
 85  MOTL/MANNERISM
 54  EGOD/DEPERSONALIZATION
 53  EGOD/DEREALIZATION
 25  THGT/INCHOERENCE
 33  DFLU/DEL. MOOD
 24  THGT/BLOCKING
 75  AFCT/AMBIVALENCE
 59  AFCT/PERPLEXITY
```

OBSESSION-PHOBIAS (OBSP)

```
 65  AFCT/ANXIETY
109  OTHS/OBJECTIVE ANXIETY
 69  AFCT/INNER RESTLESS.
105  OTHS/TENSION
106  OTHS/TENDENCY TO DRAMATISE
108  OTHS/SOCIAL ANXIETY
107  OTHS/ANT. ANXIETY
```


PARATHYMIA (PARA)

```
 68  AFCT/IRRITABILITY
 67  AFCT/DISPHORIA
 94  OTHD/AGGRESSIVE
 27  PHOR/SUSPICIOUSNESS
 99  OTHD/UNCOOPERATIVE
```

ANXIETY (ANXI)

```
 70  AFCT/COMPLAINTIVE
 86  MOTL/HISTRIONIC
112  OTHS/SEXUAL UNSATISFACTORINESS
 78  AFCT/AFFECT. INCON.
 77  AFCT/AFFECT. LABILITY
 21  THGT/PRESSURED THINKING
115  OTHS/SOCIAL MALADJUSTMENT
 79  AFCT/AFFECT. RIGIDITY
```


EMOTIONAL DISTURBANCES (EMOD)

```
 30  PHOB/OBSESS. THOUGHT
 31  PHOB/COMP. IMPULS
 32  PHOB/COMP. ACTION
 29  PHOB/PHOBIAS
```


Figure 4

PSYCHOPATHOLOGICAL SYMPTOMS   AMDP - 4   (FORM 246)   AREA LISTING

PAT	PERIOD	RTR	CONS	ORNT	ATTN	THGT	PHOB	DELU	PRCP	EGOD	AFCT	MOTL	CIRC	OTHD	GROUP
001	00 0	01	0.0	0.0	0.33	0.33	0.0	0.0	0.0	0.0	1.10	0.44	1.00	0.11	1
001	30 2	01	0.0	0.0	0.0	0.08	0.0	0.0	0.0	0.0	0.29	0.0	0.33	0.0	1
002	00 0	01	0.0	0.0	0.17	0.25	0.0	0.0	0.0	0.0	1.67	0.78	0.67	0.56	1
002	30 2	01	0.0	0.0	0.0	0.08	0.0	0.0	0.0	0.0	0.81	0.22	0.33	0.11	1
003	00 0	01	0.0	0.0	0.50	0.25	0.0	0.0	0.0	0.0	1.19	0.56	0.33	0.11	1
003	30 2	01	0.0	0.0	0.0	0.08	0.0	0.0	0.0	0.0	1.19	0.56	0.67	0.33	1
004	00 0	01	0.0	0.0	0.50	0.08	0.0	0.0	0.0	0.0	1.05	0.33	0.67	0.11	1
004	30 2	01	0.0	0.0	0.17	0.08	0.0	0.0	0.0	0.0	0.71	0.11	0.0	0.0	1
005	00 0	01	0.0	0.0	0.0	0.25	0.0	0.0	0.0	0.0	0.76	0.44	0.33	0.33	1
005	30 2	01	0.0	0.0	0.0	0.08	0.0	0.0	0.0	0.0	0.29	0.11	0.33	0.11	1
006	00 0	01	0.0	0.0	0.0	0.33	0.33	0.0	0.0	0.0	1.19	0.56	0.67	0.11	1
006	30 2	01	0.0	0.0	0.0	0.08	0.0	0.0	0.0	0.0	0.29	0.11	0.0	0.0	1
007	00 0	01	0.0	0.0	0.33	0.17	0.50	0.0	0.0	0.0	0.95	0.44	1.00	0.22	1
007	30 2	01	0.0	0.0	0.0	0.08	0.17	0.0	0.0	0.0	0.52	0.11	1.00	0.11	1
008	00 0	01	0.0	0.0	0.0	0.33	0.50	0.0	0.0	0.0	1.00	0.78	1.00	0.22	1
008	30 2	01	0.0	0.0	0.0	0.08	0.17	0.0	0.0	0.0	0.38	0.67	0.33	0.11	1
009	00 0	01	0.0	0.0	0.50	0.17	0.33	0.0	0.0	0.0	1.14	0.56	1.00	0.56	1
009	30 2	01	0.0	0.0	0.0	0.08	0.17	0.0	0.0	0.0	1.29	0.56	1.00	0.67	1
010	00 0	01	0.0	0.0	0.0	0.33	0.67	0.0	0.0	0.0	1.52	0.78	1.33	0.78	1
010	30 2	01	0.0	0.0	0.0	0.08	0.17	0.0	0.0	0.0	0.81	0.44	0.67	0.33	1
011	00 0	01	0.0	0.0	0.0	0.25	0.50	0.0	0.0	0.0	0.90	0.67	0.67	0.11	1
011	30 2	01	0.0	0.0	0.0	0.08	0.0	0.0	0.0	0.0	1.29	0.89	0.67	0.56	1
012	00 0	01	0.0	0.0	0.0	0.42	0.50	0.0	0.0	0.0	1.38	1.00	0.67	0.44	1
012	30 2	01	0.0	0.0	0.0	0.0	0.0	0.0	0.0	0.0	0.43	0.22	0.33	0.11	1
013	00 0	01	0.0	0.0	0.0	0.25	0.17	0.0	0.0	0.0	0.95	0.22	0.67	0.11	1
013	30 2	01	0.0	0.0	0.0	0.0	0.0	0.0	0.0	0.0	0.24	0.11	0.33	0.11	1

Figure 5

PSYCHOPATHOLOGICAL SYMPTOMS   AMDP - 4   (FORM 246)   FACTOR LISTING

PAT	PERIOD	RTR	ORGD	DEPR	MANI	DELU	DYSP	OBSP	PARA	ANXI	EMOD	TOT.	GROUP
001	00 0	01	0.13	1.80	0.0	0.0	0.0	1.86	0.0	0.25	0.0	0.46	1
001	30 2	01	0.0	0.40	0.0	0.0	0.0	0.43	0.0	0.13	0.0	0.10	1
002	00 0	01	0.06	2.45	0.10	0.13	0.0	1.71	0.20	0.38	0.0	0.60	1
002	30 2	01	0.0	1.15	0.0	0.0	0.0	0.57	0.0	0.13	0.0	0.24	1
003	00 0	01	0.19	1.50	0.20	0.0	0.0	1.43	0.40	0.50	0.0	0.44	1
003	30 2	01	0.0	1.40	0.30	0.06	0.0	1.00	0.60	0.63	0.0	0.41	1
004	00 0	01	0.19	1.20	0.10	0.0	0.0	1.71	0.20	0.38	0.0	0.38	1
004	30 2	01	0.06	0.50	0.10	0.0	0.11	1.14	0.0	0.38	0.0	0.21	1
005	00 0	01	0.0	1.15	0.0	0.06	0.0	1.43	0.20	0.25	0.0	0.33	1
005	30 2	01	0.0	0.35	0.0	0.0	-0.0	0.43	0.0	0.13	0.0	0.10	1
006	00 0	01	0.0	1.70	0.10	0.0	0.0	1.57	0.60	0.38	0.25	0.47	1
006	30 2	01	0.0	0.55	0.10	0.0	0.0	0.43	0.0	0.0	0.0	0.13	1
007	00 0	01	0.13	1.40	0.20	0.06	0.0	1.43	0.0	0.38	0.0	0.43	1
007	30 2	01	0.0	0.75	0.10	0.0	0.0	0.57	0.0	0.13	0.0	0.21	1
008	00 0	01	0.06	1.75	0.20	0.0	0.0	2.29	0.20	0.25	0.0	0.52	1
008	30 2	01	0.0	0.85	0.20	0.0	0.0	1.71	0.0	0.0	0.25	0.28	1
009	00 0	01	0.19	1.70	0.30	0.06	0.0	2.00	0.0	0.25	0.25	0.53	1
009	30 2	01	0.0	1.80	0.20	0.13	0.0	2.29	0.0	0.25	0.25	0.53	1
010	00 0	01	0.0	2.65	0.10	0.19	0.0	1.57	0.0	0.50	0.25	0.66	1
010	30 2	01	0.0	1.15	0.10	0.19	0.0	0.86	0.0	0.38	0.0	0.33	1
011	00 0	01	0.0	1.05	0.20	0.0	0.0	2.00	0.60	0.38	0.50	0.42	1
011	30 2	01	0.0	1.45	0.30	0.0	0.0	2.00	1.20	0.63	0.0	0.50	1
012	00 0	01	0.06	1.80	0.30	0.0	0.11	2.29	0.80	0.63	0.0	0.61	1
012	30 2	01	0.0	0.55	0.30	0.0	0.0	0.29	0.0	0.63	0.0	0.19	1
013	00 0	01	0.06	1.05	0.0	0.0	0.0	1.71	0.20	0.50	0.25	0.38	1
013	30 2	01	0.0	0.40	0.0	0.0	0.0	0.57	0.20	0.13	0.0	0.12	1

Figure 6

PSYCHOPATHOLOGICAL SYMPTOMS   AMDP - 4   (FORM 246)   MEANS OF AREAS

VAR.NO. 10 -   AFCT

	GROUP	GRP 1	R.T.
PERIOD			
DAY 00	N	13	13
	MEAN	1.14	1.14
	S.D.	0.26	0.26
DAY 30	N	13	13
	MEAN	0.66	0.66
	S.D.	0.39	0.39
C.T.	N	26	26
	MEAN	0.90	0.90
	S.D.	0.41	0.41

Figure 7

PSYCHOPATHOLOGICAL SYMPTOMS   AMDP - 4   (FORM 246)   MEANS OF FACTORS

VAR.NO.   3 -   DEPR

GROUP PERIOD		GRP 1	R.T.
DAY 00	N	13	13
	MEAN	1.63	1.63
	S.D.	0.50	0.50
DAY 30	N	13	13
	MEAN	0.87	0.87 -
	S.D.	0.48	0.48
C.T.	N	26	26
	MEAN	1.25	1.25
	S.D.	0.61	0.61

Figure 8

PSYCHOPATHOLOGICAL SYMPTOMS   AMDP - 4   (FORM 246)   PRE VS. POST FACTORS

VAR.NO.   3 -   ORGD   VAR.NO.   3 -   DEPR

- GROUP 1   - GROUP 1

PRE POST		ABSENT	MILD	MOD.	SEVERE	EXT.SV	R.T.
ABSENT	N	4	8	0	0	0	12
MILD	N	0	1	0	0	0	1
MODERATE	N	0	0	0	0	0	0
SEVERE	N	0	0	0	0	0	0
EXT.SEV.	N	0	0	0	0	0	0
C.T.	N	4	9	0	0	0	13

PRE POST		ABSENT	MILD	MOD.	SEVERE	EXT.SV	R.T.
ABSENT	N	0	0	0	0	0	0
MILD	N	0	6	5	1	0	12
MODERATE	N	0	0	1	0	0	1
SEVERE	N	0	0	0	0	0	0
EXT.SEV.	N	0	0	0	0	0	0
C.T.	N	0	6	6	1	0	13

Figure 9

PSYCHOPATHOLOGICAL SYMPTOMS   AMDP - 4   (FORM 246)   PRE (II) AND POSTTREATMENT (==) BAR GRAPH

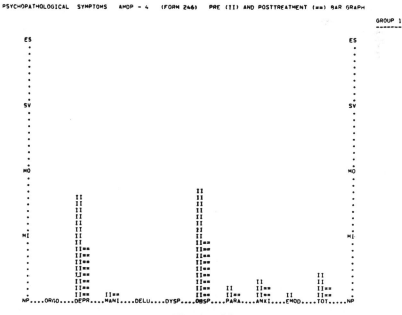

Figure 10

VARIABLE   9

PAGE   9

PSYCHOPATHOLOGICAL SYMPTOMS AMDP - 4   ANALYSIS OF VARIANCE (REPEATED MEASURES)

ANALYSIS OF VARIANCE
DISTURBANCES OF AFFECT

	DF	SUM OF SQUARES	MEAN SQUARES	F-RATIO	SIG(.05)	SIG(.05)-(GREENHOUSE/GEISER)
ANOVA ERROR 1 - BETWEEN	12	1.5603	0.1300			
ANOVA ERROR 2 - WITHIN	12	1.0912	0.0909			
PERIOD	1	1.5072	1.5072	16.5752	*	(*)

LEVEL MEANS OF TREATMENT COMBINATION

	"N"	"MEAN"	"STD.DEV."	"VARIANCE"

PERIOD

LEVEL 1	13	1.1385
LEVEL 2	13	0.6569

Figure 11

THE BIOMETRIC LABORATORY,GWU - AVACOV - UP TO 4 WAY CLASSIFICATION   PAGE   1
SYCHOPATHOLOGICAL SYMPTOMS AMDP -4   ANALYSIS OF VARIANCE (REPEATED MEASURES)
PROBLEM NUMBER   1
VARIABLE   1   PSYCHOPATHOLOGICAL SYMPTOMS AMDP -4 ANALYSIS OF VARIANCE (REPEATED MEASURES)

ANALYSIS OF VARIANCE
ORGANIC DISTURBANCES

	DF	SUM OF SQUARES	MEAN SQUARES	F-RATIO	SIG(.05)	SIG(.05)-(GREENHOUSE/GEISER)
ANOVA ERROR 1 - BETWEEN	12	0.0423	0.0035			
ANOVA ERROR 2 - WITHIN	12	0.0294	0.0025			
PERIOD	1	0.0392	0.0392	16.0058	*	(*)

LEVEL MEANS OF TREATMENT COMBINATION

	"N"	"MEAN"	"STD.DEV."	"VARIANCE"

PERIOD

LEVEL 1	13	0.0823
LEVEL 2	13	0.0046

Figure 12

This kind of work leads to a real international integration of approaches to the assessment and documentation of psychopathological data derived from clinical trials. In a subseqent phase of this work the Scandinavian Comprehensive Psychopathological Rating Scale-CPRS (ASBERG et al., 1978) will also be integrated into the BLIPS/BDP system.

Some advantages of the integrative process between AMDP and BLIPS/BDP systems follow.

The PAS of the AMDP added to the standard forms of the BLIPS/BDP brings into clinical trials with psychotherapeutic drugs a detailed and descriptive assessment of psychopathology with a clinical diagnostic approach. It includes in the documentation process a more analytic mental status examination for each patient and is intended to meet the needs of clinical investigators who wish to obtain an adequate diagnostic definition for each patient and in order to assess changes of discrete symptoms as well as global psychopathological changes.

This may be considered an important step toward the integration and reciprocal potentiation of the two systems which should lead to unifying the effort toward a continous enhancement of the level of clinical standard routine. Data processing for the PAS is now feasible by means of the BLIPS/BDP procedures. This allows better utilization of the PAS for which there is finally available a systematic and comprehensive evaluation of the collected data.

The deficiencies in clinical trials commonly adopting non standard systems for diagnosis and cross-sectional assessment and data analysis which are often quite simplistic are in fact clearly apparent. An advantage is also derived from the fact that the data collected with the PAS are now easily correlated, integrated and compared with the set of information obtained with standard instruments and analyses of the BLIPS/BDP so that cross-sectional PAS evaluation can be completed with demographic (APDI,PTR, ...), psychosocial (SAS II), dosage and side effect data (DOTES, TWIS, SAFTEE,...) as well as data from other psychopathological scales (CGI, HAM-D, HAM-A, BPRS, SADS, CPRS, ...).

An additional advantage is the possibility (given by the BLIPS/BDP) to store the data of the PAS in a storage/retrieval system, which is now available for any investigator in Pisa, and which will allow subsequent analyses of PAS data (alone or together with other assessment instruments) derived from single and/or multiple trials.

The combination and integration of the philosophy and language of the two documentation systems is aimed at producing a progressive enlargement of data users parallel with a continous improvement of communication. This unification process is a continuously evolving one on the basis of the scientific contribution of each culture though maintaining specific needs of the different cultural settings.

The enhancement of the level of data documentation will influence the quality of the planning as well as the conduct of the clinical trials and should lead to the definition of a common set of methodologies, instruments and analyses common to trials performed in different countries. At the same time such a unification process, on the basis of the characteristics of the BLIPS/BDP, a modularly constructed integrated series of computer programs which produces a documentation for a variety of scientific data imput (GUY, 1976), meets the needs of individual investigators by offering analyses and integration of a large set of instruments into a comprehensive system.

This progress toward an adequate development and unification of the methodologies of data documentation in different countries is nowadays supported by the European Community and WHO as well as by the NIMH and FDA. The widespread use of the BLIPS/BDP data analysis and documentation formats would greatly simplify the work of investigators, companies, and reviewers since each would not have to develop and interpret different data documentation formats. The integration of the PAS of the AMDP with the BLIPS/BDP system may be considered an initial step of a wider integration of the two systems. The progress in this process is strictly related to the cooperation between the CCPDD and the AMDP-users. Since the major objective of the Center is to improve the quality of clinical trials in psychopharmacology the integration of the AMDP and BLIPS/BDP systems would be a wasted effort if the whole system is not utilized globally in single and particularly in multicenter international clinical trials. Besides, most of the BLIPS/BDP standard forms, such as demographic, dosage, global assessment, etc., are complementary to the AMDP system so that the use of the integrated system is strictly in keeping with the international harmonization of clinical trials.

A further integration of the two systems will derive from the development of such cooperation. Only a wide utilization will make possible the development of a documentation program for the other AMDP scales beginning with the Somatic Symptoms Scale. In the development of these documentation programs we will certainly need assistance, suggestions and comments as well as criticism from investigators with deeper knowledge and experience with the AMDP system.

REFERENCES

Assberg M., Montgomery S., Perris C., Schalling D. and Sedvall
    G., CPRS. The Comprehensive Psychopathological Rating Scale.
    Acta Psych. Scand., Suppl., 271, 1978.
Guy W., ECDEU Assessment Manual for Psychopharmacology. DHEW
    Pub. No. (ADM) 76338, Washington, D.C. 1976.
Schooler N.R., Hogarty G.E. and Weissman M., Social Adjustment
    Scale II. In: Hargraves W.A., Atkinson C. and Soresens J.E.:
    "Resource Material for Community Mental Health Program
    Evaluation". AMD79: 328-303, Printing Authors, Washington,
    D.C., USA, 1979.

THE ENGLISH ADAPTATION OF THE AMDP SYSTEM

William Guy and Thomas A. Ban

Vanderbilt University School of Medicine and
Tennessee Neuropsychiatric Institute
Nashville, TN

The English AMDP Manual, published in 1982, had its roots in
work performed under the WHO training program in Montreal during
1974. Juri Saarma, a Visiting Professor in that program, undertook
the task of preparing a verbatim translation of all six parts of
the second edition of the AMP System with the collaboration of Drs.
Lehmann and Ban. The work was undertaken in order to provide a
comprehensive assessment system suitable both for diagnostic classification as well as for the assessment of change over time (1).

Following the initial translation, the six AMP-2 forms were
then prepared and formated for insertion into the Biometric Laboratory Information Processing System (BLIPS) which was then part of
the Early Clinical Drug Evaluation program (ECDEU) of the Psychopharmacology Research Branch of the U.S. National Institute of
Mental Health. The six forms, i.e., General Anamnesis, Psychiatric
Pathology Anamnesis, Medical Record, Psychopathological Assessment,
Somatic Findings and Termination Record, could then be processed
and analyzed by the BLIPS System and comprehensive documentation
provided to investigators (2)

This initial translation encountered a number of difficulties.
A major problem involved the item definitions which were somewhat
ambigious to those not familiar with their antecedent descriptive
psychopathological concepts. In the USA, a large number of psychiatrists have received their training in the context of psychodynamic psychopathology--particularly within a psychoanalytically-
oriented framework--and, hence, were not as conversant with the
structural psychopathology upon which the AMP system was based.

187

Consequently in 1978, Jamieson and Ban began to construct a glossary in which the descriptive definitions for the psychopathological items were supplemented with operational definitions in an effort to simplify the rating process. At approximately the same time, however, the third German edition--now called AMDP-III--was published (3). The changes in this new version were significant enough to warrant a new English translation.

The present English translation of the AMDP System (4) is the product of an intense collaborative effort on the part of American and Canadian psychiatrists and psychologists in consultation with the AMDP International Secretariat. The major task of the Secretariat was to promote an official and fully compatible English adaptation of the System. Consequently through its chairman, D. P. Bobon, it was instrumental in bringing together both Canadian and American professionals in this effort. The collaboration was facilitated by the fact that the recently-published French AMDP was then being adapted for use in bilingual Canada. The present English adaptation, therefore, had the advantage of both the basic German as well as the newer French versions in its development-- resulting in a degree of compatibility among the three versions that might otherwise not been attained (5).

A completely literal translation was not possible, although such deviations from the original German version as were necessary are very few. Many of them occurred in the anamnesic sections where North American convention dictated different categorizations. Designation of levels of education, for example, were necessarily different. Where cultural differences made it difficult to construct exactly parallel scale points, the nearest North American equivalent was used. In other cases such as diagnoses, the European (ICD-9 System) and the U.S. System (DSM-3) were both included in the English form. For the most part, however, the demographic material in the anamnestic sections of the system are compatible.

An especially intensive effort toward compatibility was undertaken for Parts IV and V (i.e., Psychopathological Symptoms and Somatic Signs). Figure 1 presents the rating form for Psychopathological Symptoms. This format is identical--language aside--with the German and French forms since it was produced directly from the French masks. This fact makes encoding for computer-readable input a much simpler process since it overcomes language barriers. It can be seen that a five-point intensity scale, i.e., "Absent," "Mild," "Moderate," "Severe" and "Extremely Severe" has been used rather than the four-point German scale. Further, nine additional symptoms derived from the French version; i.e., P1-P9, have been added to the English version. It was felt that the five-point scale and these additional items provided additional discriminatory power.

PSYCHOPATHOLOGICAL SYMPTOMS

AMDP - 4

PATIENT INITIALS _____ _____ PT. NO. _____
                1st   Last

SEX: M___ F___

BIRTH DATE: _____

RACE: W__ B__ I__ O__ OTH_____

DATE OF EXAMINATION: ____/____/____
                   M   D   Y

|_|_|_|_|_| Patient Number

|_|_|_|_| Study Number

|_| Sex (M = 1; F = 2)

|_|_| Age

|_| Race (W=1, B=2, I=3, O=4, Oth=5)

|_|_|_|_| Date of Examination

|_|_| Period

INTELLECTUAL DEFICIT

1	2	3	4	5	(9)
AB	MI	MO	SV	EX	NA

Inherited _____   Acquired _____

	0 AB	1 MI	2 MO	3 SV	4 EX	(9) NA
None						
DISORDERS OF EGO						
51 Derealization	□	□	□	□	□	□
52 Depersonalization	□	□	□	□	□	□
53 Broadcasting	□	□	□	□	□	□
54 Withdrawal	□	□	□	□	□	□
55 Insertion	□	□	□	□	□	□
56 Other symptoms	□	□	□	□	□	□
None DISTURBANCES OF AFFECT						
59 Perplexity	□	□	□	□	□	□
60 Loss of feeling	□	□	□	□	□	□
61 Blunted affect	□	□	□	□	□	□
62 Loss vitality	□	□	□	□	□	□
63 Depressed mood	□	□	□	□	□	□
64 Hopelessness	□	□	□	□	□	□
65 Anxiety	□	□	□	□	□	□
66 Euphoria	□	□	□	□	□	□
67 Dysphoria	□	□	□	□	□	□
68 Irritability	□	□	□	□	□	□
69 Inner restless.	□	□	□	□	□	□
70 Complaintive	□	□	□	□	□	□
71 Inadequacy	□	□	□	□	□	□
72 Exag. self-esteem	□	□	□	□	□	□
73 Feeling of guilt	□	□	□	□	□	□
74 Feel. impoverish.	□	□	□	□	□	□
75 Ambivalence	□	□	□	□	□	□
76 Parathymia	□	□	□	□	□	□
77 Affect. lability	□	□	□	□	□	□
78 Affect. incon.	□	□	□	□	□	□
79 Affect. rigidity	□	□	□	□	□	□
None DISORDERS OF DRIVE AND MOTILITY						
80 Lack drive	□	□	□	□	□	□
81 Inhib. drive	□	□	□	□	□	□
82 Inc. drive	□	□	□	□	□	□
83 Motr. restless.	□	□	□	□	□	□

	0 AB	1 MI	2 MO	3 SV	4 EX	(9) NA
84 Parakinesia	□	□	□	□	□	□
85 Mannerisms	□	□	□	□	□	□
86 Histrionic	□	□	□	□	□	□
87 Mutism	□	□	□	□	□	□
88 Logorrhea	□	□	□	□	□	□
None CIRCADIAN DISTURBANCES						
89 Worse AM	□	□	□	□	□	□
90 Worse PM	□	□	□	□	□	□
91 Better PM	□	□	□	□	□	□
None OTHER DISTURBANCES						
92 Soc. withdrawal	□	□	□	□	□	□
93 Exc. soc. contact	□	□	□	□	□	□
94 Aggressive	□	□	□	□	□	□
95 Suicide	□	□	□	□	□	□
96 Self-mutilation	□	□	□	□	□	□
97 Lack. feel. ill	□	□	□	□	□	□
98 Lack insight	□	□	□	□	□	□
99 Uncooperative	□	□	□	□	□	□
100 Lack self care	□	□	□	□	□	□
None OTHER SYMPTOMS						
P1 Loss desire live	□	□	□	□	□	□
P2 Asthenia	□	□	□	□	□	□
P3 Accel. thinking	□	□	□	□	□	□
P4 Tension	□	□	□	□	□	□
P5 Inc. libido	□	□	□	□	□	□
P6 Sex dysfunction	□	□	□	□	□	□
P7 Altered sexuality	□	□	□	□	□	□
P8 Thought echo	□	□	□	□	□	□
P9 Pseudohalluc.	□	□	□	□	□	□
P10 _____	□	□	□	□	□	□
P11 _____	□	□	□	□	□	□
P12 _____	□	□	■	□	□	□
P13 _____	□	□	□	□	□	□
P14 _____	□	□	□	□	□	□
P15 _____	□	□	□	□	□	□

	0 AB	1 MI	2 MO	3 SV	4 EX	(9) NA
None DISORDERS OF CONSCIOUSNESS						
1 Lowered	□	□	□	□	□	□
2 Clouded	□	□	□	□	□	□
3 Narrowed	□	□	□	□	□	□
4 Expanded	□	□	□	□	□	□
None DISORDERS OF ORIENTATION						
5 Time	□	□	□	□	□	□
6 Place	□	□	□	□	□	□
7 Situation	□	□	□	□	□	□
8 Self	□	□	□	□	□	□
None DISTURBANCES OF ATTENTION & MEMORY						
9 Apperception	□	□	□	□	□	□
10 Concentration	□	□	□	□	□	□
11 Memorization	□	□	□	□	□	□
12 Retention	□	□	□	□	□	□
13 Confabulation	□	□	□	□	□	□
14 Paramesias	□	□	□	□	□	□
None FORMAL DISORDERS OF THOUGHT						
15 Inhibited thinking	□	□	□	□	□	□
16 Retarded thinking	□	□	□	□	□	□
17 Circumstant. think.	□	□	□	□	□	□
18 Restricted thinking	□	□	□	□	□	□
19 Perseveration	□	□	□	□	□	□
20 Rumination	□	□	□	□	□	□
21 Pressured thinking	□	□	□	□	□	□
22 Flight of ideas	□	□	□	□	□	□
23 Tangential thinking	□	□	□	□	□	□
24 Blocking	□	□	□	□	□	□
25 Incoherence	□	□	□	□	□	□
26 Neologisms	□	□	□	□	□	□

	0 AB	1 MI	2 MO	3 SV	4 EX	(9) NA
None PHOBIAS AND COMPULSIONS						
27 Suspiciousness	□	□	□	□	□	□
28 Hypochondriasis	□	□	□	□	□	□
29 Phobias	□	□	□	□	□	□
30 Obsess. thought	□	□	□	□	□	□
31 Comp. impulse	□	□	□	□	□	□
32 Comp. action	□	□	□	□	□	□
None DELUSIONS						
33 Del. mood	□	□	□	□	□	□
34 Del. perception	□	□	□	□	□	□
35 Sudden del. idea	□	□	□	□	□	□
36 Delusional ideas	□	□	□	□	□	□
37 Systematic del.	□	□	□	□	□	□
38 Del. dynamics	□	□	□	□	□	□
39 Del. reference	□	□	□	□	□	□
40 Del. persecution	□	□	□	□	□	□
41 Del. jealousy	□	□	□	□	□	□
42 Del. guilt	□	□	□	□	□	□
43 Del. impoverishment	□	□	□	□	□	□
44 Hypochon. del.	□	□	□	□	□	□
45 Del. grandeur	□	□	□	□	□	□
46 Oth. delusions	□	□	□	□	□	□
None DISORDERS OF PERCEPTION						
47 Illusions	□	□	□	□	□	□
48 Verbal halluc.	□	□	□	□	□	□
49 Oth. aud. halluc.	□	□	□	□	□	□
50 Visual halluc.	□	□	□	□	□	□
51 Bodily halluc.	□	□	□	□	□	□
52 Olf/gust halluc.	□	□	□	□	□	□

Unreliability	□	□	□	□	□	□

AB 0	MI 1	MO 2	SV 3	EX 4	NA (9)

A recent acquisition with the potential to enhance reliability of the English adaption has been provided by Lapierre and the Canadian group. They have translated the Leige semi-structured interview for the Psychopathological Symptoms section into English and the interview is currently being issued to new users as part of the training procedure (6).

Figure 2 presents the recording form for Part 5 - Somatic Signs. Again, the French mask was utilized in developing the English form. A standard Somatic Inquiry from the French AMDP has also been printed on the scale to provide a semi-structured aspect to the scale. Four items, i.e. S1-S4, were also added to the scale--again from the French AMDP.

At present time the English AMDP is playing a central role in two major projects at Tennessee Neuropsychiatric Institute. The first project, funded through NIMH, is designed to develop a clinically meaningful classification of a cross-cultural hospitalized chronic schizophrenic population (approximately 1500-2000 patients) on the basis of manifest psychopathological symptoms and to test the hypothesis that such psychopathological symptoms and derived symptom profiles are similar and occur with approximately the same frequency among different cultures; i.e., Africa, Asia, Europe, Latin America and North America. Along with the collection of detailed demographic, diagnostic and treatment data, an expanded version of the AMP-II Psychopathological Assessment Form--the version available at the initiation of the project--serves as the primary rating instrument. The scale was supplemented with items derived from the Present State Examination, the Schedule for Affective Disorders and Schizophrenia and from consultation with project members in order to cover the special needs of the chronic population which was to include both adult and "geriatric" schizophrenics. A structured interview procedure and a glossary of definitions were developed to enhance the consistency and reliability of assessment. Despite its variance with the current version, the scale fortunately includes all of the items of the AMDP-III Psychopathological Symptoms and, through extraction, compatible data can be obtained for comparative purposes.

One aspect of this project will be an effort to derive sufficient data for our analysis of the Leonhard classification system. This system is clearly one of the most comprehensive attempts to delineate subcategories of chronic schizophrenia and to postulate etiological differences as well as long-term outcomes among these subcategories. Concurrent with the project, a rating schema--based on the work of Fish and Astrup--has been developed at Tennessee Neuropsychiatric Institute (7). Through the use of a set of algorithms it should be possible to classify patients into Leonhard's subtypes with the data obtained from the psychopathological ratings.

190

HOSPITAL/CLINIC:

RATER:

PATIENT INITIALS ___ ___ PT. NO._____
                 1st Last

SEX: M____ F____

BIRTH DATE:_____

RACE: W__ B__ I__ O__ OTH_____

DATE OF EXAMINATION: ____/____/____
                       M   D   Y

| | | | | | | Patient Number
| | | | | Study Number
| | Sex (M = 1; F = 2)
| | | Age
| | | | | Race (W=1, B=2, I=3, O=4, Oth =5)

| | | | | Date of Examination
| M | D | Y |
| | | | Period

0	1	2	3	4	(9)	0	1	2	3	4	(9)	0	1	2	3	4	(9)	0	1	2	3	4	(9)
AB	MI	MO	SV	EX	NA	AB	MI	MO	SV	EX	NA	AB	MI	MO	SV	EX	NA	AB	MI	MO	SV	EX	NA

None ▢ SLEEP/VIGILANCE DISTURBANCES | **None** ▢ CARDIO-RESPIRATORY DISTURBANCES | **None** ▢ NEUROLOGICAL DISTURBANCES | **None** ▢ OTHER SYMPTOMS

	0	1	2	3	4	9		0	1	2	3	4	9		0	1	2	3	4	9		0	1	2	3	4	9
101 Diff. fall. asleep	▢	▢	▢	▢	▢	▢	117 Breathing diff.	▢	▢	▢	▢	▢	▢	132 Hypertonia	▢	▢	▢	▢	▢	▢	S1 Dreams/Nightmares	▢	▢	▢	▢	▢	▢
102 Interrupted sleep	▢	▢	▢	▢	▢	▢	118 Dizziness	▢	▢	▢	▢	▢	▢	133 Hypotonia	▢	▢	▢	▢	▢	▢	S2 Allergic reactions	▢	▢	▢	▢	▢	▢
103 Shortened sleep	▢	▢	▢	▢	▢	▢	119 Palpitations	▢	▢	▢	▢	▢	▢	134 Tremor	▢	▢	▢	▢	▢	▢	S3 Tardive dyskinesia	▢	▢	▢	▢	▢	▢
104 Early wakening	▢	▢	▢	▢	▢	▢	120 Cardiac pain	▢	▢	▢	▢	▢	▢	135 Acute dyskinesia	▢	▢	▢	▢	▢	▢	S4 Dependent edema	▢	▢	▢	▢	▢	▢
105 Drowsiness	▢	▢	▢	▢	▢	▢								136 Hypokinesia	▢	▢	▢	▢	▢	▢	S5	▢	▢	▢	▢	▢	▢

None ▢ APPETITE DISTURBANCES | **None** ▢ AUTONOMIC DISTURBANCES | 137 Akathisia | S6

| | | | | | | | 121 Blurred vision | ▢ | ▢ | ▢ | ▢ | ▢ | ▢ | 138 Ataxia | ▢ | ▢ | ▢ | ▢ | ▢ | ▢ | S7 | ▢ | ▢ | ▢ | ▢ | ▢ | ▢ |

106 Decr. appetite	▢	▢	▢	▢	▢	▢	121 Blurred vision	▢	▢	▢	▢	▢	▢	139 Nystagmus	▢	▢	▢	▢	▢	▢
107 Inc. appetite	▢	▢	▢	▢	▢	▢	122 Inc. perspiration	▢	▢	▢	▢	▢	▢	140 Paresthesia	▢	▢	▢	▢	▢	▢
108 Exc. thirst	▢	▢	▢	▢	▢	▢	123 Seborrhea	▢	▢	▢	▢	▢	▢
109 Decr. libido	▢	▢	▢	▢	▢	▢	124 Micturition diff.	▢	▢	▢	▢	▢	▢
							125 Menstrual diff.	▢	▢	▢	▢	▢	▢

Laterality N ▢   Y ▢
Convulsions N ▢   Y ▢

None ▢ G.I. DISTURBANCES | **None** ▢ OTHER SOMATIC DISTURBANCES

110 Hypersalivation	▢	▢	▢	▢	▢	▢							
111 Dry mouth	▢	▢	▢	▢	▢	▢	126 Headache	▢	▢	▢	▢	▢	▢
112 Nausea	▢	▢	▢	▢	▢	▢	127 Backache	▢	▢	▢	▢	▢	▢
113 Vomiting	▢	▢	▢	▢	▢	▢	128 Heaviness in legs	▢	▢	▢	▢	▢	▢
114 Gastric discomfort	▢	▢	▢	▢	▢	▢	129 Hot flashes	▢	▢	▢	▢	▢	▢
115 Constipation	▢	▢	▢	▢	▢	▢	130 Chills	▢	▢	▢	▢	▢	▢
116 Diarrhea	▢	▢	▢	▢	▢	▢	131 Conversion symptoms	▢	▢	▢	▢	▢	▢

Weight (lbs) | | | | | |
Temperature (°F) | | | | | |
Pulse (/mn) | | | | | |
BP, sitting, dia. | | | | | |
BP, sitting, sys. | | | | | |
BP, standing, dia. | | | | | |
BP, standing, sys. | | | | | |

STANDARD SOMATIC INQUIRY (from the French AMDP)

How have you been feeling physically in the last few days?
Sleeping well? (101-104) Bothered by dreams/nightmares?
(51) Sleeping during the day? (105)
Appetite good? (106,107) Drinking more water than usual?
(103,111)
Problems with digestion? Changes in defecation or
urination from normal? (112-116, 124)
Difficulty breathing? (117) Dizziness? (118) Blurred
vision (121)
Heart pounding or beating faster? (119,120)
Legs feel heavy? (128) Ankles swelling? (87)
Feeling warm (hot flashes)? (129) Chills? (130) Perspir-
ing (sweating more than usual? (122) Problems with skin
(rash)? (23,52)
Any aches or pains? (114,126,127) Any tingling? (140)
Periods regular? (135) Sexual difficulties (frigidity,
ejaculation)? (109)
Any other physical symptoms or signs?

COMMENTS

©1981 Association for Methodology and Documentation in Psychiatry (AMDP)

Given the cross-cultured nature of the project, the data should provide an opportunity to estimate the relative frequencies of occurrence of Leonhardian subtypes both within and across cultures. Since the same psychopathological data will serve as the basis for statistically derived subtypes, comparisons with the Leonhard as well as other classification schema can be accomplished.

The second project involves the psychometric analysis of a new adverse reaction scale developed by NIMH--the Systematic Assessment of Treatment Emergent Events (SAFTEE). SAFTEE has been designed to document fully the occurrence of adverse events during the course of a clinical trial. Its uniqueness lies in the methods of eliciting information--particularly the structured series of questions comprising the systematic inquiry. The project involves the collection of multiple ratings of both "live" and videotaped interviews to serve as the bases of the estimations of both reliability and validity for multidisciplinary raters, e.g., psychiatrists, residents, psychologists, nurses. The AMDP-Somatic Signs has been chosen as the "standard" or comparative instrument. As a consequence, it will be possible to pursue psychometric analysis for this instrument as well.

Data from both projects will provide a base for the development of a data bank at TNI. The capability already exists in the BLIPS system to provide a degree of standard documentation.

With a sufficient accumulation of data, non-specially-tailored documentation can be then developed and specific statistical analyses can proceed.

REFERENCES

1. Ban, T. A., 1978, The AMDP System in English, in: "Neuropsycho-pharmacology," Deniker et al., eds., Pergamon Press, Oxford, 1575-1579.
2. Guy, W. and Ban, T. A., 1983, The AMDP System and NCDEU/BLIPS Systems: Similarities and Differences, in: "The AMDP System in Pharmaco-Therapy," Bobon et al., eds., Mod. Prob. Pharmacopsychiat., Karger, Basel.
3. Arbeitsgemeinschaft fur Methodik und Dokumentation in der Psychiatrie, 1979, Das AMDP System: Manual zur Dokumentation Psychiatrischer Befunde, 3rd Ed., Springer Verlag, Berlin.
4. Guy, W. and Ban T. A., 1982, The AMDP System: Manual for the Documentation of Psychopathology, Springer Verlag, Heidelberg.
5. Bobon, D. P., 1983, Foreign Adaptations of the AMDP System, in: "The AMDP System in Pharmacotherapy," Bobon et al., eds., Mod. Prob. Pharmacopsychiat., Krager, Basel.
6. Lapierre, Y. D., 1983, Personal Communication.
7. Ban, T. A., 1982, Chronic Schizophrenia: A Guide to Leonhard's Classification, Comp. Psychiat. 23: 155-165.

THE AMDP - SYSTEM

SCANDINAVIAN ADAPTATION

Marianne Kastrup and Per Bech

Psychiatric Department P
Hillerød General Hospital
Hillerød - Denmark

INTRODUCTION

As we have heard today the AMDP-System was founded in 1965
by a group of psychiatrists from Germany, Switzerland, and Austria
in order to develop a uniform system for the documentation of information to be useful in both clinical practice and in research.
Whereas the earliest version emphasized the medical-biological
viewpoints, the more recent versions have comprised sociological
and demographic variables. The system has proven useful and has
later been translated into a number of languages with the Scandinavian Adaptation as the last version.

The Scandinavian Adaptation

The Scandinavian version is now on the way and will hopefully
be published very soon, and we have brought along a few preliminary copies. We have chosen to let AMDP be an abbreviation for
'almen klinisk metode og dokumentation i psykiatrien', i.e.
'general clinical method and documentation in psychiatry'. Translating from one language to another is a difficult task. In our
case it has been very successfully carried out thanks to our
German born research librarian. The Scandinavian adaptation is
primarily based upon the German edition, but a literal translation has not been possible. In certain points we have deviated
from the original edition and chosen the English edition, when
this was judged to be of greater consistency with Scandinavian
concepts.

It has been our ultimate aim to let the Scandinavian adaptation of the System be of greater practical use in daily clinical

work, as well in hospitals as in general practice, than the already existing adaptations. Compared with those the Scandinavian edition has been revised and supplemented in certain areas.

Alterations in the Scandinavian edition range from minor changes to the addition of new chapters

As an example of a minor alteration may be mentioned the change made in the chapter concerning instructions for the raters.

Here, in the German edition, the grading of symptoms takes place on a four point scale. In the Scandinavian edition, as in most other translations, symptoms are graded along a five point scale. In the latter scale, 1 comprises symptoms that are present only to a very limited degree, and this means that the AMDP system becomes more sensitive with regard to the less severe conditions. The five point scale is consequently of greater value in general practice, where such conditions are more prevalent.

Besides such minor alterations we have added the chapter on basic concepts such as reliability, validity, interview technique, diagnostic sensitivity and specificity. We have considered this edition important, as the AMDP-System is a clinically based method developed to improve the reliability and the validity of psychiatric diagnoses. With this addition we provide the reader with a more comprehensive manual for assessment thus increasing its practical use. We have not yet investigated the reliability and the validity of the Scandinavian translation, but from other studies the system has been reported to be of sufficient reliability, whereas knowledge about the theoretical validity of the scales is still lacking.

Other Scales

Over the last decades a number of other scales have been developed all with a similar purpose, namely, to standardize the many data and variables collected in clinical work as well as research. The presence of a large number of scales may - contrary to the intention - inhibit rather than facilitate international communication.

The introduction of the AMDP-System in Scandinavia shall not be seen as a step further in that direction. On the contrary, we have used this opportunity to coordinate the existing subscales into one system, and have chosen the AMDP-System because of its multiaxial structure. From the item combinations of the AMDP-System it is possible to derive subscales that are practically equivalent to the item combinations from the well known scales already existing. In the following slides I have selected a few examples of this transformation. The first slide shows the Hamilton Depression Scale with certain original items and the corresponding items derived from the AMDP III version.

The next slide shows, in a similar way, the 10 original items of the Newcastle Diagnostic scale and the corresponding AMDP III items.

In the next slide the AMDP III system is used for a Mania Scale, i.e. the Bech-Rafaelsen Mania Scale, with the 11 original items and the corresponding AMDP III items.

In a similar way, the scales may be constructed by deriving the relevant item combination from theAMDP system. It is our intension that the Scandinavian Adaptation serves as a handy manual in both clinical work and research. The system has not yet proven useful in Denmark, but we are now using it for the first time in re-search in a project on Narcolepsia. We hope that the Scandinavian Version may be widely used as a manual for the transformation of items. Ultimately this helps to facilitate comparisons between different existing subscales and thus to improve international communication.

THE JAPANESE ADAPTATION OF THE AMDP-SYSTEM

Hitoshi Itoh

Department of Neuropsychiatry, School of Medicine
Keio University, Tokyo 160, Japan

INTRODUCTION

The International Committee on AMDP has long had an intention
to put "Das AMDP-System" to worldwide usage as an instrument for
assessment and documentation of psychopathology. On committee
members' recommendation I have made efforts to complete the Japanese adaptation of this system. In the late 1970's we finished a
translation into Japanese of the first edition of "Das AMDP-System,
Manual zur Dokumentation." In 1978, when we were just about to
publish the Japanese version, the third edition of the book was
published.[1] Finding this edition considerable different in contents
from the first one, we started translating the manual third edition
into Japanese once again.

As known to you all, an English version of the manual was
completed by Guy and Ban in 1982.[2] Through the courtesy and with
permission of these authors, we used part of this English version
as a reference in making our Japanese version. In this way our
Japanese adaptation of the AMDP-System was brought into the world
in 1983. It is my great honor and pleasure to have an opportunity
of speaking at this Symposium on "Translation of the AMDP-System."
Here, I should like to comment on what we became aware of while
we were making the Japanese version of AMDP and present the results
of a preliminary trial use of the system for the clinical assessment of drug therapy.

PROBLEMS POSED WHEN MAKING THE JAPANESE VERSION OF THE AMDP-SYSTEM

In order for it to be used successfully and properly as a

197

common instrument for documentation of clinical data in international cooperative studies, the AMDP-System must be translated beforehand accurately in detail. As well known to us all, the Japanese language philologically is entirely different from Western languages. It took a much longer time than expected for us to put the manual of AMDP and data sheets correctly into Japanese, accordingly.

On the other hand, however, it is an undeniable fact that a psychiatric knowledge acquired by Japanese psychiatrists is based, to a more or less extent, on Kraepelin's psychopathological investigations and the nosology of mental disorders developed by him. Experts in psychiatry of Japan are well familiarized with making clinical records using methods in the Kraepelin style for describing psychopathological phenomena.

Generally speaking, the recording sheets of the AMDP-System are therefore rather easy for Japanese psychiatrists to use in spite of their enormous contents. Nevertheless, there are some likely problems to be picked up for discussion.

About Part 1 (Anamnesis - Demographic Data), Part 2 (Life Events) and Part 3 (Psychiatric History)

Concerning Part 1, it should be recognized that there are considerable differences between countries in social scheme, laws, etc. Taking "native language" on Column No. 7 as an example, the Japanese language which is spoken by more than one hundred million persons as well as the Chinese language spoken by more than a billion of people should be handled as distinct categories as are English, German, and French; otherwise inconvenience would inevitably occur in the conduct of a cross-national cooperative study. As regards "Religion" on Column No. 20, the number of categories needs to be increased. With respect to Part 2 (Life Events) and Part 3 (Psychiatric History) no noteworthy difficulties were encountered during translation and in actual recording.

About Part 4 (Psychopathological Symptoms) and Part 4 (Somatic Symptoms)

The number of symptom items is markedly reduced in the current revised edition (1979) as compared with the first edition of "AMP Psychiatrischer Befund." This deletion seems to have been made on deliberation by the authors of the original edition who were assigned to the revision. It seems to us, however, that when used for the routine documentation of hospital admission, the first edition allows more detailed recording of symptom evaluation to be made.

There is a discrepancy in the method of severity assessment. Thus, a 4-point scale was used in the original German edition, whereas its French and English versions are adopting a 5-point scale.

This latter scale apparently is more sensitive and preferable. It is highly recommendable, therefore, to standardize the severity rating scale throughout nations.

APPLICATION OF AMDP TO ASSESSMENT OF DRUG EFFICACY

We are now conducting a trial of haloperidol decanoate in schizophrenia. In preliminary study 20 hospitalized schizophrenics are receiving haloperidol decanoate given by intramuscular injection once every 4 weeks. The drug dosage is set at around 20 times the ordinary daily oral dose and actually 100-200 mg are being administered at one time.

Used for symptom assessment are Global Clinical Judgment, BPRS, Keio University Psychiatric Rating Scale (for schizophrenia) and AMDP-System in combination. Although this clinical trial is in progress, data obtained for the initial 8 weeks of treatment were compiled and subjected to statistical analysis to serve as a topic for discussion at this symposium on AMDP. It should be mentioned, however, that because detailed information about the statistical methods used by investigators of German speaking countries in the analysis of AMDP data was not available to us and also because we were not as yet well prepared for data processing by means of a

Table 1. Changes of AMDP Factor Scores (by Bauman & Angst) during Haloperidol Decanoate Treatment (N=20)

AMDP-Syndrome	Syndrome Scores* 0 W		8 W	
	$\bar{x}$	S	$\bar{x}$	S
F.1. Apathy (Apathisches S.)	50.6	± 4.7	49.0	± 3.9
F.2. Hallucinatory syndrome (Halluzinatorisch-desintegrative S.)	49.9	± 4.3	48.1	± 3.9
F.3. Hostility (Hostolitats-S.)	49.2	± 4.6	45.1	± 5.0
F.4. Manic syndrome (Manisches S.)	49.6	± 3.6	47.9	± 1.9
F.5. Somatic depressive syndrome (Somatisch-depressives S.)	50.7	± 3.7	49.3	± 2.9
F.6. Paranoid syndrome (Paranoid S.)	48.8	± 5.2	45.3	± 4.6
F.7. Catatonic syndrome (Katatones S.)	49.7	± 5.5	47.0	± 4.8
F.8. Retarded depressive syndrome (Gehemmt-depressives S.)	49.8	± 4.9	46.5	± 3.6
F.9. Hypochondriasis (Hypochondrisches S.)	50.5	± 4.1	48.8	± 2.4
F.S₁ Manic-depressive syndrome (Manisch-depressives S.)	51.0	± 4.4	48.8	± 2.2
F.S₂ Schizophrenic syndrome (Schizophrene S.)	48.2	± 4.7	45.3	± 4.4

Table 2. Changes of BPRS Factor Scores during
Haloperidol Decanoate Treatment   (N=20)

BPRS Factor		Factor Scores			
		0 W		8 W	
		$\bar{x}$	S	$\bar{x}$	S
F.I.	Anxiety-Depression	2.1 ±	1.1	1.5 ±	0.6
F.II.	Angergia	3.5 ±	0.9	2.9 ±	1.0
F.III.	Thought Disturbance	3.1 ±	0.9	2.5 ±	1.1
F.IV.	Activitation	2.7 ±	1.0	2.1 ±	1.0
F.V.	Hostile-Suspiciousness	2.7 ±	1.1	2.2 ±	1.1
	Total Score	50.7 ±	13.2	40.3 ±	14.9

large-sized computer, statistical analyses of the data to be
presented here had to be carried out by myself using a portable
calculating machine.

From data on the BPRS calculated were the total score and 5
factor scores by the method described in the ECDEU Assessment
Manual for Psychopharmacology (Revised, 1976) published by NIMH,
USA.[3] AMDP data, on the other hand, were translated into scores by
two technics, i.e. 9 factor solution devised by Bauman[4] and 2
factor solution ("manic-depressive syndrome" and "schizophrenic
syndrome") described by Woggon and others.[5,6]

Table 1 shows mean AMDP factor scores of the schizophrenic
patients before and at the 8th week of treatment, indicating
that improvement of Factor 3 (Hostility) and Factor 6 (Paranoid
syndrome) was noticeable after treatment. Table 2 shows 5 factor
scores and total score on the BPRS recorded simultaneously.

An attempt was then made to examine for correlationship
between changes of Manic-depressive Syndrome Score, Schizophrenic
Syndrome Score and BPRS Total Score before and after 8 weeks'
treatment and Clinical Global Judgment (5 points). Table 3 gives
values of Spearman rank correlation coefficients thus found,
indicating that BPRS Total Score best correlated with Clinical
Global Judgment and AMDP Schizophrenic Syndrome Score did second
best. For the purpose of reference the degrees of correlation
between the BPRS and AMDP factors at the start of treatment were
determined. As shown in Table 4, a striking correlation was noted
to exist between AMDP Manic-depressive Syndrome and BPRS Factor 2
(Anergia) and Factor 3 (Thought Disturbance) and also between AMDP
Schizophrenic Syndrome and BPRS Factor 3 (Thought Disturbance).

Table 3. Correlation Coefficients between Clinical Global Judgment and Charges of AMDP Rating Scales during 8-W Depot-Haloperidol Treatment (Spearman Rank Correlation Coefficient: N=20)

	AMDP Manic-depressive Syndrome Score	AMDP Schizophrenic Syndrome Score	BPRS Total Score
Clinical Global Judgment (5 points)	0.42	0.51	0.69

Table 4. Correlation Coefficients between AMDP 2 Factors and BPRS 5 Factors (N=20, Schizophrenics)

BPRS Factor \ AMDP Factor	Spearman Rank Correlation Coefficient	
	F_1 Manic-depressive syndrome	F_2 Schizophrenic syndrome
F.1. Anxiety-Depression	0.49	0.17
F.2. Anergia	0.69	0.37
F.3. Thought Disturbance	0.63	0.57
F.4. Activitation	0.48	0.23
F.5. Hostile-Suspiciousnes	0.24	0.39
BPRS Total Score	0.72	0.48

Table 5. Correlation Coefficients between AMDP 9 Factors and BPRS 5 Factors (Spearman Rank Correlation Coefficient: N=20, Schizophrenics)

BPRS Factor \ AMDP Factor	(F-1) Apathy	(F-2) Hallucinatory syndrome	(F-3) Hostility	(F-4) Manic syndrome	(F-5) Somatic dep. syndrome	(F-6) Paranoid syndrome	(F-7) Catatonic syndrome	(F-8) Retarded syndrome	(F-9) Hypochon-driasis
(F-1) Anxiety-Dep.	0.19	0.10	0.48	0.21	0.61	0.32	0.40	0.52	0.48
(F-2) Anergia	0.80	0.35	0.50	0.34	0.44	0.30	0.81	0.57	0.59
(F-3) Thought-Dis.	0.61	0.53	0.48	0.46	0.43	0.51	0.59	0.42	0.58
(F-4) Activitation	0.44	0.16	0.82	0.67	0.29	0.37	0.74	0.31	0.19
(F-5) Hostile-Sus.	0.42	0.39	0.47	0.41	0.25	0.48	0.54	0.15	0.33

201

Table 5 tabulates correlations between 9 AMDP factors and 5 BPRS factors. As can be seen, a distinct correlation was observed between AMDP Factor 1 and BPRS Factor 2, between AMDP Factor 2 and BPRS Factor 3, between AMDP Factor 3 and BPRS Factor 4, between AMDP Factor 4 and BPRS Factor 1 and between AMDP Factor 7 and BPRS Factor 2 and Factor 4.

SUMMARY

The author gave a brief account of the Japanese adaptation of "Das AMDP-System." The Japanese version of the AMDP is well suited for the routine documentation of psychopathology of various psychiatric patients and seems to prove of aid in education of postgraduate resident physicians. On the other hand, we have used the BPRS and other rating scales as a means of assessing symptoms in therapeutic studies. In order to make use of the AMDP-System as an assessment instrument in the evaluation of drug efficacy, further research efforts need to be made to establish those methods of statistical analysis which are able to yield highly reliable results from data recorded on AMDP recording sheets without requiring cumbersome operations. All in all, in order to serve the purpose of a cross-national cooperative study successfully, such methods of data analysis must be internationally standardized.

REFERENCES

1. H. Helmchen, Das AMDP System, Manual zur Dokumentation psychiatrischer Befund, 3rd. ed., Springer-Verlag, Berlin, Heidelberg, New York (1978).
2. W. Guy and T. Ban, The AMDP System Manual for the Assessment and Documentation of Psychopathology, Springer-Verlag, Berlin, Heidelberg, New York (1982).
3. W. Guy, ECDEU Assessment Manual for Psychopharmacology, U.S. Department of Health, Education and Welfare, Public Health Service, Rockville (1976).
4. U. Baumann and J. Angst, Methodological Development of the AMP System, in: "Neuropsychopharmacology," J.R. Boissier, H. Hippius and P. Pichot, ed., Excerta Medica, Amsterdam (1975).
5. B. Woggon und A. Dittrich, Konstruktion übergeordneter AMP-Skalen: "manisch-depressives" und "schizophrenes Syndrom," Int. Pharmacopsychiat. 14: 325 (1979).
6. B. Woggon, J. Fleischhauer und A. Widmer, Der Einfluss von Diagnose, Klinik und Geschlecht auf die Wirkung von Bromperidol, Int. Pharmacopsychiat. 14: 213 (1979).

THE PORTUGUESE ADAPTATION OF THE AMDP-SYSTEM

M. Paes de Sousa

Clinica Psiquiatrica Universitária
Hospital de Santa Maria
Lisboa, Portugal

In Portugal, the need of quantification in Psychopathology has been slowly established and was mainly underlined after the year 70's. In our case, we felt the need of using multifactorial psychopathologic scales and the elaboration of Portuguese versions.

However, there was some difficulty to handle these scales, influenced by the anglo-american psychopathology, specially when the purpose was not the clinical trial, but rather the diagnosis and the training of the younger doctors.

These reasons explain our enthousiasm for the AMDP system, mainly the psychopathologic sub-scale, which seemed to us more adapted to the psychopathology which we have learned and used, since Portuguese psychiatry has a strong influence of the German psychopathology.

Included in the French-speaking group of the AMDP, we started using this instrument and tried a Portuguese version; this has been just reached, since the Portuguese manual of the AMDP is already being printed.

The Portuguese adaptation of the AMDP system is essensially based on the 2nd French edition (Bonbon, D.P., 1981), although the common base of both the Portuguese adaptation and the French version is the 3rd German edition (Das AMDP system; 3- Aufl. Springer, Berlin, 1979). Since we do not know the German language, the Portuguese adaptation was carefully compared with the 3rd German edition by Prof. Barahona Fernandes, distinguished psychopathologist who has a deep knowledge of the German language. Wishing to follow closely the spirit of the original version, the German one, we tried in this way to be faithful to the underlying concepts of the corresponding items;

therefore, the general plan of our work was also that of the original version.

Although it is not a literal translation, our version is however more closely related with the French adaptation; thus we adapted many of its particularities, but we have disagreed with some other ones. In case of disagreement, we tried to explain it by a note.

The Portuguese adaptation, as the French one, is constituted by the edition of the complete AMDP scales and by the corresponding manual, by the sub-scales for mania, depression and schizophrenia, and by the anamnestic data with the changes introduced in the French version.

We also adapted the psychopathologic and somatic reserve items of the French edition, as well as the syndromatic scale, originated by the studies of factorial analysis from Liège; these were made after the 2nd French edition, therefore not yet included in that handbook.

We also adopted the number of answer degrees of the French edition, which has one unit more than the German edition, since the category "marked" was sub-divided in "marked" and "very marked".

Also, the identification heading of the various scales is the French one, since it seemed to us to be simpler than the German one.

Other particularities adapted by us were those concerning the recommendations for the examiner and the raters, was well as the model for certifying the share of the medical secret, in case of video rating and diffusion of the audio-visual recording.

We should refer now some of the particularities of the 2nd French edition which were not adapted in the Portuguese version and the changes made, when compared with both the French and the German versions, in order to reach a better adaptation to the Portuguese reality; these changes are indicated and explained in our manual.

Contrarily to the French edition, we kept the item 20 (present religion) of the anamnestic documents of the German edition, although with changes in the ranking of the religion, which seemed closer to the Portuguese reality; for similar reasons, we also made little changes in the following items: 1 - admission criteria; 7 - mother tongue; 15 - military duty; 36 - admission diagnosis.

The Portuguese version had some semantic and conceptual problems; this can be seen by the titles of some items of the psychopathologic scale which are different from the corresponding ones of the French version and are generally closer to those of the German manual as shown in Table 1.

Table 1. Difficulties of translation and/or concept

2.	Turvação da consciência	Bewusstseinstrübung
24.	Pensamento bloqueado/interrompido	Gesperrt/Gedankenabreissen
33.	Humor delirante	Wahnstimmung
39.	Auto-relacionação delirante	Beziehungswahn
46.	Outros temas delirantes	Andere Wahninhalte
53.	Desrealização	Derealisation
55.	Difusão do pensamento	Gedankenausbreitung
61.	Indiferença afectiva	Affektarm
62.	Perturbações dos afectos vitais	Störung Der Vitalgefühle
64.	Pessimismo	Hoffnungslos
78.	Incontinência afectiva	Affektinkontinent
79.	Rigidez afectiva	Affektstarr
2.	Bissolution de conscience	Clouded consciousness
24.	Pensée barrée	Blocking of thinking
33.	Pressentiment délirant	Delusional mood
39.	I.D. de référence	Delusions of reference
46.	I.D. fantastiques	Other delusions
53.	Etrangeté	Derealization
55.	Dévinement de la pensée	Thought broadcasting
61.	Anesthésie affective (observée)	Blunted affect
62.	Troubles de l'éprouvé vital	Loss of vitality
64.	Perte d'espoir	Hopelessness
78.	Hyperémotivité	Emotional incontinence
79.	Monotonie affective	Emotional rigidity

For instance, the item 2, called in French "Dissolution de la conscience", does not seem correct in Portuguese, since dissolution
refers to a homogeneous process, like in chemistry the dissolution
of fluids; thus, we preferred "clouded" in the sense of opaque, not
limpid, lacking clarity, as agitated water, which we believe to be
closer to the psychopathologic fact. Naturally, we understand that
"trouble" would be a term too ambiguous to be chosen for the French
version.

Item 24 was translated as "blocked thought" which explains better the
psychopathologic fact and is more correct in Portuguese, since
"barrer" means "cover" or "coat" in our language and not "interrupt".

Item 33 rises many problems. We chose "delusional mood" since it is
the classical term usually used in the Portuguese speaking countries.

On the other hand, we do not agree with "delusional foreboding", as
in the French version, as we believe it has a restricted concept
regarding the psychopathologic fact.

Regarding item 46, we adopted the German version, since it becomes
more general, enabling to rate other themes, as for instance
afilliation and not only the fantastic and imaginary ones as in the
French version.

The item 55 "thought broadcasting", seems to us a broader concept,
covering all the possibilities of that peculiar experience; the
thought ceases to belong to the person itself; "devinement" is only
one of the possibilities since it can exist reading, transmission,
sounding, etc.

We translated item 61 as "affective indifference" since it is exactly
what is observed; indifference and not anesthesia which is a feeling.

Regarding item 62 we wrote "vital affects", because it is familiar
to us the notion of "vital affects" or "vital feelings" in the sense
of Max Scheller, who classified feelings in sensorial, vital, animic
and spiritual; vital feelings correspond rather well to the definition of this item.

Items 39, 53 and 64 were translated by more usual words in Portuguese.
We could say the same for items 78 and 79; we used very common words
in our language which correspond rather well to the glossary.

"Incontinence", for instance, gives more the sense of lack of control
than hyperexcitability and hyperemotivity which can be voluntarily
caused. The same for "rigidity" which give well the idea of reduction
of the capacity of affective modulation. Monotony is the appearance;
one can have a monotonous affect by its own will; here there is an
impassibility which is different from the monotony by difficulty
of modulating the affects.

Because there is rigidity, ones becomes monotonous: although rigidity refers to the mechanism, it is the disregulation of the mechanism which is observed in the mental disease.

We also changed the title of one of the rubrics: "Night particularities" was replaced by "Circadian variations" which we found to be more correct, since circadian refers to a period of 24 hours.

Regarding the somatic scale, we adopted several medical terms, contrarily to the French version, in this case closer than ours to the German manual. We think however that the scale is used mainly by doctors, knowing the chosen terms.

The use of the AMDP scales, mainly the psychopathologic one, made by us and our coworkers, has shown to be very useful as a means of training, since it motivates the younger ones - usually not familiar with the details and precision of the psychopathologic observation - to have a more exact and concise understanding of the psychopathologic concepts, the rating of each item forcing to its concrete knowledge.

Besides, we think that this scale is also useful in the diagnosis (Sousa, M.P., 1982).

We also found that the use of this scale has several difficulties. In this sense, a structured - type interview saves time and enables a better filling of the scale, but disturbs the possibility of a spontaneous dialogue and probably the psychotherapeutic aspects which interviews must have.

Anyway, if the examiner does not have a great experience of the AMDP, it is preferable to make a semi-structured interview.

Problems have arisen on the simultaneous interview by several examiners; and even when performed by a single one - as it is the rule - but there are several raters attending and rating. This last difficulty is not only due to the fact that the patient feels less at ease and criates more resistences, but also to the fact that the raters are more dispersed.

This is why it is advantageous to have the interviews made by the patient's assistant physician.

The best inter-raters reliability is reached when, besides the interviewer, there are only one or two raters; the great advantage of the video-rating is exactly the fact that avoids this inconvenience.

On our side, we also have tried to assess the psychometric, clinical and research qualities of the AMDP scales, mainly of the AMDP-4.

For instance, we performed a determination of inter-raters reliability in 60 out patients with various pathologies; we obtained good reliability as well in the total sample as in the sub-samples the lowest refering to delusional states (Sousa, M.P., 1982).

We performed studies of reliability in diagnosis, in which we found agreement between diagnosis made by raters not knowing the patients and those made by their assistant physicians (Sousa, M.P., 1982). There was also agreement between the diagnosis of schizophrenia (paranoid states) made by the AMDP and by the criteria of the ICD-9 (Simões et al., 1983).

Our AMDP adaptation was also used in studies of nosological classification; this was the case in one separating, through correspondence analysis, endogenous from involutional depressions with the AMDP-4 (Sousa et al., 1983); and in another one in which, with the same statistical method, 6 timoleptics were discriminated when used in the treatment of 160 depressed patients, some inhibited, others agitated (Sousa et al., 1983).

Also, AMDP-4 was used in another similar study using the discriminant analysis (Figueira et al., 1983).

We are also presently trying to assess the concurrent validity of the AMDP-4 with other compatible instruments of measure, like PSE, SCL-90 and the "test-retest" reliability with in-patients.

We think that the AMDP system is a good working instrument, as well for teaching as for psychiatric research, for instance in psycho-pharmacologic studies and, particularly in the psychopathologic investigation; although it demands a prolonged training in its use and clinicians with great experience and good knowledge in psycho-pathology.

Having this opinion, we hope that the AMDP system will prove to be useful for the Portuguese speaking physicians especially for those initiating their training in psychiatry, mainly if we think that there is more than 100 millions of persons speaking Portuguese.

References
1. Arbeitsgemeinschaft für Methodik und Dokumentation in der Psychiatrie: Das AMDP-System; 3. Aufl., Springer, Berlin (1979)
2. Bobon, D.P., (ed.),"Le Système AMDP", 2e. Ed.,Mardaga, Bruxelles (1981)
3. Bobon, D.P., Mormont, C., Doumont, A., Mirel, J., Bonhome, P., Ansseau, M., Pellet, J., Pull, C., De Buck, R., Gernay, P., Mormont, I., Lang, F., Lejeune, J., Bronckart, C., et von Frenckell, R., Analyse factorielle de la révision française de l'échelle AMDP. Résultats d'un étude internationale de 388 cas, Acta psychiat. belge., 82: 371, 1982

4. Figueira, M.L., Costa, N.F., et Sousa, M.P., 1983, Analyse des-criminante de la symptomatologie dépressive évaluée par l'AMDP-4 (in preparation)
5. Simões, M., Vieira, C.R., Tropa, J., e Sousa, M.P., 1983, Valor das escalas AMDP-4 e AMDP-Sc na validação do diagnóstico da esqui zofrenia paranoide (in preparation)
6. Sousa, M.P., 1982, A tradução portuguesa do sistema AMDP e proble mas afins, Actas Luso-Esp. Neurol. Psiquiat., 10, 6 (extra): 445
7. Sousa, M.P., Figueira, M.L., and Nicolau, M.H., Classification Analysis of depression through AMDP-4, in: "Mod. Probl. Pharmaco-psychiat., vol. 20, D. Bobon, U. Baumann, J. Angst, H. Helmchen, H. Hippius, ed., Karger, Basel (1983)
8. Sousa, M.P., Figueira, M.L. and Nicolau, M.H., 1983, Discrimina-tion of anti-depressive drug patterns through factorial mathe-matical methods (in preparation).

METHODOLOGICAL PROBLEMS IN THERAPEUTIC RESEARCH

INTRODUCTION

H. Luccioni
Clinique Univ. de Psych., Hopital de la Timone
F-13385 Marseille Cedex 05, France

Only for the past 50 years or so have the authorities bothered to set the conditions by which the commercialization of new medicaments may be permitted. Today, regulations and practices nearly everywhere have imposed the same methodology, the so-called "controlled" trial. In reality, it is doubly controlled, for it concerns not only a comparative study with a "control" group but also an effort for "controlling" the variables of the situation on the experimental model.

Some undoubtedly think back with nostalgia to the period of discoveries when one disregarded what they deem to be petty administrative interference. But rather that dwell upon these precautional excesses which are all the same justified, particularly in the field of psychiatry, the fact that, at the end of long and costly manoeuvres, we haven't really learned much seems to me to merit reflexion: we have learned little about the medicament itself, for which indications, impact, and conditions of utilization must be specified through this "clinical experiment" whose so-called lack of "objectivity" was challenged when the more simple question concerning its efficacity was raised. We have learned little about the clinical reality and biochemical mechanisms of illness, whereas these therapeutic trials constitute that which Claud Bernard called the "passive experiments", the only ones which deontology authorizes to be carried out on man and which appear all the more necessary seeing that one stresses the uncertainty of animal "models of mental illnesses". I think that it is impossible to hunt two hares at the same time, to cite a french proverb.

It is legitimate that the collectivity verify the therapeutic interest of a product before it is marketed, doing so by means of a strategy which puts the product's purported intentions on the "defensive". To this end one must learn to define a reasonable procedure more precisely, giving the indispensable assurances as to the advantages and disadvantages of the product.

It is no less legitimate that psychiatrists consider the practical and theoretical consequences following upon the discovery of psychotropic medication and that a double interogation be developped with appropriate rigorosity: the one as to the best condition of utilization in concrete clinical situations, the other as to the reappraisal of the descriptions and explanations of psychopathology, with particular attention paid to that which takes place in the "black box". And in these two cases, the methodology, this time "offensive" in order to <u>find out,</u> cannot be that of the controlled trial.

Fortunately, much has already been thought and tried. We felt it proper to ask convinced researchers to give proof of their necessary awareness, more difficult than one may imagine, that we have entered the therapeutical era of psychiatry.

INTERRELATIONS BETWEEN METHODOLOGICAL

AND ETHICAL BASIC CONDITIONS IN PSYCHIATRIC THERAPY RESEARCH

Hanfried Helmchen

Psychiatrische Klinik und Poliklinik
Freie Universität Berlin
Eschenallee 3 - D-1000 Berlin 19 - FRG

BASIC CONDITIONS

Therapeutic research in psychiatry cannot be done without patients. The main reason is that therapeutic effects can be established only against diseases, but adequate disease models of most
human specific psychiatric diseases do not exist. Furthermore,
knowledge gained from pre- or extraclinical investigations can be
applied to psychiatric patients, particularly to those with more
severe psychiatric diseases, only to a rather limited extent.This
is valid not only for
a) the results of animal pharmacology, but also for
b) observations with psychotherapy on nonpsychiatric people, e.g.
   psychoanalytic experiences in healthy persons, or results of
   behaviour modification in smokers or obese clients, or even for
c) sociological hypotheses such as the labelling theory, the ir-
   relevance of which has been shown for some psychiatric diseases.
But the validity of results from investigations with psychiatric
patients themselves is limited too. Their generalizability will
be the less the more reductionistic the research approach is, e.g.
a) by a high selection of patients,
b) by quasi experimental standardization of the setting, or
c) by short duration of controlled clinical trials.
And the less the generalizability of results the more clearly the
question must be answered whether such trials are still justified
ethically. From this comes the demand for developing research
methods that will be less difficult ethically and yet justified
scientifically. Examples are methods for research
a) in "natural" settings, or
b) with outpatients, or
c) on long terms.

213

Insofar as therapeutic research in psychiatry cannot be done without patients it is related to therapeutic practice and it has to recognize the impact of personality.

Psychiatric diseases involve the personality of the ill more than other medical diseases. Furthermore, the personality of the physician may exert a much greater and even therapeutic influence on the patient than in other doctor-patient relationships. The stronger individuality of this special interhuman relationship means that both the psychiatrist's image of the patient as a person and the reductionism of research become more relevant in psychiatric research. The researcher has to be aware that the principally necessary reductionistic approach of research may be dangerous for the patient as well as for himself: the patient may loose personal values, the researcher may be biased to generalize partialities. In this respect the scientific obligation to avoid such bias and the ethical obligation to preserve the personal dignity of the patient should and may parallel each other.

Clinical research should not be seperated too much from clinical practice. Otherwise

a) it could be difficult to translate the results of research into practice,
b) the principal identity of ethical problems could be concealed, and
c) the work of different clinicians and researchers with the same patient could cause psychological and organizational problems and irritate the therapeutic process.

THE BASIC PROBLEM

The basic obligation of each physician is to give his patient the best therapy available. But what is the best therapy available? Ideally it is the therapy with the highest, most specific and most speedy efficacy and with no side-effects, risks or disadvantages. Unfortunately, in most cases such an ideal therapy does not exist. Therefore the physician has to know the balance between benefits and harms of therapies in general and furthermore he has to balance possible benefits and harms of therapy in respect to the individual patient, his own personal therapeutic experience and abilities,and the particular situation. Almost never will he have an unequivocal and sound knowledge of all these elements and their weight in the special case to influence his choice of therapy. Therefore, each therapeutic decision and its outcome are affected by the uncertainty of personal and probabilistic estimations. In this respect it can be said that each therapeutic decision is an experiment. From this can be deduced as follows:

a) Every therapeutic decision implies the ethical obligation of balancing between benefits and harms.
b) Every such balance is uncertain to some degree.
c) This uncertainty depends on the knowledge and competence of the physician.
d) Thus it is an ethical obligation for the physician to be in-

formed of the current knowledge in order to make the best choice, i.e. to maximize the benefits and to minimize the harms in each individual case. And it is also an ethical demand to improve one's general knowledge.

It is the aim of therapeutic research to improve and extend knowledge on the efficacy and safety of therapy. As far as such knowledge is scientifically proven today at least in respect to its generalizability, it is supraindividual in nature: i.e. it is gained from more than one patient and it surmounts the experience of each individual physician. Due to the comparability of individual observations this kind of scientifically gained knowledge implies stereotyping of observations and of therapeutic measures, and for testing hypotheses an experimental design often is necessary - as in controlled clinical trials, a major tool in modern therapy research. All these measures, obligatory from a methodological point of view, may bring inconveniencies, disadvantages or risks to the involved research patient.

This seems to oppose the ethical obligation of the physician to minimize the possible harms of therapy in the individual case. But this in turn opposes the ethical demand for scientifically based improvement of therapy for all ill people. We called this the paradox of the clinical trial. WING explained that it is really not a paradox but rather a complication of the everyday therapeutic decision based on balancing between good and harm.

Thoughts for overcoming these complications are as follows:

a) The only reasons for an investigational therapy are that there is no efficient therapy for a special disease, or that the therapeutic range of standard therapies has to be improved. Therefore its higher degree of uncertainty and perhaps disadvantage may be counterbalanced by the chance of the patient under investigation to receive a therapy which is better than the existing ones. From this follows that the balance between advantage and disadvantage has to be more explicit than in the everyday therapeutic decision.

b) Although it is ethical to give the individual patient the best therapy available as well as to improve therapy by research there is a difference: the first is an unconditioned obligation, the second is an obligatory demand. To put the benefit of the individual patient on the highest rank is reasoned by the experience that this in general will be more unequivocal, more stable in time, and less open to misuse. From this order follows that the requirements of information and consent must be stricter with research therapy than in the everyday therapeutic decision.

Thus ethically there is no principal difference between therapeutic decisions in clinical practice and in research. But there are gradual differences both in respect to the accurate explicitness of balancing between benefits and harms and the degree of informed consent. These are the ethical norms as stated in the declaration of Helsinki/Tokyo 1964/75. A special problem should be mentioned here. The uncertainty of each individual therapeutic decision may

create innovations. This brings up the question where clinical practice becomes research. The answer must be threefold: In respect of
the ethical dimension there is no principle difference between an
innovative variation of a standard therapy and an investigational
therapy in the framework of a research project. But methodologically
there is a difference insofar as the former is based on individual
observations, or on ideas alone, or on serendipity, whereas the
latter tries to answer a question in a controllable way. And especially from a practical point of view there seems to be a rather
big difference: an investigational therapy declared as research
is more or less under control of the scientific community and ethical committees whereas this is often not the case with "innovative"
therapies.

SPECIAL PROBLEMS IN PSYCHIATRIC RESEARCH

Informed Consent
Informed consent should not be misunderstood as a purely technical
measure in order to minimize risks. It should rather give the patient the opportunity of choice and selfdetermination in order to
realize the dignity of his person as a basic element of the therapeutic relationship. But even in this respect there are some problems in psychiatry.
The declaration of Helsinki/Tokyo requests the sufficient information of the patient on the aim, the mode, the expected benefits,
risks and possible inconviencies of the trial. But what does "sufficient" mean with a psychiatric patient? The validity and extent
of the informed consent may be restricted either by the patient's
reduced ability to understand or to consent, by a therapeutic pri-
vilege in respect to a patient's limited endurance capacity, or by
methodological necessities, e.g. the use of a placebo.
Information of patients will be insufficient or even impossible with
patients with severe psychiatric disorders such as delirious states
or dementias: the same will be true for the consent of patients with
states of excitation, anxiety, dependency, aggressiveness, or suicidality. However, for just such patients there is a strong need
to improve existing therapies by research. This problem cannot be
solved by the implementation of a legal guardian because possible
negative social consequences of such a procedure may score rather
high in considerations of the risk-benefit-ratio.

Not only in everyday practice but also in clinical therapy research
it is necessary to balance the risks and benefits of informed consent. Thus it seems to be unethical to increase the anxiety of patients by detailed information on possible inconviencies or complications or to get informed consent from patients with retarded
depressions who could also develop feelings of guilt after having
consented or not.

Informing the patient on details of blind or placebo designs may both increase his subjective suffering and contradict the purpose of the study. It may cause not only a high drop-out rate but may be considered as a scientific absurdity, because the supposition to exclude a subjective bias is to keep the patient (and the doctor) ignorant of the application of such techniques. BOBON in Belgium "successfully supported the view that, in psychiatry, the informed consent ... is contrary to research neutrality, inducing uncontrollable placebo or nocebo effects." Others, however, argue that not giving full information to the patient on the use of a blind technique or a placebo is a fraud that will destroy a trusting doctor-patient-relationship. In any case it can be said that "recognizing the existence of ethical dilemmas is a necessary prelude to the quest for objective solutions." With respect to research it must be made very clear that empirical knowledge on the consequences of informed consent is rather lacking. Research should answer at least the following questions:

a) What are the consequences of information and consent on therapy, e.g. on compliance or outcome?

b) What role does informed consent play as a selection factor, particularly in a psychiatric population? What are, in that case, the consequences of research results on comparability and generalizability?

Controlled Trials

Control groups, randomization, blind techniques, and the use of placebos are the major elements of controlled clinical trials carried out with the aim of eliminating unspecific known or unknown, objective or subjective influences. Especially in psychiatry the elimination of the latter is essential because of high level of unspecific personality-dependent influences on the therapeutic outcome with respect to both the experience of the patient and the observation and interpretation of phenomena by the physician.

The use of placebos poses not only the already discussed contradictive methodological difficulty. There is also the problem of giving a supposedly inefficient therapy. But it is a misunderstanding that placebo treatment has no efficacy. The percentage of up to 40 % of a positive placebo response is an argument against this view. This is, of course an unspecific but nevertheless a therapeutic effect. Therefore it seems ethical to use a placebo where a specific therapy with evident efficacy does not exist or where the disease has no dangerous or life-threatening intensity or acuteness. It may be mentioned that there is a rather broad variety of views on the ethical admissibility of placebos. An example: placebo-controlled investigations on the relapse prophylactic efficacy of Lithium were already considered unethical in the Scandinavian countries in the late sixties whereas at the same time in England they were still called for. Practical problems may arise from the formalized structure of the research design, e.g. the restriction of individualized or additional therapies or the randomization. Sometimes the care personnel may exert a subliminal prescreening of patients, if they are not

well informed of the aims and justification of the investigation
and if they are unconvinced that there will be no real disadvantages for the patient. Therefore information on aims, procedures,
and results of research and corresponding training of all personnel
involved in clinical research is an often neglected but nevertheless
important task.

Reference

Helmchen, H., 1982, Ethical and practical problems in therapeutic
        research in psychiatry.
        Compreh.Psychiat., 23: 505-515

DISCUSSION : INTERRELATIONS BETWEEN METHODOLOGICAL AND ETHICAL

BASIC CONDITIONS

David Wheatley

Psychopharmacology Research Group

Twickenham, TW2 5AX, U.K

The guiding principle in research as in clinical practice must always be the answer to the question: "What is best for the patient?"

I have been involved for many years in conducting clinical trials of psychotropic drugs in general practice. These have posed particular ethical problems, since the patients are of course unsupervised, and in many instances, continuing with their normal daily lives. These involve interrelationships with other individuals both at work and socially, driving motor vehicles and the physical hazards of certain occupations such as: operating machinery, working at heights, etc., and most importantly, inter-actions with alcohol.

In these circumstances, adverse side-effects may constitute a much more acute problem than in a hospital or clinic setting. And yet, just because the majority of psychiatrically ill patients are treated in their home environments, it is essential to investigate not only the beneficial effects of new drugs but also the impact of their side-effect potential. For example, dry mouth is a side-effect that would pass unremarked upon by either psychiatrist, nursing attendant or patient, when that patient is lying in a hospital bed. But imagine the patient at work who is constantly using the telephone and this seemingly minor side-effect becomes of such paramount importance as to oblige the patient to stop taking the drug. Under these circumstances, an alternative drug even although it might be therapeutically inferior but does not produce this side-effect, may become the drug of choice.

The use of placebo controls in clinical trials constitutes another problem, but nevertheless there must always be an ethical obligation to determine that the patient really needs a potent drug, particularly in the long-term. As Professor Helmchen has emphasized, potent drugs are usually accompanied by potent side-effects, which may well be justified in life-endangering illnesses and when no other effective forms of treatment are available. To condemn a patient to a "life sentence" of drug taking with possible serious adverse effects in the long-term, cannot possibly be justified unless the effectiveness of the drug has been fully determined as a result of placebo controlled trials.

I have been mainly involved in investigating the effects of drugs in the affective disorders, namely depression and anxiety. These provide two useful contrasts in relation to these ethical problems.

In the case of depression, since reasonably effective anti-depressant drugs are available, it would be extremely difficult to justify a placebo controlled trial in general practice at the present time, in view of the danger of a fatal termination to the illness consequent upon suicide. The current range of anti-depressant drugs has been extensively evaluated in many thousands of patients worldwide and their properties are indisputably documented. Their main disadvantages are the slow onset of effect (10-14 days), and the proportions of patients who either do not respond or respond incompletely, necessitating prolonged treatment. It is therefore of paramount importance to assess new antidepressant drugs that may overcome these problems, and this would be in the best interest not only of the individual depressed patient but all other patients with this illness. Nevertheless, it should be possible to undertake trials in comparison to established anti-depressant drugs rather than run the ethical risks involved by using a placebo.

In trials of anxiolytic drugs, on the other hand, it might be considered almost obligatory to include a placebo. In this condition there is undoubtedly a strong placebo effect and the alternative might be to produce drug dependence (as in the case of the benzodiazepines) with continuing long-term risks from side-effects, and in particular drowsiness. The extent to which an individual patient may respond to placebo can only be determined by administering a placebo to that patient, and so to do must therefore be totally justifiable for the purposes of a clinical trial.

As Professor Helmchen has emphasized, the doctor-patient relationship is paramount in clinical research and in any properly conducted clinical trial it is essential to take into account this relationship. In studies undertaken by our group we have demonstrated the beneficial effect on drug response of an optimistic attitude on the part of physician and patient alike in anxiety, although no such relationship exists in depression. The occurrence of life events, both adverse and beneficial during the course of the trial must also be fully documented, since both can influence the response to anxiolytics and adverse events the response to antidepressants.

In conclusion, may I emphasize the importance of assessing drug effects in the milieu in which they will be subsequently used, namely general practice.

LIMITS AND USEFULNESS OF CLINICAL PSYCHOPHARMACOLOGY

Bruno Musch and Paolo L. Morselli

Clinical Research Department
L.E.R.S. Synthelabo
58, rue de la Glacière Paris, FRANCE

INTRODUCTION

The discovery of psychoactive drugs has followed different historical phases. Initially attempts were made to utilize natural compounds capable to modify behaviour or to synthetized analogue chemical structures. Later on the discovery "by chance" of therapeutic effects of drug developed in other indications has represented a quite frequent event in psychopharmacology,underlying the difficulty in finding adequate animal models to predict a therapeutic effect in psychiatric illness. Subsequently to the discovery of "mile stone" psychoactive drugs the developmental strategy has followed an "indirect" comparative methodology by modifying molecules known to have a psychotropic action and comparing in animal selected models the activity of the new molecules to the activity of the known ones. A moderne and more challenging approach is the one which tries to infere from the understanding of possible mechanism of action a molecular structure which could fit the ethiopatogenetic hypothesis.

ANIMAL PHARMACOLOGY

Adequate animal models for human psychiatric disorders do not exist as human psychopathology is unreproducible in animals. The conventional approach to the development of a psychotropic durg is based on a number of animal tests and related investigations which are selected according to a given biological model. This leads to the restriction of the detection of psychotherapeutic agents to similar molecular structures acting through the same mechanism with a scanty possibility to discover really innovative drugs. Further-

223

more drugs inactive in this screening battery risk to be lost for
further development anly because they do not comply with biological
model taken into consideration.

CLINICAL PHARMACOLOGY

Although a compound screened by means of sophisticated pharmacological tests can possess a clear-cut central activity, when it
reaches the humans, its clinical usefulness and even its psychotropic effects are still to be defined and demonstrated. This
implies that a classical approach of research in volunteers, aimed
to assess merely whether the compound is well tolerated and which
kind of noxious effects can produce, is scarcely informative in
terms of prediction of specific clinical efficacy. Acute single dose
studies are classically implemented by repeated dose studies which
can provide further information on short term safety without increasing the predictivity for long term safety. This step is generally
followed by open clinical trials in patients "fishing" for clinical response with the consequence that a large number of patients
needs to be exposed to the experimental drug before reaching some
evidence of clinical activity and of possible therapeutic dose to
justify further clinical development. It becomes evident that clinical pharmacology with psychoactive drugs needs to be more accurate
and comprehensive of all investigable areas of CNS activity in order
to narrow the gap between animal pharmacology and clinical pharmacology by integrating all possible informations from volunteers in
a human pharmacological profile which can be utilized for its predictivity. The aim of phase I studies in volunteers can be reformu-
lated for psychopharmacology purposes as : to test drug effects on
CNS activity by measureing different variables in volunteers in a
given experimental situation in order to achieve results which can
be considered predictive of clinical response in patients.

STUDIES IN VOLUNTEERS

In an usual laboratory setting one can monitor in unselected
volunteers many different behavioral, psychomotor and physiological
effects induced by single or repeated doses of a given compound.
The single reporting of any newly perceived symptoms by the subject
can be quantitized by the use of visual analogue scales as proposed
by Aitken[1] or adjective check lists[2] and integrated by the observer
reporting. The utilisation of Personality Inventories such as MMPI
and the IPAT is mandatory to better describe the sample population
and to possibly utilize some subject personality traits as a tool
for interpretation of drug effects. Another important variable to
be measured is the level of emotional arousal of the subject (i.e.
by means of the Spielberger State Trait Anxiety[3]) as this can strongly interfere with drug response both in safety evaluation and in

quality and quantity of behavioral and psychomotor effect. Physiological variables (blood pressure, pulse rate, sweating etc.) are useful not only to evaluate noxious effects but also to use them as markers for measuring psychic reactions assuming that these variables reflect something about subject's level of arousal or mood state.

PHARMACOKINETICS

As far as pharmacokinetic studies are concerned it has been assumed for long time that the definition of the pharmacokinetic profile is sufficiently informative for a better or more rational use of the drug : however recent data have shown that in most cases with high liposoluble psychoactive drugs, data obtained on absorption, bioavailability, protein binding, plasma half life and clearence are not superimposable for the patient where, very frequently, the tested drug is administered in association with other drugs capable of modifying the pharmacokinetic profile . Furthermore in this type of studies, where pharmacokinetic is studied as such, no information can be obtained on the possible therapeutic and toxic thresholds and consequently on the possible blood concentration/clinical effect relationship. The last inconvenient could be partially avoided by applying, already during studies in volunteers, an integrated approach where modifications of physiological variables and side effects are related both to drug plasma levels and to personality profile of the subject[4]. With this approach if we cannot for sure identify the therapeutic indication we can at least more accurately forecast the range of active dose. However even with this approach it is difficult to fully understand the information on the various factors capable to modify the kinetic profile and the therapeutic response of patients undergoing chronic treatment. In this respect even kinetic studies in patient are not informative and the only way to really achieve a rationale drug administration is to perform "biological monitoring" during phase II and III studies[5].

EVALUATION OF COGNITIVE FUNCTIONS

Techniques to evaluate cognitive functions are extensively used but they result to be often insensitive to drug induced changes, inconvenient to replicate, only partially assessing a given function and consequently leading to an overinterpretation of results from a single test. Furthermore it is fundamental to stress that the mode and level of activity of central nervous system in influenced by personality[6,7,8,9], motivation[10] and learning abilities[11], which vary from subject to subject and within the same subject according to different situations. It is also true that most of the effects detected by psychomotor techniques reflect a response along the axis "stimulant-sedative." Usefulness of these techniques is undoubtful, but they can be psychologically relevant only if the study of the drug induced effects in integrated in a well defined model where one can clearly identify what is measured by which technique in a given experimental situation, as proposed by Hindmarch[12] .

PHARMACO-EEG

The need for a more objective and quantifiable measurement of central effects has lead to the utilisation of EEG in the development of psychoactive drugs (pharmaco-EEG). This technique has gained an important role especially with the application of computer analysis[13] -. Supporters of this methodology are claiming such a superior predictive value towards all other existing techniques that pharmaco-EEG should be considered as the "method of choice" in psychopharmacology. More realistically, although the usefulness of this type of study is undoubtful, some limitations should be taken into account to avoid misleading extrapolations. The meaning of changes in electrical activity of the brain is unknown and any attempt to predict psychotropic properties by means of the measure of an electrophysiological phenomenon should be regarded as an overinterpretation. Moreover pharmaco-EEG is a complex and expensive procedure which still lacks of an international convention. The drug classifications proposed by mean of pharmaco-EEG can be done only by indirect comparison within limited models. Finally effective doses on EEG patterns and duration of effect are not predictive of therapeutic doses and of clinical effect duration.

SLEEP-EEG

Efficient and reliable sleep laboratories are now available where all sleep parameters are extensively studied. These studies are mandatory in the development of hynoptic compounds[14]. Another important information which can be achieved in these laboratories is the impact of a given drug on the electrical organization of sleep patterns. As some sleep-EEG patterns abnormalities have been correlated with specific psychiatric disorders[15], it has been proposed to consider in terms of prediction of therapeutic activity the capability of a drug to counteract these abnormalities. At present this approach is still speculative. Finally the attempt to classify drugs according to sleep-EEG characteristics faces the same problem of quantitative-EEG.

NEUROENDOCRINOLOGY

It is well known that biogenic amines and other neurotransmitters play a role in the modulation of anterior pituitary hormone secretion (APHS) . This means that if drugs which have therapeutic actions do so because of their effects upon neurotransmitters it is possible that these effects would be associated with changes in APHS which could be used as an index of clinical effects. As far as neuroleptics this approach appear to be particularly meaningful as their administration leads to a reproducible and dose-dependent elevation of PRL secretion in the individual subject [16], within a given dose range ; furthermore a positive relationship has been shown between the antipsychotic effect of neuroleptic and the associated elevation of PRL as well as between extrapyramidal symptoms, neuroleptic serum levels and PRL level after neuroleptic administration[17]. These results however were not confirmed. The administration of other class of psychoactive drugs does not lead to consistent hormonal changes nor to endocrinological side effects. Unfortunately there are several limitations to the study of APHS as an index of more central events : APHS varies in relation with temporal factors, feedback effects from target hormone secretion play an important role, it exists a wide variation in normal levels of these hormones,non specific stimuli can interfere with APHS and finally the systematic administration of psychoactive drugs provides little evidence as to their site of action.

INDUCED STATE MODEL

More specific behavioral techniques have been studies to over-come the gap between drug effects in normal subjects and clinical effect in patients and to give to the former a predictive value. Two main behavioral strategies have been followed: the use of so called symptomatic volunteers and the use of induced state models. In the former, volunteers are characterised as far as their person-ality traits. A specific effect of a drug in a particular person-ality group or on a particular personality trait can be interpreted as a predictive effect in a certain clinical situations or on par-ticular symptoms[18] assuming that, within a limited range of illness severity, it exists a continuum between "normality" and "psychopa-thology." The latter approach have been extensively tried in the past but results are equivocal[19].

CONCLUSIONS

On the basis of the above considerations we think that the pre-dictive value of phase I studies can vary according to the different classes of drugs to be tested.
Only for anxiolytics and hypnotics a certain degree of predic-tivity can be achieved in phase I studies, whereas the chance to predict an antipsychotic or antidepressant effect at an early stage is very low. In conclusion predictive value of clinical pharma-cology in volunteers and in early clinical studies is not satisfac-tory : none of all experimental techniques is "per se" predictive of a specific clinical response leading to the risk of overinter-pretation based on partial and inaccurate assessments. In parti-cular in volunteers an "integrated model" should be pursued aiming to achieve a human pharmacological profile which takes into account in all different areas to be explored the interaction between exter-nal factors (drug pharmacological characteristics, experimental

conditions) and internal factors such as subject's personality,
constitutional factors (age, social and cultural background) and the
emotional state at the time of the experiment.   In patients we
underline the need for a better quality of phase I studies which
are at present neglected because they are considered to be less
informative than phase II double-blind trials.   If the working
hypotheses towards to move are better defined thanks to more informative data from volunteers, early studies in patients can play an
important role.   Attention should be payed in patients to describe
the clinical characteristics of the experimental samples in order
to correlate the clinical response to the clinical situations.
Clinical evaluation appropriate for this type of studies should be
implemented by the use of some of the techniques utilized in volunteers such as psychomotor tests, quantitative-EEG, neuroendocrinology, together with the proposed model of "biological monitoring".
In fig. 1 we have tried to draw the idea of an "integrated approach"
for the developmental process of a psychotropic drug in modern
clinical pharmacology.

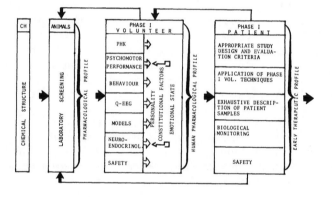

Fig. 1.   The integrated approach

Three principle steps are to be recognized before entering the extensive phase II : the animal screening of a chemical structure to
obtain the pharmacological profile, than a comprehensive phase I
in volunteers which should take into account all the possible interactions between the experimental situation, the drug and the subject's psychophysiological characteristics in order to achieve a
human pharmacological profile as predictive as possible.
The early clinical studies will follow this step : they will adequately compare the preliminary results in patients to the ones in
volunteers to build up an early therapeutic profile which will
allow a rational approach to extensive clinical trials.   Finally
we think it is important to underline that an unceasing feed-back
should exist between clinical pharmacology and animal pharmacology
which can allow a better understanding of the mechanism of action
of the drug under study.

REFERENCES

1. R.C.B. Aitken, Measurement of feeling using visual analogue scales, Proc. Roy. Soc. Med., 62:989 (1969).
2. V. Nowlis, Research with the mood adjective check-list, in :"Affect, Cognition and Personality" S. Tomkins, and C. Izard, Eds. Springer, New York, pp. 352 (1965).
3. C.D. Spielberger, R.L. Gorsuch, and R.E. Lushene, " Manuel for the State-Trait Anxiety Inventory", Tallehasse, Florida State University (1968).
4. P.L. Morselli, G.F. Placidi, C. Maggini, R. Gomeni, M. Guazelli, G. de Lisio, S. Standen and G. Tognoni, An integrated Approach for the Evaluation of Psychotropic Drug in Man, Psychopharmacologia (Berl.), 46:211 (1976).
5. P.L. Morselli, Chairman's Introductory Remarks, in :"Neuro-psychopharmacology" B. Saletu et al., Pergamon Press (1979).
6. H.J. Eysenck, "Experiments with drugs", Pergamon, Oxford (1963).
7. G.S. Claridge, "Drugs and Human Behavioural", A.Lane, London (1970).
8. A. Malpas, N.J. Legg and D.F. Scott, Effects of hypnotics on anxious patients, Br. J. Psychiat., 124:482 (1974).
9. M. Tansella, C. Zimmermann-Tansella, and M. Lader, The residual effects of N-desmethyldiazepam in patients, Psychopharmacologia 138:81 (1974).
10. F.J. Ayd, Motivations and rewards for volunteering to be an experimental subject, Clin. Pharm. Ther. 13:771 (1972).
11. K. Taeuber, M. Badian, H.F. Brettel, Th. Royen, W. Rupp, W. Sittig, and M. Uihlein, Kinetic and dynamic interaction of clobazam and alcohol, Br. J. Clin. Pharmac. 7-91s (1979).
12. I. Hindmarch, Psychomotor function and psychoactive drugs, Br. J. Clin. Pharmac. 10:189 (1980).
13. W.M. Herrmann, Some examples for the possibilities and limitations of pharmacoelectroencephalography as a method in clinical pharmacology, Meth and Find Clin. Pharmacol., 3 (supp. 1), 55S (1981).
14. I. Oswald, Sleep studies in clinical pharmacology, Br. J. Clin. Pharmac. 10:317 (1980).
15. P. Coble, F.G. Foster and D.J. Kupfer, Electroencephalographic sleep diagnosis of primary depression, Arch. Gen. Psych. 33:1124 sleep diagnosis of primary depression, Arch. Gen. Psych. 33:1124
16. G. Langer, G. Sachar, E.J. Nathan and R.S. Tabriezi, Dopaminergic factors in human prolactin regulators a pituitary model for the study of a neuroendocrine system in man, Psychopharmacology, 65:161 (1979).
17. T. Kolakowska, D.H. Wiles and A.S. McNeilly, Correlation between plasma levels of prolactin and chlorpromazine in psychiatric patients, Psychol. Med., 5:214 (1975).
18. A. Dimascio, R.E. Meyer, and L. Stifler, Effects of imipramine on individuals varying in level of depression, Amer. J. Psychiat., 124:55 (1968).
19. R.C. Pillard and S. Fisher, "Psychopharmacology : A generation of Progress", A. Lipton, ed., Raven Press, New York (1978).

BIOLOGICAL MARKERS AS MEASURES OF CHANGE

A. Villeneuve and C. Lajeunesse[*]

Dept. of Psychiatry, Faculty of Medicine
Laval University
Quebec G1K 7P4, Canada

I- INTRODUCTION

The ever increasing technological developments and refinements have made possible, in biological psychiatry, to attempt to delineate more precisely the diagnoses and the underlying mechanisms involved in psychopathological states. Research has also aimed, not only at enlarging our therapeutic armamentarium, but also at a better utilization of the available psychotropic drugs. Therefore, correlations have been tried between biological modifications, psychiatric diagnoses and prediction of response to treatment. It is in the field of affective disorders that such an approach of identifying biological markers has shown more successful. Such biological markers ideally could be used as investigational and diagnostic tools, as well as for the prediction of response to treatment and the measurement of change during therapy. The literature in this field is extremely abundant and only a very brief overview can be given here.

II- BIOLOGICAL MARKERS IN AFFECTIVE DISORDERS

Several parameters have been considered as being possibly representative pathophysiological markers of melancholia (Greden, 1982):

a) <u>Neuroendocrine tests</u>

1. Dexamethasone Suppression Test (DST)

[*] Interne, Service du Prof. T. Lempérière, Hôpital Louis Mourier, Colombes, France.

231

2. Thyrotropin (TRH) Stimulation Test
3. Growth Hormone Stimulation Test
4. Prolactin Response to Morphine
5. Melatonin/Cortisol Ratio
6. Luteinizing Hormone (LH) Response to LHRH
7. Urinary Free Cortisol (UFC) levels

b) Sleep electroencephalography

1. Decreased REM latency
2. Increased REM density
3. Reduction in delta sleep
4. Impaired sleep efficiency
5. Discriminant function scores

c) Psychomotor markers

1. Increased Speech Pause Time (SPT)
2. Limb motility
3. Facial electromyography during states of affective imagery

d) Biochemical measures

1. Urinary MHPG
2. Platelet Monoamine Oxydase (MAO) activity level
3. In vitro lithium RBC transport
4. Alpha-2 presynaptic platelet binding levels
5. Impaired immune response (lymphocyte mitogen stimulation tests)

III- DISCUSSION

a) Neuroendocrine tests:

Neuroendocrine abnormalities have been reported in major depression (Extein et al., 1982) and in this respect two tests are more particularly used, the dexamethasone suppression test (DST) and the thyrotropin-releasing hormone test (TRHT).

1. Dexamethasone Suppression Test (DST):

The most extensive series of studies on this test have been carried out by Carroll et al. (1981) in attempting to standardize and validate it. The test which allegedly possesses a high degree of sensitivity, specificity and diagnostic confidence (Carroll et al., 1981; Mendelwicz et al., 1982; Green and Kane, 1983) is useful in confirming or helping to make the diagnosis of some types of major depressive disorders (endogenous depression, unipolar or bipolar primary affective disorders).

It has been reported that age, sex, severity of depression, menopausal status or benzodiazepines at usual therapeutic doses did not influence the results. However, the test should not be performed in women pregnant or administered high doses of estrogens, in patients receiving some drugs (reserpine, opiates, hepatic enzymatic inductors), in conditions influencing weight (marked gain weight, anorexia nervosa, malnutrition), in diabetes mellitus, in Cushing syndrome or during steroid treatment, and in all severe physical illnesses (Zarifian et Lôo, 1982). Recently, in a study exploring the prevalence of an abnormal response to DST with respect to diagnosis, such an occurrence was found in 20% of a sample of schizophrenics, in over 25% of abstinent alcoholics, in 40% of neurotics (including neurotic depressives) and in almost 50% of senile dements (Coppen et al., 1983).

From a methodological standpoint, it has been pointed out lately that the major concern in the review of DST literature has been the issue of diagnostic homogeneity and that recently a major source of confusion has been the wide variation in abnormal response rates in the control groups that were chosen for comparison with the depressed patient group (Green and Kane, 1983).

As a measurement of change, the DST has an interesting application. Indeed, the test normalizes with recovery of depression and, when it remains abnormal, it has been speculated that this is an ominous prognostic sign (Green and Kane, 1983). In a limited number of patients, it has been suggested lately that nonsuppression on the DST could predict a good response to noradrenergic antidepressants, whereas suppression would predict a good one to serotoninergic antidepressants (Fraser, 1983). If the test shows considerable promise in helping to define new subgroups of depressed patients, doubts have been cast with respect to its value in predicting treatment response to adequate somatic therapy (Green and Kane, 1983). It seems however useful in helping determine treatment duration.

2. Thyrotropin-Releasing Hormone Test (TRHT):

It has been established that the TRH-induced TSH response is blunted in some depressed euthyroid patients and that this blunting may occur in some alcoholic or manic patients, but not in schizophrenics. Thus, this response to TRH has been reported (Extein et al., 1982) decreased in major unipolar depression, with discrepant findings in bipolar depression (increase or no difference). Blunted response can be induced by hyperthyroidism, increased glucocorticoids, alcohol, some drugs and advances age in males (Extein et al., 1982).

With regard to this test, the aspects of frequency, specificity, definition of blunted response, technique, prediction of outcome, amongst other factors, have been discussed recently (Loosen and Prange, 1982), as well as retest reliability (Loosen et al., 1983). It is estimated that the sensitivity, specificity and prediction value of the TRH test is comparable to the DST in the diagnosis of major depression (Extein et al., 1982). The utility of the TRHT in the assessment of the response and outcome of treatment requires further validation.

Of some unipolar patients administered both TRHT and DST, some showed a blunted response to TRH only, others to DST only, some to both, others to none of the tests (Extein et al., 1982). Therefore, the two tests may be complementary in the neuroendocrine exploration of the identification of possible unipolar depression (Extein et al., 1982; Chabrol et Moron, 1983).

b) Sleep Electroencephalography:

Although valuable for research purposes, this technique does not constitute a practical adjunct for the clinical psychiatrist.

c) Psychomotor markers:

Psychomotor function abnormalities (including speech deceleration) are fundamental features in the diagnosis and classification of affective disorders. Using speech pause time (SPT), it has been reported that melancholics have a significantly longer SPT than normal controls, schizophrenics and non-endogenous subgroups, with bipolar melancholics having the longuest values (Greden, 1982). It has been suggested that STP measures constitute a relatively simple, inexpensive, noninvasive, practical test that could supplement a neuroendocrine test like DST (Greden, 1982).

d) Biochemical measures:

The studies of brain monoamine metabolites, particularly urinary MHPG and CSF 5-HIAA, have also revealed that depressive syndromes are not homogeneous, and these findings can have some therapeutic impact. Indeed, depressions characterized by a low CSF 5-HIAA value might respond better to antidepressants inhibiting serotonin reuptake, but lumbar puncture is a deterrent procedure. On the other hand, a low urinary MHPG could indicate a better response to antidepressants inhibiting noradrenaline reuptake and a normal MHPG, a better one to those inhibiting serotonin reuptake (Lôo, 1981). With respect to the modifications of the platelet MAO activity in depressive disorders, it might be a reflexion of a serotoninergic dysfunction or of a membrane pathology (Lôo et Zarifian, 1982). Attention has been drawn on the limitations of this approach, its methodological flaws, and against a simplistic interpretation of the results (Lôo and Zarifian, 1982).

234

The other biochemical measures will not be discussed here.

IV- CONCLUSION

Various biological markers have been investigated in recent years, as diagnostic tools, as predictors of treatment response and as measures of change helping to determine treatment duration, particularly the dexamethasone suppression test (DST) in depression. However, there exists some controversy surrounding the clinical routine use of such biochemical tests devised to identify affective disorders and to monitor treatment response (Hill, 1983). These tests have indeed limitations, but are helpful particularly in research for developing a better understanding of some psychiatric disorders, and in eventually leading to better diagnostic methods and more specific therapeutic approaches. For the clinician in psychiatry, they still have a restricted routine application.

REFERENCES

Carroll, B.J., Feinberg, M., Greden, J.F., Tarika, J., Albala, A.A., Haskett, R.F., McIdames, N., Kronfol, Z., Lohr, N., Steiner, M., de Vigne, J.P. and Young, E., 1981, A specific laboratory test for the diagnosis of melancholia, Arch. Gen. Psychiatry 38: 15-22.

Chabrol, H. et Moron, P., 1983, Diagnostic biologique de la dépression par le test à la TRH et le test à la dexaméthasone, Encéphale 9: 1-22.

Coppen, A., Abou-Saleh, N., Miller, P., Metcalfe, M., Harwood, J. and Bailey, J., 1983, Dexamethasone suppression test in depression and other psychiatric illness, Brit. J. Psychiat. 142: 498-504.

Extein, I., Pottash, A.L.C. and Gold, M.S., 1982, Neuroendocrine abnormalities in affective disorders, Encéphale 8: 203-211.

Fraser, A.R., 1983, Choice of antidepressant based on the dexamethasone suppression test, Am. J. Psychiatry 140: 786-787.

Greden, J.F., 1982, Biological markers of melancholia and reclassification of depressive disorders, Encéphale 8: 193-202.

Green, H.S. and Kane, J.M., 1983, The dexamethasone suppression test in depression, Clinical Neuropharmacology 6: 7-24.

Hill, T., 1983, Psychiatrists argue value of tests, The Medical Post 19: 23.

Lôo, H., 1981, Implications thérapeutiques de la caractérisation biochimique des dépressions, Encéphale 7: 429-440.

Lôo, H. et Zarifian, E., 1982, Abord critique des facteurs biochimiques au cours des syndromes chimiques et prescription d'antidépresseurs, Ann. Méd. Psychol. 140: 240-251.

Loosen, P.T. and Prange, A.J., Jr., 1982, Serum thyrotropin response to thyrotropin releasing hormone in psychiatric patients: a review, Am. J. Psychiatry 139: 405-416.

Loosen, P.T., Kistler, K. and Prange, A.J., Jr., 1983, Use of TSH
    response to THR as an independant variable, Am. J. Psychia-
    try 140: 700-703.
Mendlewicz, J., Charles, G. and Franckson, J.M., 1982, The dexame-
    thasone suppression test in affective disorders: relation-
    ship to clinical and genetic subgroups, Brit. J. Psychiat.
    141: 464-470.
Zarifian, E. et Lôo, H., 1982, "Les Antidépresseurs. Aspects
    biologiques, cliniques et thérapeutiques," Editions Printel,
    Roche, France.

BIOLOGICAL MARKERS AS MEASURES OF CHANGE

DISCUSSION

Henri Dufour and Jean-Michel Azorin

Department of Psychiatry
Timone Hospital
13005 Marseille - France

From the 20 markers mentioned by A. Villeneuve, a general definition can be given: "all quantifiable indexes of an abnormality in the biological organization (-biological personality-) of a patient".
This presentation, and particularly the example concerning the Dexamethasone suppression test (D.S.T.), underlines the theoretical and practical interest of the "marker", in various fields of biological psychiatry: it is a sign of a biological disturbance, which enables selection of the treatment and the follow-up.

I/   All biological markers do not raise the same interest. They can be
       classified in the following way.

Biological markers
-       the monoamine metabolites (5HIAA, MHPG, DOPEG, HVA) and
        more recently neuropeptides.
-       enzymes playing a role in the neuro-transmitter pathways (MAO,
        DOMT, Tyr-bety Hydroxylase). For each of them, dosage can be
        preferentially made in one or several biological milieux.
-       The more recent and sophisticated binding techniques allow us to
        quantify the receptors affinity for a given substance.

Endocrinological markers
Most of these markers are dynamic tests. In addition to the D.S.T., T.R.H., G.H. and D.R.L. must be cited.

Physiological markers
Electro, psycho and neuro physiological indexes have to be differentiated. All do not have the same significance: E.E.G., quantitative E.E.G., sleep E.E.G. and psycho galvanic responses are

spontaneous indexes whereas evoked potentials, P 300 waves, and negative contingent variation (N.C.V.) are provoked indexes.

Some of these parameters are considered as chronobiological markers owing to ther biorythm (pulse, temperature, blood pressure).

General and immunological markers
Blood group A.B.C., daltonism, H.L.A. system and immunoglobulins.

Psychomotor markers (increased speech pause time-SPT-, Limb motility, Facial electromyography during states of affective imagery) mentioned by Villeneuve.

In a more general way, all biological characteristics of a patient can be classified, for example the ability of metabolizing a psychotropic drug, or the lithium ratio, which explores the membrane exchange. Thus, the list of biological markers progresses parallel with biological psychiatry.

II/ The characteristics of biological markers

1/ The information they give concerns a particular level of the biological organization. This level is infra-cellular with enzymes and monoamines. Others (D.S.T. for example, psycho physiological markers) give information already corresponding to the integration of several biological systems.

2/ - Some measure a transitory biological abnormality ("symptom markers"), e.g. Monoamines metabolites, R.E.M. phase in Sleep E.E.G., likely to be modified after treatment;
   - Other will provide a "vulnerability index" and will not evolve with clinical change (e.g. Platelets M.A.O., Eye tracking, H.L.A. system, D.S.T.). They are rather "structure markers" which allow a group of patients to be situated in relation with the mean of each index.

Sensitivity, spedificity, technical conditions, financial possibilities, and ethical limits (E.G. repeated lumbar punctions) are as many differentation elements among them.

The example with D.S.T. shows what the difficulites may be when technical conditions remain ill-defined.

The difficulites concern at least three aspects:

1/ The dose of Dexamethasone
   CARROLL at al. have compared the results in 368 patients. One half had received 2 mgr, and the other half 1 mgr. The dose of Desamethazone influences the test sensitivity (- 58 % with 1 mgr, 29 % with 2 mgr). Conversely, specificity is unaltered. It remains equal to 96 %.

2/ Blood sample schedule
   CARROLL et al. have determined the respective efficacy of the different blood sampling times:

- At Day 0, a blood sample is taken at 8 a.m., prior to dexamethasone administration;
- At Day 1, the results obtained from three different samples are compared:
  - 24 % of the positive tests are detected by the 8 a.m. sampling,
  - 78 % at 4 p.m.;
  - 71 % at 11 p.m.

As the 4 p.m. and 11 p.m. tests together detect 98 % of the positive results, CARROLL advises elimination of the 8 a.m. sampling. GOLDBERG proposed another method of symplin which increases the test sensitivity:
- No sampling on D 1
- Only one sampling on D 2, 9 a.m.

The non suppression is defined by a corisol level 7 µg/dl on D 2, 9 am, while CARROLL's technique gives a limit of 5 µg/dl on D 1, 4 or 11 pm.

The GOLDBERG's technique this has the advantage of only one sampling.

3/ Cortisol dosage technique

The critical thresholds to define non suppression may vary with the technique used (radio-immunology or proteic binding). In the field of endocrinology, maximum sensitivity falls down to around 10 to 25 µg/dl cortisol level: often, laboratories cannot measure values below 5 µg/dl and give extrapolated values. MELTZER et al. therefore underline the need for an agreement between physicians and laboratories on corisul critical values in psychiatry.

In France, the most currently used procedure is that standardized by CARROLL: intake of 1 mgr dexamethasone on DO at 11 p.m. On D 1, two samplings at 4 pm and 11 pm. The test is positive when one of the two cortisul levels exceeds 5 µg/dl.

III/ The choice of the biological markers will therefore depend on the type of therapeutic trials.

In drug comparison studies (Phase III), the usual target is to prove the statistical similarity between the two products only. The introduction of biological markers is desirable. Indeed the collection of data based only on clinical rating scales has reached its limits, since the results are more often than not identical: it is likely that the same clinical symptomatology hides a biological heterogenity.

In trials aiming to test the drug action mechanism, biological markers will become more and more indispensable for identifying the treated patients as well as testing the work hypothesis.

IV/ In this situation, biological markers have a new function, in the field of drug trials.

The exceed the scope of therapeutic trials. Indeed:

- they allow the development of biological hypothesis in psychiatry and form their foundation. Hence, they confirm a biological disturbance in a particular field and they established a vulnerability index within populations.
- when these markers are applied to a group of patients, they evidence correlations between biological and clinical disturbance: correlation does not however mean causality.
- some biochemical markers may orientate the choice of treatment, provided its action mechanism is well known.

Our clinical classifications probably have not their equivalent ones in the biological field. The choice of biological markers will be oriented more through the biological hypothesis envisaged and the characteristics of each marker, rather than through the clinical classification.

PROBLEMS IN THE USE OF GLOBAL SCORES OF RATING SCALES IN PSYCHIATRIC RESEARCH

H. Katschnig

Psychiatric Clinic, University of Vienna

Währinger Gürtel 74-76, A-1090 Wien

The word "rating scale" is used in at least two different ways. In the strict sense a "rating scale" is concerned with the measurement of different degrees of severity of a single item, such as "mildly, moderately, severely depressed". However, a list of such single rating scales has also come to be called a "rating scale", which is a somewhat improper use of the word. Usually the "measurement" coming out of such a list (of single rating scales) is a total score.

Rating scales are used to judge the presence and/or intensity of complex phenomena in such widely differing areas as psychopathological symptoms, tardive dyskinesia, social adjustment, or expressed emotion. In psychiatric research rating scales are employed for selecting a study sample, for attaining a diagnosis, for monitoring the course of a disease, and for measuring outcome, to name just a few possible applications.

Rating scales have had an enormous impact on psychiatric research. However, their merits do not reside in the realm of quantification, but in their contribution to a more precise definition of the phenomena rated, i.e. to qualification. The authors of psychiatric rating scales, although having quantification in mind, first had to define what they wanted to measure. Thus, Overall and Gorham (1962) first had to give definitions of the 18 items included in their "Brief Psychiatric Rating Scale"; for quantification in the narrow sense, i.e. for identifying degrees of severity, in fact no rules are given and this task is obviously left to the judgment of the rater. Hamilton (1960) likewise gave definitions of the items included in his depression scale, although his definitions are more geared to real quantification.

Whereas it is true that the introduction of rating scales into psychiatry has promoted an empirical, scientific and objectifying approach to psychopathological phenomena, the developments which have taken place in the last 15 years and the practial ways of using rating scales have become a cause for concern.

I shall concentrate on two areas which seem problematic to me:

(1) the explosion of the number of rating scales
(2) problems with global scores

THE EXPLOSION OF THE NUMBER OF RATING SCALES

The last edition of the CIPS rating scales contains more than 35 different scales and, as the editors state, this is only a selection of psychiatric rating scales available nowadays. Rating scales for measuring "Social Adjustment" are equally numerous (Katschnig, 1983).

One reason for introducing rating scales was the improvement of communication and comparability of different studies. However, the sheer number of rating scales available nowadays for measuring one and the same phenomenon, e.g. depression, undermines this aim. A bable of more or less precise but differing formulations and instruments, which is comparable to the babel of diagnostic formulations for the functional psychoses (Brockington et al.,1978), is likely to reduce comparability between different research results. Not only the definition, number, and coding of items but also the method of data collection itself may be very different: a rating scale may be used for selfrating or for expert rating, where information may be obtained from carrying out an interview (which may or may not be standardised) or from observation.

It is not improbable that different rating scales pretending to quantify a given concept in fact measure different phenomena. It seems therefore advisable to use several rating scales simultaneously or to construct "comprehensive rating instruments" from which all rating scales for a specific concept could be deducted. One example of work in this direction is Endicott et al's (1981) study, who tried to extract the Hamilton Depression Rating Scale from the SADS-C (change version) and, with the exception of one item (insight), succeeded. Likewise Bech (1981) tried to extract the "Newcastle Scale" from the WHO depression rating scale but was less successful. Such exercises are very useful and should be carried out more frequently. Also cross validation studies between rating scales pretending to measure the same concept should be undertaken. The usefulness of such comparisons can be demonstrated by data from our studies on attempted suicide and depressed patients (Katschnig,1980; Katschnig, in press), comparing two methods for measuring life stress, the London Life Event and Difficulty

242

Schedule (LEDS; Brown,1974) and the Social Readjustment Rating Scale (SRRS; Holmes and Rahe,1967). Although on a group level similar results were obtained (a rise in life stress before onset), the two instruments had a practial non-correlation on the single patient level ($r_B=0,11$). In carrying out such cross validation studies the differing basic conceptions and methodological procedures of different rating scales could become more transparent.

PROBLEMS WITH GLOBAL SCORES

For many of those who are using rating scales, ticking a checklist and summing the scores to a total score has become to be thought of as a kind of automatic procedure. However, any collection of items, however scientifically derived it may be, does not have an automatically built-in guarantee for precise and reliable measureements. This usually depends on the judgmental abilities of the person carrying out the rating and not on the rating scale itself. It is frequently overlooked that both the Hamilton Depression Rating Scale and the Brief Psychiatric Rating Scale suggest that two clinicians should rate one and the same patient and come to a kind of agreement rating. The Hamilton Depression Rating Scale even derives its total score by adding the ratings of two clinician, a procedure seldom adhered to. Usually a single clinician makes the rating, which, paradoxically enough, is then doubled. Thus, whereas the creators of these rating scales were well aware of the importance of the abilities of the rater, this is very frequently forgotten.

It is well documented that the reliability of the total score of a rating scale is much higher than the single item reliability. For instance the Hamilton Depression Rating Scale has a global score reliability of up to 0,9, whereas the individual items have a much lower reliability of between 0,35 and 0,83. In our study on life events in attempted suicides (Katschnig,1980) a very high correlation for the global scores of the Social Readjustment Ratings Scale was found between two ratings carried out within a two weeks' interval. The correlation coefficient was 0,9. On the individual item level, however, only a little more than 50% of the items were rated on both occasions identically (KAPPA = 0,14).

To show the consequences of including low reliability items in a rating scale yielding a global score, I will draw on some data we have collected in a study on depression (Katschnig et al.,1981; Katschnig,1984), using among other diagnostic tools the "Newcastle scale". The two problems which arise will be dealt with under the headings of "pseudo-preciseness" and "pseudo-homogeneity".

Pseudo-preciseness

The Newcastle scale (I) has been empirically derived by

Carney et al.(1965) by applying a multiple regression analysis
to depressed patients who had been divided into an endogenous and
a neurotic group by the clinicians. The items which best discriminated between these groups were given rounded weights and were put
together into the so-called "Newcastle scale" (see table 1). A
score of 5 or less assigns a patient to the neurotic group, a score
of 6 or more leads to labeling the patient as "endogenous".

Table 1: The Newcastle Scale I (Carney et al.,1965)

adequate personality	+1
no adequate psychogenesis	+2
distinct quality	+1
weight loss	+2
previous episode	+1
depressive psychomotor activity	+2
anxiety	-1
nihilistic delusions	+2
blame others	-1
guilt	+1

When the Newcastle scale was applied to a sample of 176 inpatients, 108 were classified as neurotic and 68 as endogenous. As
can be seen in figure 1,very slight changes in those items which
have a low reliability - "adequate personality" and "no adequate
psychogenesis" - lead to very large differences in the diagnostic
assignments. If a rater were to have classified all patients as
having an adequate personality, 83 would have been called endogenous; if he were to have classified all as having no adequate
personality, only 48 would have been called "endogenous". The situation becomes even more dramatic with the item "no adequate psychogenesis": 116 patients would have been called endogenous if "no
adequate psychogenesis" were to have been judged as present and
only 39 would have received the "endogenous" label if for all
patients an "adequate psychogenesis" were to have been found by
a rater.

It follows that the consequences of rating one single item as
present or not present may be considerable. Thus when global scores
are used, the inclusion of items with low reliability may become
very problematic. If the list of items is rather long, the inclusion of one or the other low reliability item is obviously not so
problematic as in short scales, such as in the Newcastle Scale.
This conclusion is of considerable practical importance, as the
Newcastle Scale is widely used for identifying biological correlates of endogenous depression. Similar considerations apply also
to other rating scales. For instance 20 out of 55 items of the
"Comprehensive Psychopathological Rating Scale (CPRS)" are reported
to have a reliability coefficient (KAPPA) of lower than 0,6 and 6
thereof one of lower than 0,4 (Kuny et al.,1982).

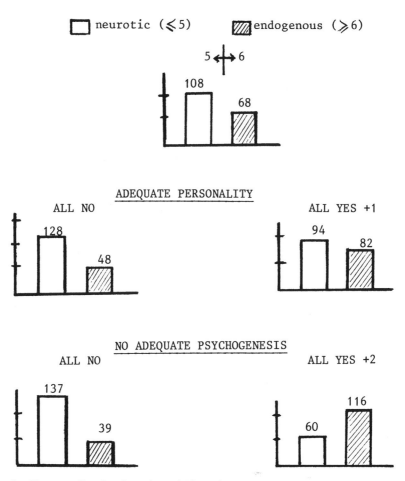

Fig.1: Newcastle Scale classification of 176 depressed patients

Pseudo-homogeneity

The second problem to be discussed here, is that of "pseudo-homogeneity", which is also connected with classifying patients into those below and above a certain score, either for the purpose of diagnostic assignment or for dividing patients into improved and non improved groups. The Newcastle Scale can serve as an example for illustrating also "pseudo-homogeneity".

As can be seen in the tables 2 and 3, psychopathological pictures which are very different from one another can belong to the same diagnostic group, whereas syndromes which are very similar to each other can belong to different diagnostic groups.Thus, theoretically, a patient showing distinct quality of depression, weight loss and nihilistic delusions, would be called neurotic (table 2), whereas a depressed patient with an adequate personality, a previous episode and no adequate psychogenesis suffering just from weight loss would be labeled "endogenous"; if showing also anxiety, the same patient would slip into the "neurotic" group (table 3).

Table 2: Examples for Newcastle Scale

+1 Adequate Personality	+1 Distinct Quality	+1 Distinct Quality
+2 No Adequate Psychogenesis	+2 Weight Loss	+2 Weight Loss
+1 Previous Episode	+2 Nihilistic Delusions	+2 Nihilistic Delusions
+2 Depressive Psychomotor Activity	+1 Guilt	
Σ=6 (Endogenous)	Σ=6 (Endogenous)	Σ=5 (Neurotic)

Table 3: Examples for Newcastle Scale

+1 Adequate Personality	+1 Adequate Personality	+1 Adequate Personality
+2 No Adequate Psychogenesis	+2 No Adequate Psychogenesis	+2 No Adequate Psychogenesis
+2 Weight Loss	+2 Weight Loss	+2 Weight Loss
	+1 Previous Episode	+1 Previous Episode
		-1 Anxiety
Σ =5 (Neurotic)	Σ =6 (Endogenous)	Σ=5 (Neurotic)

This heterogeneity has to be kept in mind when comparisons are carried out between different studies using dichotomized global scores of rating scales in diagnosing patients or in evaluating treatment outcome. One way of coping with this problem would be the use of data analysis techniques which consider also the qualitative and structural differences between groups (e.g. profile analysis).

CONCLUSION

Quantification has come to be regarded as the basic and essential step of science. The term "quantitative" is frequently used synonymously with "scientific". The process by which quantification occurs is called measurement. Campbell (1938) has defined measurement as the "assignment of numerals to represent properties of material systems other than number, in virtue of the laws governing these properties". This definition is governed by the assumption of an isomorphism between properties of objects which are not our invention, and the properties of the relationship between the numerals which are our invention.

This classical definition of measurement has been expanded to include those "measurements" where the relationship between numerals does not find a corresponding relationship in the objects. Stevens (1951) therefore defined measurement as "the assignment of numerals to objects or events according to rules". These rules may, but need not, imply the principle of isomorphism. Any other rule agreed upon is sufficient.

In psychiatry "measurement" is primarily concerned with this broader second definition, which refers to a less differentiated level of "measurement", meaning frequently just the reliable naming of a phenomenon; here the terms "quantification" as well as "measurement" are misleading. The term "qualification" meaning the presentation of the qualities of an object or event in a reliable verbal manner, seems more appropriate here. If qualification is not guaranteed, quantification is useless and even misleading.

There are two practical conclusions to be drawn from the results presented, which may seem obvious but are, nevertheless, frequently disregarded:

First, psychiatric rating scales should not include items with low reliability. This may, however, lead to a substantial loss of information and, consequently, to a loss of possible insights. The only way out obviously consists in trying to increase the interrater reliability for individual items in providing training courses, which should be organised both on a national and international scale, in order to assure comparability across different studies. Just making sure that two raters show good agreement in a specific study is not enough.

A second conclusion is that, whenever global scores are calculated, also individual item analyses should be carried out. There are statistical techniques available for measuring structural differences (such as profile analysis), which take into account the single item ratings.

If the advantages of rating scales as a method for objectifying complex phenomenon is to be retained, such rating scales must not be regarded as having the properties of thermometers. A continuing effort is necessary both in preparing raters for data collection and in the analysis of the data to assure this objectivation.

References

Bech, P.,1981, Rating Scales for Affective Disorders: Their
Validity and Consistency, Acta Psychiat.Sand.,64:Spl 295

Brockington,I.F., R.E.Kendell, J.P.Leff, 1978, Definitions of
schizophrenia: concordance and prediction of outcome,
Psychological Medicine, 8: 387-398

Brown, G.W., 1974, Meaning,measurement and stress of life events,
in: "Stressful Life Events: Their Nature and Effects",
Dohrenwend, B.S. and Dohrenwend, B.P., eds., Wiley,New York.

Carney, M.W.P., Roth, M., Carside, R.F., 1965, The diagnosis of
depressive syndromes and the prediction of ECT response.
Brit.J.Psychiat.,111: 659-674

Campbell, N.R., 1938, Symposium: Measurement and its Importance
to Philosophy, Proc.Arist.Soc.Suppl. 17: 121-142
Harrison, London.

Endicott,J., Cohen, J., Nee, J., Fleiss, J., Sarantakos, S.,
1981, Hamilton Depression Rating Scale, Arch.Gen.Psychiatry
38: 98-103

Hamilton, M., 1960, A rating scale for depression. J.Neurol.
Neurosurg.Psychiat. 23: 36-62

Holmes, Th.H., Rahe, R.H., 1967, The social readjustment scale,
J.psychosom.Res. 11: 213-218

Katschnig,H., 1980, Measuring Life Stress: A Comparison of Two
Methods. in: Farmer,R. & St.Hirsch (Eds.): The Suicide Syndrome. Croom Helm, London

Katschnig,H., 1983, Methods for Measuring Social Adjustment, in:
"Methodology in Evaluation of Psychiatric Treatment",
Helgason,T. Ed., Cambridge University Press, Cambridge

Katschnig,H., 1984, Inferring Causes: Some Constraints in the
Social Psychiatry of Depression. Commentary to the article
by P.E.Bebbington. Integrative Psychiatry 2: 77-79

Katschnig,H., (Ed.): Life Events and Psychiatric Disorders -
Controversial Issues. Cambridge Unviersity Press, Cambridge,
in press

Katschnig,H., A.Brandl-Nebehay, G.Fuchs-Robetin, P.Seelig,
G.Eichberger, R.Strobl, P.P.Sint, 1981, Lebensverändernde
Ereignisse, psychosoziale Dispositionen und depressive
Verstimmungszustände. Psychiatrische Universitätsklinik, Wien

Kuny, S., Maurer, M., Dittrich, A., Woggon, B., 1982, Interrelia-
bilität der deutschsprachigen Version der Comprehensive Psychopathological Rating Scale (CPRS), Int.Pharmacopsychiat. 17:
354-369

Overall, J.E., Gorham, D.R., 1962, The Brief Psychiatric Rating
Scale. Psycholog.Rep. 10: 799

Stevens, S.S., 1951, Mathematics, measurement and psychophysics.
in: Handbook of Experimental Psychology, Stevens, S.S. ed.,
Wiley, New York

SOME METHODOLOGICAL COMMENTS DERIVED FROM

FACTOR ANALYSES OF THE AMDP-SYSTEM

Daniel Bobon and Benoit Troisfontaines

Dept of Psychiatry, University of Liège Med. School

(Rue St-Laurent, 58, B-4000 Liège, Belgium)

The objective of any factor analysis (further abbreviated FA) is to reduce the number of variables by studying the correlation of items in building factors like the clinician studies the relationships between symptoms and syndromes.

The revised version of the AMDP-System, elaborated by a German-Swiss-Austrian Association for Methodology and Documentation in Psychiatry (Arbeitsgemeinschaft für Methodik und Dokumentation in der Psychiatrie, 1979, 1983) Bobon et al., 1983; Guy and Ban, 1982) is made of three forms on anamnestic data and of two forms on present state. The psychopathological form AMDP-4 contains 100 items common to all translations and 15 write-in items; the somatic form AMDP-5 contains 40 common items and 7 write-in items; all items can be pooled in FAs since the rating of severity is the same for all (0-4: absent-mild-moderate-severe-extremely severe + a nominal category "not ascertained"). The French section of the AMDP agreed on the reserve items for the purpose of covering fields insufficiently covered in the German version, such as anxiety and sexuality (Bobon, 1981).

In a Franco-Belgian multicentre study, the AMDP-4 and -5 forms have been completed in 337 patients representing a large nosological spectrum (Bobon et al., 1982). The present comments are based on this study and on an unpublished extension of the sample to 492 patients.

Despite differences in scale versions, in raters and in samples, the factor structure of the AMDP psychopathological form is extremely stable: 7 factors are common to the French FA and to all German FAs (Apathy-Retardation, Delusions, Depression, Mania, Hostility, Obsessions-Phobias and Psycho-organic Syndrome),

1 factor is consequent to the higher number of rotated factors in the French FA (Dissociation-Depersonalisation) and 2 factors are generated by the additional French items (Anxiety, Dramatization).

On the extended sample of 492 patients, a 13-factor solution confirms the stability of these 10 psychopathological factors and demonstrates three "somatic" factors distinct from the German analyses: a factor on Somatic Complaints (including the item on Hypochondriasis), a factor on Anticholinergic Symptoms (corresponding to the German "autonomous" or "vegetative" factor) and a factor on Insomnia (combined with Depression in all German FAs). Despite lower factor solutions, the factors on somatic complaints and on anticholinergic symptoms remain independent, which might be of great interest in psychopathological and drug trials.

One classically considers that the number of subjects should be superior to the number of items in the ratio of at least 3:1 for the sake of intercorrelations. In the case of small samples such as the present one, this ratio can be improved by excluding items. We have demonstrated (Bobon et al., 1982) that unfrequent items contribute little to the factor structure of the AMDP because of low loadings in major factors or high loadings in minor factors. The somatic items may be excluded too (for example in case of videotaped ratings of the AMDP-4 form only): they do contribute to somatic factors but they have low loadings in the psychopathological factors.

We confirm previous observations in the literature on FA: the least factors are submitted to rotation, the more the functions are hierarchized (e.g. intrication of Depression and Retardation, of Delusions and Hallucinations etc); the more factors are rotated, the better the functions are differenciated (e.g. Delusions subdivided in Delusions, Hallucinations, Dissociation and Syndrome of Alien Influence).

The homogeneity vs. heterogeneity of the sample depends on the aim of the FA, i.e. on the aim of the measuring instrument. If one looks for a screening instrument, one should select an heterogeneous sample as we did; if one looks for the differenciated factor profile of depressives, one should factor-analyze an homogeneous sample of depressed patients.

Comprehensive scales such as the AMDP-4 and -5 are time-consuming but they have three definite advantages over more specific short scales: 1) establishment of a syndromic diagnosis (which precludes the nosological diagnosis); 2) detailed description of a patients' sample before treatment; 3) eventual demonstration of syndrome shifts (manic shift under antidepressants etc) and of significant differences between two active drugs, where the total score of a short scale would show no difference.

References

Arbeitsgemeinschaft für Methodik und Dokumentation in der Psychiatrie
(Ed.), 1979, Das AMDP-System, 3rd ed. Springer, Berlin.

Arbeitsgemeinschaft für Methodik und Dokumentation in der Psychiatrie
(Ed.), 1983, Testmanual zum AMDP-System. Springer, Berlin.

Bobon D.P.(Ed.), 1981, Le Système AMDP, 2e éd. Mardaga, Bruxelles.

Bobon D., Mormont C., Doumont A., Mirel J., Bonhomme P., Ansseau M.,
Pellet J., Pull C., De Buck R., Gernay P., Mormont I., Lang F.,
Lejeune J., Bronckart C., von Frenckell R., 1982, Analyse
factorielle de la révision française de l'échelle AMDP.
Résultats d'une étude internationale de 388 cas. Acta psychiat.
belg. 82: 371-389.

Bobon D., Baumann U., Angst J., Helmchen H., Hippius H.(Eds.),1983,
The AMDP-System in pharmacopsychiatry. Karger, Basel.

Guy W., Ban T.(Eds.), 1982, The AMDP-System. Springer, Berlin.

THE ROLE OF 'INTERVENING VARIABLES' IN CLINICAL RESEARCH

D. Widlöcher

Professor of Psychiatry

Salpêtrière Hospital - Paris

The study of the relationships between behavioural variables and drugs has two distinct purposes. The firts purpose is to specify drug indications and efficacy. The second purpose is to better characterize the relationship between cerebral structures and behaviour on the basis of the known mode of action of drugs. To serve either purpose, we use several behavioural variables (several items on a scale or several scales). The action of a drug is thus usually studied on one or two dozen variables. The recourse to a variety of variables is justified on several grounds. Firstly due to our very unprecise means of observation and criteria for description and quantification of behavioural data, an evaluation based on only one item would be very unreliable. By using a relatively high number of traits, the risk is minimized : thus an inadequate rating of one item is compensated by a better rating of the others. The second reason lies in the fact that actions are subject to multiple determinations. Each behavioural trait is the result of several factors and drugs do not necessarly act on all of them. In other words, one behavioural trait cannot be considered as a sufficient index of drug action and as representing the behavioural target of the drug.

This is why we always presuppose that there exists between observed behavioural indices and the drug a non-observable intervening variable to which both dependent and independent variables are correlated. In operational terms, if M is the drug variable (presence or absence, dose, treatment duration, etc.) and $S1, S2 ... Sn$ the symptoms observed, instead of $S1 = f(M)$, $S2 = f(M)$, $Sn = f(M)$ the formulation will be $S1,2,n = f(X)$ and $X = f(M)$, X corresponding to a state directly caused by M and more or less closely correlated to variables $S1, 2 ...n$. Also from an operational point of view, the intervening variable accounts for the fact that the various symptoms are not equally dependent on the independent variable 'drug' and that the variance of rated symptoms is not accounted for by the sole target-object of drug action. From a psychobiological point of view the independent variable corresponds to the neurophysiological state directly dependent on drug action. On the other hand the fundamental question is whether such a state of the brain also corresponds to a psychological object, i.e. a behavioural or mental event lending itself to observation. This is like asking whether there is any meaning to statements such as : drug A is antiagressive or drug B is antidepressive.

This question lies at the heart of the methodology of clinical psycho-pharmacology studies. It corresponds to an ambiguity inherent to the concept of intervening variable. In fact, two different ways of defining the status of the intervening variable can be opposed. The first definition rests on the idea that this initially unobservable and hypothetical variable corresponds to an object which inserts itself between the object represented respectively by the independent and the dependent variables. In order to test this hypothesis, an additional value is needed. In other words, observable indices giving it an objective existence must be elicited. In this manner, a causal track may be established, this creating a link between three series of observable variables. From that point of view, the hypothetic variable constitutes a provisional construction which will be verified only when it can be reduced to a new observable variable. The second definition of the status of the intervening variable rests on the idea that such a variable does not represent an unobservable object but corresponds to a law governing the observable dependent variables. To test this hypothesis, the explanatory and predictive value of such a law has to be specified. New hypotheses and predictions about previously observed data must be derived from it and their objective verification must be sought.

Let us illustrate these opposite definitions with examples. In the first instance, an intervening variable susceptible to become a new observable variable has to be defined. This is what takes place in studies searching for psychophysiological or biological indices of a behavioural state. For example, between the action of an anxiolytic drug and traits considered as anxiety-correlated indices or states, the existence of a condition of the organism that defines anxiety proper will be presupposed, and certain physiological indices making it possible to observe this condition will be established. Such indices and the variable which can be measured through them are no longer an intervening variable but a new, observable variable. The object it measures, the physiological anxiety state, enters the causal track by linking mechanisms between nervous structures which are the target of the drug and the various behaviours more or less correlated to anxiety.

254

Another example concerns the relationship between 5 H.I.A.A.
level in CSF, depression and suicide. Suicide rate in depressed
patients seems to be linked to a low level of the serotonin metabo-
lite (M. Asberg and coll.). But research along the causal track
leads, through complementary experiments, to establishing between
5 H.I.A.A. level and the suicide variable the insertion of another
intervening variable, the aggressive dimension, as distinct from
depression.

Most quantitative psychopathology studies do not lead to the
discovery of such indices. They identify a dimension, a factor
accounting for the fact that a group of traits are partly correlated
to one another and covary under the influence of the drug. When
experts observe an 'increase of I.Q.' or an 'improvement of intellectual development' under the influence of the drug in some children,
they observe nothing else but how a group of test responses covary on account of the drug. Intelligence, an intervening variable,
is not an unobservable object. It is the law which says that when
a child answers a certain type of problem correctly, he will also
answer correctly any problem on the same type. The intervening
variable 'intelligence' cannot be considered as a potential observable object which would enter the causal track existing between
the state of the brain and the capacity to answer all the problem
submitted. Similarly, when the group of symptoms which are the best
predictors of a favorable outcome of imipramine (progressive onset,
weight loss, anorexia, insomnia and retardation) are described,
hypothesis can be formulated (R.J. Bielski and R.O. Friedel) that
these organic symptoms are the nucleus of endogenous unipolar
depression. Indeed, multivariate analyses suggest that there is a
common factor to these variables as opposed to others. The term
'endogenous unipolar depression' corresponds here to a law organizing depressive traits together, suggesting either that these traits
correspond at least partially to a structural and functional unit
or that they are in a causal relation to one another. Further
research should prove which of these hypotheses is valid by refining,
for instance, the study of the possible dependence relation between
sleep disorder and retardation. This dependence relation might well
be accounted for by retardation causing sleep disorder, ore more
likely by sleep rhythm alteration being a precipitating factor of
retardation onset. If the causal relation hypothesis is not sustained, one can maintain the existence of a structural and functional
relationship depending on the same neuro-physiological mechanism.
But the hypothesis that all these traits are dependent on a still
unobservable trait which would remain to be identified through new
indices is excluded by all these complementary studies.

Such a distinction seems all the more important as a number of studies do not make clear which strategy has been chosen. When it comes to classifying groups of patients and no longer defining groups of traits, then ambiguity is apparent. Sometimes, the nosological class is considered as a law accounting for the coexistence of traits because of their structural and functionnal coherence (G. Klerman). At other times, the nosological class is seen as the expression of a particular process, an autonomous disease with its specific etiology. In the first instance, categorization corresponds to a law. In the other, it suggests the existence of a specific causality and invites the search for objects and their indices entering the causal track. In the second perspective, we are invited to search for the primary disorder, at the behavioural level, which could cause all other observable traits.

We do not mean that a choice has to be made between the two approaches. It should only be emphasized that according to the chosen hypothesis, different strategies will be needed for further investigations. In one case, hypotheses have to be validated. In the other case, indices must be sought which would make it possible to turn the intervening variable into a new dependent variable.

ON SOME TRAPS OF INTERVENING VARIABLES

COMMENTS ON D. WIDLÖCHER'S PAPER

Marc N. Richelle

Psychological Laboratory

University of Liege, Belgium

Widlöcher's paper clarifies, in a very relevant way, an essential distinction in the use of the words and concept of intervening variables. On one hand, intervening variables appear as a sort of missing link in a causal chain of events, some of which only are known. In this case intervening variables refer to events awaiting for explicit description. On the other hand, intervening variables have the status of a law, as Widlöcher calls it, or, as we would prefer to call. it, in a somewhat more vague and less ambitious manner, a construct. In this case, one will not expect to uncover events formerly inaccessible to inquiry, but only to disprove or to confirm a more or less consistent set of relationships.

The following comments will bear upon two points : 1) the distinction though an important one, is not always easy to draw practically; 2) no one can dispense with intervening variables in scientific reasoning, but no one should cease mistrusting them.

It should be reminded that the notion of intervening variables came into favour, in psychology, after Tolman, unable to explain the performance of rats in a maze, in terms of direct relations between independant and dependant variables, resorted to a cognitive map - in other words to some mediating level of internal representation, or of information processing as one would say today. The intervening variables in this sense, hold a central place since then in so-called cognitivist psychology. The latter gives special attention to the stage of elaboration that must be inferred to account for such phenomenon as the organisation of words in semantic clusters in a memory task. What used to be an intervening variable has become the very subject matter of that field of research. I should be noted that the issues are phrased in strictly psychological terms

- organisation, accessibility, hierarchisation, and the like.

The situation is quite different in the examples discussed by Widlöcher, taken from psychiatric research concerning drug effects. At one end, an independant variable, the compound, is clearly identified; at the other end, behavioral data, the symptoms, are described, with variable degrees of precision. Between the two, some causal sequence is assumed, the chemical compound altering neural structures in some way, with these changes being, in their turn, responsible for the changes observed in behavior. The missing link is first looked for at the neurochemical or at the neurophysiological level, and if one succeeds in describing the mechanism of action of the drug, one will have the feeling of having elucidated the intervening variable.

There is not doubt that we know more after we have shown that a given substance has a given action on serotoninergic neurons. But has the intervening variable been changed into an observable variable? We are left, of course, with the problem of the relation between the serotoninergic system(s) in the brain and behavior. The gap remains fantastically wide, and the variables to be disclosed hardly less difficult to deal with than before. The gap is often bridged, lightly enough, by putting between the newly discovered link and the dependant variable a link that is derived from the relation first observed between the drug and the symptoms, rather than it helps in explaining that relation. For instance, if the drug X changes the symptoms of depression, and if it is shown that X acts via the system S in the CNS, it will be concluded that S underlies, determines, explains the symptoms of depression. It is clear that the intervening variable is, in fact, only very partially elucidated, and what remains to be explained might very well fall into the second category proposed by Widlöcher, at least as long as the relatioship between behavioral and neuronal data will remain as mysterious as they are nowadays.

In consequence, we shall have to live, at least fo some time, with the second type of intervening variables. This is all right if we are aware of the risks involved. Ideally, we should, as suggested by Widlöcher, treat them as hypotheses - asking such questions as : is a given set of psychological and behavioral manifestations a structural and functional entity that can be clearly related to some nosological category ? In current research, however, they are often mistaken as unquestioned explanations. It is especially flagrant when the intervening variable is termed as a psychological function - intelligence, memory, agressivity, anxiety, and the like... If one neglects to characterize precisely such entities, - with means specifying corresponding behavior - it will always be possible to give them an explanatory power in favour of one's prefered interpretation. If I define anxiety, agressivity, memory, etc.. from a limited behavioral event, and if I use this definition to characterize the effects of a given drug, I dispense myself with investigating other possible factors responsible for the observed effect. A pseudo-explanation, putting an end to fruitful research, has taken the place of heuristically useful hypothesis. Psychiatric research is still sufficiently plagued with that kind of intervening variables to make a warning advisable.

EXPECTED AND UNEXPECTED PROBLEMS IN HOSPITAL CLINICAL TRIALS

Ole J. Rafaelsen

Psychochemistry Institute & Department of Psychiatry
Rigshospitalet
9, Blegdamsvej
DK - 2100 Copenhagen, Denmark

Clinical trials in hospital - and outside - are major under-takings. In the 1950's and even 1960's they were regarded as easy assignments for ambitious younger staff members and a gentleman-like hobby or pastime for the senior clinician. But that has all gone with the wind. Both clinicians and the drug companies feel it increasingly difficult to carry out such studies to the extent that it often seems to be an obstacle for the progress in clinical psycho-pharmacology.

So what are the expected and unexpected problems in hospital clinical trials?

I will like to discuss the problems under 3 headings:
1. Staff ambivalence
2. Patient ambivalence
3. Patient disappearance

STAFF AMBIVALENCE

This may again be divided into 4 problems:
1. Ethics
2. Competing and conflicting views on psychiatry
3. Non-science attitude to psychiatry
4. Work load

Ethics

The ethical problems of drug trials are nowadays made quite explicit and open via the obligation in many countries to get the

261

approval of the local, regional or national ethical committee. I will only mention two aspects of importance for psychiatry: It is accepted by the Declaration of Helsinki (1964, revised 1975), that there may be situations where it is not in the best interest of the patient(s) to obtain full information, but in such cases the researchers must be able to explain the specific reasons to the ethical committee which then must decide whether this is acceptable or not (§II.5).

I should also like to bring to your notice the very diplomatic way in which the problem of informed consent is phrased. The Helsinki Declaration states that "informed consent should be obtained, preferably in writing". This was a compromize in order to satisfy those countries where the law profession has managed to make it obligatory to obtain informed consent in writing. To me this is an encroachment of legal points of view on the doctor-patient relation- ship, and in my part of the world we have till now been able to repel such influence and I - in my country - advice never to have patients giving their consent in writing.

Competing and conflicting views on psychiatry

It is evident that psychiatry has to - or tries to - contain some very different, contradictory, and sometimes openly belligerent views on psychic disorders and that this has obvious and far-reaching consequences for treatment and research. Even when the medical staff manages to respect that major differences in approach exist between staff members, the biologically oriented psychiatrists accepting psychotherapy - and even practising it themselves - and the psychoanalytically oriented accepting psychopharmacology - and even making use of it - the major problem is the nursing staff (and in some cases the psychologists and social workers). Nursing staff attitudes - positive and negative - may show that armistice between the psychiatrists may be less solid than hoped for.

The nursing profession is also at a crossroad, where the more ambitious or advanced or adventurous claim that the less ambitious are accepting an old-fashioned female submissive role, as slaves for ambitious male doctors.

So some nurses turn to philosophical discourse reading Habermas, while others will undertake own research, have their own research programs focussing on individual and community health and patient resources - opposed to the medical doctors with their emphasis on disease processes and patients' inborn or acquired vulnerability.

Non-science attitudes to psychiatry

This leads us to the bordering problem of non-scientific atti- tudes. Many doctors and nurses are attracted to psychiatry due to its involvements outside the natural sciences; some will even claim

that only a minor part of psychiatry is related to the natural
sciences, and this of course have consequenses for their views on
research which could take two directions: one that the approaches
of the humanistic disciplines should be employed, e.g., hermeneutic
rather than positivistic; the other that research with quantification
and falsification in its banner is useless or even damaging and in-
humane.

Anti-psychiatry writers have sometimes managed to influence
hospital staff that did not realize that antipsychiatry basically
was part of a more generalized move against authority, profession,
and intellect.

Work load

It is bad if a researcher does not realize how much work a
certain project involves for himself, but it is even worse if he does
not realize how much work it involves for others, perhaps especially
the nursing staff. I am afraid that the nursing staff sometimes is
not properly informed before the start of a project, is not properly
supported during the project, and is not properly recognized when it
is all over.

PATIENT AMBIVALENCE

1. Time loss
2. Uncertainty
3. Non-compliance

Patient ambivalence will often be thought of as a problem
whether the patient trusts the doctor or not, and therefore accepts
to enter a study or refuses to do so.

Time loss

Even if the research program has a choice between two treatments
believed to have the same wanted effect(s), qualitatively and quantitatively, and therefore easily acceptable by the patient, time loss
may be a definite problem. Most clinical trials require a wash-out
period, and the length of that period always generate heated debate
during the research planning, as 2 to 4 weeks would be ideal for
pharmacokinetic reasons, but such a hurdle would clamp down patient
entry very considerably.

In some places it has been attempted to solve this problem by
having an obligatory 7 to 14 days placebo period (which then also
serves as a wash-out period), but it means that some doctors and
nurses tell some 'white' lies in this introductory period.

Uncertainty

Even if it is often heard these days that patients want complete information to enable them to make their own choices, it is my firm impression that many patients want to lean on the authority of their doctors, the more so when the disease is serious or even life-threatening. So even though a patient intellectually can accept a certain clinical research program, he or she is deprived of denial as a psychological defense mechanism in the case of doubt whether his or her treatment is the right one. And patients in doubt of the right or wrong treatment respond less favourably than those who are full of trust.

Non-compliance

A wealth of studies have indicated that non-compliance is a serious problem in pharmacotherapeutics inside and especially outside hospitals. Research programs can include measures that minimize non-compliance, but even so researchers often become surprised or discouraged by non-compliance; the research setting reveals what is often hidden or neglected in every-day practice.

PATIENT DISAPPEARANCE

1. Stricter criteria
2. Change in hospitalization pattern
3. Over-optimism or bio-statistical ignorance

It comes quite often as a great surprise to researchers - ready to start after having toiled with the more and more cumbersome preparations - that there are no suitable patients around. This may at least have 3 reasons.

Stricter criteria

Assessment in psychiatry has become more sophisticated during recent years. This is valid both for diagnostic assessment systems and for quantificatory tools, i.e., rating scales. A rating scale can in a standardized way give a naturalistic measure of this clinical picture. The research criteria can exclude most patients. In daily practice we rarely realize the variation in clinical pictures that we accept without becoming too worried about diagnosis, but in clinical trials the researchers are often surprised how few patients fulfil the inclusion criteria.

Change in hospitalization pattern

In all medical specialties in developed countries patients hospitalized have more and more psycho-social problems complicating and blurring earlier 'classical' pictures; this trend is very marked in psychiatry.

Long-term treatment of affective and schizophrenic disorders will keep many patients out of hospital; those still being admitted represent a skewed subsample in relation to therapy resistance and to non-compliance. Such patients are less than optimal for a clinical trial.

Over-oprimism or bio-statistical ignorance

It is nowadays relatively simple to predict the number of patients needed to test an O-hypothesis, if it is decided what difference one is looking for and what certainty one will demand regarding type one and type two errors.

And still researchers embark on projects where it is highly improbable that the necessary number of patients will turn up within the next 3 to 5 years. It is perhaps the most frequent unethical involvement of patients when they enter studies that will never be completed and thus have participated without any benefit for themselves or for mankind.

PROPOSALS FOR THE FUTURE

So, how can we minimize the expected and unexpected problems of clinical hospital trials in the future?

I believe that one important factor is to construct better protocols. The introduction of ethical committees has led to an improvement of research protocols, as these now always have to be submitted to extramural inspection.

As a tool in the preparation of research protocols we have worked out two check-lists, skeletons or aide mémoires: one for clinical trials together with Dr. Per Bech and one for biological psychiatry (other than drug trials) together with Dr. Annette Gjerris. These tools are at the present being tried out at various research centres under the aegis of WHO.

REFERENCES

Kramp, P., Shapiro, R.W., and Rafaelsen, O.J., 1980, Multi-axial classification system of affective disorders (Multi-Clad), in: "Psychopathology of depression", Achte, K., ed., Psychiatria Fennica, Suppl: 321.

Rafaelsen, O.J., 1977, Objectivity in psychiatry. The viewpoint of biological psychiatry, in:"Danish year-book of philosophy. 4th Panel Discussion", Objectivity in Psychiatry, Munksgaard, Copenhagen, 14:187.

Rafaelsen, O.J., 1979, Ethics of Psychopharmacological Research, Prog Neuropsychopharmacol, 3:281.

Rafaelsen, O.J., and Bech, P., 1982, Protocol aide-mémoire for clinical research trials in psychopharmacology. Phase III studies. A proposal submitted to WHO.

Rafaelsen, O.J., and Gjerris, A., 1981, Aide-mémoire for investigations in biological psychiatry. A proposal submitted to WHO.

WHO / CIOMS, 1982, Proposed international guidelines for biomedical research involving human subjects, Geneva, WHO/CIOMS.

DISCUSSION : EXPECTED AND UNEXPECTED PROBLEMS SEEN

DURING CLINICAL TRIALS IN HOSPITAL SETTING

Dick Pierre

University Psychiatric Institutions

CH 1225 Chene-Bourg / Geneva

These last years, the growing difficulties seen during clinical trials in the industrially developed western countries have reached such a preoccupying level that serious fears are entertained about their probable impact upon our knowledge widening and future therapeutic possibilities.

There should be no major objections to O. Rafaelsen's clear analysis of the present state of affairs. Yet, considering the different unfolded problems, that they were expectable and expected or unexpected is now irrelevant compared to their actual consequences, in particular, the relative importance of the exercised pressions and of the resulting hindrances upon the clinical trials. This situation probably is not identical everywhere, but it seems to follow the same course.

With the social evolution during the second half of our century, a complete change of laymen's ideas and attitudes towards medicine in general and psychiatry in particular seems to have taken place. The medical role, more or less hidden, relatively mysterious, has been "desacralized". Foregoing the rules of a would-be-constructive criticism, the discussions and disputes have degenerated; contradictory opinions are tainted by ideology or even fanatism, aiming first of all at hegemony.

As a result, pressure groups have formed, using antipsychiatry and antichemisty-natural-ecology amongst other movements as banners.

The formulation and application of ethical rules in clinical trials have reduced their number and lead clinicians and manufacturers to respect a more rigorous methodology. Yet, through excessive red-tape or self-interested ethical commissions' manipulations, it is not impossible to hamper research to a point where chances for a future development are compromised.

Another difficulty comes from the changes in psychiatric wellfare methods, with the result among others to considerably modify the number and the characteristics of hospitalized patients. Is or will it still be possible to recruit representative groups of patients within this population suffering from the pathology one would like to study, since so many stay outside ? Transposing these trials in outpatient practice offers only a partial solution and could only be done with a suitable adjustment of the methodology, taking into account the risks and the obligations of a thoroughly different situation. And last but not least, the various impediments to clinical trials serve to emphasize a paradox : when the amazing progress of biological (chemical, pharmacological) research these last years would imply a more direct cooperation between pharmacologists and clinicians, the latter might be missing !

Failing an adequate animal model, many original hypotheses can only be corroborated in clinical trials, thereby making it possible to widen our knowledge in the physiopathology of mental diseases and the means to treat them in the future.

Surely the future of psychiatric therapeutics will be compromised if the actual restrictive ideological, political and social pressures worsen. Devising standard protocols and refined methodologies, necessary as they are, could yet be insufficient if the international organisations moral authority does not answer for them.

This problem's importance and complexity would fully justify that W.H.O. and the International Psychiatric Association attend to it and propose general rules as a reference and model.

Maybe this could help us prevent imposition of excessive and restrictive rules by an administrative power generally more interested in legal than ethical matters, making the clinical trials necessary to therapeutical progress impossible.

NATURALISTIC STUDIES : FEASABILITY AND INTEREST

Alain Spriet* and Pierre Simon**

* Laboratoires Hoechst, 3, avenue du Général de Gaulle
92800 Puteaux, France
** Département de Pharmacologie Clinique,
La Pitié-Salpétrière, 75013 Paris, France

If the controlled trial is the best tool to test a well defined, unique and a priori defined hypothesis, it is a poor way to describe peculiarities, originalities and preferred indications of new medicines.

Extensive uncontrolled studies by practitioners could be better used than usually without bearing suspicion of purely "promotional" or "seeding" purposes.

They should be designed as heuristic (hypothesis generating) methods (in contrast to controlled trials limited to test an unique well defined hypothesis).

We suggest the following rules :

- broad patient selection (within recognized indications) in order to approach "representativeness";

- minimal interference with normal follow-up of patients by their doctors : usual environments, routine follow-up and interviews, investigational material (case record forms, scales, samples) looking as little "experimental" as possible;

- concern about risks and benefits in natural use (eventually with non-optimal prescribing habits[1]);

- obviously when the trial is initiated by the manufacturer, free samples of the drug should be given. Solutions have

to be found to make this feature as "natural" as possible
(intervention of pharmacist ? agreement with social security ?)

- large sample size to give some interest to subgroups[2]

- relative freedom in prescription schedule provided any
  details are reliably recorded;

- follow-up visits at fixed dates but with some tolerance range
  (or even several options to visit schedules)

- outcome evaluation by broad, simple, multifactor rating scales.
  Even for simple scales, minimal training of raters should be
  considered. Use of video tapes as training material can be the
  solution to train many raters for a multi-investigators study.

- essentially descriptive statistics with feed-back from the
  results on the choice of methods : subgroups, item weightings,
  use of prior covariates (social environment, personality,
  therapist features) as well as variates known after
  initiation of treatment : adherence, life events;

- backward thinking from results to initial features using
  methods to "discriminate" responders from non-responders;

- attempt to validate "prediction" by split-sample methods, by
  prospective prediction in further cases, or N calculations
  of prediction functions from N - 1 cases, with application
  to N-th case;

- awareness of very large probability of chance finding from
  multiple and flexible statistical methods, and need of
  confirmation of any important results by specific controlled
  trials.

FEASIBILITY

The problem of data collection by many investigators of simple
data with a simple protocol faces a formidable handicap : doctors
are used with old pratices of non-strict studies aimed to simple
"calculation of percentages" in which no rigor was expected. The
old bad habits are long to abandon. Intention to do better studies
does not imply, in this context strict adherence to a strict
protocol but reliable information.

Training sessions prior to the trial improve considerably
data collection. Discussions of protocol, taking into account
objections and suggestions from participants, are also necessary.

Checking data in order to pinpoint inaccuracies, contradictory
informations, and missing data, is necessary.

The system of clinical trials technicians (clinical research associates) visiting participants for controlled trials seems unrealistic for extensive studies.

We have experienced a system of mailed feed back with good response rate but it should be further improved.

Costs of extensive studies are still difficult to evaluate and are largely conditioned by the fees that doctors expect from participation.

It is generally calculated per case record filled, and on the basis of the fees per visit. Therefore the total number of cases is limited by available budget. It is conceivable that doctors can participate for modest fees in the case of a study not initiated by a drug company.

Two studies aimed specifically to prediction and presented as so to participants, were coordinated by us in the recent years, respectively with 958 and 509 cases using procedures recommended here. The second study was done in order to take into account problems in the first [3,4,5]. Both studies were done by psychiatrists with the antidepressant Nomifensine.

One recently completed extensive study with the anxiolytic drug Clobazam [6], done by general practitioners included 11242 out-patients. It allowed, for instance, calculation of frequencies of side effects separately for each dose and each type of co-therapy. Data from this study can now be used for descriptive "heuristic analysis".

INTEREST

It is still too early to know which practical results will be actually obtained from so planned and analysed studies.

We can only speak about hopes. The preliminary attempts mentioned earlier, done by psychiatrists, brought essentially confirmation of the role of prognostic variables already known as possibly playing a role.

But more analyses, or more data from more patients treated by other doctors (general practitioners) with longer treatments are probably necessary to go farther.

It is hardly conceivable that drugs having different impacts on brain amines yield qualitatively the same effects and that the same patients can take benefit from any of them. The differences must lie somewhere and we should try hard to find them. We hope that positive interest will be demonstrated by other studies.

REFERENCES

1. L. LASAGNA, A plea for the "naturalistic" study of medicines, Europ. J. Clin. Pharmacol., 7:153-154 (1974).
2. R. SIMON, Patient subsets and variation in therapeutic efficacy, Br. J. Clin. Pharmac., 14:473-482 (1982).
3. GROUPE COOPERATIF D'ETUDE, Résultats d'un essai prédictif de réponse à la nomifensine chez les malades ambulatoires, Nouv. Presse Méd., 7:2323-2330 (1978).
4. A. SPRIET, D. BEILER, J. DECHORGNAT, C.D. CHIGOT, M. ROSSNER, P. SIMON, Méthodologie d'une étude coopérative des prédicteurs de réponse dans des syndromes dépressifs ambulatoires traités par la nomifensine, Nouv. Presse Méd., 7:2317-2322 (1978).
5. A. SPRIET, J.C. LEMARIE, J. DECHORGNAT, P. SIMON, Facteurs pronostiques chez des déprimés ambulatoires traités par la nomifensine, Psychologie Médicale, 14:1741-1755 (1982).
6. A. BERGMAN, K. PAHNKE, Bericht über eine offene Studie Clobazam, Internal report Hoechst A.G., Frankfurt.

THE NECESSITY OF NATURALISTIC STUDIES

René P. De Buck

Clinical Psychopharmacology Research Unit
Institute of Psychiatry, Brugmann University Hospital
Brussels

Spriet and Simon have discussed quite a few very important points and I am in agreement with most of their attitudes towards naturalistic studies. However, as a clinician, I should like to go a little further in this naturalistic direction.

Nobody would dare to pretend nowadays that phase 1, A and phase 3 - controlled studies could be avoided or even reduced. We can understand that before marketing a drug, some undisputable data should be collected as to clinical efficacy and side effects. These data are also exacted by the various administrations. But what do we really know about a drug when it is marketed ? What can we really expect from it ?

The present methodology used in planning clinical trials leaves us with much ignorance and frustration. I have conducted myself quite a number of clinical trials, mostly double blind comparisons with a reference drug, as well with neuroleptics, with anxiolytics as with antidepressants and what kind of results did we get after filling in hundreds of forms... almost always the same: no statistically significant difference between the two drugs !

We should admit that our present procedures tend to level off any new, original, interesting features of the drug on trial.

We seem to have forgotten that one interesting case report may bring along more progress than ten controlled studies and that the main discoveries of the past thirty years in clinical psychopharmaco-logy have been made by chance, by serendipidity or thanks to the talentuous observation of a skillful clinician.

In this respect, naturalistic studies appear to be a true necessity. Here we have big numbers of patients, natural conditions of observation and we have also time. Time is important for in quite a few instances, new indications, new dosage schedules, new side effects such as dependance, new interactions with other drugs only appear after a few years of use.

Who should organize these postmarketing studies ?
The drug company ? Government agencies ? My personal opinion would be in favour of leaving this to the practitioners themselves. Even if some financial support by the manufacturer might be needed for the organisation of such studies, they should originate independen-tly to avoid any suspicion particularly in the present negative climate towards the pharmaceutical industry.

In the process of organizing such a naturalistic study, one has immediately to face an important contradiction: one has to obtain, as Dr Spriet and Simon have pointed out, rigorous and relia-ble data which means respect of some protocol but one has also to interfere as little as possible with the usual therapeutical setting of the practising psychiatrist or general practitioner.

The protocol should be simple, open to spontaneous observations. It should not include too many heavy scales but offer much blank space for comments.

The clinician should be able to work exactly as usual, with nothing experimental in the atmosphere. He should devote to the patient the usual time. Nothing unfamiliar should interfere. That is why we should advocate that the doctor prescribes the drug in the usual way and that the patient should buy it from the pharmacist. At this stage no biological evaluation should routinely be asked for. This might make the patient anxious.

It is difficult in such a short time to discuss the various aspects of these naturalistic studies but I shall add an important point. In such a natural setting, we should be aware that many other factors besides the drug can play a role, the main ones being life events and the personality of the doctor. These impor-tant variables should be evaluated in some way in order to define the impact of the drug itself. Life events should be carefully recorded.

Before the start of the trial, the participants should be extensively interviewed on their background conceptions, motivations, drawbacks, opinions about drugs and so on, so that the coordinators might have a profile of the doctors involved. They should also be completely informed about the purpose of the study, the scales used and encouraged to detailed observation of individual cases.

Provided all these precautions are taken, naturalistic studies could be an unvaluable complement to phase 1 and 2 and phase 3 - controlled studies. Only with the help of such projects shall we be able to assign to a new drug its real profile of indications and limitations and, still more important, to raise new hypotheses. This might allow clinical psychopharmacology to come out of the present routine and make new progress.

STATISTICAL METHODS IN PSYCHIATRY - VIRTUAL MODELS

J.R. Barra

University of Grenoble

1- The statistical methods actually used in therapeutic trials do not seem satisfactory for many reasons :

a) When they are based upon classical statistical inference, these methods demand a probability model define a priorie i.e. "n independent observations from a same theoretical patient". This model is difficult to justify and the rules intended to insure its credibility lead to conditions of homogeneity which are sometimes excessive and result in a small number of observations.

b) When they are based upon Data Analysis it is the computing procedure that is fixed and the rigidity of the model is replaced by the "computing dictature". The methodological bases no longer exist and therefore the conclusions are uncertain.

c) They are directly taken from statistical methods used in the therapeutic trials in medicine and do not take into account the specificity of the statistical function in psychiatry.

An excellent criticism of this situation can be seen in [4] and in [2].

2- Classical statistical inference

The following diagram represents the usual process of a classical statistical approach :

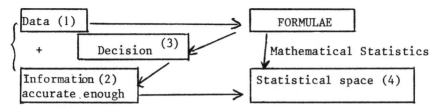

In the therapeutic trials :

(1) The number of observations is generally small (30 to 50).
(2) We are speaking here of the rules of controlled trials where we need experimental conditions (homogeneity between and within groups) so that the statistical space correspond to one or more samples.
(3) The decision is to accept or to reject the medicine
(4) The statistical space is the product of samples (cf. [5]) that means independent groups of independent observations of a same theoretical patient representative of the group.

The classical statistical inference has :

a) The advantage of an error whose probability is controlled (level of significance).

b) The following disadvantages :
   1. Small number of observations
   2. Exclude the taking into account of factors
(psychiatric...) that we would expect to be very interesting
   3. The fundamental role played by the statistical space : we do not discover anything, we confirm or we invalidate sub-hypotheses within a set of a priori hypotheses.

3- Exploratory data analysis

The following diagram represents the usual process of exploratory data analysis :

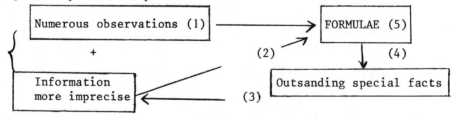

where :

(1) More open trials with less strict rules.
(2) The choice of formulae is empirical enough and can be guided by pre-conceptions of the psychiatrist.
(3) Conjections, that is to say the most often, correlations between factors and effects of the medicine.

Data Analysis has the following advantages :
1. One can take into account a large number of different trials.
2. The protocol of these trials can be more flexible.
3. One can more easily integrate in the analysis the experimentalist's intuition.
4. One can take into consideration quite a large number of factors.

But the fundamental disadvantage is that it does not lead to conclusions with measurable risks.

4- Virtual models

The two preceeding approaches of statistics are more complementary than in opposition and only differ by the role attributed to the model which is chosen a priori and unchangeable in classical statistical inference, eluded but concealed in data analysis.

In fact one can easily see that the majority of formulae of data analysis can be obtained by the methods of classical statistics according to the choice of an adequate fundamental statistical space.

Then it is natural enough to propose as methodological basis of data analysis the notion of a virtual model. We are speaking about a statistical model that does not correspond well with any reality but which is fictive and we do not seek to justifiy it a priori ; we introduce this model momentarily with the hope that the results of the observations behave as if the model were acceptable.

This notion of virtual model seems satisfactory to fill the methodological gap that for example VICTOR in [4] deplores in data Analysis ; moreover this virtual model is a good guide for choosing the formulae that we use.

According to this point of view, data Analysis can be considered as a statistical analysis relatively to virtual models eventually variable ; so the credibility of the results are mainly correlated to the stability of these results when the observations or the virtual model change.

5- Suggestion for an iterative methodology

The above mentioned leads to the binging into operation by iteration a combination of two families of statiscal methods.

For the therapeutic trials in psychiatry :
a) Maintain the actual procedure of therapeutic trials on a small number of patients carefully selected but only with an administrative inference without purpose of research.

b) Introduce a new procedure having an exploratory character based upon a very large number of observations ; we will take into account

b) Introduce a new procedure having an exploratory character based upon a very large number of observations ; we will take into account many factors without any pretention of objective inference but only with the purpose of researching some conjectures on the medicine's efficacity.

It is essential to be very strict with the ontology and to recall that no inference with measurable risks can be possible. Moreover it is clear that such studies certainly demand a quite sophisticated computing logistic.

In conclusion we can test the conjectures which are given by 2), using therapeutic trials of type 1) ; in this case the observations will be evidently different in 1) compared to 2 and the rules will be as strict as now but adapted to the tested conjectures.

REFERENCES

[1] FISHER, Statistical Methods for Research workers. Oliver and boyd, 1956.
[2] SCHNEIDER, The role of hypothesis testing in clinical trials. Methods of information in meicine, Volume 20, n° 2, Avril 1981.
[3] J.W. TUKEY, Exploratory data Analysis. Addison Wesley, 1977.
[4] VICTOR, Exploratory data analysis and clinical research. Methods of information in Medicine, Volume 21, 1982.
[5] J.R. BARRA, Mathematical basis of statistics. Academic Press, 1981.

DISCUSSION OF: STATISTICAL METHODS IN PSYCHIATRY:

VIRTUAL MODELS

H. Luccioni
Clinique Univ. de Psych., Hopital de la Timone
F-13385 Marseille Cedex 05, France

Victor, whom Prof. Barra cited, took a stand against the tendency to believe that there is "automatically good science" if results are based on tests of statistical significance. In effect, these presuppose a univocal hypothesis and specific conditions. Now in psychiatry, on the one hand, the state of knowledge requires above all that research proceed step by step as one would explore a poorly known continent and, on the other hand, the pre-requisites of strictly decisional statistics are not respected in the investigations owing to the practical difficulties that they raise. This is why the first "Meeting of Methodology of Research in Psychiatry" in Marseille in 1971 took these "new" statistics represented by data analysis as its theme. They were just becoming known then and have since enjoyed an extraordinarily wide diffusion penetrating all those disciplines which CANGUILHEM qualified as "formless" in opposition to the methodologically constituted sciences. They are in effect "statistical instruments", the application of which is particularily seductive because of the few constraints they place on the collection of "phenomena" and at the same time because of all they enable to reveal concerning structures or inapparent regularities. But in our workshop, which had decided to carry on its reflective effort, the same questions cropped up time and time again asking whether precisely this facility was not dangerous and this fecundity illusory.

Evidently, the computor does not possess the powers of a mysterious alchemy capable of turning common lead into pure gold, and we recognize even better the necessity of applying a critical wisdom both "upstream" and "downstream" from the "current" under statistical analysis in order to avoid coming out with just anything. But above all it was our good fortune to have in our midst specialists of mathematical statistics ill-disposed to go along with the pragmatic complacency of the researchers "in the field". Barra especially stressed the existence of a "methodological gap" and reminded us that statistics having no mathematical bases are unreliable. Today he

281

proposes an iterative methodology combining both families of statistical techniques through the application of this notion of "virtual model" which appears well adapted to the reality of research in psychiatry.

But he does not hide from us that these studies he proposes will require a rigorous deontology and new computor logistics.

RESEARCH STRATEGIES AND TACTICS IN PSYCHIATRIC RESEARCH

INTRODUCTION

H. Luccioni
Clinique Univ. de Psych., Hopital de la Timone
F-13385 Marseille Cedex 05, France

During the last two decades psychiatric theory and practice has been shaken by two series of earthquakes, of variable magnitude, whose epicenters lie precisely at the antipodes. One series, known by the rather vague epithet "antipsychiatry", trends to separate psychiatry from medicine by denying the reality of "mental illness". The other, arising with the discovery of psychotropic medication, medicalizes it to the extent that one wonders if the traditional specificity of the discipline - the "psyche" will be forgotten. This latter seismic phenomenon, to me more devastating to traditional thought and action, has already succeeded in upsetting research by working an ever-increasing number of disciplines into its field: phenomenology, biochemistry, psychophysiology, statistics, and also pharmacokinetics, electrophysiology, neuropsychology, etc.

It would be foolish to deny the great progress of knowledge achieved by this "biological" psychiatry; however, a careful and critical witness cannot avoid being disappointed and irritated by the <u>uselessness</u> of much of the mass of work being done. It looks as if one "pretends" to do research, with a luxury of instrumental manuevers and recourse to statistical significances - all in an experimental proceedings which does not seem to have been seriously thought out . . . . .

Will one retort the subject matter is complex and thus a complete description and coherent explanation is not possible? To be sure, a so-called "classic" epistemology has defined scientific procedure according to two requirements: the first is that of the <u>quest for a linear causality,</u> made possible by the <u>experimental structure</u> wherein all variables other than those under consideration are effiectively neutralized; the second is that of a logic according to which a statement can only be true or false, evidently in keeping with the principle of non-contradiction. Now, it was clearly impossible for psychiatric research to satisfy these requirements.

Nevertheless, the progress of knowledge in the sciences - an extraordinary progress - has imposed a new methodology. This turning-point occurred exactly 50 years ago, when, through an astonishing conjuncture from the formal point of view, Godel and Tarski introduced the notion of the "value of truth" and, from the experimental point of view, Heisenberg introduced the principle of uncertainty . . . . . and since then many others have contributed, such as Prigogine, for whom Tissot is justified in underlining the serendipitous importance.

A conclusion? It is fitting here in Vienna to quote Popper. His opinion carries clout, undoubtedly owing to the numour with which he defends the idea that science is a controlled convention.

But this is not the place to give a lecture. Besides, methodology is not a framework of precise constraints encompassing creative wealth. The essence of this "open" epistemology lies in what Gonseth called the "philosophy of re" reflect, recommence, rectify - and of these imperatives reflect is the most important. This is what those giving lectures and taking part in discussions on nine important questions invite us to do.

GENOTYPE, PHENOTYPE ET REGULATIONS EPIGENETIQUES

Tissot René

Institutions Universitaires De Psychiatrie

CH 1225 Chene-Bourg / Geneve

D'aucuns se demanderont au nom de quelle aberration on a pu confier ce sujet à un clinicien, même s'il est quelque peu mâtiné de biologiste, et plus encore au nom de quoi le clinicien sollicité a pu accepter cette tâche ! Bonnes raisons ou non, au sens gidien du terme, on peut en citer plusieurs. La pratique médicale, et mieux encore la pratique psychiatrique permettraient à elles seules de réfuter les théories reçues qui, encore trop souvent, relient génotype et phénotype par une causalité linéaire et univoque. Nombre de spécialistes qui ont le plus contribué à établir la complexité de la construction du phénotype à travers l'interaction du génome et de l'environnement restent, par conventionnalisme ou inertie métaphysique, des champions de ces idées reçues. Ainsi MONOD qui écrit : ... "Ce système, par ses propriétés, par son fonctionnement d'horlogerie microscopique, qui établit entre ADN et protéines, comme aussi entre organisme et milieu, des relations à sens unique, défie toute description dialectique. Il est foncièrement cartésien et non hégélien : la cellule est bien une machine". LEDER, après avoir montré que les recombinaisons du génome se poursuivent au niveau des lymphocytes B durant toute la vie afin de produire l'énorme diversité des anticorps, conclut qu'elles procèdent du hasard. Plus grave est l'extension de ces mêmes notions à la biologie générale des comportements. Comme l'écrit DOBZHANSKY, "pour un darwiniste social, il est indiscutable que des problèmes sociaux tels que le crime, la pauvreté, l'ignorance sont issus, non de quelques défauts d'organisation de la société mais simplement d'une déficience des gènes". Au contraire, les antidarwinistes voulaient "que la réforme sociale et l'environnement fussent tout puissants. Ils en venaient à rejeter tout conditionnement génétique des caractères de l'indi-

285

vidu. Si bien que la position adoptée... n'était plus que le simple
reflet d'opinions politiques". Malheureusement, depuis l'impression
du livre de DOBZHANSKY, cette querelle ne s'écrit plus au passé. On
voudrait pouvoir négliger le darwinisme social et l'antipsychiatrie.
Mais notre discipline à maille à partir avec ces idéologies dans sa
pratique de tous les jours. Elle ne saurait oublier que, dans l'his-
toire, des querelles semblables ont précédé la mise en oeuvre de
certains génocides. A. HOCHE, distingué neuropsychiatre qui a large-
ment contribué à la description de la dégénérescence transsynapti-
que, n'écrivait-il pas, avec BINDING, un juriste, en 1920, dans un
opuscule intitulé "Die Freigabe der Vernichtung lebensumverten Lebens", "un jour viendra où assez mûris, nous estimerons que la mise
de côté de ces individus à l'esprit mort n'est pas un crime mais
bien un acte permis, un acte utile".

Venons aux faits. Nous examinerons succinctement : la crise du
néo-darwinisme ou de la théorie synthétique de l'évolution; les problèmes posés par l'épigenèse, aussi bien au niveau de l'embryologie
que du développement postnatal; les isomorphismes de l'épigenèse à
ces différents niveaux; les leçons de la clinique psychiatrique;
pour conclure à l'inanité de l'opposition de l'inné et de l'acquis
et à la nécessité d'un tertium pour lequel beaucoup de données de
faits sont déjà acquises mais au développement duquel s'opposent les
paradigmes traditionnels des sciences positives.

La crise du néo-darwinisme et de la théorie synthétique de l'évolution

La théorie synthétique, comme chacun le sait, comporte deux
aspects principaux :

1) les mutations géniques d'origine aléatoire sont la source des variations des organismes; l'évolution des espèces résulte des changements du pool génétique d'une population; ces derniers provien-
   nent eux-mêmes de l'accumulation de mutations; autrement dit,
   l'accumulation de micro-changements évolutifs rend compte de la
   macro-évolution;

2) la direction des changements est le fait de la sélection naturel-
   le portant sur chacune de ces petites variations.

Le noeud de cette conception, la micro-évolution rend compte de la
macro-évolution, est fortement contesté. Les paléontologistes estiment que les séries de fossiles dans lesquelles s'observe l'apparition d'espèces nouvelles ne sont pas compatibles avec cette théorie.
Le plus souvent une espèce reste identique à elle-même pendant de
très longues périodes (milliards d'années) puis brusquement dispa-
raît pour être remplacée par une autre très différente mais qui dérive manifestement de la précédente. L'évolution paraît donc comporter

des sauts dont les aléas de la fossilisation souvent incriminés ne
sauraient rendre compte. La stabilité des espèces suppose donc une
organisation du pool génétique capable de ramener tous les changements intermittents à la position moyenne commune. Pour expliquer les
modifications brusques de la macro-évolution, certains évoquent l'i-
nitiative de populations pionnières qui auraient changé de milieu.
Elles seraient alors en déséquilibre, menacées d'extinction, ou sus-
ceptibles de donner naissance à une nouvelle espèce. Il ne s'agit
encore là que de coup de pouce à la théorie synthétique. Certains
embryologistes et biologistes moléculaires s'en écartent davantage.
Ils estiment que de nombreuses directions nouvelles évolutives peuvent être attribuées non pas à un changement intrinsèque de un ou
plusieurs gènes par mutation aléatoire mais à un réarrangement du
pool génétique. Un réarrangement suppose qu'il y avait avant lui un
arrangement, donc une organisation génique stable dont les relations
entre les différents éléments qui la composent sont aussi importantes que les propriétés intrinsèques de chacun d'eux. Les embryologistes insistent encore sur le fait que les contraintes de l'épigé-
nèse imposent des canaux au programme génétique. N'importe quelle
construction n'est pas possible. Les instructions du génome seraient
filtrées par les contraintes du développement de façon à aboutir à
un phénotype donné. Ce filtrage ne porte pas sur le phénotype achevé
mais opère tout au long de son développement. Ceci nous amène au problème central des

Régulations de l'épigenèse

Tout est encore à faire pour l'oeuf fécondé qui vient de rece-
voir son génome. L'épigenèse, aussi bien celle de l'embryon que du
développement postnatal, va constituer une vaste entreprise de maîtrise des phénomènes aléatoires de l'environnement.

Schématiquement, les embryologistes distinguent trois grandes
périodes dans l'ontogenèse : une première pendant laquelle l'embryon,
s'il est mutilé, est capable d'une régénération totale. Une deuxième
de différenciation des tissus et des organes avec des possibilités
d'induction variées mais sans cette capacité de régénération totale.
Une troisième de réintégration où les tissus et les organes différenciés sont à nouveau soumis à une organisation globale, en particulier sous l'influence du système nerveux, pour parvenir à un fonctionnement intégré. Pendant ces trois périodes fonctionnellement très
différentes, le génome de l'embryon devrait être identique selon la
théorie synthétique. Rien n'empêche d'admettre qu'il comporte lui-
même la programmation de ces diverses étapes et qu'en conséquence il
construise l'environnement auquel il va répondre différemment à chaque période. Pour être lui-même au départ du milieu intérieur caractéristique de chacune d'elles, sa réponse (première période, régéné-

rescence totale; deuxième période, régénérescence différentielle) n'en varie pas moins en fonction de cet environnement tissulaire. Il existe donc, à tout le moins, entre le génome et son environnement tissulaire, une organisation de type systémique dont une causalité à sens unique ne saurait rendre compte. Pour WADDINGTON, l'environnement cytoplasmique : "agit différentiellement sur les noyaux en activant certains gènes dans une région et d'autres gènes dans une autre". A la deuxième période en particulier, l'activité du génome est canalisée. Cette canalisation, pour laquelle WADDINGTON a forgé le terme de "créode" (chemin nécessaire) peut résulter aussi bien de l'autorégulation de la population des gènes entre eux, que du milieu intérieur (facteur cytoplasmique), que d'événements survenant dans le milieu environnant extérieur au sujet. La créode réalise une homéorhésis qui est beaucoup plus qu'une homéostasie puisque, en dépit des changements de condition du développement, elle maintient la direction d'évolution d'un système. L'embryogenèse est d'abord caractérisée par des adaptations qui permettent de maintenir l'homéorhésis grâce à la propre organisation interne de l'organisme. On peut parler d'adaptation endogène mais elle ne saurait tenir à l'action unilatérale du génome. La transplantation d'une ébauche de rétine plus petite que la normale entraîne le développement d'un cristallin adapté. Si l'on veut encore parler de sélection, il s'agit de ce que déjà BALDWIN nommait la sélection organique (effet Baldwin, systèmes régulateurs et téléonomiques du milieu intérieur).

Après la naissance, les interactions du génome avec l'environnement vont dominer la situation. Mais on conçoit de moins en moins l'action du milieu comme une sélection par élimination ou conservation d'un phénotype achevé. Le milieu agit certes sur le phénotype mais tout au long de son développement, et en particulier par la sélection organique, en modifiant le milieu intérieur dans lequel se déroule le programme génétique. L'homéorhésis de structuration anatomique se poursuit. L'ouvrage récent, bien informé, de CHANGEUX en donne de nombreux exemples. Rappelons les différences de l'agencement synaptique de crustacés isogéniques, la régression postnatale du nombre des jonctions synaptiques des cellules de Purkinje du cervelet du rat et de la souris, la réduction du nombre des neurones médullaires de l'embryon du poulet, l'organisation postnatale des jonctions neuromusculaires liée à leur activité, comme celle du cortex visuel du chaton qui, s'il est aveuglé, ne se développe pas. Quelles que soient les vertus explicatives de la sélection stabilisatrice qu'affectionne CHANGEUX, nous sommes loin de comprendre les mécanismes intimes de ces régulations épigénétiques qui se manifestent tout au long du développement du gamète fécondé à la mort. Elles témoignent à tout le moins que les relations à sens unique génome / phénotype auxquelles reste fixé un MONOD ne peuvent en rendre compte. Avec PIAGET et WADDINGTON nous dirons "que le génome doit être conçu comme un système actif de réponses et de réorganisation faisant face au milieu sans le subir sans plus, mais utilisant ses informations au lieu de l'ignorer et de lui imposer son programme".

Certaines études de biochimie moléculaire approchent ces mécanismes de plus près. Nous retiendrons l'exemple du contrôle génétique de la production des immunoglobulines (LEDER). Il montre que les réorganisations du génome dans les lymphocytes B se poursuivent toute la vie, et il aborde leur description au niveau moléculaire. La conception génétique traditionnelle atomistique faisait appel à la causalité linéaire, supposant qu'à chaque anticorps formé correspondait un gène programmeur. Or on sait que le système immunologique peut produire de 10^6 à 10^8 anticorps spécifiques. L'auteur montre que cette énorme variété d'anticorps peut correspondre à la recombinaison de "régions" constantes du génome au nombre de quelques-unes, avec des chaînes variables en plus grand nombre comportant un gène régulateur. De cette façon, quelques centaines de lieux géniques rendent compte de la production de 10^6 à 10^8 variétés d'anticorps. Il s'agit d'un principe d'économie un peu comparable à celui des langues naturelles qui, avec quelques phonèmes, permettent d'engendrer un nombre de signes ouvert à l'infini. Le signal de la mise en production de l'anticorps est bien sûr la présence d'antigènes. Pourtant l'auteur conclut, en fidèle néo-darwiniste, que les réorganisations géniques en cause se produisent au hasard et que seules seraient fixées, du fait de la présence d'antigènes, celles qui sont utiles. Une loterie vertigineuse de recombinaisons serait donc sans cesse à l'oeuvre au niveau du génome pour qu'à l'arrivée de l'antigène, la combinaison gagnante soit à disposition et se stabilise. C'est conférer au seul hasard un pouvoir téléonomique bien puissant.

Les isomorphismes de l'épigenèse organique et psychologique

Limitons-nous à quelques exemples : la réduction du nombre des contacts synaptiques entre neurones ou entre neurones et fibres musculaires trouve son pendant dans la diminution du nombre des "syllabes" du chant du moineau des marais, de la naissance à l'âge adulte. De même on sait, après JAKOBSON, que le bébé émet tous les phonèmes constitutifs des différentes langues naturelles du globe. Les débuts de l'apprentissage du langage sont marqués par une réduction importante des phonèmes émis, précédant le réapprentissage laborieux de ceux de la langue maternelle.

Le développement cognitif a ses chemins obligés, ses créodes comme le développement embryologique. Avant 4 ou 5 ans on peut apprendre aux enfants à compter jusqu'à 20. Cela n'entraîne pas la maîtrise de la numération. Même après les avoir comptées, ces enfants n'admettent pas l'égalité de deux collections d'objets (oeuf et coquetier par exemple) en dehors de leur correspondance spatiale biunivoque. La maîtrise de la numération implique le chemin obligé de la synthèse des opérations de classifications et de sériations qui est plus tardive.

Les réorganisations du génome telles celles décrites par LEDER, ne sont pas sans rappeler la productivité du raisonnement logico-mathématique qui, comme les précédentes, ne trouve à s'insérer dans le réel qu'une fois consolidée la synthèse de ses nouvelles structurations. Créode encore que le développement divergent et décalé des divers invariants physiques, longueur, quantité de matière.

Selon PIAGET, les processus cognitifs "apparaissent comme la résultante de l'autorégulation organique dont ils reflètent les mécanismes essentiels et comme les organes les plus différenciés de cette régulation au sein des interactions avec l'extérieur". La psychogenèse, comme l'organogenèse, comporte une organisation séquentielle de stades. "Ceux-ci ne se définissent pas simplement par une propriété dominante, mais par une structure d'ensemble en équilibre caractérisant les régulations et les conduites de l'organisme, régulations et conduites auxquelles il est sans cesse ramené jusqu'à l'apparition d'un nouveau stade". Toute dérive dans cette organisation séquentielle est rapidement corrigée ou entraîne des anomalies importantes.

Les leçons de la clinique

Qui voudrait nier l'origine héréditaire de la chorée de Huntington, l'origine environnementale de la paralysie générale ? Il n'est pas davantage question de négliger la composante héréditaire des grandes psychoses naturelles de l'homme après tant de travaux patients et pertinents. La faille tient à l'extension consciente ou non du modèle dichotomique chorée de Huntington / paralysie générale, endogène / exogène, à la physiopathologie de l'ensemble des syndromes psychiatriques. Depuis KRAEPELIN, face à un malade dépressif, la psychiatrie prétend décider s'il s'agit d'une dépression endogène ou exogène. Les plus éclectiques d'entre nous souhaitent peser les composantes endogènes et exogènes. Les autres ont tendance à tout ramener au génome ou à l'environnement. Or tous les critères successivement essayés ont été successivement invalidés, le dernier d'entre eux, la réaction de la sécrétion de cortisol à la dexaméthasone comme les précédents (CARROLL, MENDLEWICZ). Après les travaux des classiques, de KETY et de bien d'autres, il est toujours des irrédentistes pour affirmer que la schizophrénie n'est qu'une sociopathie. Les arbres généalogiques les plus aveuglants, l'évolution de jumeaux élevés séparément, rien ne peut les dessiller, tant dans certaines circonstances, comme le disait PASCAL, "trop de clarté éblouit". Mais, par ailleurs, la catatonie avait pratiquement déjà disparu des hôpitaux scandinaves, bien pourvus en personnel, avant la psychopharmacologie; l'école anglaise nous a montré qu'un schizophrène stabilisé, exposé à un milieu stressant, rechute s'il ne reçoit pas de neuroleptiques, alors que s'il bénéficie d'un entourage dont l'expression émotionnelle est adéquate, il peut le plus souvent se passer de thérapeutiques pharmacologiques. Même si l'on ne veut pas prendre en compte les observations d'enfants sauvages, que dire des dépressions anaclitiques de SPITZ et des singes à mère "fil de fer" de HARLOW !

La seule observation clinique, même si le cercle des sciences ne nous offrait aucun début d'explication des mécanismes en cause, permettrait d'affirmer, avec PIAGET, que "le développement épigénétique... n'est pas un simple mélange d'éléments innés et acquis mais une organisation cherchant son équilibre"; que ce développement repose sur trois grands facteurs : "la programmation due au génome, les influences du milieu, et les facteurs d'équilibration ou autorégulation qui ne sont ni proprement héréditaires (puisqu'ils s'imposent motu proprio en fonction des situations), ni acquis de l'extérieur (puisqu'il s'agit de régulations internes").

Ceci suffirait pour conclure à l'inanité de l'opposition de l'inné et de l'acquis. Comment se fait-il que la plupart d'entre nous ne l'admettent pas et que, même quand nous l'admettons, nous nous comportons encore comme si l'organisme et l'environnement étaient deux choses séparées ? C'est le poids des paradigmes décrits par KUHN. Notre pensée reste marquée par deux traditions honorables qui, toutes deux, sont réductionnistes. Conformément à la démarche du cartésianisme, plutôt qu'à celle de DESCARTES, nous croyons pouvoir rendre compte du complexe par la composition additive du simple et, conformément à la physique du XIXe siècle, nous n'arrivons pas à nous dégager de la causalité linéaire et à sens unique du déterminisme laplacien et du principe de Clausius et Carnot. Enfin, avec le positivisme, nous tenons le développement de la connaissance pour une accumulation de faits empiriques interprétés par une logique tautologique immuable. Rien de plus anachronique : "la raison elle-même ne constitue plus un invariant absolu" (PIAGET); l'universalisme de la causalité linéaire est mort avec l'action instantanée à distance infinie de NEWTON, l'augmentation généralisée de l'entropie n'est plus qu'un mauvais rêve caractéristique des structures fermées. Avec PRIGOGINE, nous savons que loin de l'équilibre entropique le monde physique comporte des structures qui perdurent et qui sont porteuses d'ordre et de néguentropie tant qu'elles peuvent dissiper de l'énergie au dépend de l'augmentation de l'entropie générale du milieu sur lequel elles sont ouvertes. Avec BRILLOIN et SZILLARD, le démon de Maxwell est exorcisé. Dès le niveau élémentaire de la biologie moléculaire, la causalité repose sur des relations répétables allostériques codées qui mettent en jeu des quantités d'énergie quasi nulles. Comme y insiste MONOD, ce code est "chimiquement arbitraire en ce que le transfert d'informations pourrait tout aussi bien avoir lieu selon une autre convention". Puisque ces codes, comme celui de la langue, sont capables de glissements sémantiques ou, comme dit CHAPEVILLE, de lectures différentes, il n'est pas irréaliste d'affirmer que le démon de SAUSSURE-MONOD est également exorcisé. Pour les structures ouvertes, qu'elles appartiennent au monde inanimé, comme les structures dissipatives de PRIGOGINE, ou au monde vivant, organique ou psychologique, la condition sine qua non de leur permanence comme de leur développement est leur capacité d'assimiler l'environnement en s'y accommodant. Structure, organisme d'une part et milieu nourricier ne sont pas séparés mais organisés en un système de régulations dont les propriétés tiennent davantage aux relations entre les éléments qui le composent qu'aux propriétés intrinsèques de chacun d'eux (BERTALANFFY).

LITERATURE

1. BALDWIN, J.M., 1896, A new factor in evolution, American naturalist, 30, 441-451 et 536-553.
2. BERTALANFFY von, L., 1980, Théorie générale des systèmes, Dunod, Paris, 1 vol., 298 p.
3. BINDING, K. und HOCHE, A., 1920, Die Freigabe der Vernichtung lebensunwerten Lebens. Ihr Mass. und irhe Form, Felix Meiner, Leipzig, 1 vol.
4. BRILLOIN, L., 1963, Science and information theory, Academic Press, New York, 1 vol., 351 p.
5. CARROLL, B.J., 1982, The dexamethasone suppression test for melancholia, Brit. J. Psychiat., 140, 292-304.
6. CHANGEUX, J.P., 1983, L'homme neuronal, Fayard, Paris, 1 vol., 419 p.
7. CHAPEVILLE, F. et NINIO, J., 1979, Darwinisme et biologie moléculaire, In : Le darwinisme aujourd'hui, Seuil, Paris, 1 vol., 93-110.
8. DEVILLERS, C., BLANC, M., 1981, La crise du néo-darwinisme. Recherche, 12, 1154-1156.
9. DOBZHANSKY, T., 1969, L'hérédité et la nature humaine, Flammarion, 1 vol. 182 p.
10. HARLOW, H.F. and HARLOW, M.K., 1965, The effects of early social deprivation on primates. In : Désafférentation expérimentale et clinique,2ème Symposium de Bel-Air, Genève, septembre 1964, Georg, Genève et Masson, Paris, 67-77.
11. JAKOBSON, R., 1942, Kindersprache, Aphasie und allgemeine Lantgesetze, Uppsala, Uppsala Universitets, Arsskrift, 1 vol. 83 p.

12. JAKOBSON, R., 1949, Les lois phoniques du langage enfantin et leur place dans la phonologie générale. In : Troubetzkoy, N., Principes de Phonologie, Klincksieck, Paris, 367-379.
13. KUHN, T.S., 1972, La structure des révolutions scientifiques, Flammarion, 1 vol., 246 p.
14. LEDER, P., 1983, Genetic control of immunoglobulin production, Hospital Practise, 18 (2), 73-82.
15. LEWIN, R., 1980, Evolutionary theory under fire. Science, 210, 883-887.
16. MENDLEWICZ, J., CHARLES, G. and FRANCKSON, J.M., 1982, The dexamethasone suppression test in affective disorder : relationship to clinical and genetic subgroups, Brit. J. Psychiat., 141, 464-470.
17. MONOD, J., 1970, Le hasard et la nécessité, Seuil, Paris, 1 vol., 197 p.
18. PIAGET, J., 1974, Adaptation vitale et psychologie de l'intelligence, Hermann, Paris, 1 vol., 109 p.
19. PIAGET, J., 1967, Biologie et connaissance, Gallimard, Paris, 1 vol., 420 p.
20. PRIGOGINE, I. et STENGERS, I., 1979, La nouvelle alliance, Gallimars, Paris, 1 vol., 302 p.
21. SPITZ, R.A., 1945, 1, 1946, 2, Hospitalism : an inquiry into the genesis of psychiatric conditions in early childhood, Psychoanal., Stud. Child, 53-74 et 113-117.
22. TISSOT, R., 1979, Introduction à la psychiatrie biologique, Masson, Paris, 1 vol., 170 p.
23. TISSOT, R., 1974, Thérapeutique médicamenteuse au long cours des psychoses, In : Traitement au long cours des états psychotiques, Privat Ed., Toulouse, 49-100.
24. VAUGHN, C.E. and LEFF, J.P., 1976, The influence of family and social factors on the course of psychiatric illness. A comparison of schizophrenic and depressed neurotic patients, Brit. J. Psychiat., 129, 125-137.
25. WADDINGTON, C.H., 1957, The strategy of the genes, G. Allen and Unwin, LTD, London, 1 vol. 262 p.

WHY SHOULD THE PSYCHIATRIST BE INTERESTED IN NEURO-CHEMISTRY?

Helmut Beckmann

Zentralinstitut für Seelische Gesundheit
Mannheim
6800 Mannheim 1, FRG

The concept of biochemical disturbances underlying psychic disorders is a very old one. It has first been formulated by Hippocrate. He was of the opinion that certain mental diseases derive from a specific interaction of various body humors. Under this impression he defined i.e. depressive disorders as melancholia.

From this height of ancient Hippocratic thinking psychiatry went into medieval darkness until the end of the 18th century. At that time Pinel was the first to consider the insane as a sick person in the medical sense and pleaded for adequate therapeutic methods. Later, clinicians as Wilhelm Griesinger and Emil Kraepelin postulated a mainly biological etiology of mental illness. In a few european psychiatric institutions a rigorous quest for biochemical aberrations in psychic disorders began.

Kraepelin together with W. Wundt studied systematically the influence of psychotropic compounds such as alcohol, tea and paraldehyde on normal psychic functions. His book on "The influence of certain drugs on basic psychic phenomena" from 1882 may be called the beginning of modern scientific psychopharmacology.

Further endeavors in this particular field were greatly stimulated by the discovery of biological substrates of various neuropsychiatric disorders.

The greatest breakthrough of biological thinking in psychiatry of that time was the discovery of etiology, the unspecific and finally the specific cure of general paresis which was one of the major neuropsychiatric diseases of the last centuries. The identification of Treponema pallidum by Schaudinn and their identification in the brains of afflicted patients by Noguchi and Moore (1913) was paralleled by the finding of Wassermann (1906) that both syphilis and general paresis had identical serological tests. Wagner von Jauregg (1918) decisively improved the effectivenes of therapy by malarial fever treatment for which he finally received the Nobel Prize. However, the battle was not entirely won until 1940 when penicillin was introduced.

Whereas general paresis proved to be of infectious origin, pellagra was shown to be due to a vitamin deficiency. This psychosis consisted of affective symptoms as delusions, hallucinations and dementia. It was an illness of high incidence in certain endemic European and American areas. Guided by pertinent observations Goldberger (1914) postulated a role for dietary deficiency or imbalance in the etiology of pellagra. By providing a more balanced diet pellagra was defeated and a method for its prophylaxis demonstrated. This opened the possibility of identifying a neurochemical lesion as an etiologic factor of one major psychosis and spurred the hopes of psychiatrists for further discoveries in psychoneurochemistry.

Another example of the successful implementation of the neurochemical paradigm in neuropsychiatry is exemplified by the therapy of the seizure disorders by the bromides in 1857 by Locock and phenobarbital by Hauptmann in 1912. Diphenylhydantoin, although synthesized in 1908 was not used until 1938 when Merritt and Putnam reported its effectiveness as an anticonvulsant. The relationship between psychiatric symptoms and seizure disorders, particularly those of the temporal lobe emphasized further the fundamental relationship between biological and psychological aspects of behavior.

Unfortunately, neither the bromides or barbiturates nor the vitamins or the antibiotics proved to be efficacious in the endogenous psychoses. Although introduction of insulin coma therapy by Sakel in 1936 and the electric convulsive therapies by Meduna (1937) and Cerletti and Bini (1938) was one important stride forward decades of disappointment and scepticism seized a considerable amount of leading clinicians. Philosophical and social disciplines without therapeutic impact gained much weight.

Modern psychopharmacology with more specific drugs began in 1952 when Delay and Deniker discovered the antipsychotic effects of clorpromazine. A few years later the similar effects of reserpine, the anti-depressant effect of monoamine oxidase inhibitors and imipramine, and the antianxiety effects of meprobamate and the benzodiazepines were discovered and introduced into clinical practice.

Within one decade clinical psychiatry had changed grossly from a institutional supportive care with mainly philosophically oriented physicians to a medical science. Meanwhile, psychopharmacology as a basic science has developed tremendously. Knowledge about these drugs' biological mechanisms may often exceed that of other substances in clinical use. This has provoked an entirely new research paradigm in that many scientists now - instead of only understanding their effects - use psychoactive drugs as tools to elucidate basic functions of the nervous system.

Against this background neurochemistry emerged as a special branch of biochemistry. Its objectives are to investigate the molecular events which subserve activity of the CNS and which account for organ activities in the brain. Great progress has been achieved in the description of the general metabolism of various chemical constituents, as the proteins, the nucleic acids, the cyclic nucleotides, neuroendocrine effects on and of the CNS, further of specific qualities of neural membranes, engergy yielding pathways etc.

However, the most rewarding and heuristically fruitful concept for the understanding of psychic disorders was that of neurotransmitters. These substances are released in packets from the presynaptic endings into the synaptic cleft and, by binding to specific receptors, stimulate the postsynaptic neurones. Neuro-transmitters are inactivated by specific enzymes, by reuptake of the transmitter or by diffusing away from the synapse. They may be excitatory or inhibitory depending on their specificity or their specific localization within the central nervous system.

Until now three large classes of neurotransmitters - amines, amino acids and polypeptides - have been described. However, for the majority of these compounds only the name putative transmitters is justified as many uncertainties concerning their exact function continue to prevail. Psychotropic agents act primarily to alter synaptic transmission by enhancing or retarding the synthesis, storage, release or inactivation of the neurotransmitters. During the last decades it became evident that they are the direct means in the psychiatrist's hand to alter and to modify neurochemical processes within the CNS of the mentally ill. Because of the exponentially growing progress of both psychoparmacology and neurochemistry the psychiatrist feels not only a vivid interest but rather a tremendous task and duty to keep informed and experienced for the welfare of his patients.

Furthermore, the importance of the model psychoses for the development of psychiatry must be emphasized. The fact that chemical substances as mescaline or amphetamine provoke a psychosis which resembles partly the endogenous psychoses has initiated much debate on the identity of these models with the endogenous psychoses. For the majority of clinicians this issue is settled: psychic disturbances caused by hallucinogens are symptomatic, exogenous psychoses. They can be identyfied by experienced clinicians. However, great difficulties of diagnosis can occur. For the scientist, it is amazing that chemotherapeutic agents influence largely the same symptoms in the exogenous as well as in the endogenous psychoses. One may speculate that at least some of these therapeutical analogies suggest a pathogenetic analogy. From this it is expected that the model psychoses are one major pathway for research into the endogenous psychoses.

The neurochemical quest for metabolic aberrations of neurotransmitter functions has so far not yielded a sufficient insight into the basic mechanisms of the endogenous psychoses. However, can we expect to get sound information on biochemical processes in the brain by measuring metabolites in plasma, urine or even cerebrospinal fluid? Or, can we evaluate central receptor properties on blood platelets or lymphocytes? Presently scientists develop more refined strategies and powerful instruments to measure neurochemical events within the central nervous system of both healthy man and psychiatric patient. The positron emission tomography is one beginning of visibilizing chemical events within the living human brain.

Eclectic application or combination of strategies
which search for peripheral markers of central events,
use of psychoactive drugs with defined pharmacological
properties as tools and instruments like positron
emission tomography will yield more profound understanding of psychochemic processes. Hypotheses on the
etiology of normal and pathologic behavior can be
generated, refused or verified. Finally, better treatment methods can be developed.

It is my conviction that psychic phenomena and neurochemical events are one entity and only two sides of
the same medal. However, the gap in the understanding
of both sides may never be closed by our endeavors and
lastly prove to be incomprehensible and unsurpassable
for human mind.

It was Freud who wrote in the beginning of this century:
'We are interested in psychotherapy in that it works
by psychological methods and, for that moment, we do
not have others. In the future, we possibly shall learn
to exert more direct influences with special chemical
agents on the energy and their distribution in the
psychic apparatus'. Would Freud himself - being still
with us - have admitted that future has already begun?

THE TASKS OF THE PSYCHIATRIST BEFORE THE BIOCHEMICAL CONTRIBUTIONS

C. Ballús

Departamento de Psiquiatría
Facultad de Medicina
Universidad de Barcelona. España

We must not forget that human personality constitutes a total
ity comprising its biological levels -including the neurochemical
one- up to the psychological and social ones. We mean that human
personality and, with it, man's behaviour, constitute a complex
bio-psychological quality.

On the other hand, man is in continuous interaction with the
environment in which he must be duly integrated under normal and
healthy conditions.

Also, within his internal structure, he must reach a good
integration between his different components and we must not
forget the influence from external stimuli on the functioning of
such internal structures.

In this sense, the neurochemical level is determined and
determines in a certain way the behaviour and with it the biographical facts of man: historical-social-cultural. This mutual
action between "Ego and the world" starts at the beginning of
life and keeps on throughout the whole evolutive process.

I am fully in agreement with the relevant paper of Professor
Beckmann regarding the chemical point of view, but I would only

dare underline the need to consider human behaviour, normal or pathological, within an anthropological and holistic context.

The neurochemical level is at times a departure measure of the ways of behaviour related to it. At others it is the arrival point of influences from the external world. Neither its study nor its knowledge can be disconnected from other behaviour levels (psychological and social) in the human being.

Let us not forget that phrase by the Spanish philosopher X. Zubiri: "Our brain is the organ which places us in the situation of having to think". We can add that our brain places us also in the situation which allows us to define and makes us love. This gives the personality to man, of which the brain is a part and it also handles the total role of our behaviour.

The great scientific discoveries of our time in brain neurochemistry would be determined by a centralization of the psychiatrist on the same, forgetting the human being as a totality with its historical-social-cultural dimensions.

A great Spanish doctor and philosopher -J. de Letamendi- wrote last century: "Medicine today lacks men and exceeds frog".

The mission of our psychiatric generation and of the future ones consists in the integration of the 1983-frog to the holistic totality of man.

WHY SHOULD PSYCHIATRISTS CONCERN THEMSELVES WITH THE RESULTS OF PSYCHOPHYSIOLOGICAL RESEARCH ON PSYCHOLOGICAL DISORDERS?

Hans Heimann

Nervenklinik Tübingen

Osianderstr. 22, D - 7400 Tübingen

At present, scientific theory on psychological disorders is governed by monocausal concepts. Schizophrenic syndromes, for example, are explained by the dopamine hypothesis on the one hand, by psychoanalysts as the consequence of pre-oedipal disturbances of the mother-child relationship, or by learning theorists as an acquired paradoxical style of communication in the double bind hypothesis on other, just to name a few extreme positions. Arguments can be found for each of these pathogenetic concepts, but they have not remained uncontradicted. Schizophrenic syndromes are on a level of complexity that they reveal different facets to each observer according to his standpoint and perspective. Each of these aspects, taken for itself appears to have certain justification, without being able to explain and interpret the phenomena in their entirety, and above all without leading to satisfactory treatment on a secure empirical basis with capacity for further developments.

The situation sketched here for the schizophrenic syndromes also applies to the affective psychoses as well as to the psychogenic disorders in the broadest sense. Only in the case of psychoses on an organic basis does the situation appear to be simpler, although substantial incongruencies are uncovered by quantitative comparisons - for example in the degenerative aging processes - of the demonstrable cellular degeneration of the brain to the psychopathological alterations.

Viewing our habits of theorizing in the field of psychological disorders from a distance, as if to arrive at a general overview of methodological orientation, we see the same picture emerging again and again: The attempt is made on a psychopathological level to define syndromic or nosological entities by drawing boundaries based on various criteria. These entities are then related to either neuropathological, neurophysiological, or neurobiochemical results on the one hand, and to ontogenetic psychodynamic or socio-communicative systems on the other. The relationship between the psychopathological level on the one hand and the neurobiological, psychodynamic, or sociodynamic niveau on the other is, as a rule, considered to be monocausal; that is, a specific disturbance is sought on other levels as well which can be made responsible for the syndromes on the psychological level.

The logic of research leads consistently to the increasingly differentiated quantitative assessment of psychological phenomena on the psychopathological level on the one hand - and this has already resulted in the multidiagnostic use of a wide variety of diagnostic systems - and on the other hand to the development or theoretical deepening and broadening of the methodological approaches with respect to conditional circumstances. In this re-gard, neurobiology is presently advancing through the development of new envisualising techniques which allow more differentiated insight into central nervous processes; furthermore, through neuro-endocrine stimulation methods and through the discovery of the significance of different neurotransmitters and their metabolites.

What, then, is the role of psychophysiology, and why is it important for psychiatric research? By psychophysiology we mean, first of all, measurable changes in peripheral autonomic parameters under systematic variation of psychological, situational conditions. Two factors which have been investigated as independent variables in connection with psychopathological states are the pathology-in-duced changes in psychoautonomic systems and, more recently, the event-related slow potentials of the central nervous system. Thus, psychophysiological investigations initially fit into the monocausal thought patterns already described above. In other words, it is postulated that specific changes in the area of psycho-autonomic functioning or in the event-related potentials of the central ner-vous system underlie a certain psychopathologically distinguishable syndrome.

This theoretical model is so self-evident that differences in psychophysiological reactivity found in patients with a certain syndrome, as compared to a healthy control group, become less interesting as soon as they are found in another syndrome as well. When, for instance, schizophrenic patients have to press a key in reaction to an imperative stimulus after a warning signal, and when a slow negative baseline shift (so-called post-imperative negative variation or PINV) appears in the EEG after the key had been pressed, then this is first of all interpreted as being specific to schizophrenia. When the same phenomenon appears in depression, as demonstrated by a number of studies, the phenomenon forfeits

its interest because it only seems to distinguish between "psychotic" and "nonpsychotic" subjects.

This methodological approach, by the way, can also be found in psychophysiological investigations from the previous century. Auguste VIGOUROUX, for instance, in his Paris dissertation from 1890, studied the electrical skin resistance level of melancholic patients and found it to be raised; a result which has been demonstrated repeatedly in more recent times. VIGOUROUX discussed it only from the standpoint of diagnostic differentiation of states of melancholia, and thus as an extension of the psychopathological approach. Apart from methodological problems of reliability and comparability in measuring electrical skin resistance at rest, the problem of the nonspecificity of such an activation measure remains, and in terms of discriminating psychopathological analysis it has a random effect. It would be wrong, for instance, to draw the conclusion that melancholic patients are generally desactivated, because they are over-activated in other psycho-autonomic systems; for instance, they generally have an increased pulse rate, an elevated plasma level of cortisone, and higher body temperature.

Even when so-called multiconditional causation of psychological disorders is postulated for everything from the organic psychoses to the psychogenic disorders in the field of psychosomatics and especially for the endogenous psychoses, in actual research this formulation proves to be something of a smoke-screen. The researcher is forced to accept certain theoretical models which promise him clear answers in his empirical investigations. He concentrates on one nosological category and, starting from the psychopathological level, he tries to find specific changes on the aforementioned level of causal relationships. This corresponds to habits of psychiatric thinking that are very difficult to overcome.

In so doing, it is overlooked, for example, that in internal medicine, genuine advances in the pathophysiology and treatment of internal diseases were achieved only when a pathophysiological, system-oriented view had been accepted in addition to the descriptive nosological entities. This is demonstrated, for instance, by the discovery of the significance of immune systems in a variety of nosological disease entities or by the stress research started by SELYE, which focuses particularly on "nonspecificity". One could cite similar examples from the field of endocrine diseases. In internal medicine, this altered view has led away from rigid focus on descriptive, nosological differentiations, which can continually be refined and justified on a symptom level toward consideration and investigation of pathophysiological aspects of systems operating in a variety of nosological areas.

It is my conviction that the psychophysiological investigation of the organism under the pathological conditions of psychological disorders necessarily demands analogous steps of the researcher.

It is entirely conceivable that the biological substrate of psychic disorders, which manifests itself psychophysiologically in the organism's various adaptive systems with respect to environmental conditions, is relatively independent of our descriptive nosological categorization criteria. This means that similar protective mechanisms for counterbalancing pathological impairment may be operative in different nosological areas.

This is suggested by our own systematic psychophysiological investigations of depressive and schizophrenic syndromes, gathered over approximately 10 years. The results have forced us to add a supplemental pathophysiological point of view to the one-sided, strictly nosological research strategy, as already postulated by KRAEPELIN in 1920. In the following section I will summarize these findings and will then point out some resulting perspectives for future research.

The core of symptoms of depression are a triad which includes psychological and somatic symptoms, but also contains symptoms of loss (as a necessary but not specific category) which characterize the relationship of the depressed individual to his environment. This symptomatology of loss consists of the loss of interest, the loss of ability to experience pleasure, and the loss of performance ability. It corresponds to a tendency of the depressed patient to withdraw and, as we could demonstrate, to a depression-induced, active repulsion of informational intake.

On a psychophysiological level, in the investigation of the orienting response to an irregular series of ten 80 dB tones in depressive syndromes, the skin resistance orienting reflex was absent in approx. 40 % of patients. Furthermore, we were able to demonstrate that acoustically evoked potentials are reduced up to 25 % in these patients, and that the expectancy wave (CNV, that is: the slow negativity between a warning stimulus and a subsequent imperative stimulus signalling the patient to press a key) is 50 % less than in a matched group of healthy controls. Finally, our depressed patients exhibited a raised PINV, which is especially marked under conditions of lacking or impeded control of a relatively aversive stimulus. If one views the psychophysiological results on the orienting response as the manifestation of the organism's reaction to external stimuli, then it is justified to conclude that depression can be equated with the repulsion of information intake and withdrawal. The absence of an orienting reaction in skin resistance is most marked in the group of inhibited endogenous depressed patients.

If one concludes that these results are specific to the nosological entity of endogenous depression, then one would fail to recognize the meaning of this finding. This absence of the orienting response is also found in 40 % of acute schizophrenic patients, and we could demonstrate both the reduction in evoked potentials and expectancy wave between warning signal and imperative stimulus as well as the increased post-imperative negative variation in schizophrenics. However, it is significant that among both the New York and the Tübingen schizophrenics, the nonresponders in the orienting reaction situation are those patients who show a stronger withdrawal tendency and increased depression on the psychopathological level.

This congruence of psychophysiological findings for depressed and schizophrenic patients - that is, the demonstrated nonspecificity - should not lead us to the conclusion that we must fall back into the notion of the so-called homogenous psychosis ("Einheitspsychose"). Rather, it suggests a pathophysiological view in which similar compensatory mechanisms are set in motion in different nosological areas in some patients. Emotional withdrawal, avoidance behaviour, and repulse of informational intake in depressive syndromes are the organism's answer to an imbalance in the limbic reward- and punishment-systems, favoring the punishment-system, which robs anything and everything of pleasure. In a subgroup of schizophrenics, the same protective mechanisms are mobilized as defense measures against the flooding of information-processing centers.

I believe that with this view we are reviving a conception of psychological disorders that was already anticipated in the previous century. For instance, similar thoughts can be found by the Belgian psychiatrist GUISLAIN, who described the so-called "phrenopathies" in the 1830's: namely, that the pathological process of psychological disorders leads to a reaction of the organism which in turn is responsible for a part of the phenomena on the psychopathological level. GRIESINGER also carried this thought further, and it reappears with a somewhat different clinical connotation in Eugen BLEULER's conception of the primary and secondary symptoms of schizophrenia. Today, we can hope that psychophysiological methods will help us to undertand more precisely the organism's compensatory mechanisms in its relation to the environment under psychopathological conditions, and perhaps even to influence them therapeutically according to the demands of the pathological situation. The psychophysiological methods and their existing results, therefore, are not only an extension or explanation of our nosological descriptions, but they also force us to take a new perspective - namely, a pathophysiological perspective - which gives the concepts of multiconditionality a new and concrete meaning.

It remains for us to mention that the investigation of various psychophysiological systems - skin resistance, pulse amplitude, EEG - under psychopathological conditions reveals yet another aspect. It provides us with an answer to the question what pathological behavior means with respect to the psychophysiological organism in its totality. It is not hyperactivation or hypoactivation, that is, not a general arousal shift, that determine the pathology of the organism in its relation to the environment, but the fact that the psychophysiological systems in the area of autonomic functioning as well as of the cortical potentials either do not respond or, in contrast to the healthy organism, exhibit no differential or situation-specific modulation. We have been able to prove that in both the schizophrenic and the depressed patient, these different systems sometimes correlate highly with each other, which is not the case for healthy individuals under the variation of situational conditions. Thus, we are dealing psychophysiologically in the pathological state with an all-or-nothing principle and, in contrast, with a differentiated, situation-specific reaction in the healthy person. I have attempted to place the results of psychiatric research on psychophysiology into a larger context, simplifying the issue in order to stimulate new strategies of research. I am well aware that we will encounter serious methodological difficulties in this area and that there is a danger of psychophysiologists losing themselves in the technical problems of their research methods. It was my intention to point out the broad outlines in order for psychiatric research to leave an overly narrow descriptive-nosological viewpoint at last, and to consider mutual pathophysiological mechanisms and systems of the various nosological areas, which are probably more significant for treatment than the nosological conceptual boundaries. Psychopharmacological research, as far as I overlook it today, provides me with the most important arguments in this effort.

PSYCHOPHYSIOLOGY AND PSYCHIATRY: A DISCUSSION

Y.D. Lapierre

Royal Ottawa Hospital & University of Ottawa

1145 Carling Avenue, Ottawa, Ontario, Canada, K1Z 7K4

In the range of investigational approaches to the human psyche, psychophysiology is the bridge discipline between biochemical and cellular levels and on the other hand, behaviour be it internal or external, and social interactions. Psychophysiology allows the monitoring of physiological processes of organ systems which would otherwise be inaccessible. The electrical potentials thus recorded are either of the slow event-related variety arising directly from the central nervous system or indirectly via the neurovegetative systems. Another type of potentials recorded are those related to fast potentials emanating from the brain or muscle.

The sources of electrical activity reflects central or autonomic nervous system activity in its tonic or phasic state. Generally, it is considered that tonic activity reflects the structurally-based function of the brain whereas the phasic potentials reflect the functional response pattern of brain activity. Whether these are directly related to psychopathology or an epiphenomenon of different psychic states is not clear. The present understanding is that it is most probable that these outcome measurements are the resultant of a series of ill-defined variables such as age, sex, personality type as well as psychopathological state.

The basic reflex, i.e. the orienting response (OR), does indeed appear to vary in different psychopathological states such as schizo-phrenia, depression and anxiety. This variation is not limited to increased or decreased arousal but, as pointed out previously, may have some features characteristic of certain pathological states.

The number of variables intervening and interacting prior to the output of these electrical potential patterns makes it all the more

309

difficult to attribute a variation in pattern to any specific pathology. This problem of interpretation which was mentioned in Prof.
Heimann's paper, remains and may only be solved with a new approach
to the problem. At the present time, the traditional method of
relating psychophysiological events to psychopathological condition
is to initially make the diagnosis and then establish the psychophysiological profile of this a priori diagnosis. Clinical diagnosis
in conditions such as anxiety, depression and schizophrenia is
fraught with intangibles and a lack of objectivity whereas the ultimate purpose of psychophysiological evaluation is to objectify and
clarify this diagnostic problem. As the initial sample is not homogeneous, the variance involved in the interpretation of the resulting
profile is inevitably greater and less interpretable. It may be more
appropriate to initiate the process more broadly and more generically
in diagnostic group selection. Subsequently, the elaboration of a
psychophysiological profile could contribute to the more precise
definition of the clinical entity and its specific subgrouping.

Psychophysiology is presently at a cross-roads. A number of
studies have gathered an unlimited amount of data which still
lacks cohesiveness in the clarification of the underlying psychopathology. Unless new approaches are taken, psychophysiology will
stagnate and will not provide us with the clinical applications for
the definition, or understanding and treatment of psychopathological
entities.

IS BEHAVIOR STILL A RELEVANT VARIABLE ?

Marc N. Richelle

Psychological Laboratory

University of Liege, Belgium

The title of the present paper, being in the interrogative
form, suggests that those currently doing psychiatric research sometimes dispense themselves with any reference to behavior. I shall
contend that such a trend, if it really exists, might, among other
consequences, result in not giving the recent achievements in
various fields all the impact they could have. The question raised
bears on clinical research as well as on fundamental or preclinical research, though I shall refer only to the latter, and more
specifically to experimental psychopharmacology, for illustrative
examples.

BEHAVIOR AND PSYCHIATRY : A BRIEF RETROSPECT

It might seem advisable first to agree on some definition of
behavior. It turns out that this is not as simple as might seem,
because of semantic drifts and because the term has been contaminated by the theories with which it has been associated, or by the
(mis)interpretations of these theories. To state it briefly, let
us admit that behavior covers active interactions in which an individual organism engages with his environment.

The place given to behavior by psychiatrists, be it in their
descriptions of mental diseases or in their attempts to explain
them, has changed, throughout the history of the field, with
changes of emphasis in psychopathological theories on one hand,
and with the vicissitudes of the notion of behavior in psychology
on the other hand.

It will be reminded that early in the century psychologists,
almost unanimously if not always enthusiastically, adopted behavior

311

as the subject matter of their science, instead of consciousness or mental life. Indeed, this revolution bore on method rather than on subject matter. Psychologists, aware of the many inadequacies of introspection, turned to observable events as providing safer ground for scientific inquiry; and, as scientists in other fields traditionally do without any frustration, they postponed the exploration of many areas until they become accessible to observation.

Nineteen century psychiatry, through its remarkable effort in describing and classifying psychiatric symptoms, had in some way anticipated behaviorism, in giving observable events obvious priority, and in distrusting introspection, the limits of which clearly appear to those who study organisms with whom communication is not always easy to establish.

In a quite different orientation, none more radically than Freud has contributed to a general distrust of introspection as a valid way to know human beings, by disclosing the totally unconscious factors that determine many of their actions.

However, despite its attention to the analysis of behavior, psychiatry has looked at it mainly in terms of symptoms, along the traditional lines of clinical medicine : symptoms are interesting, essentially, in so far as they reveal an underlying pathological state, the origin of which is to be found at another level. In the organicist tradition, some anatomo-physiological anomaly is assumed, while in the psychoanalytic tradition, the dysfunctioning is to be traced to the psychic apparatus. In both cases, behavior has but an accessory status. Explanation, and eventually intervention, are located at another level.

This still prevalent view has not favoured a behavioral approach to psychiatry. Behaviorism logically leads to consider behavior in its own right, but attempts to reformulate psychopathological disorders were slow to emerge. With the exception of a few forerunners, it was not before the nineteen fifties that proponents of behavior therapy or modification developped techniques based on a conception of symptoms, not as revealing some deeper problem, but as the very locus of the disorder. This by no means implies discarding a search for the variables responsible for the behavior being considered. But priority will be given to the interaction of the individual with his/her environment, that is, to a functional analysis that does not take for granted that the final explanation is to be found at another level, be it material or conceptual.

It is difficult to measure the influence of behavioral concepts on psychiatry through the therapeutic practices. Admittedly, these have been, at least in their earliest phase, oversimplifying and, occasionally, triumphalistic. They undoubtedly have underestimated developmental factors in the understanding of mental disorders, they have ignored structures, as well as the distinctive features and consequences of symbolic behavior, they have, more often than not, indulged into inconsistent eclecticism. They did not adequately reflect the more subtle views of a modern science of behavior.

COGNITIVISM AND BEHAVIOR

Two currently expanding trends tend to present behavior analysis as an outdated stage of psychology and psychopathology. One has developed within psychology itself, under the label cognitivism. The other, biological psychiatry, is flourishing within psychiatry, as a modern form of organicism, enriched with the impressive achievements of basic biological sciences. Much could be said on the cognitivist paradigm, as some authors call it, in its relation with psychopathology. The word cognitivism has many different meanings in contemporary psychology, somewhat artificially confused by the use of a common unifying term. To many psychologists, it points to a real change of the subject matter of their science, behavior making the stage free for a new version of mental life, made of information processing, strategies, cognitions, competences, and the like. In its most coherent aspects, cognitivism aims at infering properties of the mechanisms involved in processing sensory, perceptual, mnesic or linguistic information from experimental operations which, unavoidably, bear on behavioral data. It defines, in a purely abstract way (not by refering to specified neural mechanisms in the C.N.S.) the conditions to be fufilled by the mental or neural device if it is to generate or control the observed behaviors. It covers a number of research areas traditionally concerned with higher levels of conducts, grasping and processing of information, problem solving, knowing, symbolic representations, and the like. Many cognitivists would also include, as a logical extension of their territory, at least to their own eyes, supposedly cognitive mechanisms which, by inference, are said to underly as well any complex regulation of behavior, such as an athlete adjusting his arm movement toward a target or migrating birds finding their way from one continent to another.

By claiming to offer models of processes located beyond observable behaviors or identifiable stimulations, cognitivism seems to present itself as a kind of psychology better prepared to meet the concern of CNS specialists. It emphasizes internal processes, possible candidates for a neurophysiological or neurochemical redefinition - through it should be emphasized again that cognitivist models are, as a rule, purely abstract, and have, until now, hardly produced any really valuable neurophysiological counterpart (whatever their heuristic significance for psychological research proper).

There is no doubt that cognitivism has reinstated terms and explanations very close to mentalistic formulations that were strongly rejected by a functional analysis of behavior. A famous example is the notion of <u>linguistic competence</u> as developped by Chomsky and, after him, by a generation of psycholinguists. Infered from the formal properties of a speaker's utterances, this mental entity has turned out to be of no great help in psycholinguistic research and has been progressively left aside, especially by specialists of language development. What is wrong with such notions is not, as Skinner observed, that they are <u>mental</u> (as such they would simply raise a problem of accessibility that psychology, cognitive or not, is currently solving step by step) but that they are oversimplifying and offer the illusion of explanation. We shall come back to this point in a moment.

BIOLOGICAL PSYCHIATRY AND BEHAVIOR

The attitude of biological psychiatry towards the analysis of behavior is of a more subtle and, sometimes, paradoxical nature. Let us first state that, in our view, there can be no real antagonism between the two approaches; there is on the contrary, continuity and complementarity since the behavioral approach unambiguously inscribes the analysis of behavior within biology. This implies a biological theory decisively open to successive levels of analysis and prpared to recognize its specificity to each level in a integrating hierarchy quite alien to crude reductionism. This view has been endorsed by most great biologists today but it is not, by far, part of the thinking habits of all those who practice biological research.

Biological psychiatry, being heir to the organicist tradition, is not totally free from a reductionist conception of mental disorders. Be it in neurochemistry and neuropharmacology, or in genetic studies, the search for univocal organic causal factors is often implicit, if not overtly stated. Pathological behavior is viewed as the by-product of neural dysfunction or of genic disorder. It is given its status of symptoms, in the most classical sense, the origins of which are not to be looked for, and not to be found anywhere else. The success of psychopharmacological treatment gives some support to this reductionism, at least at first sight.

As far as methods are concerned, one would expect that biological psychiatry would resort to the same degree of sophistication when it deals with behavior as it does when it deals with neurochemical or neurophysiological aspects of research. One is struck, however, by the discrepancy between exceedingly refined neurochemical techniques and, for instance, the uncritical use of categories in the description of clinical symptoms, or the choice of crude experimental tools for animal behavior studies, an admittedly necessary link between preclinical research and therapeutic essays on psychotropic compounds.

Let us mention a few examples of such oversimplification in

current psychopharmacological research. A unique test, such as passive avoidance, is said to measure memory, so that any compound that will alter performance in that test will be said to act upon memory capacities. A simple motor test, such as the duration of immobility of rats in water or the locomotor hyperactivity of rats raised in isolation,is taken as valid in checking for antidepressive effects in experimental psychopharmacology. In the first case, one is, curiously enough, back to an old psychology of mental faculties, that looked definitely abandoned years ago. This anachronism might result from two sources. First, the cognitivist trend mentioned above has reinstated terms that behaviorists had learned to avoid, because they are misleading. If it is fair to say that cognitivist psychologists do not use terms such as memory, attention, anxiety, as they were used in the nineteenth century, it is true also that the neurochemist, the neuroendocrinologist, the pharmacologist, when they talk about behavior, make a second hand use of that vocabulary, not distinguishable from prescientific use. Secondly, a central notion that emerged from behavioral studies in pharmacology and eventually became familiar to all psychopharmacologists in the sixties, the notion of drug-behavior interaction, seems to be overlooked by many contemporary researchers. It essentially refers to the fact that behavior is not only a dependent variable the variations of which are to be recorded as a function of pharmacological agents, but that is has also the status of independant variable; pharmacological action is to be described as a function of the behavior being studied, i.e. as a function of a set of environmental contingencies and of modalities of interactions between the organism and its environment. This notion could not possibly have emerged if behavioral psychopharmacologists in the fifties and sixties had not explored a wide variety of such modalities (under the label of schedules of reinforcement for instance). It is easily neglected when one single behavior is taken as a valid "model" of anxiety, depression, memory, etc.. or when behavioral research attempts to keep up with the rapid progresses of neurochemical studies. It is, of course, incompatible with one-way causal explanations, since it implies that external variables are taken into account. At the clinical level, it gives social, historical and cultural factors the place they deserve in the analysis of mental disorders, besides organic factors, and it precludes any a priori anticipations as to the causal relations involved. Curiously, enough in this respect, the cognitivist approach, essentially concerned with disclosing the mental structures of the subject, favours the reductionist revival typical of certain trends in biological psychiatry.

In de second example mentioned above, namely the locomotor hyperactivity of rats raised in isolation, a simple behavior is taken as reference for characterizing drug affects. But this is done in a patent circularity, where the relations between neurochemical, behavioral and clinical levels are juggled away. The behaviour used as reference in animal experimentation has been chosen only on the ground that it is altered by a category of compounds that are known to exert a given therapeutic action. More often than not, it is easy to show that another behavior might be used just as legitimately, that would not be modified in the same way by the category of drug being considered.

Coming back to behavior would also dispense experimental research in psychiatry with all the detours and blind-alleys in which it is periodically led by more ambitious "models" such as the learned helplessness model of Seligman, offered as a model of depression. It could be shown easily, after several authors, that interpretations of experimental data are in cases like this exceedingly frail, and far from legitimating extension to human pathology. The drift from experimental data, certainly not without interest in themselves, to more and more farfetched interpretations is often done by resorting to cognitivist concepts.

Finally, a precise analysis of behavior is still strongly desirable in the description and classification of clinical data. In spite of more than a century of symptoms description, and of recent attempts to refine and harmonize the inventory of patients behavior, nosological categories still lack precision in many respects. Some categories retain the imperfections of knowledge in the days when they first emerged, and have not really been critically revised since them. The classical distinction between endogenous and exogenous depression is a case in point. Though not all psychiatrist agree about the distinction, or, if they do, about the criteria on which to ground it, it is so familiar that it is used as a reference, without any questioning, in many pharmacological and genetic researches. These terms, loaded as they are with etiological connotations, implicitly bring support to causal hypotheses adopted in these fields of biological psychiatry. Looking for other possibilities is discarded, or left to approaches totally alien to scientific rules, with little chance for a really integrative synthesis. The contribution of biological psychiatry, in the long run, will find its true significance if it gives behavior the place it deserves and if it faces its complexities, as they appear to both the experimenter and the clinician.

THE NATURE, ORIGIN AND TREATMENT OF NEUROSES

Hans J. Eysenck

Institute of Psychiatry
University of London

I have for a long time maintained the view that for the future development of behaviour therapy, a proper theoretical basis is absolutely essential (Eysenck, 1976). I have equally maintained that such a theory must be neo-behaviouristic, i.e. based on concepts of conditioning and extinction (Eysenck, 1982). Only on such a basis can we hope to build up a model of treatment for neurotic disorders that is anything other than purely pragmatic, serendipic and ultimately haphazard and accident-prone (Eysenck, 1983). Science demands more than accidental therapeutic success; it demands a proper understanding of the dynamics of the nature and origin of neuroses if their treatment is to be successful to an altogether higher degree than it is today. Cognitive theories have recently received much applause, but there is no evidence that the methods used have any proper theoretical underpinning, that specific methods of therapy can be derived from these theories, or that they are more successful than, or even as successful as the methods of behaviour therapy originally deduced from conditioning principles (Eysenck, 1960, 1964; Eysenck & Rachman, 1965).

As an example of the successful application of scientific principles to the treatment of neurotic disorders, consider our latest set of experiments on the treatment of obsessive-compulsive disorders, particularly compulsive handwashing (Rachman & Hodgson, 1980). These large-scale studies were undertaken, and the target behaviour determined, because of two vitally important factors. In the first place, these disorders are known to be difficult or impossible to treat by means of psychotherapeutic or psychoanalytic principles; as Rachman and Hodgson point out, this is even admitted by psychoanalysts themselves. In the second place, there is a good animal analogue in the work of Solomon et al. (1965), leading directly to a method of treatment which is in good accord with the writer's theoretical conceptions (Eysenck, 1983). The results of applying this analogue to human patients gave extremely satisfactory results, with something like 85% to 90% of patients finding cure or considerable relief, without relapse or symptom substitition during follow-up. It is difficult to discover corresponding success attending deductions from cognitive theories or principles.

In essence, the writer's theory is based on the original Watson and Rayner (1920) paradigm, namely that neurotic symptoms are acquired by means of Pavlovian conditioning, and that treatment can only be successful if it incorporates Pavlovian extinction (Eysenck, 1979). However, there are many obvious criticisms to be made of Watson's original theory, and these have made necessary a number of modifications and changes which have effectively changed the theory and brought it into line with modern work in the fields of conditioning and clinical psychology (Eysenck, 1983). One of these changes relates to the unfortunate tendency of early behaviourists like Watson to disregard evidence of genetic factors in the causation of behaviour, and thus to postulate entirely environmental causes for neurotic symptoms. There is strong evidence of such genetic factors in the personality make-up of prospective victims of neurotic disorders (Fulker, 1981), and even in the symptomatology shown by sufferers. Heritabilities of specific phobic tendencies, as calculated from MZ and DZ twin differences (Rose &Ditto, in press), are sufficiently high not to be disregarded. Seligman (1971) has suggested the concept of "preparedness" as an intermediate stage between direct inheritance of specific phobic avoidance behaviours, and purely environmental conditioning mechanisms; "prepared" stimuli, in his theory, condition more readily, and extinguish less readily, than stimuli not so prepared through evolutionary developments.

Accepting that heredity makes an important contribution to the development of neurotic disorders overcomes some of the difficulties created by Watson's environmentalism. We can now explain the highly specific nature of phobias, by denying Pavlov's principles of "equipotentiality" among conditioned stimuli; we can see why some of the studies attempting to replicate Watson's experiment in conditioning fear of rats in little Albert failed (the experimenters used non-prepared stimuli); and we can see why the criticism that laboratory conditioning experiments demand very precise parameter values for, e.g., CS-UCS timing, which exactitude is not to be found in normal life events, is ill-founded; it is not required for prepared stimuli where conditioning occurs even with degraded input.

But there are many more telling criticisms of the Watson model. It requires a traumatic event to initiate the conditioning sequence, but in peace-time neuroses at least such traumatic events

318

are not to be found in most instances. This might possibly be
explained away in terms of "preparedness" or direct inheritance,
but other criticisms remain. As Kimmel (1975) has pointed out,
conditioned responses should extinguish when presented without
reinforcement, but neurotic symptoms frequently do not. Again,
neurotic symptoms seem to have an insidious onset, and grow stronger in a kind of positive feed-back cycle, rather than extinguish.
This well-known feature of peace-time neuroses is impossible to
explain on Watsonian principles.

Eysenck (1968) has suggested a theory of the incubation of
fear/anxiety conditioned responses which is based on the postulation
that these responses are not acquired by means of Pavlovian A
conditioning, but rather Pavlovian B conditioning (Grant, 1964.)
These two paradigms are very different, with Pavlovian B conditioning showing two important features which make it a much more reasonable analogue for the acquisition of neurotic symptoms. Put
briefly, in Pavlovian B conditioning the US provides the motivation,
whereas in Pavlovian A conditioning this has to be present before
the beginning of the experiment. Also, in Pavlovian B conditioning,
the CS is similar to or identical with the US, whereas in Pavlovian
A conditioning the CS is often quite unlike the US. It would seem to
follow that when a CS of the Pavlovian B type is presented without
apparent reinforcement, it so much resembles the US that identical
URs are produced by the animal, and hence reinforcement is experienced.
This would lead to incrementation of the CR (incubation), rather
than to extinction, and that is of course precisely what is found
in the acquisition of neurotic symptoms, and also in many animal
experiments quoted elsewhere (Eysenck, 1982). Eysenck also shows
under what conditions Pavlovian B conditioning produces extinction,
and under what conditions incrementation of the CR; it is suggested
that these results are of great importance and direct relevance
to the treatment of neurotic patients (e.g., Eysenck, 1978).

It is suggested further that this remodelled theory presents
a paradigm for the genesis of neurotic disorders, and their nature;
it also accounts for such successes as different methods of treatment
have had for their cure. Pavlovian extinction has been shown to
be involved, not only in the major types of treatment subsumed
under the heading of "behaviour therapy" (desensitization, flooding,
modeling), but also in the many varieties of psychotherapy and
psychoanalysis; indeed, even the successes subsumed under the
heading of "spontaneous remission" can be so accounted (Eysenck,
1980). The theory can not only account for these successes of
treatment; it also accounts for the greater success of some
treatments as compared with others, and for the fact that some
treatments (notably psychoanalysis - Strupp et al., 1977) often
make patients worse. These are strong claims to make for any
theory, and such claims can only be judged by detailed reference
to the various empirical studies and theoretical elaborations on

wnich it is based (Eysenck, 1982.)   The theory may be considered
a Kuhnian paradigm, in that it accounts for much if not all of
the empirical knowledge we have accumulated in this field, and
also suggests many testable deductions which can be used to
support or refute it.   Best of all, it presents a challenge to
what Kuhn calls the "puzzle-solving" abilities of practitioners
of "ordinary science", i.e. their ability to detect anomalies,
and to study these in sufficient detail to make it possible to
assimilate them to the theoretical model, or else to infer the
need for a revolutionary change of model.

It might be thought that the cognitive model presents such
a revolutionary change, but such a belief cannot be sustained.
Cognitive psychologists have never taken the trouble to study
the conditioning and extinction paradigm in sufficient detail to
point out anomalies so serious as to threaten its very existence;
their objections have usually been based on preconceptions and
principles not supported by empirical evidence.   They have never
demonstrated by experiment that their results cannot be explained in
terms of Pavlovian conditioning, particularly when it is remembered
that the Pavlovian system incorporates a <u>second signalling system</u>,
i.e. that of language, and that according to Pavlov, Staats and
many others <u>words can be conditioned stimuli and conditioned</u>
responses.   This extension of the principles of conditioning is
almost entirely disregarded by cognitive psychologists.

The conditioning paradigm outlined above is not the only
model available at the moment, and two others deserve explicit
mention.   The first of these is the model suggested by Gray
(1981, 1982), based on the hypothesis that specific phobias are
in fact directly inherited;   as we have seen, there is some
evidence available to suggest strong genetic involvement in the
genesis of phobic reactions.   If this be so, then treatment
would consist, not of Pavlovian extinction, but of <u>habituation</u>.
This in fact has been the suggestion of Watts (1971) who indeed
treated behaviour therapy as a case of habituation (see also
Lader and Wing, 1966.)   "If much of the behaviour of the
dysthymics is an innate reaction to stimuli to which he is
particularly sensitive, it follows naturally that the disappearance
of such reactions is due to habituation of the kind described by
Sokolov (1960) . . . And if habituation underlies behaviour
therapy, the key variable would be expected to be - as it is -
total exposure time;   although Watts (1971) was also able to
identify other likely variables and to show that these too
affected treatment outcome as predicted". (Gray, 1981, p. 266).
This certainly is a tenable hypothesis, but the substitution of
habituation for extinction does not change in principle the
predictions which can be made for treatment outcome.

In criticism, one must doubt the extent to which it is

320

feasible to inherit behaviour as such (Delgado, 1979). There is always interaction with the environment, and Gray's "innate reaction to stimuli to which (the dysthymic) is particularly sensitive" is not all that dissimilar to Seligman's notion of "preparedness". It is theoretically difficult to distinguish between "habituation" and "extinction", and it may not be easy to devise crucial experiments to decide between these two theories. Genetic factors are undoubtedly important, but it seems more likely that they act in such a way as to sensitize a person to form specific conditioned responses more readily, to react more strongly (in terms of the autonomic system) to such stimuli, and to extinguish them less readily. Note also that the heritabilities in Table 1 fall far short of unity; the Gray and Watts theory does not attempt to account for the environmental part of the variance, as the Eysenck model does.

The second alternative theory is due to Kimmel and Burns (1977). Their model is based on the distinction between phasic and tonic emotional reactions, the former referring to brief reactions to sporadic brief stimuli, such as the reactions commonly studied in laboratory research on conditioned fear, and the latter to those longer-lasting conditions characteristic of neurosis. An example of this distinction is taken from Asratyan's (1965) work on transswitching. If a given CS signals shock to the dog's left hindleg during the morning, but to the right hindleg during the afternoon, the dog learns to lift the appropriate leg at the appropriate time. The CS is a phasic stimulus, and the conditioned leg-lifting a phasic response. At the same time, EEG recordings showed a focus of heightened activity in the anterior parietal region of the cortex, ipsi-lateral to the locus of the shock; this tonic activation is present throughout the experimental session, and thus controls an ongoing state rather than a discrete response.

Kimmel and Burns go on to suggest that the distinction between a Pavlovian CS and a Skinnerian S[D] also exemplifies this distinction between a phasic and tonic stimulus, and go on to suggest an outline of a theory of operant conditioning of anxiety, based on the experimental work of Greene and Sutor (1971) on humans, and some work on monkeys of their own. They suggest that the typically phasic CRs obtained by Pavlovian conditioning cannot be used to mediate tonic anxiety reactions of the kind observed in neurosis, and that operant conditioning alone is capable of producing the tonic reactions required. They also suggest some ways of deducing methods of treatment from their model, but this is not sufficiently worked out to make critic-ism in detail useful. Clearly their criticism of the Watson model has substance, but these criticisms apply only to Pavlovian A conditioning, not to Pavlovian B conditioning, and hence leave the Eysenck (1982) model unaffected.

It is not suggested here that this new model can answer all our questions, or be used to generate methods of treatment which will work in all cases. It is suggested that it constitutes a paradigm, in the Kuhnian sense; it can account for the majority, if not all, the known facts, it makes testable predictions, and it offers opportunities for the puzzle-solving abilities of scientists working along the lines of "normal science". The existence of alternative theories, such as those of GRay and Watt, or of Kimmel and Burns, should make possible the devising of crucial experiments which should enable us to reject the less successful contender. It is along these lines, and along these lines alone, that I believe behaviour therapy will be able to advance, and to become truly scientific, rather than being an art, dependent on personal inclinations of the therapist, and for ever cut off from the degree of certainty in its application which only laboratory-based research and genuine theoretical elaboration cn grant. At the moment cognitive theory does not present a proper alternative to the model because it does not really exist, or is capable of making specific and testable predictions; should it advance to the status of a proper fully developed theory, it may of course present a challenge to the model here suggested which it does not do at present. However that may be, little advance in application is likely to occur without advances in theory, and the experimental study of theoretical issues in the laboratory remains the inescapable source of knowledge and further improvement in therapy.

REFERENCES

Asratyan, E.A., 1965, Compensatory Adaptation, Reflex Activity and the Brain. New York: Oxford University Press, 1965.
Delgado, J., 1979, Triunism: A transmaterial brain-mind theory. Ciba Foundation: Brain and Mind, Pp. 369-394. Excerpta Medica, Ciba Foundation Series 69, Amsterdam.
Eysenck, H.J. ed., 1960, Behaviour Therapy and the Neuroses. Pergamon Press, Oxford.
Eysenck, H.J., ed., 1964, Experiments in Behaviour Therapy. Pergamon Press, Oxford.
Eysenck, H.J., 1968, A theory of the incubation of anxiety/fear responses. Behav. Res. & Therapy, 6: 309-321.
Eysenck, H.J., 1976, Behaviour therapy - dogma or applied science? in: Theoretical and Experimental Bases of the Behaviour Therapies, M. Feldman & A. Broadhurst, eds., Wiley & Son, London.
Eysenck, H.J., 1978, What to do when desensitization goes wrong? Australian Behav. Therapist, 5: 15-16.
Eysenck, H.J., 1979, The conditioning model of neurosis. The Behav. & Brain Sci., 2: 155-199.

Eysenck, H.J., 1982, Neobehavioristic (S-R) theories, in:
    Contemporary Behavior Therapies, G.T. Wilson & C.M. Franks,
    eds., Guilford Press, New York.
Eysenck, H.J., 1983, Classical conditioning and extinction:
    the general model for the treatment of neurotic disorders,
    in: Perspectives on Behavior Therapy in the 'Eighties, Vol. 9,
    pp. 77-98, M. Rosenbaum, C.M. Franks & Y. Jaffe, eds.,
    Springer Publishing Co., New York.
Eysenck, H.J. & Rachman, S., 1965, The Causes and Cures of Neurosis,
    Routledge and Kegan Paul, London.
Fulker, D., 1981, The genetic and environmental architecture of
    psychoticism, extraversion and neuroticism, in: A Model for
    Personality, Pp. 88-122, H.J. Eysenck, ed., Springer, New
    York.
Grant, D.A., 1964, Classical and operant conditioning, in:
    Categories of Human Learning, A.W. Melton, ed., Academic
    Press, New York.
Gray, J.A., 1981, A critique of Eysenck's theory of personality,
    in: H.J. Eysenck, ed., A Model for Personality, Springer,
    New York.
Gray, J.A., 1982, The Neuropsychology of Anxiety, Oxford University
    Press, New York.
Greene, W.A. and Sutor, L.T., 1971, Stimulus control of skin
    resistance responses on an escape-avoidance schedule.
    J. Exper. Anal. Behav., 16: 269-274.
Kimmel, H.D., 1975, Conditioned fear and anxiety, in: Stress and
    Anxiety, Vol. 1, C.D. Spielberger & I.G. Sarason, eds.,
    Wiley, New York.
Kimmel, H.D. and Burns, R.A., 1977, The difference between
    conditioned tonic anxiety and conditioned phasic fear:
    implications for behavior therapy, in: Stress and Anxiety,
    Vol. 4, Pp. 117-131, C.D. Spielberger and I.G. Sarason,
    eds., Wiley, New York.
Lader, M. and Wing, L., 1966, Physiological measures, sedative
    drugs, and morbid anxiety, Oxford University Press, London.
Rachman, S. and Hodgson, R., 1980, Obsessions and Compulsions,
    Prentice-Hall, New Jersey.
Rose, R.J. and Ditto, W.B., in press, A developmental-genetic
    analysis of common fears from early adolescence to early
    adulthood, Child Devel.
Seligman, M., 1971, Phobias and preparedness, Behav. Ther., 2:
    307-320.
Sokolov, Y.N., 1960, Neuronal models and the orienting reflex,
    in: The Central Nervous System and Behavior, Pp. 187-236,
    M. Brazier ed., Third Conference, Josiah Macy Jr. Foundation
    New York.
Solomon, R., Kamin, L. & Wynne, L. 1953, Traumatic avoidance
    learning: The outcomes of several extinction procedures with
    dogs, J. abnorm. & soc. Psychol., 48: 291-302.
Strupp, H.H., Hadley, S.W. & Gomes-Schwartz, B., 1977, Psycho-
    therapy for Better or Worse, Jason Aronson, New York.

Watson, J.B. & Rayner, R., 1920, Conditioned emotional reaction,
J. exper. Psychol., 3: 1-14.

Watts, F., 1971, Desensitization as an habituation phenomenon:
Stimulus intensity as a determinant of the effect of
stimulus length, Behav. Res. & Ther., 9: 209-217.

DISCUSSION OF H. J. EYSENCK'S REPORT

Jean Sutter

Faculté de Médecine de Marseille (France)

Professor Eysenck clearly showed how important differences of
personality and motivations in psychiatric practice are.
But the theme of our symposium oblige us to look at the role of
these differences in the strategy and tactics of research and
there, we must state that they are the origin of considerable
complications and difficulties.
Schematically, one may distinguish two eventualities, according as
individual pecularities constitute permanent or on the contrary
varying features.

1 - <u>Fixed traits</u> are appreciated in terms of presence or absence,
rather than of importance or intensity. They are countless and it
is not possible to make use of more than a few ones. Typology
tries to palliate this difficulty: each type joins together
several traits, whose observations has proved interdependence. So
it is possible to constitute 2 or 3 groups of individuals, hardly
more, because when the number of groups increases, they become
less and less significant.
Ideal should be that all authors refer to the same typology.
Unfortunately that is a quite inaccessible ideal: traditional
psychiatrists will intend to use Kretschmer's typology,
psychoanalysts will describe their patients as hysterical or
obsessional, cardiologists will refer to patterns A and B, and so
on. Moreover it must be said that, according to the aim of the
research, it is not always the same traits that are to be chosen.
Inevitably, many individual differences cannot be retained. One
must be attentive to these circumstances. On the way, it will
often appear that a trait at first neglected is to be taken in
consideration, while another, which proved less significant will
be removed.

2 - <u>Individual differences whose intensity varies</u> from an
individual to another: they are to be utilised as variables, from
a statistical point of view.
It is possible only when these traits may be measured or at least
located on an intensity scale. So is it for instance in the case
of numbers memory or reaction speed.
Once more, of course, the number of characters retained has to be
moderate, on pain of making data exploitation impossible.

3 - Following remarks concern the both categories we have
mentioned above.
- Owing to the lack of precision of vocabulary, it is always
necessary to describe with utmost precision the individual
peculiarities retained. The modifications they may present during
evolution also are to be closely observed, especially during the
course of therapeutics.
- it is preferable not to be satisfied with a sketchy description
but on the contrary to do one's best for understanding the origin
of traits, their mechanisms of production and their significance.
The best seismology is always the one which leans on
psychopathology.

I shall conclude with a formula which is nothing more than a
statement of obviousness: strategy and tactics of research cannot
avoid considering individual differences and they must treat them
so that their disadvantages would be reduced and on the contrary
they turn them to account. So will be improved understanding and
weight of experimental process.

PSYCHIATRY AND THE SOCIETAL SCIENCES

Yves Pelicier
Chef du Service de Psychiatrie Adultes
Hopital Necker
149, rue de Sèvres, F-75015 Paris, France

The sciences of the human environment are mainly represented by social psychology, sociology and ethnology, to which may be added human geography, political science, law, economic sciences, etc., but these sciences can be integrated within the framework of an overall sociology.

The methods permitting the clinician to gain some knowledge of the environment are indeed numerous; they can be grouped in the following categories:

1. The Social Inventory

There is need to collect precise information concerning the patient directly. When such an inventory has been achieved, one has socio-clinical correlations associating with a type of morbidity or a clinical situation from a collection of items.

The most important items to be collected include:
1. the upbringing
2. education
3. family
4. the profession
5. the economic status
6. daily life:
   6.1. the habitat
   6.2. leisure
   6.3. the social supports.

These socio-clinical correlations can be treated in two ways:

1. for monographic utilisation, for a better knowledge of the patient and the elaboration of therapeutic strategies,
2. the epidemiological and statistical utilisation of these data, permitting with prudence an exploration of the sociogenesis of mental diseases. That use is largely facilitated by informatics.

2. The Cultural Balance

In this area there is need to explore the cultural contents of accessible milieux by the observation of behavior, of works and productions of all kinds. To be complete, the cultural balance should deal with the dominant culture, but also the sub-cultures (according to the era, the socio-economic level, the ethical or geographic origin).

This balance permits a description of the characteristic traits in the following fields: family life, profession, interpersonal relations, economy, politics, religion, arts, etc.

The methods used for the development of this balance originate in various fields: sociological analysis, institutional analysis, ethnological, etc.

The cultural balance includes an ensemble of data and valid information for very large, but also very small (marginal) groups. It characterizes ways of existence, of behaving and of perceiving, at the origin of attitudes, of action schematics, of roles and of statutes.

3. Biographical Analysis

This part of any clinical inquiry, but from the perspective individual/environment, it has to be very attentive to everything that illustrates these relationships within a life history. In the way, in which the social inventory basically establishes a verification (statement), the biography describes an evolution and a movement. A biography is therefore what an individual produces in function of its environmental conditions and of the circumstances.

One of the aspects of biographical analysis is presently represented by the theory of "life events", completed by the inclusion of the social supports. Biographical analysis is a path of access to a special and individual sociogenesis.

4. The Study of Interaction

The three preceding levels do not relieve of the study of the social actor and of his proper relational strategies.

One can envisage various approaches in this: study of scenarios, transactional analysis, observation of social behavior (directly or by video recording), using codes for decoding (like the Basle categories), observation of small groups, sociometrics, etc.

Starting out from the cultural balance, going on via the social inventory and biography, it is possible to collect data of partly general, partly individual kind, concerning the patient and his milieu. One of the risks of this kind of research is its extent and the heterogeneity of the contributions. The systemic concept allows the operation of a synthesis in specifying on the one hand, where the sick isolated individual does not exist, and, on the other hand, where it is not recognizable, except in the perspective of the system, in which it participates. At that moment, the clinician disposes of a series of complementary and non-contradictory informations concerning: the body, its status and history; the psychism, its state, its history and its way of expression in a personality; the milieu, its general characteristics and the particular modality, according to which it is implicated with regard to the given individual.

The clinical job here consists in refusing as always linear causality.

The problem of milieu/patient interaction can be reviewed by a series of interventions, possible at different levels, leading to variable psychological and psycho-pathological consequences:

1. During the formation of the "I" and the "Me" on the base of early family - and of "self" experiences (i.e. the "reflexive me") by the development and the generalisation of relationships with others. This refers to the controversial but indispensable notion of the base personality.

2. During the consolidation of personality construction by means of experiences, events and changes in the biography or of characteristic crises of the whole life-cycle (from puberty to old age).

3. At any moment, when at whatever level of the system, tensions, conflicts, frustrations or transformations appear.

But the richness of socio-clinical data does not make its great relativity: there is nothing in the milieu, nothing which

would make sense, but in resonance with the personality and its
history.

That is why sociology and socio-biology cannot operate
without reference to individual experience. The milieu, by the
richness of its stimulations, by the frustrations or the
gratifications, to which it gives rise, exercises an unceasing
influence on the psychism, but the event or the situation develops
their sense of individual experience. What the clinician observes,
is therefore a resultant: we are concerned with transplanted
situations, with cultural changes, with problems linked to work, to
racism, to aging, the veritable measure of the psychopathological
impact gives significance, which a fact carries for a given
individual. Unable to understand this, there is a risk of massive
simplification, Inversely, precisely because individuals are no
islands, because they are permanently implanted in systems, the
sense of milieu has much to tell with regard to the clinical
treatment of mental diseases.

ABOUT PROFESSOR PELICIER'S INTERVENTION

J.C. Scotto

Chef du Service Hospitalo-Universitaire
de Psychiatrie d'Adultes
Hôpital Sainte Marguerite - 13277 Marseille Cédex 9

The relationship between surrounding and mental pathology appears the most clearly among migrant people. Migration is very frequent today. It begins with moving inside the own country : inside migration (BERNER) bring us close by the same phenomenas than transcontinental one. For us, living in Marseille, the best example comes from transmediterranean migration, from south to north, from Nord-Africa to France. This moving belongs to "acculturation" movement actually increasing in maghrebian countries. Each migration is really a "transplantation" with his two risks : anomy (with consequences such lack of organisation, and lack of morality) and alienation (since migrant feeling drives many times to loose of identity).

The most important, as a pathogenic factor, is not the geographical distance but the restriction of ability, often complicated by going down on social scale. Result is always a lack of adaptation.

However, in our psychiatric practice, we need a good information about all historical and geographical characteristics of the patient's biography : we cannot understand his living experiences when having not such knowledge. So, too many students and young physicians are unable to get a good interpretation of these problems because they do not interest themselves to these dimensions of life : they have quite no information about history and geography, language and customs, etc. Lack of culture, sure, but also and may be more, lack of technics : each medical practice, and psychiatric one most of all, proceeds from capacity to imagine the patient in his own context. Building a relationship, evaluating a pathological situation, conceiving a therapeutic strategy, how could be possible to do all these without a good perception of patients original surroundings ?

331

THE RELIABILITY AND VALIDITY OF DIAGNOSTIC CATEGORIES

Gerald L. Klerman
Professor of Psychiatry, Harvard Medical School
Director of Research, Stanley Cobb Research
Laboratories, Department of Psychiatry
Massachusetts General Hospital
Bulfinch 3
10 Fruit Street
Boston, MA 02114

INTRODUCTION

Once a nosologic class has been generated, whether by theoretical inference, clinical description or other modes, the
next set of tasks involve validation of the class.

It should be emphasized that the existence of a nosologic
class is not given the truth of a nosologic class, or its
validity is not established merely by description, or by
assertion of authority or inclusion in official governmental or
professional nomenclatures. Rather, establishing the validity
of a diagnostic class requires the development of relevant
empirical data. Moreover, these data must be evaluated in some
framework of the scientific process. Within the current
positivistic philosophy of science, the process of generating
nosologic classes would be the phase of research otherwise
considered hypothesis-generating. The process of validating
nosological classes would be "hypothesis-testing." The
hypothesis being tested is that the given class has correlations
with other relevant domains or variables either concurrent,
antecedent, or predictive.

Within such a framework, the current consensus is that
establishment of the validity of a diagnostic class requires a
series of steps in which a major task is the development of
operational criteria.

Operational Criteria

The transformation of these descriptions into precise definitions is highly desirable before efforts at reliability and validation can be successfully undertaken. Definitions are most useful when they have both theoretical and conceptual clarity. The definitions are of two types: they describe the observed signs and symptoms of the manifest psychopathology, and they list the criteria for inclusion and exclusion. Examples of this in recent years have been the criteria of the St. Louis group described by Feighner (1972) and the Research Diagnostic Criteria developed by Spitzer, Endicott and Robins (1975).

Assessment of Reliability

The term "reliability" is derived from psychological research, particularly psychometric formulations. In psychometrics, reliability refers to the internal consistency of individual measures or of the items comprising a scale or test. For example, items in an anxiety scale should assess anxiety and not depression or paranoia. However, reliability in medical diagnosis refers to interjudge agreement or concordance. There are two levels of such agreement. One is the reliability of the judgments of the individual signs and symptoms, and second is the reliability of the assignment of patients to particular classes (i.e. diagnosis).

Reliability may refer to the concordance between an interviewer and observer in the examination of a single patient, between multiple observers of a videotape of a clinical interview, or between independent interviewers of the same patient at different times.

Depending on the type of measure, two statistics are considered most appropriate. The intercrest correlation is used for the judgment of dimensional variables such as degree of anxiety or level of impairment. The statistic kappa has been developed to assess the interjudge reliability for categorical judgments such as assignment to a diagnostic class or the presence or absence of a salient feature such as delusions or non-delusions.

Spitzer has investigated sources of "unreliability" in the diagnostic process. The largest source of variance is in the criteria used by different clinicians for the same disorder. This source is much more common than subject variance (a patient having different conditions at different times); occasion variance (having different conditions at different times that are part of the same disorder); information variance (information gathered from a family rather than an interviewer); an observer variance (different clinicians having

different opinions about specific signs and symptoms observed
during a single interview.

Demonstration of Validity: The Role of Etiology
    Ideally, validity of nosologic classes should be based on
knowledge concerning etiology and causation.

    Many critics of the diagnosis in psychiatry (Szasz, 1961)
have based their criticism on the allegation that the etiology
of psychiatric conditions remains unknown and that given this
situation, classification is premature. However, this radical
attitude ignores some very important facts. The etiology of a
number of important psychiatric conditions is in fact known;
for example, vitamin B deficiency leads to pellagra, organic
brain syndrome is caused by specific drug intoxications such
as, bromism, and some psychoses are related to CNS syphilis.
In the field of mental retardation, considerable progress has
been made in delineating those conditions resulting from
chromosomal anomalies, such as Down's syndrome, or amino-
aciduria, such as phenylketonuria. For the disorders of
pellagra, bromism, and syphilis, current mental health
practitioners tend to be ignorant of these conditions because
the success of previous generations of psychiatrists in
diagnosing, treating, and preventing these disorders has made
them rarities in current clinical experience.

    These successful efforts at demonstrating etiology for
psychiatric syndromes have rested upon the concept of a single
necessary, but not always, sufficient antecedent factor. The
classic approach to etiology in medicine and extended to
psychiatry has searched for some factor which is necessary, but
not always, sufficient, and an antecedent in temporal sequence
to the occurrence of the clinical syndrome. This model of
causation has proven most successful with infectious disease
and nutritional deficiencies. For example, the exogenous
pathogen, tuberculis bacillus, is a necessary but not sufficient condition for the diagnosis of tuberculosis. In the case
of tuberculosis, it is informative because its history indicated that up until the discovery by Koch of the tuberculis
bacillus, there were multiple theories, what we today would
call psychosomatic concepts. Moreover, while tuberculis
bacillus is a necessary condition for tuberculosis, other
factors play important contributory roles; factors such as the
nutritional status of the individual, housing, social
background, and the level of sanitation in the community.
While the necessary but sufficient approach has been highly
successful, it appears to have its limits; not only in
psychiatry, but in other fields of medicine. As an alternative, a multifactorial model of causation has been advocated,
particularly for chronic non-infectious diseases. The most

successful application of multifactorial approaches seems to be that of cardiovascular disease, hypertension and arterio-sclerosis. In these conditions, no one factor appears to have emerged which is necessary or sufficient. The evidence indicates that a combination of contributing factors either by addition or interaction is necessary. For example, in hypertension, there are important contributions from factors such as, genetics, salt in the diet, and exposure to stressful events. Applied to arteriosclerosis, the multifactorial mode has identified the role of genetic background, fat in the diet, exercise, cigarette smoking, and Type A personality.

In principle, the multifactorial approach should be well suited for psychiatric disorders such as, depression, schizophrenia, and alcoholism. For many of these disorders, genetic and environmental factors have been identified. However, it is not clear in psychiatric disorders whether these factors are additive or interactive. Moreover, the level of evidence in support of the individual factors for psychiatric disorders has not been established with the degree of precision and certitude as that which has been developed for cardiovascular disorder and other medical conditions.

Given this situation, the etiology of the majority of psychiatric disorders must be speculations as to etiology. Various schools of psychiatry differ as to the importance they give to various factors; more significantly, the level of certitude they apply towards the available evidence. This situation has created a serious problem due to the tendency for different schools with varying ideological commitments to reach premature closure concerning the quality of available evidence, and the certainty regarding the etiologic basis of certain conditions.

This situation has been particularly noteworthy with regard to hypotheses as to etiology derived from psychoanalytic theory. For example, in the early decade of the twentieth century, a number of diagnostic classifications were developed which specified the predisposition to adult disorders on the basis of fixations at levels of psychosexual development in childhood. Thus, Glover (1956) and Fenichel (1945) in their texts on psychoanalysis describe schemata in which various adult psychiatric disorders were based upon fixation at oral, anal or phallic stages of development. These hypotheses were not substantiated and required either modification or abandonment. Similarly, efforts to develop classification of psychiatric disorder based upon ego functions or other intrapsychic mechanisms have thus far been unsuccessful.

Another example of premature closure is to be found in the

336

area of psychosomatic medicine. Franz Alexander and his colleagues attempted to relate specific medical disorders such as arthritis, hypertension, peptic ulcer, and hyperthyroidism to specific intrapsychic conflicts. While these formulations were intellectually attractive, the evidence in support of their validity was lacking, and this approach to the classification and etiology of psychosomatic disorders has had to be abandoned as premature and lacking empirical foundation.

The tendency to premature closure is not limited to hypotheses as to etiology generated by psychoanalysis. Many formulations of biological factors as causative for schizophrenia or other conditions, had to be abandoned after initial optimism and ethusiasm. While the quality of recent research in schizophrenia and bipolar manic-depressive illness is considerably better than the quality of genetic and biological research in previous decades, the evidence in support of any specific hypothesis remains inconclusive at this time. Given this situation, a preponderance of researchers have come to rely upon descriptions of psychopathology, including current and past manifestations as criteria for defining nosologic classes.

Current signs and symptoms are assessed primarily by interview, past psychopathology, review of records, and data from family and other informants.

Nosologic classes defined by descriptive psychopathology have been found to have high reliability in facilitating communication among clinicians. This approach has advantages in that it involves minimal etiologic assumptions, minimal level of inference, and can be applied in clinical decision-making. With regard to pharmacotherapy, for example, depressed patients with endogenous symptom complex have been found to respond best to tricyclic antidepressants, and patients meeting criteria for bipolar affective disorders are most likely to respond to lithium carbonate therapy.

It is recognized that an approach that relies so heavily on descriptive psychopathology in formulating syndromes is limited in the long term; it is far from the ideal. However, the justification for current reliance upon this method is two-fold. First, because the present state of knowledge does not allow us to state with certainty the etiologic basis of most psychiatric disorders, reliance upon descriptive psychopathology renders the decision-making process least contaminated by theoretical presumptions as to the outcome of further research. Second, it is hoped that the definition and delineation of nosologic classes based upon descriptive psychopathology will result in the selection of increasingly homogenous groups of patients, with further research to verify hypotheses related to etiology. One of the sources of criticism of previous research attempting to demonstrate etiology, has been that heterogenous groups of patients have been studied and that failure to find consistent etiological evidence is due to heterogenous populations and unreliable diagnostic criteria.

The Validity of Etiologic Classes Based on Non-Biological Factors

Most, but not all of the examples used to illustrate the principles enunciated in this paper have come from hypotheses related to genetic or biological causation. Given the history of psychiatry as a field of medicine, such emphasis is understandable. In medical thinking, outside of psychiatry, almost all concepts of etiology refer to some biological factor such as genetic, nutritional, or bacteriological. Psychiatry is almost unique in the field of medicine in proposing non-biological etiologies. This has been related to the development of new schools of psychiatry. For example, the psychoanalytic schools emphasize early developmental achievement and intrapsychic personality conflicts as etiologic for psychiatric disorders, particularly the neurosis. Similarly, the behavioral schools have proposed learning experiences both based on classical Pavlovian conditioning or Skinnerian conditioning as the basis for learned maladaptive conditions as exemplified in obsessive-compulsive states, phobias, and learning difficulties in childhood. Social learning explanations have also been recently extended to include disorders such as depression and alcoholism, and drug addiction.

It is unclear what types of evidence would satisfy both the proponents and critics of these hypotheses. At times, the radical critics of psychiatry, particularly Szasz, seem to take the position that nothing other than structural pathology demonstrated at autopsy would be a satisfactory criterion for etiology. I am not aware that anyone has enunciated the criteria for evidence that would satisfactorily demonstrate the etiology of some non-biological factors such as, early childhood parenting or some learning exposure.

Internal Validity

By internal validation, I refer to correlation with information as to clinical signs and symptoms available to the clinician or researcher at the time of the current episode. In psychological testing framework, such correlations might be said to contribute concurrent validity. The standard mode of accomplishing this is to compare a proposed set of diagnostic criteria with those of established clinical interviewers.

With the availability of new psychometric techniques

utilizing multivariate statistics, and the development of high
speed electronic computers, intrinsic validity efforts often
involve determining the extent to which the symptoms and
behavior observed to go together do, in fact, coincide. This
is achieved by correlational techniques such as, factor
analysis, cluster analysis, multivariate and discriminate
function, and other techniques. Eysenck asserts that factor
analysis is the sine qua non of validity. Recently, other
statistical approaches such as, cluster analysis and multiple
discriminant function have been used to test the validity of
diagnostic classes by investigators such as, Lorr (1962),
Overall (1962), and Paykel. These approaches, however, have
been criticized by Kendell and by Paykel.

Correlation with External Criteria
      The most powerful forms of validity are those that involve
correlation with external criteria. These criteria are listed
on Table I and include familial aggregation for genetic evidence, and laboratory studies that use chemical, morphological
and radiologic findings.

      For example, the current interest in the dexamethasone
suppression test for possible correlation with endogenous
depression has been reported by Carroll (1982) and others.
Similarly, the radiologic findings from the CAT scan have
suggested the existence of a subgroup within the larger group
of chronic schizophrenics, a finding emphasized by Weinberger
(1979) and others at St. Elizabeth's Hospital, NIMH.

                              TABLE I

ANTECEDENT VARIABLES	CONCURRENT VARIABLES	PREDICTIVE VARIABLES
Familial and Genetic Developmental Factors	Biological Abnormalities Psychosocial Conditions	Outcome Variables
.premorbid personality	.cognitive responses	.response to treatment
.epidemiologic factors	.autonomic nervous responses	.duration of episode
.psychosocial conditions	.intrapsychic problems	.probability of relapse
	.current psychosocial conditions	.probability of changing conditions

Follow-up studies are valuable to determine whether or not those patients originally diagnosed with one condition, were actually suffering from another condition, or whether or not there is predictive validity.

By far, the most important determinant of validity is the existence of correlates of a nosologic class from domains of variables other than those that were used to define the disorder. Thus, if a syndrome based on signs and symptoms can predict course and probability of relapse, it is more powerful than one that cannot.

Boundaries Between Disorders
The discussion thus far has summarized current thinking about internal and external validation for individual nosologic groups. Recently, however, Kendell has proposed an additional criterion for the validity of a diagnostic group other than correlation. Kendell (1982) proposes that the existence of a diagnostic group requires demonstration, that the individual's with this disorder can be separated from other disorders in some multidimensional space. He points to the common clinical observation that there are many cases which seem to lie in the area of overlap between separate disorders. For example, there is considerable overlap between anxiety states and non-psychotic depressions. Moreover, the overlap between affective illness and schizophrenia has been the most troubling area of investigation and has contributed to the development of concepts such as, schizoaffective psychoses.

Kendell proposes that in order to establish the true independence of a disorder such as, schizophrenia, it is necessary to show that it is possible to separate groups of individuals that meet the criteria. Efforts have often been made to demonstrate bimodality of distribution of samples of patients on some diagnostic measure. For example, Roth and his associates in the Newcastle school have argued for the bimodality of distribution between endogenous and neurotic depression and also between depressive states and anxiety disorders. Other investigators have not been able to confirm the findings of the Newcastle group with regard to the separation of endogenous versus neurotic depressions. However, using discriminant function techniques, two investigative groups in the United States, Rickles and Downing and associates in Philadelphia and Prusoff and Klerman, have shown the separation of anxiety states from depressive conditions using patient self-report. Kendell's criteria has itself generated considerable controversy as summarized by Guze. The types of validity are shown in Table II.

TABLE II

Types of Validity

I. Internal Consistency (or descriptive validity)

The extent to which the characteristic features of a
disorder are unique to that disorder or are shared also by
individuals with other disorders or without any disorder.

II. Correlation with External Criteria

A. Biological correlates

(1) autopsy and histopathological data
(2) microbiological and immunological data
(3) morphological (including chromosomal) data
(4) electrophysiological (EEG) data
(5) biochemical data

B. Familial association and genetic transmissions

C. Psychosocial and personality variables

(1) personality patterns
(2) personal development and familial interaction
(3) life events and stress

D. Response to treatment

E. Clinical course and outcome subsequent to index episode

(1) degrees of impairment
(2) stability of diagnosis over time
(3) causes of death including suicide
(4) occurrence of medical illnesses

F. Epidemiological: systematic variation of rates
(incidence, prevalence, morbid risk) by time, place,
age, sex, social and economic status, etc.

III. Statistical Separation from Other Disorders in
Multidimensional Space

CONCLUSIONS

The current period is of considerable optimism within the
various fields relevant to diagnosis and classification:

Psychopathology, clinical psychiatry, biology, epidemiology. Considerable progress has been made in overcoming many of the difficulties that have plagued the field since World War II. The development of techniques such as operational criteria, improved modes of training, techniques for the assessment of reliability and a growing consensus as to the nature of validity have contributed to a period of renewed interest for important issues that have concerned the field for over one hundred years. It is hoped that the next decades will witness further progress in clarifying these issues and that the growing consensus within the research community will lead to the generation of new knowledge relevant to the better diagnosis and classification of mental disorders.

REFERENCES

Carroll, B.J. Clinical application of the dexamethasone suppression test for endogenous depression. Pharmacopsychiat. 15:19-24, 1982.

Feighner, J.P., Robins, E., Guze, S.B., Woodruff, R.A., Winokur, G., and Munoz, R. Diagnostic criteria for use in psychiatric research. Arch Gen Psychiatry. 26: 57-63, 1972.

Fenichel, O. The Psychoanalytic Theory of Neurosis. New York: Norton, 1945.

Glover, E. On the Early Development of the Mind: Selected Papers on Psychoanalysis, Vol 1. New York: International University Press, 1956.

Kendell, R.E. The choice of diagnostic criteria for biological research. Arch Gen Psychiatry. 39:1334-1339, 1982.

Lorr, M. et al. Inpatient Multidimensional Psychiatric Scale (IMPS). California: Consulting Psychologists Press, 1962.

Overall, J. and Gorham, D. Brief psychiatric rating scale. Psychol Reports. 10:799, 1962.

Spitzer, R., Endicott, J., and Robins, E. Research diagnostic criteria rationale and reliability. Arch Gen Psychiatry. 35:773-782, 1978.

Szasz, T. The Myth of Mental Illness. New York: Harper and Row, 1961.

Weinberger, D.R., Torrey, F., Andreas et al. Lateral cerebral ventricular enlargement in chronic schizophrenia. Arch Gen Psychiatry. 36: 735-739, 1979.

DISCUSSION ON G. L. KLERMAN'S PAPER

"THE RELIABILITY AND VALIDITY OF DIAGNOSTIC CATEGORIES"

C. B. Pull

Centre Hospitalier de Luxembourg
4 Rue Barblé
1210 Luxembourg

The discussant fully agrees with G. L. Klerman's position on operationalized criteria as a necessary condition for investigating the validity of nosological classes. In addition to the strategies proposed by Klerman for determination of validity by internal and external criteria, the potential of two French diagnostic instruments is presented in the following.

L.I.C.E.T.-S[1] is a List of Integrated Criteria for the Evaluation of Taxonomy in the field of non-affective psychoses which assembles all specific criteria for schizophrenia, acute delusional states and chronic delusional states proposed in 9 different classification systems. The list, which presents a set of 70 internationally recognizable criteria was used in a nation-wide investigation[2] in France to elucidate the criteria relied upon by French clinicians to assign patients to either one of the following nosological classes : schizophrenia, bouffée délirante, chronic hallucinatory psychosis and chronic delusional psychosis. For each of the preceding categories, the descriptions of cases provided through L.I.C.E.T.-S were almost identical in what concerned age of onset, duration, symptom pattern and exclusions. The results emerging from the investigation consequently provided all major elements required to operationalize each one of the four diagnostic classes.[3,4] The procedure would thus appear to have at least some potential for generating empirical diagnostic criteria and might be considered among additional strategies for determination of validity by internal criteria.

L.I.C.E.T.-D[5] is a List of Integrated Criteria for the Evaluation of Taxonomy in depression, which assembles 7 alternative sets of criteria, presented in their exact original formulation. Results from a preliminary investigation[6] which compared French clinical diagnosis of psychotic depression with 6 alternate sets of criteria for possibly related categories, revealed significant differences in the proportion of patients defined by each set of criteria. The French diagnosis "psychotic depression" and the DSM III diagnosis "Major depressive episode with melancholia" identify the same patients. On the other hand, only three out of four psychotic depressions are endogenomorphic cyclo-thymic axial syndromes (Vienna), two out of three are endogenous depressions (Newcastle) or endogenomorphic depressions (Klein) and less than half are primary depressions. Only one out of four French psychotic depressions would meet the criteria for all of the six other concepts. This very narrowly defined group of "primary-psychotic-melancholic-endogenous-endogenomorphic" depressions, we propose to call "a concordant group of depressions". L.I.C.E.T.-D is currently used, in several investigations, to compare different definitions of psychotic depression in relation with the AMDP-system, the Pichot Depression and Mania Rating Scale and Inventory, the dexamethasone suppression test and response to treatment.

REFERENCES

1. C. B. Pull, M. C. Pull, P. Pichot, LICET-S : Une Liste Intégrée de Critères d'Evaluation Taxinomiques pour les Psychoses Non-Affectives, J. Psych. Biol. Thérapeut., 1, 33 (1981)
2. C. B. Pull, M. C. Pull, P. Pichot, Etude Nationale sur les Critères de Diagnostic des Psychiatres Français dans les Psychoses Non-Affectives : Premiers Résultats. Comptes rendus du Congrès des Psychiatres et Neurologues de langue Française, P. Sizaret, ed, Masson, Paris (1981)
3. C. B. Pull, M. C. Pull, P. Pichot, Comparing French and International classification systems. I. Schizophrenia Pr. VII World Congr. Psychiat. (1982)
4. C. B. Pull, M. C. Pull, P. Pichot, Comparing French and International classification systems. III Paranoid disorders Pr. VII World Congr. Psychiat. (1982)
5. C. B. Pull, M. C. Pull, P. Pichot, LICET-D : Une Liste Intégrée de Critères d'Evaluation Taxinomiques pour les dépressions, Psychologie Médicale (in press)
6. C. B. Pull, M. C. Pull, A. Stauder, P. Pichot, Comparing French and International Classification Schemes : II. Depression Pr. VII World Congr. P(1982)

THE IMPORTANCE OF MULTICAUSALITY FOR THE CLINICIAN

P. Berner

Psychiatric University Clinic
Vienna
Austria

Classical psychiatry distinguished between environmental and somatic sources of mental abnormality. In doing so, it supported the tenet of unicausality, to wit: each mental illness has a unique cause. During the course of the first half of our century this reductional point of view was gradually replaced by the hypothesis that mental disorders result from the interaction of various factors. This has led to the creation of pathogenetic model consisting of four different areas or 'spheres', within which the factors lying behind the appearance of a given mental illness may be distributed.

TABLE 1

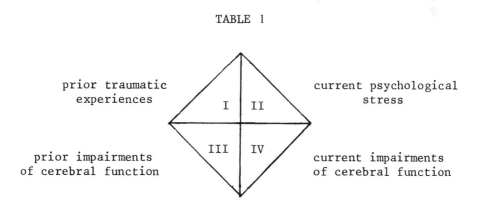

prior traumatic experiences — I, II — current psychological stress
prior impairments of cerebral function — III, IV — current impairments of cerebral function

Two of these spheres concern psychogenesis: Prior traumatic experiences and current psychological stress. The two other spheres concern somatogenesis, which can be genetically determined or acquired embracing impairments of cerebral functions prior to and coinciding

345

with manifestation of morbidity. Sometimes etiology is restricted to only one of the spheres, but far more often causal factors are distributed among several of them.

Numerous investigations confirm that the distribution of partial causalities such as past or present impairment of cerebral function of infectious, metabolic, toxic, or traumatic origin; prior sensitizing experiences; and current stress may differ from one case to the other. Such factors may be implicated to varying degrees of probability when a hereditary disposition becomes morbidly manifest. Any clinician knows that such multiple causality does not restrict itself to the appearance of hereditary illnesses but should be suspected for a large number of other psychic disorders as well. Abnormalities in the four spheres should therefore be considered to be risk factors whose concurrence will determine the appearance, course and phenomenology of morbidity.

The clinician is called upon to detect these risk factors and evaluate their pathogenetic importance at each stage of the illness. This is a difficult task because each factor has a qualitative and a quantitative aspect and their interactions are not easily unmasked. The observer is confronted by a seeming imponderableness of an abnormal mental state which he can describe and even perhaps classify on the syndromatological level; however, it is difficult for him to determine to what extent the various factors he may have unearthed are endowed with etiological weight. In such situations the instrument of documentation and classification, even those covering several spheres of information (so-called 'multiaxial' systems), are only of relative 'pathogenetic weights' or interactions. The clinician would be in a better position to evaluate these weights and interactions if he were to consider the patient as a subject whose behaviour and past experience are to be approached with an attitude of 'comprehension' and an effort at 'interpretation', and not be simply content with a 'causal explanation' approach of the psychopathological phenomena presented.

Jaspers, who characterized these three approaches, remarks that one can submit certain phenomena which appear together regularly and are followed by certain consequences to a causal explanation. Among the various modes of comprehension, which cannot be treated extensively here (see Jaspers' 'General Psychopathology'), rational and genetic comprehension are particularly important for the clinician. The first mode has to do with a deliberated understanding of the rational material divulged by the individual (for example, comprehension of the logical connections in a delusional system). The second enables us to grasp, with the aid of intuition, how psychic material is sequentially interrelated i.e., how one psychic element leads to another (for example, thought content from affectivity). Finally, one invokes interpretation when only a few stray signs enable a likely extrapolation to the case in question of the connection between phenomena which have been understood through experience acquired from previous cases. In the natural sciences causal

346

explanation is the only possibility; in the psychological realm, comprehension and interpretation have their place as well. We shall now show, by means of a case presenting a delusion of prejudice, how these different approaches can contribute to the clarifying of pathogenetic connections

A 51 year old woman raised in a burgeois setting in the north of Germany and married to a Viennese lawyer of modest origin, feels herself to be the victim of a slander campaign undertaken by a childhood friend of her husband. She is convinced that this friend is intent on ruining her marriage because of the harm it has done from the very beginning to the friendship between the two men and is setting the rumour afloat that she is an undercover prostitute in order to achieve this end. She admits to having always been opposed to the friendship because she never felt at ease in such vulgar surroundings. Her certainty dates back to an incident which occurred in 1981, when the friend had called up and invited the couple to go for a walk. She turned down the invitation, claiming that she was too tired. The friend supposedly replied, 'yes, we are too old for indulging in light activities'. His insinuation came to her in a flash: She was engaging in adulterous activities. From that moment on, unequivocal experiences (people avoided her, regarded her with curiosity, etc.) were to reinforce her conviction that a systematic intrigue was afoot. When she would attempt to discuss this matter with her husband, he would not believe her and change the subject. This led to an escalation of quarreling between the two, from which the patient became convinced that her husband was implicated in the plot and wished to get rid of her.

As time passed, she became more and more convinced that these calumnies started in 1979. At that time the wife of her husband's friend would phone her often, proposing that they go to town together. Previously, she had believed that this woman was inviting her to go window-shopping in downtown Vienna, now she was sure that the woman wished to let her know that she was wise to her participation in the prostituion which took place in the center of town. Since then, more evidence added to the patients convictions.

When psychiatric consultation took place, the following was divulged. Since the beginning of the couple's relationship, sexual life had been constantly marred by premature ejaculation. Menopause set in in 1980. The telephone call in 1981, mentioned above, occurred when the patient had been suffering for a few weeks from a mild endogenous depression. This depressive state subsided without treatment about five months later. In 1971 the patient had suffered from a similar state, albeit without delusional symptoms, which lasted six months and was treated with antidepressants.

If one limits oneself to pure description, this case presents a delusion of prejudice at the moment of consultation in 1983, an endogenous depression in 1971, and a combination of both elements in

347

1981. In order to grasp the origin of the delusion of prejudice, one need follow the path of rational comprehension indicated by the patient. This put enables the psychiatrist to establish a dialogue. However, following it solely and to its logical conclusion would implicate not only the refusal to establish any diagnosis whatever but also lead to the development of a folie à deux. Consequently, in order to arrive at a plausible diagnosis, one must also follow the path of genetic comprehension: according to Jaspers, a bona fide delusion exists when the examiner is confronted by an 'incomparable subjective conviction' which cannot be further clarified by other phenomena and is consequently incomprehensible. For Minkowski this delusional conviction is to be found when 'chance is excluded'. It exists in our patient because she rejects a priori any explanation other than her own.

For Jaspers, when comprehension reaches its limits, explanation takes over. Thus he sees real delusional ideas as arising from either a primary pathological experience or a modification of the personality. When delusional ideas first make their appearance in our patient in 1981, the exclusion of chance can be attributed to the primary pathological experience of endgenous depression, consisting in a displacement and narrowing of affectivity into the negative range. The origin of the ideas themselves, however, should be sought in another partial causality sphere indicated by interpretation: the patient's rejection of her husband's friend may have given rise to a fear of retaliation; such feeling must already have existed during the first depressive phase in 1971. Why did the delusional morbidity first appear during the second depressive phase ten years later? This question may be answered in part by the appearance of a new element: the Menopause, a period of life when sexuality often becomes an important pre-occupation. We may thus postulate partial causalities pertaining to three of the spheres in our diagram: one should consider the onset of of menopause in 1981 as having a potentializing effect on the previous traumatic experiences; but what is probably decisive for the new turn taken by the illness is the cerebral dysfunction resulting from the endogenous depression, since this impairment may be held responsible for the transformation of simple fears into delusional ideas.

The delusional conviction during the depressive phase in 1981 reinforces itself antero- and retroactively (Marchais): antero-active reinforcement leads to a broadening and a consolidation of the delusional system, even after the endogenous depressive phase subsides for the patient's behaviour provokes reactions on the part of the entourage which lend support to her ideas. Thus the patient introduces herself as an additional link into the chain of causality. Events preceding the delusion's manifestation become incorporated into the delusional system as constituting elements. This is reinforcement in the sense of a 'causality through a retractive loop' (Richelle). The patient's personality becomes progressively modified as a result of these antero- and retroactive reinforcements, for otherwise she would have begun to criticize her attitude during remission of the depressive phase. Thus new grounds for the continuation of delusional certitude successively take over as those responsible for its acute appearance (depressive focussing) subside.

Our patient has enabled us to illustrate how the clinician may gather insight into causal constellations existing at a given moment in the evolution of an abnormal mental condition. This insight is achieved through the alternative application of explanation. of the various modes of comprehension, and of interpretation. The evaluation of the pathogenetic weights of the different partial causalities as well as the knowledge of the succession of 'psycho-pathological constellations' (Marchais) which bring about a redistri-bution of these weights have an impact on diagnostic and prognostic assessment and therapeutic measures. If a system of classification attributing one diagnosis to each patient had been applied to our patient in 1981, she would have received the diagnosis of either psychogenic delusion or endogenous depression. In the former case, the depression would not have been treated, the consequences of which really took place. In the latter case, the acute appearance of delusional conviction may have been avoidable through antidepressant therapy. Failure to investigate her problems psychotherapeutically would have maintained the risk of renewed delusional manifestation upon reappearance of cerebral dysfunction (for example, upon relapse into depression). Once delusional conviction is established, all psychotherapeutic measures should aim at the resumption of its criticism, for the chances of fostering critical capacity diminish the longer the conviction is ,maintained. Experience shows that such resumption of criticism is only possible when the cerebral dysfunction responsible for the acute conviction is eliminated and personality modification leading to chronic conviction has not yet taken place. Recognition and exploitation of this optimal interval offer therapy its best chances for success. This is only possible if the clinician recognizes the partial causalities involved and appreciates their changing relations. In his psychotherapeutic endeavour he will on the one hand take into account the moment of illness onset, determined for the patient by the retroactive reinforcements, and on the other hand try to prevent the appearance of anteroactive reinforcements which promote and accelerate modifications of the personality.

REFERENCES

Berner, P. 1977, Psychiatrische Systematik, H. Huber, Bern/Suttgargt/ Vienna
Jaspers, K., 1965, Allgemeine Psychopatholige, 8 Aufl., Springer, New York
Lacan, J., 1932, De la psychose paranoiaque dans ses rapports avec la personnalité, Le Francois, Paris

Marchais, P., 1983, Les mouvances psychopathologiques. Essai de
        psychiatrie dynamique. Erès, Toulouse
Minkowski, E., 1958, Das paranoide Syndrom in athroplogischer Sicht.
        In: J Zutt u.C. Kulenkampff, 17-21. Springer, Berlin-Göttingen-
        Heidelberg
Richelle, M., 1982, Causalité et pscyholgie expérimentale. Conférence
        aux Journées de l'association pour la méthodologie de la
        recherche en psychiatrie, Marseille
Spriet, A., 1982, Discussion aux Journées de l'association pour la
        méthodologie de la recherche en psychiatrie, Marseille

DISCUSSION: CAUSAL PSYCHOPATHOLOGY - MULTICAUSALITY IN THE CLINIC - BY PROF. PETER BERNER

Pedro Polónio
Head, Lisboa Univ. Clinic of Psychiatry
Av. da Igreja, 39-11º
1700 Lisboa, Portugal

I am sure that we have all met with the patient, of whom Prof. Berner has spoken to us with all that comprehensive delicacy, considering the different ways open to treatment, even with the treatment of the husband. The classical, passive, contemplative and descriptive position of the disease development, productive of symptoms, is not at the first level of interest for the psychiatrist. He concentrates primarily on the acquisition of the knowledge necessary for healing, the most urgent and most noble task of the physician, to demonstrate the origin and the foundation of the multicausality.

In the functions of the nervous system and even more in the very complex interactions of psychological life and of the cerebral activity, it is easy to demonstrate what is at the base. The Jacksonian principle of an integrated hierarchy of functioning of the nervous system must be reviewed in the light of a multiple and dynamic, pervasive and continued interaction within a rigorous and determined organization, which is nevertheless plastic and susceptible to reorganization. Through the activity of systems with interconnection by multiple convergent and divergent links, chains of complex interaction subject to reciprocal subordination are developed. There are numerous autonomous activities, which go beyond the primary notion of reflex brain activity and the Jacksonian hierarchic activity, which one can consider as a better approximation, like a poliarchy without any rigorous determinism. In such a way, psychic life and the illness can be regarded under the sign of multi-causality.

The interaction of cerebral function and psychic life in

their autonomous activities can be explained by the emergence of new qualities, where the laws of biology related to the laws of chemistry and of psychics give remarkable results. Everything can be brought down to basic laws, but these laws do not permit us to prognosticate the new laws of emerging phenomena, which have the nature of facts.

The activity of the emergent spirit is complexly related to its biological base, of which it is the natural continuation and from which it diversifies in biological. We can describe a causal reciprocal relationship, a continuity relationship, an operational parallel relationship, an epiphenomenic relationship (the one occasionally being the appendage of the other without there being any reflection along the way), a mediate relationship.

There are psychological epiphenomena of higher nervous activity, which do not make sense, but which may acquire it due to the autonomous activity of the psychic event. Ereutophobia may be one of these expressions.

With progressively emergent character one could describe consciousness as an occasional epiphenomenon of nervous activity, whose utility has become very great thanks to the development of thought, of memory and the apparatus of thought, language and writing, which permit any person to utilize them, as if they possessed all the knowledge gained by mankind.

Clinical empirical activity overcomes with ease the insoluble conceptual contradictions between the life of the mind and the life of the body, those universes, which seem unable to meet. Internal realities and external realities are in accessible to consciousness, except by means of the interpretations possible on the basis of all the xperiences, which has made possible the construction of the universe of man. We are unable to understand the patient without understanding that reduction of the human and social universe to his own personal universe.

Due to the permanent interaction of psychology and physiology within the framework described, it was possible to avoid a rigorous determinism of psychiatric symptoms. Psychiatric symptoms are dyadic, having a beginning and an end. They are the final expression of psychological or physiological events and the source of new development with a dynamic autonomism. Physiodynamic developments can lead to organic disease and to death and psychodynamic developments can lead to an alteration of past appearances to discover truth in shining splendour. Devoid of meaning, they possess the force of revelation and of metamorphosis, texts, which permit contradictory interpretations, masks, which disguise a fatal and very sure knowlege. This psychopathology indicates the existence of biopsychological functions with subordinate reciprocal dynamism and a relative autonomy of psychological and physiological levels. The differentiated quality of sadness, of endogene depression, which blocks reactive sadness, can easily be identified with an occasional sadness. Trivial, anodyne and forgotten depressive experiences can be revived with intensity like the reactivation of past traumatic experiences that become determinant of the future.

In conclusion: the study of the pluriconditional genesis of psychic disturbances marks a step forward in the comprehension and the treatment of psychiatric diseases.

PSYCHIATRIST IN PRIVATE PRACTICE AND RESEARCH

Cyrille Koupernik

Prof. Hon. College de Médecine des Hopitaux de Paris
74, avenue Marceau, 75008 Paris (France)

INTRODUCTION. The purpose of this paper is two-fold: (a) to show that the P.P.P. can be a useful contributor to research, and (b) that participating in research will act as a psychotherapy for the P.P.P.

The first question to be asked is: Is there room at all for this type of obsolete clinician in modern psychopharmacological research? Therefore I will attempt to explain why my own answer is a cautious "yes". It is quite obvious that the P.P.P. can not be an active participant in a high-level research, not only because he may not have the required training, but also because such an involvement may prove to be detrimental to his main function, i.e. diagnose and treat individual cases. But, to use the terminology of modern brain Biochemistry, he may be a modulator and a support of memory.

His main quality is permanence. Usually research projects are carried on in large teaching Institutions where there is a continuous turn-over of junior members of the staff. Now they are the ones in charge with clinical evaluation of the patients included in the project. Therefore, not only is there an unceasing shift from one relationship to another, but also slow changes in patient's condition may well be missed. The P.P.P. (provided his patient remains faithful to him) is, on the other side, a permanent witness, a kind of chronic-writer, better and better acquainted with the destiny of the patient, his personality, the course of the disease and, last but not least, the possible iatrogenic pathogeny or incompatability with newly prescribed drugs.

In my opinion his contribution to research should run parallel to accomplishment of his main task as described before. But he must avoid subjective judgements; in other words he must be taught beforehand and provided with guidelines. I do not think that he should be asked to carry on a double-blind study; its requirements would be too time-consuming and would probably interfere with the psychotherapeutic aims. But he may answer regularly precise questions, such as:

a) - effect of the drug;
b) - tolerance;
c) - main side-effects;
d) - psychological tolerance;
e) - compliance

The P.P.P. may also be able to appreciate the possible effects of medication on family-life and professional activity. To sum up I will stress the fact that we need adequate long-term catamnestic studies of our medications and that for this type of project collaboration of P.P.P can be invaluable.

It may prove difficult for the P.P.P. to keep abreast with the progress in his discipline. He is a lonely man, often overworked, he also may have other interests and be less prone to take part in Congresses and Symposia. If he becomes a part-time member of a research-project he will feel himself stimulated and his participation will, in itself, act as a refresher. This is an important aspect, at least in my country where only too often psychiatrists with no pharmacological training or reading apply drug-treatment in a kind of passive and un-interested way. I would say that they do not define a therapeutic target when starting treatment; they often combine anti-depressants and neuroleptics, which, in my mind, is seldom justified. Some of them have had their training before the advent of biological Psychiatry; others are rather hostile to chemotherapy or use it as a placebo, or even a means of repression. I do believe that collaboration with a qualified team will show them that they are neglecting a useful therapeutic tool.

THE PRIVATE-PRACTICE PSYCHIATRIST AND RESEARCH

REPLY TO M. KOUPERNIK

Christian Müller

Clinique psychiatrique universitaire de Lausanne

Hôpital de Cery, CH-1008 Prilly

In his presentation, M. Koupernik clearly demonstrated the limits for participation in research of the psychiatrist in private practice. He spoke of a diachronic and of a synchronic aspect. I am in complete agreement with him as to the role of stimulator and critical observer which the private practitioner can play in relation to specialized research teams in institutions.

My contribution therefore does not tend to criticize M. Koupernik's point of view but rather to add a dimension differing from the one he envisages. He says quite correctly that biological research requires a rigorous methodology, that it works with cohorts of patients, uses double-blind trials and makes use of a whole range of sophisticated data processing technology -- thus going beyond the possibilities of a psychiatrist in private practice. The other dimension to which I referred relates to the functional aspect of certain psychopathological conditions. I feel it would be wrong to exclude from the field of psychiatric research the sociopsychiatric and psychological aspects of long term psychoses, such as schizophrenia for example. I maintain that the studies of Racamier and Benedetti, Searles and others, all of whom have worked in an extrainstitutional milieu, have made outstanding contributions to our thinking. The psychiatrist in private practice has the special opportunity of observing his psychotic patient over the long term, and of assessing the impact of various factors appearing during the adult life of the psychotic. Whereas the psychiatric literature of the last century was rich in "case studies", the past 60 years have been marked by the appearance of statistical methods, of applications of evaluation scales and of tests. For my part, however, I look forward to a renewal of isolated, detailed and painstaking observation, which will take into account all the parameters of our present knowledge. I am convinced that the psychiatrist in private practice can play an important role in this renewal.

TREATING WHAT? – LABELING LABILITY IN PSYCHIATRY

Robert J. Campbell

Clinical Professor of Psychiatry, New York University
School of Medicine
Director, Gracie Square Hospital, New York City

The current state of our knowledge about the diseases we treat
and the treatments we use is incomplete, tenuous, and often based
upon hypotheses that have yet to be confirmed. Accordingly, we
must continue to gather data from many levels and resist the
temptation to squeeze out observations into a foxed and rigid mold
that cannot incorporate new findings or different perspectives.
Failure to do so will make it impossible to know how to apply any
of the methods we devise to different populations, in different
countries, and by workers of different theoretical persuasions.

Evaluation depends upon a multitude of factors, and the current
emphasis on the quantifiable and the reliable perpetuates the myth
that science reveals pure truth, unsullied by the social context
from which it springs. The major elements to be considered include:
(1) definition of the illness; (2) the biopsychosocial characteristics of the person with the illness; (3) description of the
specific treatment method and its rationale; (4) efficacy; (5) side
effects; (6) comparison with other treatments including cost-
effectiveness and cost-benefit analyses; (7) the social context
within which treatment will occur; (8) the ethical ramifications
of the treatment.

Any treatment must be evaluated from the perspective of the
general goal of psychiatric medicine: to ensure the availability of
a full range of appropriate psychiatric treatments for those who
need them. Its objectives can be grouped into four major categories
- what kind of treatment is to be given; who will prescribe and
administer it; where and under what conditions will it be given;
and who will pay for the treatment?

Each of the categories, of course, interacts with all the others. Since the other presentations within this plenary session limit themselves to particular types of intervention or evaluation, I shall purposely choose examples that cut across boundaries and relate to more than a single category.

The Kind of Treatment: Issues include the right of the patient to have a say in whether he is to be treated at all; his right to a voice in planning the treatment program; preservation of a range of treatment alternatives; and, increasingly troublesome areas for us in the United States, maintaining a balance between individual and social needs; defining informed consent; and preserving confidentiality.

Within psychiatry there is controversy about diagnosis and labeling, about differentiating between variation and disease. We espouse the medical model and deny that we follow society's mandate in applying labels of sickness. Yet we now learn that tobacco addiction is illness, and we wonder if last year's smoker may have to enter a rehabilitation program to get this year's job.

We hear Szasz (1982) denounce us for "the medicalization of life" and for inventing illnesses, and then devising pseudotreatments for them. Masturbation is now therapy for the new-found condition of masturbatory orgasmic deficiency. Such criticism poses the knotty question of what is illness or disease, and how it is to be differentiated from sin, crime, creativity, or normality.

Despite our eagerness to reassert the definition of psychiatry as a medical specialty, we cannot ignore the fact that in some respects it is different from the rest of medicine. Among many other differences is that by its nature, psychiatry deals with questions of guilt and responsibility, soul and mind, attitudes and values, freedom to think and to act, the relationship of the individual to society.

In the United States, at least, designating undesirable conduct or even undesirable viewpoints as illness rather than as crime has been a major earmark of this century. The merger of the welfare state with the reforming drive of the social and behavioral sciences has produced the therapeutic state that turns our energies into prevention and rehabilitation. Those who might finally be labeled as patients are, naturally, apprehensive. They fear that in the name of therapy, society will impose upon them controls over their behavior that it ought have no concern about.

Consider, for example, the mother on welfare. Should aid to her needy children be cut off if she has an illegitimate baby after she has accepted welfare payments? Can the state tell her how to spend her welfare check? What happens if she tries to oppose the system? Will her hostility be interpreted as healthy resistance to oppression or will the examining psychiatrist, the modern day guardian of morality and the priest of the current technologic age, decress instead that her hostility is sickness or criminal?

There has been a recent emphasis in all of medicine on risk factors, but not even the scientific community has always been aware of the tentativeness of their implications. Only rarely have studies even considered the need to quantify the risk for any individual, to determine the relative importance of any one such factor to the others, to assess how many other risk factors might exist beyond those being described, to weigh the risk factors against possible protection factors.

In what has been called a "second public health revolution," programs for detection and early treatment of unrecognized disease are being mounted. Typically, they involve treatment of many persons with drugs, sometimes for life, and such drugs often have a substantial impact on the quality of life of those who take them. (Guttmacher et al., 1981)

Some strategies of prevention aim to alter specific behaviors that put people at risk and often assume that individuals are responsible for maintaining their health. A few have even suggested that those who voluntarily place themselves at greater risk for disease or injury pay a greater share of health care costs. How this would apply to persons in dangerous occupations that guard the public welfare, such as the police, firemen, or members of the armed forces, has never been made very clear.

Medical strategies aim to prevent illness through specific prophylactic treatments. A major problem in this approach is that the decision to treat is made under conditions of great uncertainty. Similar to trying to differentiate between the social drinker and the alcoholic, between schizoid or schizotypal personality and schizophrenia, in making a "diagnosis" of hypertension, for example, the clinician finds there is no method of determining whose pressure will rise, whose will fall, and whose will remain in the borderline range. So how can he justify even subtle coercion of people to change their ways of living when he can adduce nò need for such change? The public, no less than psychiatrists themselves, recognizes the clash between our dual functions of helping patients and also of helping society to run more smoothly.

Furthermore, if definitions of illness and labels for disease differ widely from center to center, how can one ever tell what treatment is best for what disorder?

Notwithstanding the foregoing, let us assume that we have somehow overcome the hurdle of diagnosis. What would be our concordance rate in picking the most appropriate treatment? Is psychotherapy the best because it is physically the least invasive? Is electroconvulsive therapy always the worst, even though it might save the patient's life and restore him more quickly to functioning? Is drug treatment the best because it is so easy, or is it the worst because of its potential for long-term side effects? What are the measures, who will apply them, who will weight them? Who has the right, or the duty, to decide what treatments to develop, and evaluate?

Given a changing subject, in a changing environment; with an illness that affects the subject's development or the acquisition of social or vocational skills and thus his way of dealing with the environment; with an illness that manifests itself in the way the subject behaves, and thus invites (or incites) a host of societal reactions and demands; with an illness that will itself change as it pursues relentlessly its natural course - it is manifestly impossible to take any from what we currently label schizophrenic disorders and pronounce that for such-and-such a subtype, treatment A is the best, B is the second best, and so on.

In the case of a chronic, recurring, irregularly progressive disorder particularly, there is the further consideration of the timing of the diagnosis. The clinician's natural tendency is to overdiagnose so that he can intervene at the earliest possible moment and prevent further deterioration. But if he is successful in preventing progression, the researcher then tells him that he did not start with that kind of disease in the first place.

Thus, it makes a great deal of difference in evaluating treatment methods if, on the one hand, borderline personality, narcissistic personality, and schizotypal personality are distinct, separable disorders and if the natural history of each is that it will remain confined to the range of personality dysfunctions, or if, on the other hand, they are indistinct and overlapping entities whose overall course tends to be progression into schizophrenia. Is the person schizophrenic and thus appropriate for the application of treatments effective in schizophrenia only when his manifestations are confined to the personality area? Is the person alcoholic only when he develops cirrhosis or brain damage? Is the person diabetic only if he falls into coma?

Who Gives the Treatment? includes a host of different problems, such as defining what a psychiatrist is. What does he do that is different from other mental health professionals? Do the best trained treat the sickest people, or do they treat those who could probably get along without any treatment?

Within this area, but spread as well throughout the others, are

362

research issues: (1) investigator bias, such as not investigating
(or advocating) a treatment that one cannot himself dispense; (2)
lack of incentive, such as drug companies not marketing or developing a product because it will give no profit; or deciding not to
seek government (FDA) approval for established treatments (such as
ECT devices), because the amount of profit to be realized from a
limited market would not justify the cost of performing the
necessary evaluations; (3) the effects of consumerism on research,
such as determining what can be evaluated; (4) the economic factors
that militate against research, and the effect of both consumerism
and economy on training, since the preceptor-student relationship
is often misinterpreted as a means of imposing inferior care.

Where Will Treatment be Given? The restriction of treatment
site to a single model is likely to deprive a significant proportion
of people in need of the help they might otherwise get. Note,
for example, the out-patient vs. in-patient controversy. Inpatient
treatment is easier to control and monitor, but it is more costly.
Outpatient treatment is more in accord with the philosophy of
community psychiatry, but it tends to blur the difference between
headaches in living and psychiatric illness, and while it is less
costly for the individual patient it also encourages overutilization
and in the end drains the economic pool that must cover all health
services, thereby restricting the care that can be given to those
who need it most.

How Will Treatment Be Paid For? Policies governing payment for
treatments tend to structure the treatment programs devised and
limit the range of treatment options provided. It is not too difficult to find clearcut instances of policy that has changed the
definition of illness as a way of denying access to treatment or to
treatment facilities, the first move in what I have elsewhere called
the numbers game. Once patients no longer are treated, there is no
way for them to be counted. If they cannot be counted, in a relatively short time the illness will have been eliminated, for there
is no longer any way it can appear in an official register. If it
does not exist, of course, there is no need to treat it - and all
the money previously devoted to treatment, research, and training
programs can be deployed in other areas. In such a way, policies
may define the diagnosis and spell out what may be considered
illness.

One of the important tasks for the future will be working out
ways of fulfilling ethical obligations to patients and health professionals without becoming so fastidious that other rights and
obligations are violated in the process. Unfortunately, it always
seems that the diseases which are the most significant in terms of
amount of human misery and economic burden are the very ones in
which the ethical issues are the most perplexing.

In Alzheimer's disease, for instance, what intensity of dysfunction must be manifested before a patient shall be deemed unable to consent freely to research procedures? Does every procedure require consent - even examinations of stool and urine, which would be flushed away in any event? If, in fact, not all procedures demand elaborate steps to insure informed consent, who will decide which procedures require it and which do not?

Finally, a note about the fruitless search for the treatment or the treatment setting for the conditions that psychiatrists treat. The staggering increase in psychiatric services that has taken place in the last 25 years in the United States has been in the outpatient modality, and it seems probable that the reversed ratio of outpatient to in-patient treatment is not a result of developing community support programs as a more appropriate alternative to inpatient care. Rather, it is the result of tapping a previously unengaged population whose needs are quite different from the hard core of disorders that will continue to need inpatient care. Indeed, there is nothing to indicate that any of the currently available modalities of care can be discarded. Despite earlier intervention, prevention efforts, and more specific treatments, some patients will still need hospitalization. Group and family therapy will help many, but others will require individual therapy. Psychotherapy may be the least intrusive or invasive form of intervention, but it alone cannot suffice for all patients; somatic therapy, including psychotropic medications, will continue to be needed by many. Behavior therapy and other innovative approaches will continue to produce dramatic results in some conditions, but others will respond only to intensive and prolonged psychoanalytic therapy.

Recent economic changes, unfortunately, have produced a shift from a funding backdrop of lavish abundance to one of parched frugality. In consequence, accountability, cost containment, and outcome studies have become the litany of the day. Yet as has often been noted, if health priorities and treatment approaches are set only on the basis of demonstrable efficacy, there will be no room for trying to find solutions to problems that have not yet been answered. How, for example, would Wagner von Jauregg's malaria treatment of general paralysis of the insane have fared under such a system?

REFERENCES

Guttmacher, S., Teitelman, M., Chapin, G., Garbowski, G., and
        Schnal, P., 1981, Ethics and preventive medicine; the case
        of borderline hypertension, Hastings Center Report, 11: 12.
Szasz, T., 1982, Dissident psychiatrist, International Herald
        Tribune, June 1:5.

THE EVALUATION OF TREATMENT METHODS BY RATING AND SELF-RATING SCALES

Detlev von Zerssen

Max-Planck-Institut für Psychiatrie
D-8000 Munich / FRG

INTRODUCTION

In spite of the widespread and still increasing use of rating as well as self-rating scales in the evaluation of psychiatric treatment methods there is as yet a lot of skepticism among clinicians as to the utility of these devices. At best, they argue, will the application of such scales confirm what good clinicians already know. But do they, indeed, know so much about the efficacy and the side effects of the various treatment methods in the large variety of mental disorders and is there always agreement among them? General experience does not concord with such assumptions! Nevertheless, in one respect clinical conceptions are thoroughly confirmed by statistical analyses of data collected by means of rating scales: If these scales include a large set of items covering, more or less, the total spectrum of psychopathological symptoms as described in textbooks of clinical psychiatry and if item scores were obtained from large and diagnostically heterogeneous samples of psychiatric patients representative of a newly admitted hospital population, then the application of various kinds of factor- as well as cluster-analyses to the data usually reveals symptom patterns that correspond very closely to the textbook descriptions of the main syndromes of psychopathology. The factors of the well-known Inpatient Multidimensional Psychiatric Scale (IMPS: 1) are a good example for this agreement between statistically and clinically conceived syndromes (2,3,4).

This excellent concordance of clinical concepts and the results of statistical analyses of data obtained by means of clinical rating scales should encourage the clinician to use these scales as tools for documenting his findings in patients under treatment and to check his impressions of the therapeutic results. He may then experience, with some surprise, that the application of scales does not always confirm preconceptions shared by the majority or, at least, a considerable and often distinguished minority of clinicians. This will be further demonstrated by contrasting some of such unexpected findings with the respective clinical prejudices.

EXAMPLES OF REFUTED CLINICAL ASSUMPTIONS

Clinical Prejudice 1:

"Self-rating is not sensitive enough for the evaluation of psychiatric treatment since the patients under study are usually too sick to make adequate statements concerning their mental conditions."

This prejudice seems to be even in accord with the results of empirical studies in which observers' rating scales were used together with selfrating scales (cf. 5). In such investigations factor analyses tend to yield independent factors for selfratings and for observers' ratings (3,6). Moreover, one particular selfrating scale, the well-known Selfrating Depression Scale (SDS: 7) often proved, indeed, much less sensitive to change during antidepressant medication than observers' rating (e.g. 8).

However, the factor analytic studies mentioned were performed on cross-sectionally obtained data whereas the evaluation of treatment has to be based on repetitive measurements. Therefore, I performed a principal component analysis of the differences in scale values obtained at admission and discharge by means of the IMPS (1) and a set of concomitantly applied selfrating scales (9,10) in as many as 420 psychiatric inpatients (10). In this case, the first component was clearly constituted by those selfrating and observers' rating scales that are closely related to depression, i.e. the IMPS subscales ANX, RTD and IMF and the selfrating scales for Depression (D-S/D-S'), general as well as somatic Complaints (C-L/ C-L'), and, in particular, the Adjective Mood-Scale (AM-S/AM-S'; in German: "Befindlichkeits-Skala" = Bf-S/Bf-S'). The fourth component was composed of selfrating-(P-S/P-S') and observers' rating-scales (PAR) reflecting paranoid thinking and only the four other components were either entirely constituted by self-ratings (component 2) or observers' ratings (components 3,5, and 6). Consequently, the scores of the selfrating scales with high loadings on the first component (AM-S/AM-S', D-S/D-S', and C-L/C-L') seem appropriate for the evaluation of antidepressants and those with high loadings on the fourth factor (P-S/P-S') for the evaluation of neuroleptics, at least in certain patient populations.

The appropriateness of the Adjective Mood-Scale for evaluating the clinical efficacy of antidepressants can be further demonstrated

by the high concordance of changes in the scores of both parallel
forms (AM-S and AM-S') with the score of the Hamilton Depression
Scale (11) during the treatment of depressives with either Amitriptyline or Trazodone (12). In this study, the SDS (7) was shown to be,
indeed, rather insensitive to change, but this finding cannot be
generalized with regard to other self-rating instruments.

In the study under consideration the most pronounced decrease
in scale values of the Adjective Mood-Scale as well as the Hamilton
Depression Scale was observed during the first week of treatment.
This is in sharp contrast to another clinical prejudice.

Clinical Prejudice 2:

"Antidepressants become clinically effective only after a
latency of two to three weeks."

This assumption is also contradicted by many other studies in
which rating- and/or selfrating-devices were used for the evaluation
of antidepressive medication. One instructive example is found in a
publication by Haskell et al. (13) on the efficacy of Amitriptyline
in a sample of 172 outpatients observed over a treatment period of
four (to six) weeks. 44% of the decrease of the total score of a clinical Depression Scale occurred during the first week while thereafter
the decrease was quite steady and less pronounced. The initial improvement after only one week of medication was most pronounced with
respect to the following symptoms: initial insomnia (75% of the total
decrease), suicidal feelings (73%), irritability (70%), and delayed
insomnia (67%). Since the steep decrease of the total score during
the first week was restricted to the subsample of patients with neurotic depression (80% of the total sample) it may be interpreted
as a placebo reaction. Even though, there was a steady decrease of
the score throughout the observation period in the residual group
of patients with endogenous depression. This observation is at
variance with the assumption of a latency of two to three weeks in
the drug response.

Further evidence against the latter assumption can be found in
Woggon's (14) correlational analyses of scale values for affective
symptomatology (derived from the AMP-documentation system, cf. 15)
in 87 patients with the diagnosis of endogenous depression. The
correlation of the total score at day 0 of a three weeks' treatment
period with the score at day 20 of antidepressive medication was
0.30; it increased to a coefficient of 0.60 after only five days
of treatment and reached a value of 0.75 already at day 10. This
increase in the score's predictive power (regarding the outcome
criterion, i.e. the treatment response after three weeks) within
the first 10 days of antidepressant medication is a very strong
counter-argument against the view held by so many clinicians (and

pharmacologists!) according to which the initial response to antidepressants is entirely due to a placebo reaction.

Clinical Prejudice 3:

"The clinical efficacy of antidepressants can be increased and
its latency can be reduced by intravenous administration."

This prejudice has markedly influenced the clinical practice
of antidepressive treatment. Results of controlled studies using
rating and selfrating scales for the evaluation of the differential
efficacy of intravenous and oral application of verum versus placebo
do not support the assumptions underlying this practice (cf. 16).
Therefore, oral administration of antidepressants should still be
the treatment of first choice, even in severe depression. The same
is true of the application of neuroleptic drugs in the acute treatment of schizophrenics which is at variance with another clinical
prejudice.

Clinical Prejudice 4:

"The clinical efficacy of neuroleptics can be increased by
intravenous administration."

This assumption is contradicted by a controlled investigation
which we performed in 29 acutely psychotic patients treated with
equivalent doses of either oral or intravenous Haloperidol in a
double-blind design (17). The combined score of seven IMPS factors
reflecting the symptomatology of acute psychoses (EXC + HOS + CNP +
MTR + GRN + PAR + PCP) indicated an advantage of intravenous administration only during the first hours of the first day of treatment
but not during the subsequent observation period of nine days. It
can be inferred that intravenous neuroleptic medication should be
restricted to the first dose in severely excited psychotics (unless
the patients are not willing to take the drug orally).

The last example of the utility of clinical and selfrating
scales in the evaluation of psychiatric treatment refers to a clinically presumed side effect of neuroleptics.

Clinical Prejudice 5:

"Depressive syndromes in schizophrenic patients are mainly
induced by neuroleptic medication."

In 1980 I published the average factor-scores of the AMP-system
(cf. 15) of 38 inpatients with acute schizophrenic psychoses before

and after four weeks of neuroleptic treatment (18). The data clearly indicated a reduction of the total scores, even with respect to the depressive syndrome (corresponding to the factor ANX of the IMPS). However, after neuroleptic medication, this syndrome prevailed in relation to factors reflecting the specifically psychotic symptomatology as, e.g., the paranoid-hallucinatory factor (corresponding to the IMPS factors PAR and PCP) so that the patients appeared relatively depressed after successful antipsychotic medication. In general, the depressive syndrome seems to be an integral part of the total symptom pattern of many schizophrenic psychoses and to respond, favourably, at least in part, to neuroleptic medication. This inference was supported by subsequent investigations performed by our group (19) and other authors (20). Therefore, the question should be raised whether depressive episodes occurring during long-term treatment with depot-neuroleptics have to be conceived as "covered relapses" rather than as side effects of neuroleptic medication.

CONCLUSION

The application of rating and selfrating scales in the evaluation of treatment methods does not always confirm the preconceptions of "experienced clinicians". These scales should be regarded as useful tools for checking the views held by clinicians and stimulate them to reconsider their preconceptions. This will hopefully lead to a correction of some biased assumptions regarding the efficacy and side effects of therapeutic interventions and thereby help to optimize evaluation research and clinical practice in the field of psychiatric treatment.

REFERENCES

1. M. Lorr, Assessing psychotic behavior by the IMPS, in:"Psychological Measurements in Psychopharmacology," P. Pichot and R. Olivier-Martin, eds., Karger, Basel - Munich - Paris - London - New York - Sydney (1974).
2. W. Mombour, G. Gammel, D. von Zerssen, and H. Heyse, Die Objektivierung psychiatrischer Syndrome durch multifaktorielle Analyse des psychopathologischen Befundes, Nervenarzt 44:352 (1973).
3. D. von Zerssen and C. Cording, The measurement of change in endogenous affective disorders, Arch. Psychiat. Nervenkr. 226:95 (1978).
4. V. Cairns, D. von Zerssen, K. H. Stutte, and W. Mombour, The stability of the symptom groupings in the Inpatient Multidimensional Psychiatric Scale (IMPS), J. psychiat. Res. 17:19 (1983).
5. D. von Zerssen, Self-rating scales in the evaluation of psychiatric treatment, in:"Methods in Evaluation of Psychiatric Treatment," T. Helgason, ed., Cambridge University Press (in press).

6. T. Fahy, Some problems in the assessment of current mental status
    of depressed patients, in:"Das depressive Syndrom," H. Hippius
    and H. Selbach, eds., Urban & Schwarzenberg, Munich - Berlin -
    Vienna (1969).
7. W. W. K. Zung, A self-rating depression scale, Arch. gen.
    Psychiat. 12:63 (1965).
8. L. Arfwidsson, G. d'Elia, B. Laurell, J.-O. Ottosson, C. Perris,
    and G. Persson, Can self-rating replace doctor's rating in
    evaluating anti-depressive treatment?, Acta psychiat. scand.
    50:16 (1974).
9. D. von Zerssen, in collaboration with D.-M. Koeller, Klinische
    Selbstbeurteilungs-Skalen (KSb-S) aus dem Münchener Psychia-
    trischen Informations-System (PSYCHIS München), Manuale.
    a) Allgemeiner Teil; b) Die Beschwerden-Liste; c) Paranoid-
    Depressivitäts-Skala. Depressivitäts-Skala; d) Die Befind-
    lichkeits-Skala, Beltz, Weinheim (1976a-d).
10. D. von Zerssen, Clinical Selfrating-Scales (CSr-S) of the Munich
    Psychiatric Information System (PSYCHIS München), in:"Assess-
    ment of Depression," N. Sartorius and T. A. Ban, eds., Uni-
    versity Park Press, Baltimore (in press).
11. M. Hamilton, Development of a rating scale for primary depressive
    illness, Brit. J. soc. clin. Psychol.6:278 (1967).
12. D. P. Bobon, Y. D. Lapierre, and T. Lottin, Validity and sensiti-
    vity of the French version of the Zerssen BfS/BfS' self-rating
    mood scale during treatment with trazodone and amitriptyline,
    Prog. Neuro-Psychopharmacol. & Biol. Psychiat. 5:519 (1981).
13. D. S. Haskell, A. DiMascio, and B. Prusoff, Rapidity of symptom
    reduction in depressions treated with amitriptyline, J. nerv.
    ment. Dis. 160:24 (1975).
14. B. Woggon, "Prognose der Psychopharmakotherapie," Enke, Stutt-
    gart (1983).
15. U. Baumann and R.-D. Stieglitz, "Testmanual zum AMDP-System,"
    Springer, Berlin - Heidelberg - New York - Tokyo (1983).
16. W. Kissling, H. J. Möller, H. Lauter, S. Kraemer, U. Binz, and
    G. Wendt, Doppelblindvergleich von Maprotilin (Ludiomil®)
    i. v. versus oral, in:"Der depressiv Kranke in der Klinik,"
    M. Wolfersdorf, R. Straub, and G. Hole, eds., Beltz, Wein-
    heim (in press).
17. H.-J. Möller, W. Kissling, C. Lang, P. Doerr, K.-M. Pirke, and
    D. von Zerssen, Efficacy and side effects of haloperidol in
    psychotic patients: oral versus intravenous administration,
    Amer. J. Psychiat. 139:1571 (1982).
18. D. von Zerssen, Psychopathometrische Verfahren und ihre Anwen-
    dung in der Psychiatrie, in:"Die Psychologie des 20. Jahr-
    hunderts," U. H. Peters, ed., Kindler, Zurich (1980).
19. H. J. Möller and D. von Zerssen, Depressive states occurring
    during the neuroleptic treatment of schizophrenia, Schizophr.
    Bull. 8:109 (1982).
20. A. Knights and S. R. Hirsch,'Revealed'depression and drug treat-
    ment for schizophrenia, Arch. Gen. Psychiat. 38:806 (1981).

EVALUATION OF METHODOLOGICAL PROGRESS IN
CLINICAL PHARMACOPSYCHIATRY

Kurt A. Fischer-Cornelssen

Senior Expert, Clin. Research, Pharma Industry, Basle
Im Lohgraben 58
CH-4104 Oberwil, Switzerland

Improvements in psychopharmacological treatment benefiting the
patients are only possible if our clinical studies achieve the
highest scientific standards in respect of logic, quality, objectivity, and validity (Fischer-Cornelssen, 1980). Therefore we have
to ask: 1) What is the state of art; 2) What were and are the
mistakes and pitfalls; 3) What progress has been made during the
last decade and what is the outlook?

THE "STATE OF THE ART"

Relevant, reliable and valid clinical results can only be
achieved by using adequate, accurate and ambitious methods of high
quality and by fulfilling statistical requirements. These requirements necessitate, in the open and double blind phase, multicenter
trials, upon which our main interest is concentrated. The pooling
of multicenter data from several homogeneous, uniform and standardized studies provides a better differentiation between similar
drugs, gives clearer and more comprehensive results, increases
objectivity and generalization by repetition in a range of treatment
settings and enhances power and evidence of statistical analyses
than data from one or more single study(ies). (Angst, Boissel a.
Klimt, Downing et al., Fischer-Cornelssen et al. 1974, Klerman,
Perris a. Jacobson, Wittenborn).

In the planning, design, execution, and evaluation of clinical
studies, the most important tasks are (Fischer-Cornelssen 1971,
74, 76, 80):

Limitation of Undesirable Variances

To keep the variability within and between the studies of a multicenter trial low, to make pooling and comparability possible and to enhance relevance, reliability and validity, the following pre-requisites are necessary for the study protocol, the execution, documentation and evaluation: uniformity, systematization and standardization, strict prescriptions and descriptions of parameters, criteria and execution, access to type and number of appropriate patients and facilities, conscientious and experienced investigators and personnel, adherence to the spirit and the letter of the protocol (quality consciousness). Some examples:

a) According to clinical experience the target patients providing the most conclusive therapeutic answers are for antidepressants, those with endogenous depressions (WHO-ICD 9: 296.1 and 296.3; DSM-III: only 296.2, 296.3, 296.5 / subtype ._3 = with melancholia), for neuroleptics those with "florid" paranoid schizophrenia (ICD: 295.3, DSM-III: 295.2, 295.3 / subtypes ._3, ._4; and, for minor tranquilizers, those patients with sub-chronic or chronic anxiety states (ICD: 300.0, .2, .4; DSM-III: groups 300.0, 300.2; 309.24). In spite of the well known cross national and transcultural differences in diagnostic labelling a determined effort should be made to obtain a homogeneous patient sample within a study and a multicenter trial. Heterogeneity of diagnoses is one of the main sources of variability in studies. In 62 % of cases inadequate guidelines seem to be the basis for variances, in 32 % inconsistency of the patient's behaviour (Ward). After the proof of efficacy in homogeneous patient groups – or parallel to it – patients with heterogeneous diagnoses can be studied.

b) Patients should show a medium to severe degree of illness because improvement or differences after drug treatments are bigger than in patients with low degree of severity (statistical significance!). A detailed multi-dimensional description of the inclusion criteria for patients in the study protocol ("operationalization") is a must and should include: the supposed diagnoses and sub-groups wanted, the target and secondary symptoms, their degree of severity, the genetics (family history), the nature of past and present episodes wanted. This has to be completed by stating thoroughly the exclusion criteria (Perris and Jacobson, adapted).

c) To limit the chances of an   – or   -error (type 1- or 2-error, a drug is found incorrectly to be effective or ineffective) the number of patients required has to be high enough. As an example: with an   -risk of 5 %, a   -risk of 10 % and a difference of expected improvement of 10 % between the investigational and the standard drug, twice 400 patients are necessary to demonstrate a relevant difference statistically (Schwartz). This does not exclude the possibility of finding, by chance, a significant difference with lower patient numbers.

Assessment of Desired Variables (Treatment Effects)

a) Statistically, a uniform fixed dosage schedule for all patients would be ideal. But extreme individual differences in pharmacokinetics, drug metabolism and reaction to treatment do not allow this. Clinically and ethically, the only acceptable standardization is a fixed starting dose and a dosage adjustment within fixed time frame (e.g. 2 weeks) to the optimal level for each patient which is then maintained till the end of the study. In phase I- as well as in phase II-studies the duration of treatment should not be less than 6 weeks. Only after reaching the "steady state" levels of the drug in blood and brain, e.g. after about 3 weeks, efficacy and tolerability have a chance to stabilize and can then be assessed reliably during the following 2 to 3 weeks (incl. safety).

b) The global or overall assessment of therapeutic benefit to the patient by the doctor remains, even today, the most important, reliable and valid variable for decision making on therapeutic effect. It has to be structured logically into its factors and scores and their criteria should be described in detail ("operationalization").

c) A thorough description of the frequency and intensity of psycho-pathological and somatic symptoms is a desired variable of main interest and an indispensable addition to the global evaluation. Most symptoms are only valid under the headline of the respective diagnosis (e.g. quality of anxiety may be different in schizo-phrenia, depression or anxiety neurosis). This profile of symptoms should be documented for each patient before the start of the treat-ment (basic description and profile of population) and systematic-ally in the course of the treatment (sample days).

d) Innumerable rating scales are available for the systematic assessment and evaluation of symptoms and signs. The long ones (more than 50 items) are impractical, unfeasible and too time consuming for daily clinical work and common psychotropic research. They have to be reserved for special institutions and basic re-search. The short ones (20 or less items) do not fulfill the quality needs and do not cover the respective spectrum of important symptoms. Only a few rating scales are used frequently and have "proven" in the past "to be useful" in clinical drug studies. For many of these "common" rating scales the proof of content, con-current or construct validity or for intrarater-consistency (test-

retest) and interrater reliability clinically often seem to be weak
(e.g. too low patient numbers, heterogeneity etc.). And, in addition to this, without high standard clinical studies and methods
relevant analyses of the quality of rating scales are impossible.
The available clinical data for most of the rating scales are not
strong enough to allow a definite judgement on their value and
benefit. Symptom check lists of medium length (30 to 50 items) are
promising if they fulfill the important practical requirements:
relevant psychiatric content, built on clinical and biometrical
experience, broad spectrum of symptoms with as many items as
necessary and as few as possible, logical structure and scoring,
resemblance to clinical practice, feasibility and practicability.

e) It is self-evident that all efforts to achieve quality in the
basic theoretical requirements and design mentioned above are sense-
less and ineffective if they are not fully transferred into practice
e.g. execution, documentation and evaluation of the respective
clinical studies. There is only one way with "sweat and tears" to
succeed: slavish attention to a myriad of details during the performance, quality consciousness and quality control (Meinert),
careful monitoring and conscientious reporting and documentation
of every detail as well as attention to analysis and interpretation
of data and results.

MISTAKES AND PITFALLS

There are no limitations on the number of ways that an experiment can go wrong (Gocka). Nothing can be taken for granted and
every detectable or discrete (undesirable) variation will affect
the success of a study (Klett and Caffey). Some examples:

a) The sometimes theoretical and artificial newly created classification systems may be more responsible for misunderstandings and
wrong or bad results than the established real cross-national or
international or transcultural differences in diagnoses. An example
is the so-called diagnosis "major depression" which cannot be translated correctly into any other language or into a common or broadly
acceptable diagnosis. Studying, for example, an antidepressant in
"major depression" one may have difficulties in proving efficacy or
establishing a different profile compared to a standard drug or even
placebo. The mixture of endogenous depressions ("melancholia" or
"endomorphic") and non-endogenous depressions in studies of antidepressants is not only contradictory to the content of hypothesis-
testing and to the principle of minimization of undesirable variances but also to clinical experience: medium to severe endogenous
depressions demonstrate the greatest improvements with good antidepressants and the smallest with placebo. For non-endogenous

374

depressions the difference antidepressant - placebo is often much
smaller, the dosage much lower, and other drug treatments show
equal, better or convincing better results (new minor tranquilizers,
somatic treatment, psychotherapy). Wrong patient selection enhances
type 1- or 2-errors substantially and may be a disaster for progress
in psychopharmacology.

b) The same applies to small patient numbers. Many (if not most)
drug studies have employed or employ sample sizes that are too small
to give sufficient statistical power for detecting or proving
effects or differences between new agents and a standard (Downing
et al., Fischer-Cornelssen 1980). There is a possibility that investigational drugs with a good or outstanding therapeutic effect
could be found by chance in spite of using low quality rating
scales (with a low content validity!). But in order to find clear
differences in efficacy and therapeutic profile high quality methods
and rating scales are necessary.

c) Because of a multiplication of variabilities and faults, logical
design and quality of identical planning, execution and analysis of
multicenter trials are far more important for the outcome and require
greater specification and care than that of single studies (Downing
et al., Klerman, Klett and Caffey, Okun). Missing data, sloppy data
processing and -analysis procedures can be at least as deleterious
to end results as carelessness in the generation of data (Meinert,
Boissel, Okun).

THE PROGRESS OF THE LAST YEARS AND THE OUTLOOK

There was and is a great increase, one could say "an inflation"
in so-called "high claiming" open and double-blind studies as well
as "multicenter trials". That will say that the idea is much more
known than years ago. And there is a growing fashion to give clinical
studies the appearance of high quality and sophistication. But in
reality only 5 to 10 % of studies fulfill, to an acceptable extent,
the mentioned requirements. Especially cross-national and international multicenter trials rarely reach, in respect of homogeneity
and standardization, strict control of conditions, procedures and
executions and statistical considerations, the necessary level which
is essential for high quality and clinically relevant outcome. There
is a great interest in the potential usefulness of ("clinical")
testing in psychiatry, but the statistical principles required for
critical evaluation of their value remain poorly integrated into
clinical thinking (Baldessarini, adapted). This seems - at least
partly - to be a result of difficulties in education, training and
advanced training of our young colleagues as well as of low interest
and drive to learn and to do the best possible for the benefit of

the patients. We have to ask ourselves whether we have done as much as possible to maintain a basic consciousness for conscientious, high quality and ethical research. At the end our question concerning the future remains open: Have We Forgotten to Observe, to Criticize Ourselves and to Learn?

References

Angst, J., Bente, D., Berner, P., Heimann, H., Helmchen, H., and Hippius, H., 1971, Pharmakopsychiat. Neuropsychopharmakol., 4:201.

Baldessarini, R.J., Finklestein, S., and Arona, G.W., 1983, Arch. Gen. Psychiatry, 40:569.

Boissel, J.P., and Klimt, C.R., 1979, Essais controlés multicentres. Principes et problèmes, Inserm, Paris, 274.

Downing, R.W., Rickels, K., Wittenborn, J.R., and Mattsson, N.B., 1971, in Levine, J., Schiele, B.C., and Bouthilet, L.: Principles and Problems in Establishing Efficacy of Psychotropic Agents, U.S. Government Print. Off., Washington, Health Serv. Publ. No. 2138:321.

Fischer-Cornelssen, K.A., Hole, G., and Abt, K., 1971, New audio-visual method, Prensa Med. Mex., Proceed. Vth World Congress Psychiat., 291.

Fischer-Cornelssen, K., Ferner, U.,and Steiner, H., 1974, Arznei-mittel-Forsch./Drug Res.,24:1706.

Fischer-Cornelssen, K.A., and Ferner, U., 1976, Psychopharmacol. Bulletin, 12:34.

Fischer-Cornelssen, K.A., 1980, Methods of Multicenter Trials in Psychiatry: REVIEW, Progr. Neuro-Psychopharmacol. 4:545 (66 ref.).

Fischer-Cornelssen, K.A., 1980, REVIEW VIDEO, Acta psychiat. scand., 61:228.

Gocka, E.F., 1978, in Clark, G.L., and Del Giudice, J., Principles of Psychopharmacol., Academic Press, New York, 420.

Klerman, G.L., 1971, Arch. Gen. Psychiat., 24:305.

Klett, C.J., and Caffey, E.M., 1978, in Clark, W.G., and Del Giudice, J., Principles of Psychopharmacol., Academic Press, New York, 435.

Meinert, C.L., 1979, in J.P. Boissel and C.R. Klimt, Inserm, Paris, 123.

Okun, R., 1978, in Clark, W.G., and Del Giudice, J., (ed.), Principles of Psychopharmacol., Academic Press, New York, 409.

Perris, C., and Jacobson, L., 1977, Drugs Explt. Clin. Res., 1:79.

Schwartz, D., 1979, in J.P. Boissel and C.R. Klimt, Inserm, Paris, 103.

Ward, C.H., Beck, A.T., Mendelson, M., Mock, J.E., and Erbaugh, J.K., 1962, Arch. Gen. Psychiat., 7:198.

Wittenborn, J.R., 1977, Pharmakopsychiat. Neuro-Psychopharmakol., 10:205.

EVALUATION OF TREATMENT METHODS: PSYCHOTHERAPY

Hans H. Strupp

Vanderbilt University
Department of Psychology
Nashville, Tennessee

Despite decades of research and a voluminous clinical literature, psychotherapy remains in an embattled state. Does it work?
Is it effective? Whom does it benefit? Should it be covered
under National Health Insurance, and if so, to what extent? How
can psychotherapeutic services be made less costly and more readily
available? Who is qualified to be a psychotherapist? What background training should be required? These are but a few of the
questions which continue to exercise the minds of proponents and
opponents alike. Complicating the situation is the Government's
recent interest in the controversy. How can legislators and
policymakers resolve the dispute among scientists, practitioners,
and third parties? How can they evaluate the scientific evidence?
How can they enact intelligent and reasonable legislation? Since
psychotherapy is now described as a billion dollar "industry", the
issues are not trivial and the stakes are high. Two things are
clear: the problems are not likely to be resolved in the foreseeable future and they will not be decided on the basis of
scientific evidence alone. The best one may hope is that political
decisions will be maximally informed by rationality and reason.

The recent past witnessed the publication of a book, titled
The benefits of psychotherapy, which is likely to have a considerable
impact on research, practice, training, and government policy.
Authored by three researchers at the University of Colorado (Mary
Lee Smith, Gene V. Glass, and Thomas I. Miller), it is a fine
demonstration of behavioral science research, employing sophisticated
methodology and techniques of statistical analysis. The authors,
moreover, have no vested interest in the field and are thus immune
from the charge of grinding axes. Their method of research, called
meta-analysis, is based on the premise that no single study can

377

conclusively answer basic questions in the field; however, by computing an index (called average effect size) based on normalized mean deviations of treated groups from control groups on a variety of measures, it is possible to combine the results of widely divergent studies, and to arrive at stable cumulative effects. A total of 475 controlled studies of psychotherapy entered into their analyses, and 112 experiments were analyzed to determine the separate and combined effects of psychotherapy and drug therapy. What were their major conclusions?

1. "Psychotherapy is benefical, consistently so and in many different ways. Its benefits are on a par with other expensive and ambitious interventions, such as schooling and medicine. The benefits of psychotherapy are not permanent, but then little is.

2. "Different types of psychotherapy (verbal or behavioral: psychodynamic, client-centered, or systematic desensitization) do not produce different types or degrees of benefit.

3. "Differences in how psychotherapy is conducted (whether in groups or individually, by experienced or novice therapists, for long or short-periods of time, and the like) make very little difference in how beneficial it is.

4. "Psychotherapy is scarcely any less effective than drug therapy in the treatment of serious psychological disorders. When the two therapies are combined, the net benefits are less than the sum of their separate benefits."

These conclusions generally support the results of previous analyses of the literature. Taken together, they lend substantial support to the field as a whole. In the following paragraphs I wish to explore some of the implications for psychotherapists and those concerned with the training of therapists.

1. Perhaps most impressive are the robust effects of a great diversity of operations grouped under the heading of "psychotherapy." Whether psychotherapy is performed expertly or imperfectly, whether patients are ideally suited or less so, whether the therapist espouses one theoretical orientation as opposed to. another, the outcomes are generally favorable. As a minimum, these findings establish psychotherapy as a useful tool in treating a variety of disturbances in living, all the more since there are often no viable alternatives.

2. Having said this, it is important to guard against the faulty inference that careful patient selection is unimportant or that careful training for psychotherapists can be dispensed with. In fact, the findings highlight the critical importance of patient variables--the person's total life adjustment, motivation for

participating in a therapeutic relationship, and a sense of responsibility. To illustrate further: Results from the Vanderbilt Psychotherapy Project (Strupp & Hadley, 1979), an intensive study of time-limited psychotherapy, showed that patients who met these criteria profited most from therapeutic work with highly experienced psychotherapists. Conversely, patients who were deficient in these areas and those who were negativistic, resistant, and hostile proved relatively refractory regardless of the therapist's skill or level of experience. This result, coupled with others, strongly suggests that (a) patient selection is crucial for optimal outcomes and (b) therapists do their best work with patients who can readily enter into a collaborative relationship with a competent professional. By analogy, many types of medical treatment are most effective if the patient possesses the requisite resources, such as good general health, absence of complicating conditions, and the like. No one faults the method of treatment or the physician if the results are poorer under less than ideal conditions. No more should be expected from psychotherapy and psychotherapists. Frequently heard disparagements, such as "the rich get richer" or "psychotherapy works best with people who need it the least," are hardly warranted.

3. All available evidence strongly supports the conclusion that factors common to all forms of psychotherapy carry greater weight in treatment outcomes than particular techniques advocated by various schools. Common factors encompass ingredients found in any good human relationship--e.g., empathy, understanding, respect--but, as noted above, there must be a patient who can profit from what a therapist can reasonably provide. Again, the data do not prove the converse, that a therapist's specialized skills in facilitating a constructive emotional experience leading to greater self-acceptance, self-esteem, and autonomy are dispensable. Parenthetically, the latter kinds of changes may be so subtle that they are not reflected in the imperfect measuring instruments on which one must necessarily rely. There may also be a difference between quantity and quality of change. As yet, there are no good techniques for measuring the latter and it may remain impossible to do so because the value placed on a particular personality or behavior change is always debatable.

4. If the "common factors" position is correct, it seems unlikely (although not impossible) that we will be able to develop specific forms of psychotherapy for treating specific disorders of the kind set forth in DSM-III. Specificity, to be sure, is a relative matter, but if it is true that the patient as a person is of greater relevance to the psychotherapist than a constellation of symptoms from which he or she may suffer, the chances of making headway in understanding and treating a person are greatly enhanced if we pay greater attention to life adjustment, ability to cope, character structure, chronicity of the problem, and the like. If marked deficiencies exist in these area, the prognosis must generally

be considered "guarded," as every clinician is aware.

5. What might be the implications for the training of therapists? I wish to advance the following recommendations:

(a) In keeping with the "common factors" position, it is
important to select trainees who are sufficiently talented to
provide an appropriately helpful and nurturant relationship to a
relatively broad spectrum of patients;

(b) Trainees should receive comprehensive and thorough
training in psychopathology, major theories of psychotherapy, and
systematic exposure to the large storehouse of clinical knowledge
rather than narrow or specialized training in a few techniques;

(c) Trainees should acquire a theoretical framework
sufficiently systematic and comprehensive to permit an understanding of seemingly discrete clinical phenomena. In short, while
an intuitive but bumbling therapist may be of some help to many
patients, a well-trained professional who can effectively cope with
a variety of clinical problems, use professional judgment, and
practice responsibly and ethically will have no peer. Let us
also remind ourselves (and society at large) that the psychotherapist is more than a "change agent"!

References

Smith, M. L., Glass, G. V., Miller, T. I., 1980, The benefits of
    psychotherapy. The Johns Hopkins University Press, Baltimore.
Strupp, H. H., & Hadley, S. W., 1979, Specific versus nonspecific
    factors in psychotherapy: A controlled study of outcome.
    Archives of General Psychiatry, 36, 1125-1136.

SOCIOTHERAPY IN THE PSYCHIATRIC

CLINICS OF GENERAL HOSPITALS

F. Alonso-Fernández

Professor-Head of the Psychiatric Dept.
University Complutense, Madrid-3

GENERAL PLANNING

In the current health conception, the traditional medical model
has been changed towards a bio-psycho-sociological model, which demands to therapies not only to deal with illness and suffering, but
also to promote well-being, life quality and social support. Nowadays
we are therefore concerned by patient's cure in the medical, psychological and social sense. In the functioning of psychiatric clinics
of general hospitals (PCGH), besides explicit sociotherapy, there
is an important implied sociotherapy. The achievement of acceptable
assistential outputs and the activity of a staff with good aptitudes
for social interactions, sensitize people which contact with them,
stimulating comprehensive attitudes towards mental patient. Between
specific sociotherapy and this implied sociotherapy, there is an integrated closed retroactive circuit of cybernetic type. It is possible to use some results of this implied sociotherapy, chiefly the
doctor's attitudes toward the mental patient, as an indicator to
evaluate the holistic functioning of PCGH.

The consolidation of the patient in his primordial family group
is nowadays a socio-dynamical constant in PCGH objectives. Frequent
interviews with family members and participation of the family and
friends in hospital care from the beginning of treatment, are duties
included in this basic familiar orientation of our general assistential program.

Family therapy is distributed in the following procedures: group
therapy centered in the interaction between the members; psychosocial therapy, extended to aspecta of family life outside to those
constructed by subjects themselves; therapy based on the systemic

381

connection between family environment and its distribution in a
series of subsystems. Above all we use the type of family therapy
described by BOLMANS[1] and PIHA, LAHTI and AALTONEN[2], where family
is used to cooperate in the therapy as the basic social institution
of our community and as the principal environmental human frame.That
means the family taken as the key symbolic system for convivence.

To evaluate the functioning of the family we take into account
its interior and exterior sectors: the relationship between its
members, mentioning their ages and parentage degree, as well as the
behavior and adjustment of individuals, roles distribution, intrafa-
miliar relations, care and education of childrens, home organisation,
social activities, economical aspects, and finally health habits and
level of cooperation with psychiatrists and social workers.

To repair the wide scope of deficiencies found in the family
taken as a cooperation structure (lack of cohesion, dispersion of
its members, inappropiate functioning, marginal situation, multiple
morbidity, etc.) and to reinforce its influences, we turn more and
more to social networks therapy, in all the structural units.

A subject's whole social net is divided into three degrees : a
primary net (family relationships, close friendships), secondary net,
(superficial relationships) and tertiary net (indirect relationships
through the members of the primary net). Within the whole of social
transactions, it matters to distinguish the pure sociological attributes from social connections which have an affective content and a
psychological function. Our preferential model of intervention on
social nets is a both reduced and dispersed version, which works
through meetings with groups of 6-12 people, taken from above mentioned three degrees and whose main objectives are to form a consulting council and to find out a tutor guide for the patient. This special technics could be named effective net method.

On the other hand, the goals and technics of sociotherapy program exhibit different aspects in the diverse structural units:hos-
pitalization, day-hospital, emergencies, consultation-liaison and
consultation.

SOCIOTHERAPY IN THE HOSPITALIZATION UNIT

The hospitalization unit is the basic axis of PCGH and it must
constitute thanks to its sociodynamic qualities the most radical alternative against the "integral or totalitarian institution"[3].

In concordance with this character of total anti-institution,
PCGH must organize hospitalized patient's life according to these
standards: identity protection,maintenance of large connections with
family and friends, outgoing from hospital in the afternoons as soon
as possible, week-end visits at home, and an enough active life regi-

me in the hospital in both spontaneous aspects and through stimulation application.

Such a sociodynamic program is based in developing freedom, movement, communication and responsibility aspects, all of them as therapeutic agents, directed to reach the main objective of the PCGH which is to reintegrate the mental patient to the free and common society in the shortest period of time, along with his settling in an enough strong familiar support.

The evaluation of therapeutic results during hospitalization based in the most reliable specific indicators (mean stay, reentry percentage, bed or year-patients' rotation) must be associated with an evaluation of sociotherapeutic functioning based on the outgoing and visiting rates and on the social variables that we shall point out later.

SOCIOTHERAPY IN THE DAY HOSPITAL

The day hospital (DH) attached to CPHG works out as a bio-psychosocial center, that is a social, psychological and medical therapeutic center, stressing with a special emphasis psycho-sociotherapeutic activities , which are distributed, in our DH, in the following sections: three permanent occupational shops, sociotherapy club, social assistance in connection with patient's home and various group cotherapy systems (group psychotherapy, systemic family therapy, couple therapy, expression and dance therapies, etc...).

In the occupational shops primordial activities are divided in labour therapy (work used as a professional activity), occupational therapy (creative and recreative activites) and a continuous evaluation of the behavior and the reactions of the patient. Among the special sociotherapic modalities used in these DH, expression techniques stand out: body expression, scenic expression, music therapy and dance therapy, whose common denominator is to stimulate chiefly the capacity of communication. This is the reason why they deserve the name of "stimulation sociotherapies".

DH offer to the patient a richer in freedom, naturality and communication environment than the classic therapeutic community. It is evidently preferable to cultivate patient's connection with the free culture than inserting him in any form of therapeutic or medical culture. Besides that, it is clear that the therapeutic community system, except for drug addicts and young people with behavior troubles, has got obsolete within the frame of social ecology and modern communitarian psychiatry.

Whereas encystment or too long hospitalization periods generally lead the patient to the institutionalism of deficit his too long stagnation in DH implies an institutionalism of abundance which can be distinguished by its overprotective character or by constituting an institutional countertransference[4],[5].

The two main objectives of these DH are: the rehabilitation or social readaptation of the patient, that means his full reinsertion in a normal communitarian and professional life, and also the increase of quality of life style. To put forth the sociodynamical productiveness of DH, we can take as a basis their freedom regime and the degree of similitude of their environment with social context, without forgetting the usual therapeutic and social indexes.

SOCIOTHERAPY IN PSYCHIATRIC EMERGENCIES, CONSULTATION-LIAISON AND OUTPATIENT-CONSULTATION

The inflation observed in crisis situations and psychiatric emergencies nowadays (crisis have a socio-familiar character and emergencies a medical or psychopathological character) is chiefly due to the lack of social solidarity and communication, lack of social support, unemployment, marginality and drug abuse. SATLOFF and WORBY[6] properly consider that psychiatric service for emergencies is an indicator of the sociocultural and clinical changes, embracing therefore the position of our cross historical psychiatry[7],[8] where we study the clinical changes observed throughout time and their correlation with sociocultural changes.

Consequently, the systematic study of socio-familiar aspects implied in emergencies is more justified nowadays than in previous times. That induces us to use this kind of techniques and social resources in emergencies integration process. All that results in a considerable improvement of obtained results and reduces very much hospitalisation rate. This evaluation is easy to do.

There is a general agreement between authors in pointing out that consultation-liaison service, where psychiatric assistance is done in cooperation with the doctors of other departments, must not take care only of the consultations demanded, but also of the training and information of the doctors from other hospital departments as to psycho-social medicine and psychiatry. Moreover it would be recommendable to devote a special program to this teaching. This clinical and educational spreading of the biopsychosocial model would bring about considerable benefits to the whole hospitalary institution, which would give rise to an increase of psychosocial care and of therapeutic results, particularly improving those parameters directly related to psychiatry, such as medical attitude towards mental patient and a greater precocity and adequacy in the demand of psychiatric consultation-liaison.

The sociotherapeutic point of view, in the form of the corresponding trends and therapeutic goals, takes a primordial and systematic participation in services administered in outpatients clinics.

Once more, we must stress the fact that it is impossible to do a good sociotherapeutic and communitarian psychiatry work, if the therapists themselves do not have an attitude of authenticity and a motivation oriented enough towards interpersonal relations.

SOCIAL INDICATORS

The most specific social indicators are related to social capacities and life quality. Using a pragmatic crierion, we can distinguish two main social capacities: assertive capacity (the capacity to play our own role) and relational capacity (the capacity of social interaction). The most systematised and·valuable exponents of both capacities are put in action both in family and work environment and during patient's stay at DH.

On the other hand, life quality evaluation can be done according to different indicators. Secondary indicatios of life quality are referred to the achievement of life preliminary goals, such as a suitable lodgment, a satisfactory ecology, the economical independence, the drug abstention or moderate consumption, etc. These data can be described in measurable terms. On the contrary, calibration of life quality taken as an ultimate goal is based on introspective evaluation of diverse personal affective and conative experiences, identified[9,10] as happiness, well-beeing, experience of autorealisation and feeling of freedom, which are not directly quantifiable.

Employment expectatives for the inveterate mental patient deserve a special mention, considering that work holds a central position in many social readaptation programs and that obtainment of a stable employment has got in a more and more difficult duty, as unemployment rate has been growing. The employability of rehabilitated mental patient chiefly depends on his forwardness to show before the employer a sufficient relational capacity (for communications and cooperation) and a good disposition to assume work in its different aspects: assertive attitude, motivation, training and perception of self-expectatives.

A severe problem underlies to the subject of social indicators: the value and legitimacy of quantitative psychopathology. The supporters at any cost of quantification stand by this methodologic orientation as the only scientific way. That hides the fact that most of empiric sciences are very scarsely quantifiable and that they cannot be disqualified because of their supposed lack of rigour. What is rigorous and scientific is to apply measures to things which admit or demand it. Heidegger suggested to reserve mathematical logic to the study of nature, whereas "spirit sciences and all the living beeing sciences should be precisely inexact to be able to be rigorous"

Though the social dimension of health is not measurable as a

whole, the introduction of mathematical logic in this field allows
to do comparative evaluations of partial data, a method which brings
about some points of objetive precision that we should not omit.
Quantifiable social parameters and indicators have therefore an evaluative usefulness as to the justified and necessary therapy, but that
does not allow us to omit neither primordial indicators of life quality and existence, nor other not quantifiable forms of social indicators, simply because they cannot be laid down as numbers. Here
numbers only get their real and deep sense in the light of psychosocial understanding of the subject and his world. Qualitative indicators are unperfect as well, due to their unavoidable connection
with value judgments.

Despite of all their inconvenients when they are handled isola-
tely, quantitative and qualitative social evaluators from a valid
experimental whole for assistential and therapeutic control; experiences exchanges and research activities, as they are mutually
complementary. The series of social evaluators used by us, comprises work activities, family and social networks functioning, social
capacities and the most relevant indexes of life quality.

Though I am not partizan at all of politisation of psychiatry,
I consider that psychiatry cannot live backwards to politic reality,
unless it gets psychotic or it takes an anetic character. Therefore,
I must articulate everything I have told here about sociotherapy
with the point of view of ideologies. Such a complicated matter can
be schematized asseverating that sociotherapic planification of psychiatry can only develop adequately in a sociopolitical context where
liberties, social justice and solidarity are in the full light.

REFERENCES.
1. W.M. Bolman, Preventive psychiatry for the family:theory,approa-
   ches and programs, Am.J. Psychiatry 125:458 (1.968).
2. J. Piha, I Lahti and J. Aaltonen, The therapy of the family
   without family, Psychiatria Fennica 133-138 (1.978).
3. E. Goffman, "Asylums", Anchot Books, New York (1.961).
4. N. Reider, A type of transference to institutions, Bull. Menninger Clin. 17:58 (1.953).
5. M. Gendel and F. Reiser, Institutional Countertransference, Am.
   J. Psychiatry 138:508 (1.981).
6. A. Satloff and C.N. Worby ,The psychiatric emergency service:
   mirror of change, Am.J. Psychiatry 126:1628 (1.970).
7. F. Alonso-Fernández, "Fundamentos de la psiquiatría actual".
   Paz Montalvo, Madrid,4th edition (1.978).
8. F. Alonso-Fernández, "Compendio de Psiquiatría", Oteo, Madrid,
   2th edition (1.982).
9. S. Naess, "Concepts and methods in a norwegian study of quality
   of life", Inas, Oslo (1.979).
10. T. Sörense, "Freedom and social support", Psych.Social Science,
    1:197 (1.981).

SYSTEMATIC PSYCHOPATHOLOGY AND SYSTEM ANALYSIS IN PSYCHIATRY

Johann M. Burchard

Psychiatrische und Nerven- und Poliklinik
der Universität Hamburg
Martinistrasse 52
D - 2000 Hamburg 20

The development of every science corresponds to the quality
of its methodology and epistemological perception. Both theoretical
aspects are depending on the knowledge of semiology and its systematic order which opens the doors for the analysis of the system.
The goal of such epistemological processes is the possibility of
manipulation of the system. Medicine as a whole is striving for a
complete analysis of the structure of the human organism by the
help of comparative systematic studies on the basic normal structures and their pathological variations.

Structural analysis of complex systems is inevitably going the
way of stepwise approximation. In the beginning there will be the
collection of single symptoms, later followed by symptomatology and
finally by systematic semiology. The final point of this development is the enlightenment of the structure or the structuralistic
stage, by which all phenomena can be explained.

Psychiatry has been going this way too, but its stage of evolution is far back compared with the other disciplines of medicine.
In psychiatry we are finding a deplorable lack of epistemic knowledge and structural cognition. The well known first rank symptoms
of K. Schneider for instance are meaning: "Schizophrenics are diagnosed following symptoms, which are typical for schizophrenic patients". We are having a nosological system with hundreds of positions, which is so primitive, that informed non-professionals are
handling it as well as professional psychiatrists (Sulz & Gigeren-
zer, 1982).

The Kraepelinean nosological system implicates the belief in nosological specificity of psychopathological signs. In clinical practice this is quite useful, but our theoretical needs are not satisfied. It is evident that the greatest part of the psychiatric diseases is exclusively defined by psychopathological findings. On the field of organic psychosis we have identified some nosological entities, but their clinical pictures are purely diagnosed by the help of the idea of psychopathological syndromes. Antipsychiatry has grown hot about the nosological pretension of classical psychiatry. Psychiatry should use time now for improving systematic knowledge i.e. the cognition of the functional language of the human brain and its systemic breakdowns and alarm states.

Historical process of psychiatry has evolved the first stages of the following classification. We will try to evaluate the missing ones by comparing the present state of psychiatry, our systematic knowledge from psychopathology and general laws of system identification as found in the development of other sciences:

1. The symptomatological phase in late 19. century. Most prominent authors have been C. Wernicke (1874) and the representatives of association psychology.

2. The syndromatological period was initiated by K. Bonhoeffer and A. Hoche (about 1910), which worked out the unspecifity of symptom complexes. They were defeated by E. Kraepelin's nosologism.

3. The defeat of syndromatologists was caused by a lack of order of symptom complexes, which was elaborated in the systematic period. The most prominent authors were S. Freud (works following 1895), E. Kretschmer (beginning 1922) and H. Ey (1948 - 54). The laws of dissolution and reconstruction have been analyzed (F. Llavero 1953). Systematic psychopathology is leading to systemically adapted stage 4:

4. Structuralistic (systemic) psychopathology is starting, where interest in separation of axial syndromes and alarm-state-like psychoses and neuroses is growing. Interest rises too in the reconstruction of the healthy-normal system, which we cannot directly derive from psychopathology. We are calling the subsystem which corresponds to axial syndromes, psychoses and neuroses

5. the reference system. Its properties can be evaluated by analysing our knowledge of systematic order of psychopathological syndromes and their general principles and laws (see: J.M. Burchard,

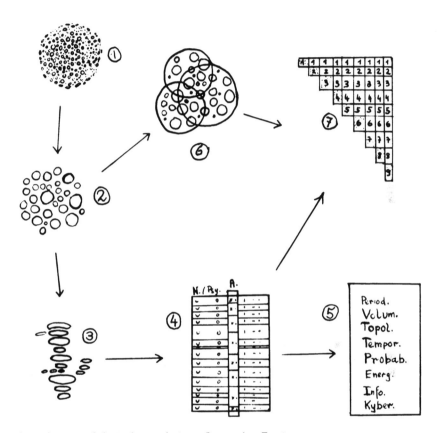

Fig. 1: Psychiatric epistemology in 7 stages.
1: symptomatological phase; 2: syndromatological period;
3: systematic psychopathology ; 4: structuralistic stage
(axial syndromes and psychoses/neuroses); 5: reference system;
6: nosological system of Kraepelin; 7: advanced nosological
system.

1980). The reference system is containing periodical, volumetric (steering personality volume), topological, temporal, probabistic, energetic, information and cybernetic functions.The investigation of the reference system may be possible on the basis of experimental work rising from psychopathological research. The reference system is only a subsystem in man. So we believe that psychopathological changes are always partial and do not concern the personality as a whole.

6. The Kraepelinean nosological system is simply the overlapping of circles of forms or syndroms.

7. On the basis of systemic psychopathology we are proposing an advanced nosological system with 9 psychiatric diseases (1 normals, 2 reactive diseases, 3 neurotic diseases, 4 psychopathic diseases, 5 monopolar depressive diseases, 6 manic-depressive diseases, 8 oligophrenic diseases, 9 exogenous-organic diseases).

Horizontally we find the typical states ($\boxed{3}$) and the pseudo-

states ($\boxed{3}$ or $\boxed{6}$). Vertically we find the abortive forms

above the typical states.

$\boxed{7}$ $\boxed{7}$ $\boxed{7}$ reads as follows: typical endogeneous schizophrenia-

oligophrenic pseudo-schizophrenia (Pfropf-schizophrenia) - exogenic pseudo-schizophrenia (hallucinosis).

Not only our theoretical needs could better be satisfied by a systematized psychopathology and a better nosological system. Especially the diagnostic capicity of psychiatrists will grow, when they adapt a model and a systematic order of syndroms in a scale of dissolution and reconstruction. Also training of students and post-graduates can be improved. Psychiatry has for a long time remained in a retarded condition compared with psychoanalysis. Systematization and model-refered diagnostic thinking are characteristic traits for psychoanalytic schools. But the model of Freud's theory is too small for clinical use. In psychiatry we need a broader spectrum of conceptions. Only the upper 10 percent of the total unconscious are defined by the Freudian terms. Apallic syndrom, Korsakow syndrom and organic brain syndrom and the refered psychoses are out of bounds of psychoanalytic terminology and area. Also the schizophrenic psychoses as well as the manic-depressiv ones need an other, more specific model, by the help of which they can be simulated and represented. Clinical work in psychiatry should become based one lucid structural thinking like psychoanalytic work, but without its narrow viewpoint.

References

In: J.M. Burchard: Systematische Psychopathologie. Bd. 1 and 2. UTB 1003 and 1004. F.K. Schattauer Verlag, Stuttgart 1980

THE DISTURBED MIND. MULTISTRUCTURAL

SYSTEMATIC MODEL OF PSYCHOPATHOLOGY

Henrique Joao Barahona Fernandes

Rua Actor António Silva, 5, 8º.D

P-1600 Lisboa, Portugal

Present problems in psychiatry imply a medico-anthropological perspective based on a pluralist methodology referring to a complex model of the personality in situations organized into multiple functional systems. What we call psychiatric anthroposciences are postulated this way. In our view psychiatry is undergoing a divergent process leading to partial and unidimensional reductionist criteria without integration of their particular supporting investigations. It was not possible to proceed beyond limited, unstructured eclectism.

It is only with difficulty that projects of overall comprehensive models become diluted into ambiguous generalities. We propose to take the model of disturbed man, departing from "normal", in his bio-psychocultural complexity as a generic reference of observable data. Figure 1 shows within its circle the area (dotted lines) of the personal functional systems, C, PC, I, etc., and their respective gradient of perturbation (the arrows). There is still no consensus on a general theory of psychiatry. Nevertheless, on the basis of clinical and therapeutical experience within the last decades it is possible to design some rules and laws as a foundation of a systematic structured psychopathology given. The well-known difficulties of nosology and classification, the formulation of an alternative type of systematics may allow a unitary and regular system of description of psychopathological phenomena and their contributing conditions (from ecological, genetic and other biological conditions to social, historical, and cultural conditions).

It is also only with difficulty that the efforts of exact

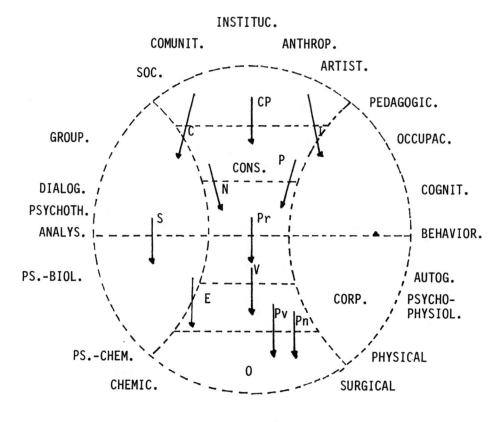

FIG. 1

evaluation which are current in natural science and the rigor which is possible in cultural science accomplish either with epistemic or other requirements a coordinated praxis of application in diagnosis and therapy. The positiristic classical definition of medical entities (displaying a chain from etiopathogenesis to symptoms) only exceptionally constitutes adequate psychopathology, even when we take into consideration those single factors without which disease will not occur (e.g., traumatic, toxic, infectious, psychic). Clinical manifestations may either be multiple for each determinant factor or the same for multiple factors - there is no psychopathological specificity. Similarly to what happens with other contructs such as "basic syndromes", "axis syndromes/ psychoses", "patterns of biological-vital ground", and "generative patterns of disturbed operationalities", we have proposed to differentiate the following constructs:

a) General ways of personality disturbance (GWD)
b) Basic psychopathological structes (BPS), (Barahona Fernandes, 1964)
c) Gradients of personality perturbation (GPP)

GWD are psychopathological forms common to normal or healthy persons. Under some circumstances it would not be human not to become anxious, depressed, fearful, suspicious, or even delusional (e.g. the way in which creative phantasy may become delusional). There is a continuum between the manner of spontaneous reactive "forms" of the average individual and his normal variants, the "episodic" and exceptional reactions, and the frankly abnormal/ psychopathological.

In the BPS there is already a discontinuity or even rupture with non-deviant structures, whereby the limits of said structures are exceeded to varying degrees, possibly reaching complete heterology, such as transitivism in schizophrenic primary delusions. The symptom which is finally observed is the result of overstructuration and modulation of its basis through BPS.

Constructs a) and b) seem to have more differentiating power than the usual distinctions - psychotic, neurotic, organic. BPS are transphenomenal modifications of different functional systems in their multiple dynamic interrelationships. They have their place between symptoms and determining conditions, all the while having foundations of their own on other pattenrs (ethological, neurophysiological, chemical, etc.) undergoing intensive research nowadays. Each BPS is identified intuitively by the peculier pregnant accentuation of some of the characteristic clinical manifestations. For example, delusional activity in melancholia is supported and moulded by the BPS's endothymic desintigration (ED) which corresponds to the functional system of the vital endothymic

ground (E). Reactive delusion corresponds to a "situative alteration" (SA) of the BPS. It is so that BPS are repeated with the same configurations whatever the GWD may be and are also thus not specific of any "disease". Constructs a) and b) should be evaluated independently of their determinant conditions. The GWD are phenomenologically apprehended through understanding personal experiences, behavioural manifestations, or acts provoked by a structured environment. There is thus a continuity of intentions with their present and preceding circumstances which is compatible with normal empathic comprehension. The intentions are also comprehensible in the frame of reference of personal situation and biography. BPS are explained on a deterministic or probabilistic mode by the set of factors mentioned above. We have defined elsewhere a glossary of 66 BPS and 11 GDP, each to be evaluated on an ordinal scale and with four degrees of entensity - "absent", "incipient", "clear", and "pregnant". Each degress of disturbance can be used to evaluate premorbid states, morbid episodes, diachronic sequences, and present states separately.

Construct c) - the GPP - consists of systematic sequences of BPS referred to each personality system (S, CP, N, C, E, P, Pr, I, Vi, Pv, Pn). Figure 2 indicates their relative hierarchical rank in a gradient ranging from psychoneurological to situational. Characteristics common to all of them are differentiated as "abnormal infant evolutions" (AIE), "variants" (V), "alterations" (A), "abnormal evolutions" (AE), "abnormal organizations "(ON), and "desintigrations" (D). The BPS may be used as indicators of syndromes. This is a systematic structural scale which offers the possibility of evaluating the complex but regularly organized mode of correspondence between gradients and the functional systems of disturbed personality. An "architecture", or if yo whish "orchestration", of disturbed man would result from our conception.

Vectors in figure 1 represent caesurae or discontinuities in each functional system of personality, allowing a global view of the whole. "So as a sparkling crystal, enduring, splitting".

These concepts can be used for different aims: (1) Techniques for more detailed, structural interviewing; (2) reference data for investigation of correlations, clusters, etc.; (3) formulation of a structured and personalized/individual diagnosis and its diagnostic and therapeutic inferences. They may serve as a contribution to the general problem of classification of mental disease (WHO); a kind of multiaxial, "graduated" (Barahona Fernandes, 1965) classification which may be considered in the discussion of international classification of mental disease.

GRADIENTS OF PERSONALITY DISTURBANCE		SYSTEMATIC SEQUENCE OF BASIC PSYCHOPATHOLOGICAL STRUCTURES (PBS)					
		MAIN BPS - SYNDROM INDICATORS					
SITUATIVE	S			SA	SAE	SAO	
CULTURAL PERSON	CP			CPA	CPAE	CPAO	
NEUROTIC	N	NAIE	NV	NA	NE	NO	
CHARACTER	C	CAIE	CV		CAE	CAO	CD
ENDOTHYMIC	E	EATE	EV	EA	EAE		ED
PARANOID	P		PV	PA	PE	PO	PD
PROPRIOM	Pr	PrAIE	PrV	PrA	PrAE		PD
INTELLECT	I	IAIE	IV	IA			ID
VIGILANCE	Vi			ViA			ViD
PSYCHO-VEGETATIVE	Pv	PvAIE	PvV	PvA	PvAE		PvD
PSYCHONEUROLOGICAL	Pn	PnAIE	PnV	PnA	PnAE		PnD

Fig. 2

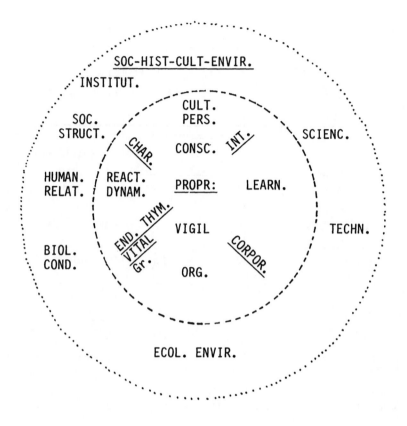

Model of personality in situation

FIG. 3

REFERENCES

Barahona Fernandes, H. J. (1968) Structuration personelle des valeurs. Créativité et Guérison. L'Espans. Scientif. Fr. 15-22.
Abnormal Personalit. Reactions. Evolution. Endothymopathies. - Foreign Psych., 1970. 72-73
(1974) Structures psychopathologiques de base et pharmacopsycho-thérapie. Annales de Psychothérapie, 5 (8) 41-53.
(1977) Dialectique de l'esprit objectif et de l'esprit personnelle. L'Evolution Psychiatrique XLII, 3 877-887
(1980) Un modèle anthropologique médical de la psychiatrie. Actualité Psychiatrique, no. 6
Ein medizinisches-anthropologisches Krankheitsmodell in der Psychiatrie. Arch. Psychiat. Nervenkr., 229 63-73
(1980) Spécificité et structures psychopathologiques de base. In Spécificité de la Psychiatrie (eds. Masson, Paris)
(1982) Classificacoes internacionais e diagnóstico individual estruturado e personalizado. O médico. Ano 33, no. 1591, Vol, 102.857-875
(1982) Some Problems of Psychiatry, I, II - Acta Psiquiatrica Portuguesa. Vol. 28, 111-116
Berner, P., (1982) Psychiatrische Systematik, Bern
Biafang, S. (1980) Evaluationsforschung e. d. Psychiatrie, Funk, Stuttgart
Burchard, J. (1980) Lehrbuch der Systematischen Psychopathologie. Vol. I und II, Schattauer.
Coentro, M., Análise estrutural dos estados limites (Borderline) pela escala de Barahona Fernandes (em public.)
Disdorfer, C., et al. (1982) Models for Clinical Psychopathology. M.T. Press, New York
Stone, M. (1981) The psychiatric clinic of North America, Vol. 4, No. 1
Janzarik, W., Neue Wege der Psychopathologie, Enke, Stuttgart, 1983

SYSTEM'S PSYCHOPATHOLOGY

J. Simoes da Fonseca
Head, Department of Medical Psychology of the
Faculty of Medicine/Chief of Service in the Department
of Psychiatry, Hospital Sta. Maria, Lisbon, Portugal

Most System's approaches to Psychopathology have been centered in
methods leading to nosological delimitation and classification,
or else in the specification of choice of observable data or still
on theoretical constructs which finally serve these same purposes.
In our view, the fact that those classifications are based on
"clinical indicators" of heterogeneous origin, is not generally
recognized. Even the references to System's Theory using surface
metephors may paradoxically obliterate the evolution that the
contribution the System's Theory may bring to Psychopathology.
Using more rigorous methods by means of which data would be
acquired in well controlled environmental, and expecially social
interactions, would provide some help to guide us in the epistemic
muddle of clinical diagnostic classifications, provide some needed
cross-validation to purely clinically oriented systems and more
important than that, help us in finding ways of explaining
psychopathological phenomena in a relational-analytic manner.
The Psychology Group of the Fac. of Medicine made during the last
nine years some experiments on interpersonal relationships which
involved the free behaviour of a single person with a restrict
group of subjects which reacted towards within strictly ritualized
form.

We were not concerned with diagnostic aims, but rather tried to
understand interpersonal relationships in a System's Theoretical
frame of reference. We used twenty classes of equivalence of
inticator variables which served to describe social interactions
of 165 subjects evenly distributed by 11 clinical diagnostic
groups.

We obtained a better inter-group diagnostic separation in

Multivariate Discriminant Analysis, using the frequency of
occurence of social phenomena than using variables extracted from
AMDP IV and V clinical scales - as we can verify comparing fig. 1
and fig. 2. Fig. 1 represents a plot of results obtained using 20
social indicator variables per subject. Fig. 2 represents results
of Multivariate Discriminant Analysis using variables extracted
from AMDP IV and V.

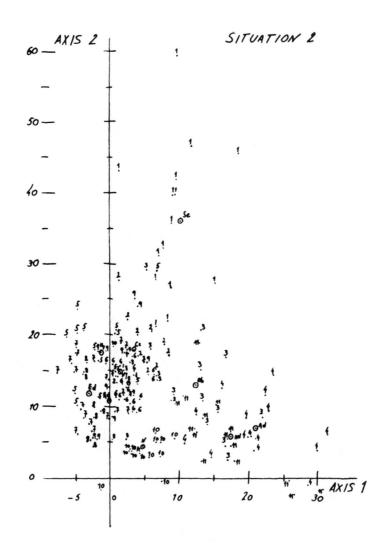

Fig. 1: Results from Multivariate Discriminant Analysis (Soc.Dat)
Code: 1) P. Schiz (Sc); 2) Centreceph.Ep. (Ce); 3) Obs.Neur.(Ob);
4) Adol.N.Help(Ad); 5) Hyst.(Hy); 6) Temp.Ep. (Te); 7) End.Depr.
(Ed), 8) React.Dep.(Rd); 9) Neur.Dep.(Nd); 10) Normal Adults (N);
11) N.Adol.(Na). Numbers 1 to 11 indicate the position of any
subject and the diagnostic group. Letters near to circles signal
group centroids.

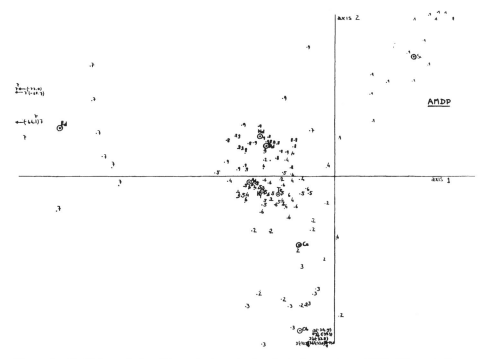

Fig. 2: Multivariate Discriminant Analyisis using AMDP IV and V
data. Code: 1) P.Schiz (Sc); 2) Centreceph.Ep.(Ce); 3)
Obs.Neur.(ob); 4) Adol N.Help(Ad); 5) Hyst.(Hy); 6) Temp.Ep.(Te);
7) End.Depr.(Ed); 8) React.Dep.(Rd); 9)Neur.Dep.(Nd); Numbers 1 to
9 indicate the position of any subject and the diagnostic group.
Letters near to circles signal centroids.

Behind this result is a series of developments - in 1970 an
attempt to develop and operational logical calculus for
"signification and intention". Between 1970 and 1975 we used
adapation to a structured environment, with four diagnostic
groups, analyzing data in terms of the concepts of Discrete
System's Theory.

What seems relevant to us, is not that these methods allowed
inter-group separations more refined than using clinical data -(or
even the fact that using the same type of analysis on 4 groups of
subjects the evaluation of speeches of politicians in a
Parliament, we were able to diagnose with accuracy a social
situtation and predict some events which were to come).
Using our indicator variables (we prefer to call either clinical
or social variables this way, because it is adequate to their real
scientific status - with some piecewise exceptions nobody has been
able to relate to analytically in a precise form the complex set
of clinical variables we have available at present - genetic,
biological, psychological, social or cultural data - and clinical

phenomena. They should therefore stay with the denotation of scientific indicators, effective for some heuristic purposes, but lacking explanatory power in many senses.

Our indicator variables do not escape this status, but as we adhered to System's Theory in the strict sense, we were able to analytically define interpersonal cost-value adaptative-maladaptive ratios, cost-value ratios within external reference systems, or else simple probability ratios of adaptative or maladaptive phenomena under different social straims.
An epistemic analysis of this type leeds us to obtain a ranking of our diagnostic groups concerning these interpersonal relationships as it can be seen in Fig. 3.

Taking now as variables, the ratios between the meam probabilities of occurrence of each of the social interactive phenomena in each group, respectively, on one hand and on the other hand respectively their mean probability of occurrance in the group of Normal Adults, we obtain characteristic patterns of ratios for each diagnostic group, as it can be seen in Fig. 4.

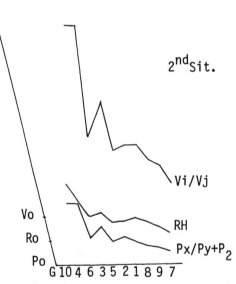

Fig. 3 - This figure shows the relative ranking of the different groups concerning (a) Probability ratios $Px/Py+Pz$ which are represented at the lowermost line; (b) "Mean Costs" (Entropy ratios RH, which are defined in the intermediated line; c) Referential adaptive values Vi/Vj which are defined in the uppermost line. Code: G1, stands for schizophrenic Paranoids; G2, Centrencephal. Epilpt; G3, Obsessive Neur.; G4, Adolescents with adaptive problem; G5, Hysteric Neur.; G6, Temporal Epileptic; G7, Endogenous depress.; G8, Reactive Depres.; G) Neurotic Depres.; G10, Normal Subjects. These data were obtained in the 2nd social interaction we studied.

404

	1	2	3	4	5	6	7	8	9	10
QUHOLF	++	++	+++	—	—	++		+	++	0
TRANSLAC	+++	++	+	+++	++	+	+	++	+	0
INCAP.	—	+++	++	++	++	+++	+++	+++	+	0
AFIRD	+	-	+	+	+	+	+++	++	++	0
MIXT	+	+++	+++	++	+++	++	—	+	++	0
AFECT-	+	+	—	—	++		+++	++	+	0
POSIÇÃO NORM		+	+	++						0
AFECT+	+	++	+		+++	+++	+++	+++	+++	0
REEEM										0
RECOMP										0

Fig. 4 - On the leftmost column are indicated the then classes of particular phenomena we did study, with their labels. On the following columns G1, stands for Schizophrenic Paranoids; G2, Centreceph.Epilept.; G3, Obsessive neurot.; G4, Adolescents with adaptation problems; G5, Hysteric Neur.; G6, Temporal Epileptic; G7, Endogenous Depres.; G8, Reactive Depres.; G9, Neurotic Depres. and G10, Normal Subjects.

This figure describes ratios observed in situtation 2, between values observed in each diagnostic group and the group of Normal subjects.

An interesting epistemic issue, relevant to clinical diagnosis, appears in figure 1. There we can note that Adolescent subjects without symptoms, denotes by.11 in fig. 1 and their group centroid are clearly separated from.10 (Normal Adults) and much closer to .3 the group of Obsessive Neurotic Patients, and from .4 Adolescents which required qualified help.

This means, in our view, that an unrecognized "Obsessional Cognitive set" is present in Normal Adolescents, but in this case without clinical symptom formation.

This relevant distinction and, on the other hand, the recovery of clinical diagnosis using data obtained in our interpersonal experimental set-up require a set of theoretical explanations. It is our hypothesis that interpersonal acts are produced by a characteristic structure of generative operators. Those operators will stochastically generate adaptive or else maladaptive phenomena.

If we go further, a step behind, a simple theoretical assumption is to admit that the characteristic structures of generative operators derive from "predecessor patterns". Each predecessor patterns by interative occurance, will converge to the same final limiting structure of generative operators which is implies by the invariance of the structure of the probability distribution of accurrance of phenomena which depend on thos operators. Through these concepts, a deeper insight may be obtained, if we assume

that symptoms are also final phenomena, produced by structures of adjoint combined operator structures, also with their own "predecessors" and interative convergence processes.
Adaptive, maladaptive phenomena, symptoms, signs, will alternate, due to the competition of the two iterative converging processes, as well as to the prepotence of the environmental solicitations. Symptomatic sets are therefore acompanied by sets of indicators which are not nosological indicators - although nosological distinctions may be recovered using them. Symptomatic and syndromatic structures are no more rigidly stable structure but rather dynamic patterns which alternate with more or less deviant structures of basically normal operators.

It is furthermore clear that the ratios of adaptive or maladaptive phenomena and the ratios of symptomatic interperonal structures that also can be used in interactions with the environment, determine what we might call "relapses", "recoveries", "defective or residual states". Symptoms, signs, appear as dependent on particularly rigid and prepotent structures of generative operators which probably will not be more than the results of mutant extreme forms of predecessor structures. How the characteristics of this "mutation" can be defined and a reparative effect can be obtained by selective competition with predominantly adaptation producing structures requires a careful model analysis behind the space of this paper.

Nevertheless, whatever the etiology of the disturbance may be, a final epistemic unification may be obtained through the use of their concept of structure of generative operators.
Even peronality structure may be defined as the result of basic genetic, constitutional, biological structures which put limits to "abilities" further modelled by maturation, learning processes, social and cultural modelling which give particular biases to the two kinds of generative and predecessor structures.
The hystorical personal tales typified in literature as well as in scientific psychodynamic currents would be not more than short-hand methaphorical characterization of the processes which lead to personal structures.

Many times they will also allow the recovery of diagnosis, but this intervetion in adaptation, maladaptation and symptom formation will occur through the "final common pathway" of structures of generative operators of adaptive or maladaptive phenomena or symptoms, or of their predecessor converging structures.
Nosological entities recover nevertheless their status not as it occurs in Internal Medicine, but rather by the "process charateristics" of the formation and functioning of those generative and predecessor structures we have been refering to.
A restrict number of limiting forms of structures will be a

"generative basis" of all mixed structures which then will
generate the variety of clinical forms we diagnose.
Paradigms for this complex structures may be listed in a tentative
form. The main problem still remains at the epistemic level of
psychophysical relationships from which we are only using the
indicators, not the phenomena.

References may be found in Act. Psychiatrica Portuguesa 1979 -
1983.

AXIAL SYNDROMES AS A NEW TOOL IN PSYCHIATRIC RESEARCH

Hans Schanda and Peter Berner

Psychiatric University Clinic Vienna, Austria

CRITICAL SURVEY

The classificatory procedure in psychiatry is - from the
theoretical as well as from the clinical standpoint - a rather
inhomogeneous and inconsistent process with a lot of disagreement
between different schools. Until now psychiatric research workers
don't give enough attention to this fact; this leads to many contradictory scientific results even after use of the same study
design.

As long as one depends on criteria such as course and outcome,
genetic findings, or therapeutic response (e.g. lithium) to test
diagnostic concepts, the nosological level seems too pretentious
to provide a basis for reproducible homogeneous results. The main
classification systems in use nowadays base themselves on the
(nosological) concepts of E. Kraepelin and E. Bleuler, which influence also systems on a pretended syndromatological level.

But aside from nosological and syndromatological considerations,
etiology and pathogenesis are also used in different ways for
diagnosis. This results in a "babel of differing formulations of
the same concept" (Brockington et al., 1978) and is one main source
for misunderstanding and disagreement. The divergencies of the
classificatory systems are mainly based on the following problems:
The selection of items, used for diagnosis can be determined on
theoretical, pragmatic, or empirical considerations. The typical
"theory-oriented" approach is E. Bleuler's concept of schizophrenia
(1911). Bleuler distinguished between "basic" (fundamental) and
accessory disturbances from a phenomenological standpoint, whereby
the basic disturbances were believed to result directly from an

underlying hypothetical somatic disorder. On the other hand, he differentiated primary and secondary symptoms according to their chronological appearance in the course of disease.

The typical pragmatic approach is exemplified by K. Schneider (1939), who established a hierarchy of first and second rank symptoms for the diagnosis of schizophrenia. Bleuler's basic symptoms seem to relate to an underlying somatic nature of the disease, but they lack exact definition, Schneider's first rank symptoms (FRS) are clear and reliable, but their specificity for schizophrenia remains questionable (Carpenter et al., 1973). The empirical approach is represented by Kasanin's concept of schizo-affective psychoses (1933) and Langfeldt's (1939) concept of schizophreniform psychoses, where symptomatical and non-symptomatical indicators for poor or good prognosis (mainly based on follow-up studies) are used as inclusion or exclusion criteria.

As a reaction to the multitude of diagnostic formulations, compromise classification systems were created with the hope that these compromises would be accepted world-wide, and consequently psychiatric diagnoses would show better agreement. The typical examples for such compromise classification systems are the "International Classification of Diseases (ICD), now in its 9th revision (1978), and the "Diagnostic and Statistical Manual" (DSM) of the American Psychiatric Association (3rd revision, DSM-III, 1980). The ICD-9 suffers from a lack of logical consistency, which allows to satisfy different directions of thought by simply adding new categories. The different use of the term "reactive psychosis" in Scandinavian and Non-Scandinavian countries is a good example for the uselessness of the compromise - the wish for better international comparability of this group of psychoses was a fallacy. The main deficiency of the ICD-9 is its uniaxiality, i.e. the impossibility to separate different aspects of psychiatric disorders.

The DSM-III, the other compromise system, is based on the principles of multiaxiality. Axis I and II include all of the mental disorders, axis III is assigned for physical disorders and conditions, axis IV serves to document social stressors, and axis V the "highest level of adaptive functioning last year". But multi-axiality alone is no guarantee for the solution of diagnostic problems. In the DSM-III, for example, the axes devoted to clinical diagnoses include algorhythms which are themselves multiaxial because they are based on information derived from different areas: course, duration, severity, and also some physical conditions, are sometimes used to varying extents for the establishment of diagnoses.

In 1912 Hoche published his paper on the importance of the so-called "symptom-complexes" in psychiatry. In his reductionistic and sceptical opinion as to the possibilities to find a biological correlary for the "clear and typical" pictures of a disease, he regarded the usual diagnostic entities as too broad and the symptom-level as too narrow for classification of psychiatric abnormalities. As a link between these two he proposed what he called "symptom-complexes". He regarded them as a component of the normal psyche as well. The symptom-complexes constitute the character of a person. In the case of a psychiatric abnormality they determine the pattern of the abnormal reaction. The clinical reality with the uniformity of certain symptom-constellations (syndromes) confirms his assumption; however, most of the classificatory attempts do not focus enough on this syndrome-level.

THE AXIAL SYNDROMES

Our research criteria emerged from studies on paranoiac and paraphrenic syndromes (Berner, 1965), which indicated that these states may occur as purely psychogenic developments as well as on the basis of an underlying manic-depressive illness, a schizophrenic, or organic process. The differential diagnosis was not deductable from the delusions as such, but only from the psychopathological symptoms accompanying them. We therefore arranged this "background-symptomatology" into what we call, following Hoche, "axial syndromes" (AS). We think that they contain,in the form of algorhythms, what we consider the most significant features of an underlying cyclothymic, schizophrenic or organic disturbance. Our term "axial syndrome" should not be mistaken for the conception of the several diagnostic "axes" in the DSM-III.

According to the literature and to our own experience the presence of symptoms constituting our AS makes MDI or schizophrenia highly probable, but not conclusive. For instance they may also be observed occasionally in organic brain diseases. We therefore prefer to classify these syndromes as "like": "endogenomorphic" or "organomorphic". A final diagnosis may only be made after we have confirmed it by means of biological and genetic factors and illness course. In contrast to Schneider's pragmatic approach our's is theoretical. Its central features are the Bleulerian concepts of associative loosening and affective blunting, and Janzarik's (1959) theoretical position, supported by the observations of the Hamburg group (Bürger-Prinz, 1961; Mentzos, 1967). The latter two positions stress the fact that disturbances of mood and drive occur in functional as well as in organic conditions and have no nosological significance. One type of mood/drive disturbance, the rapid alteration, which Janzarik called "Unstetigkeit" (unsteadiness) and the Hamburg group "Mischbilder" (unstable mixed states) are one main basis for psychotic productivity which constitutes many of the FRS (especially the delusional perceptions). But it can also be the source for some of the Bleulerian basic symptoms like ambivalence, depersonalisation, and derealisation. So we excluded these symptoms from our concept of the endogenomorphic-schizophrenic AS, stressing only those symptoms, which seem to us highly

Table 1. Endogenomorphic - Schizophrenic Axial Syndromes

Definitive: A and/or B present, probable: only C present

A) Incoherence without marked pressure or retardation of thinking or marked autonomous anxiety; at least one of the following symptoms required.
   1. Blocking: Sudden cessation in the train of thought; after a gap the previous thought may be taken up again or may be replaced by a different thought.
   2. Derailment: Gradual or sudden deviation from the train of thought without gap.
   3. Pathologically "muddled speech": Fluent speech, for the most part syntactically correct, but the elements of different thoughts (which, for the patient, may belong to a common idea) get muddled together.
B) Cryptic neologisms: The patient does not explain their private meaning spontaneously.
C) Affective blunting without evidence of marked depression, tiredness, or drug effect. This term includes flatness of affect, emotional indifference, and apathy, essentially, the symptom involves a diminution of emotional response.

correlated with the "process" itself: thought blocking, derailments, and pathologically "muddled speech" (drivelling), all summarized under the term incoherence; neologisms; and affective blunting, the typical sign for deficiency (table 1). One main disadvantage of this definition is the transitoriness of symptoms such as incoherence.

The endogenomorphic-depressive AS is characterized by marked changes in mood and drive and, as a central point, the typical biorhythmic disturbances (diurnal variations and sleep disturbances) (table 2).

In contrast, the endogenomorphic-manic AS is represented by a marked plus symptomatology in the same dimensions (table 3). The main features of the endogenomorphic-dysphoric AS are hostile tension and hostile reactions (table 4).

According to our theoretical position we also describe an endogenomorphic AS of unstable mixed states, embracing rapidly alternating swings of different mood and drive conditions. This includes a possible discordance of affectivity and drive (table 5). In all syndromes diurnal variations and sleep disturbances are obligatory. Especially in unstable mixed states psychotic symptomatology may appear (also partly in form of FRS) and mislead, in our opinion, to the diagnosis schizophrenia or at least schizoaffective disorder. Mixed states appear very often in the course of otherwise typical MDI.

Table 2. Endogenomorphic - Depressive Axial Syndrome

A and B obligatory

A) Appearance of marked changes in affectivity, emotional
   resonance, or drive following a period of habitual
   functioning. At least one of the following symptoms
   is required.
   1. Depressive mood (with or without anxiety)
   2. Emotional resonance either lacking or limited to
      depressive responses
   3. Reduced drive or agitation
B) Appearance of biorhythmic disturbances.Symptoms 1 and 2
   are required.
   1. Diurnal variations of one or more of the symptoms
      under A.
   2. Sleep disturbance. At least one of the following
      symptoms required.
      a) interrupted sleep
      b) early awakening
      c) prolonged sleep

Table 3. Endogenomorphic - Manic Axial Syndrome

A and B obligatory

A) Appearance of marked changes in affectivity, emotional
   resonance, or drive following a period of habitual
   functioning. At least one of the following symptoms
   required.
   1. Euphoric/expansive mood
   2. Emotional resonance limited to manic responses
   3. Increased drive
B) Appearance of biorhythmic disturbances.Symptoms 1 and 2
   are required.
   1. Diurnal variations of one or more of the symptoms
      under A.
   2. Shortened sleep.

By use of the AS it is possible to create very homogeneous groups
of patients regarding course and outcome, genetic findings, treatment response, and biochemical data. This was proved in a number of
studies of our clinic, mainly on delusional psychoses. For further
research on various topics the establishment of such homogeneous
subgroups is necessary. And so the use of the AS seems in our eyes
justified, not with the aim to replace widely used nosological
diagnostic systems by the concept of the AS, but to provide a
basis for psychiatric research.

Table 4. Endogenomorphic - Dysphoric Axial Syndrome

A and B obligatory

A) Appearance of marked changes in affectivity, emotional
   resonance, or drive following a period of habitual
   functioning. At least one of the following symptoms
   required.
   1. Irritable mood (dysphoria).
   2. Emotional resonance limited to hostile responses.
   3. Increased readiness to hostile acting out.
B) Appearance of biorhythmic disturbances symptoms 1 and 2
   are required.
   1. Diurnal variations of one or more of the symptoms
      under A.
   2. Sleep disturbance. At least one of the following
      symptoms required.
      a) interrupted sleep
      b) early awakening

Table 5. Endogenomorphic Axial Syndrome of Unstable
          Mixed States

A and B obligatory

A) Appearance of rapidly alternating swings in affectivity,
   emotional resonance, or drive following a period of
   habitual functioning. At least one of the following
   symptoms required.
   1. Rapidly alternating swings between depressive and/or
      anxious, euphoric/expansive, or hostile mood.
   2. Rapidly alternating and exaggerated emotional resonance
      touching various affective states (depressive, anxious,
      manic, hostile).
   3. Rapid change between inhibition, agitation, increased
      drive, and occasionally aggression.
B) Appearance of biorhythmic disturbances.Symptoms 1 and 2
   are required.
   1. Diurnal variations of one or more of the symptoms
      under A.
   2. Sleep disturbances. At least one of the following
      symptoms required.
      a) interrupted sleep
      b) early awakening

REFERENCES

American Psychiatric Association, 1980, Diagnostic and Statistical Manual of Mental Disorders (DSM-III).

Berner, P., 1965, Das paranoische Syndrom. Monographien aus dem Gesamtgebiete der Neurologie und Psychiatrie 110,Springer, Berlin.

Bleuler, E., 1911, Dementia praecox oder die Gruppe der Schizophrenien, Deuticke, Leipzig, Wien.

Brockington, I.F., Kendell, R.E. and Leff, J.P., 1978, Definition of schizophrenia: Concordance and prediction of outcome, Psychological Medicine 8: 387.

Bürger-Prinz, H., 1961, Probleme der phasischen Psychosen, Enke, Stuttgart.

Carpenter, J.W.T., Strauss, J.S.S. and Muleh, S., 1973, Are there pathognomonic symptoms in schizophrenia? An empiric investigation of Schneider's first rank symptoms. International pilot study of schizophrenia, Arch.gen.Psychiat. 28: 847.

Hoche, A., 1912, Die Bedeutung der Symptomenkomplexe in der Psychiatrie, Z.Neurol. 12: 540.

Janzarik, W., 1959, Dynamische Grundkonstellationen in endogenen Psychosen. Monographien aus dem Gesamtgebiete der Neurologie und Psychiatrie 86, Springer, Berlin, Göttingen, Heidelberg.

Kasanin, J., 1933, The acute schizoaffective psychoses, Amer.J. Psychiatry 13: 97.

Langfeldt, G., 1939, The schizophreniform states. A catamnestic study based on individual re-examinations. Munksgaard, Copenhagen.

Mentzos, S., 1967, Mischzustände und mischbildhafte phasische Psychosen, Enke, Stuttgart.

Schneider, K., 1939, Klinische Psychopathologie, Thieme, Leipzig.

World Health Organisation, 1978, Mental disorders: Glossary and Guide to their classification in accordance with the 9th Revision of the International Classification of Diseases, Geneva

SPECIFIC AND NON-SPECIFIC INFORMATION IN PATHOGENESIS OF

PARANOID-HALLUCINATORY SYNDROMES

Steffen Haas

Central Institute of Mental Health

D - 6800 Mannheim 1, I 5

In comparison to earlier years, today there is among research workers on psychoses general agreement on the fact that both genetic-biological as well as diverse environmental influences determine the kind and partly even the existence of delusion with its different types.
BURCHARD (1980) logically differentiates between a specific information on delusional syndromes resulting from prolonged conflict situations preceding the onset of psychoses or other extreme burdens which do not represent the disease itself, such as for example prodromal syndromes, and furthermore a non-specific information largely characterizing the basic disease with its cognitive and emotional disorders. Within this paper the in my opinion typical form and contents of delusional syndromes as well as conflict situations and those situations triggering off an onset of psychoses in citizens of the German Democratic Republic (GDR) shall be pointed out. They partly reflect typical social circumstances in the GDR or arise from these conditions and, thus, are to be counted as specific information.
The investigation includes patients from East Berlin who are being confronted every single day with the special political situation due to the division of Germany and above all of Berlin.
This paper is based on my dissertation which I started in East Berlin in 1967 under the direction of KARL LEONHARD and which I accomplished in 1972 under J.M. BURCHARD in Hamburg.
Medical records of 50 male and 50 female patients with the diagnosis of affective paraphrenia according to K. LEONHARD (1966), who were treated at the Charité in East Berlin, were evaluated. Only the most important statements made in this in the meantime fifteen years old dissertation shall here be repeated.
According to prevailing symptoms delusional ideas were divided into:

a) delusion of interference: which occured in two thirds of all
   cases (32 men and 35 women), (b) delusion of grandiosity: which
   was found in about one fifth of probands (11 men and 6 women)
   and (c) delusion of hypochondrical complaints: found in one
   sixth of probands (7 men and 9 women).
The occurrence of a delusion of interference, which must be understood as a central disturbance of communication probably resulting
from the loss of the hierarchy of experiences in all paranoid
psychoses according to HUBER (1983), does not deviate in frequency
from findings in other countries.
According to KRANZ (1967) the delusion of interference has been
at the top of all types of delusion in all periods under during
the last 100 years.
An interesting point is, that in about half of the patients
(35 men and 21 women) delusional ideas had above all a political
coloring.
A significant frequency in this point was only found in the delusion of interference.
Religious delusional ideas were only found in a total of 6 patients.

      Especially in men in leading positions political delusional
ideas were recorted mainly referring to their professional position. This is not surprising insofar as this groups of persons
inevitably has a positively or negatively influenced relationship to the political power from which typical conflict situations
can arise. In this group of persons the political delusional theme
occured significantly combined with the feeling of social interference.
Furthermore, in these persons the delusional theme was closer to
reality than in persons from lower social background or in patients with less intelligence. The political theme of delusion
occured independently from age and sex.
Obviously general difficulties in life and low intelligence lead
to more superficial and partly fantastic delusional ideas.

      The imagined persecution came from state agencies in half of
the patients. Persons talmig up a more negative attitude towards
the GDR imagined to be persecuted by state security police or
other police authorities. Party members in contrast felt to be
exposed to the persecution by Western secret services.
Only a total of six women felt to be persecuted by the SS or
national socialists. An interference or persecution by religious
authorities was only found in a total of 10% of all patients.
An additional delusional idea with sexual coloring - here again
mainly within the frame of a delusion of reference - occured in
almost half of the women with an average age of over 40.
Conflicts and possible situations triggering off the onset of
psychoses could be found in three quarters of all patients.
Professional conflicts were predominant in men in a ratio of

16:1, meanwhile in female patients difficulties in the private sphere prevailed in a ratio of 2:1, for example divorce in nine cases, illegitimate children in six cases and the beginning of climacterium in again six cases.

The following essential findings and considerations shall be summarized:

1. The development of delusional is definitely influenced by the Zeitgeist on the one hand, and on the other hand by general desires and hopes. Thus, it is a pathological expression of natural human feelings - a fact which was already pointed out by KRAEPELIN.

2. The total social sphere with its problems in the field of work and achievements, independently from prevailing social structures, represents an important field of tension in the human life.
It is understandable that conflicts, personal and professional difficulties can become the object of specific information by the elaboration of delusional ideas and possibly also on the development of delusion.

3. The frequent occurence of delusional ideas with political background - meanwhile those ideas with religious background are less important - can be considered as a possibly GDR-specific delusional theme mainly caused by political and social pressure being of importance above all in higher social positions. These findings are different from investigations carried out in Western countries as well as the fact that no pathological fear of the economic existence could be found in GDR-patients suffering from delusional ideas.

4. Thus, it can be summarized that delusional ideas do not develop independent from personal external factors and that every thing which influences and occupies a healthly person's mind continues to be valid for patients as well.
An understandable connection exists between prepsychotic life situation and delusional ideas.

Literature

Burchard, J.M., 1980, Lehrbuch der systematischen Psychopathologie;
2 Bd., Schattauer, Stuttgart, New York

Haas, St.,1972, Inhalt der Wahnvorstellungen in Beziehung zur
präpsychotischen Lebensstellung, Dissertation Hamburg,
1972

Huber, G.,1983, Das Konzept substratnaher Basissymptome und seine
Bedeutung für Theorie und Therapie schizophrener Erkrankungen, Nervenarzt 54: 23 - 32

Kranz, H.,1967, Wahn und Zeitgeist, Stud. Gen., 605 - 611

Leonhard, K., 1966, Aufteilung der endogenen Psychosen,
Akademieverlag, Berlin

HUMAN AUTOLINGUISTIC NATURE AND

PSYCHIATRIC DIAGNOSTIC SYSTEMS

Werner F. Pritz

Salzburger Landesregierung
Sozialmedizinischer Dienst
A-5010 Salzburg, Austria

INTRODUCTION

The purpose of this comment - and it is to be taken only as a comment - is to call attention to the significance of the self-referential, i.e. autonomous, organization of living systems in general and human individuality in particular. (Von Foerster, 1982; Loefgren, 1981; Pask, 1981.)

The major problem in this new look would not be the paucity of relevant empirical data from normal and abnormal psychology and psychobiology but the reordering of their theoretical consideration from this perspective. In this sense the present statement attempts to direct attention on the work of some scholars who have been with the investigation of the logic of organismic systems for decades and who have been - like the bulk of cybernetic thinking in this respect - largely ignored by the main stream of psychiatry.

FOCUS ON LIFE AS A HIERARCHY OF LANGUAGES

Loefgren (1981, p.237) states that "with language broadly conceived of complementary description-interpretation pairs, we reach an autolinguistic view of life", when one considers life as a hierarchy of languages (genetic, inner cerebral languages, verbal and non-verbal external communication languages). Also Pattee (1972) suggests that life implies an understanding of general language structures, and vice versa. He defines as general language structure "any coordinated set of constraints or rules by which classes of physical structures are transformed into specific actions or events (p.103)".

One universal property of languages is the self-reference

property which serves to establish hierarchical control introducing meta-language statements with respect to pertinent object languages. Any psychiatric diagnosis is at risk to confuse observations and conclusions at a meta-level with the pertinent object-language level. This is particular obvious with respect to the semantic confusion of the concepts of mood and affect. (Owens and Maxmen, 1979; Pritz, 1983)

The concept of linguistic hierarchy is intimately related to a clear distinction between description and interpretation (Or, theory and model). Loefgren (1981) as well as Pattee (1973, 1977) views the description-interpretation processes as inverse dominance relations. A biological property whether inherited or acquired can always be identified "as a biological interpretation of a biological description"(Loefgren, 1981, p. 244); and, to quote further "these interpretation and description processes, biological as they are, can accordingly be themselves identified as biological interpretations of biological descriptions".

Therefore, any psychiatric diagnostic system which goes beyond descriptive clustering must orient itself according to both the complexity of description and the complexity of interpretation (Loefgren, 1977). In this consideration of human behavior defined within a theory of action and seen as a hierarchy of languages every justification for a multi-diagnostic scheme is present.

FOCUS ON DESCRIPTION

There are various notions of description (Maturana, 1970). The connotative aspect of description, which refers to the observing relationship between an organism and its niche, can be defined with Peterson (1975, p.3) as follows: "Any thing which is inter-pretable is a description of that which is produced under the interpretation". In a more general way descriptions are to be regarded "as codings of finite procedures from which some other object may be produced in some computational environment" (p. 11).

"A description describes in extension (i.e., it predicts) and is ultimately simpler than that which is described" (Loefgren, 1981, p. 239). Evolution has led to the elaboration of higher levels of self-description in a linguistic mode. These models which we name as goals, strategies, plans, policies - conscious or unconscious - appear in an "observer included (circular, closed) epistemology like 'objects'" as descriptions of 'Eigen-functions', 'Eigen-operations', 'Eigen-behaviors', etc. (Von Foerster, 1982, p. 278). Psychiatric diagnosis is in essence the process of evaluation of such 'eigen-logics' (self-referential domains).

Conant and Ashby (1970) like Rosen (1979) emphasize the model character of all descriptions in living systems. Rosen speaks of these systems of description as "anticipatory" or "feed forward" systems. This means, that "any present change of state is determined by an anticipated future state, computed in accordance with some internal model of the world" (p. 284). Such a theorem, founding a theoretical psychobiology, changes "the status of model making from optional to compulsory" because it sees the "cause-controlled" type of behavior creation as the predominant strategy in living systems contrasted to the inferior method of "error-controlled" action. (Conant and Ashby, 1970)

This view of organisms and of mind as "hypothesis-generating and testing" (Goodwin, 1972) has far-reaching consequences and implications for psychiatric practice. Model construction of the world and of oneself and model observation in the context of a polythematic ('poly-contextural') logic (Guenther 1976, 1979, 1980) provide hope and promise for the future of a 'verstehende' psychiatry with regard to problems like delusional and compulsive - obsessive processes.
Remark: Until now no general purpose operators have been discovered within the brain, but only special purpose systems seem to give the brain its highly differentiated modular structure.

FOCUS ON THE SEMANTIC CLOSURE OF DESCRIPTION-INTERPRETATION

Pattee (1982) poses the question of how the dynamics of construction (interpretation) interrelates with the linguistics of the descriptions in actual organismic performances. The first mode is rate dependent because it is bound to the physicality of the actual instrumental implementation; the second mode is rate independent. This dependence on the part of interpretation processes on the dynamics of the underlying physical structure has far-reaching consequences for the psychiatric discussion of the depth of mood-shifts, confusional states, and so on. Lack of space does not allow further comment on this most important topic.

FOCUS ON PROBLEM CONSTRUCTION

Getzel (1979) among others focuses our attention on the fact that the world is "teeming with dilemmas", but that "the dilemmas do not present themselves automatically as problems capable of solution or even sensible contemplation" (p. 167). Despite the fact that problem finding and problem solving melt into one another "to perceive of a problem is the creative act" as Weston and Von Foerster (1974, p. 11) put it. Thus the problem of problem solving in any system, natural or artificial, must be approached first by the discussion of how contexts for understanding questions and formulating dilemmas as problems are established.

A classification of the creative procedures of problem posing must be an unavoidable element of new diagnostic conceptualizations which realize that a psychological theory of perception can be obtained "in which situations are perceived only to the extent that they can be resolved" (Weston and Von Foerster, 1974, p. 13). Hence, questions like how does a particular mood state change problem creation and problem solving, or, how does a particular neurotic attitude or a specific socio-cultural content prejudice abnormal contexts of problem formulation are not only legitimate but obligatory steps in psychiatric diagnosis.

FOCUS ON THE COMPLEXITY OF HUMAN SELF-INTERPRETATION

As apparent from the great number of emotion words in the various languages the ontological polythematic structure of human behavior is of unexplored complexity even if we meet daily this complexity in the sum total of cultural creativity and abnormal behavior generation. A part of these innumerable thematic domains is concerned with the complexity of the act of organismic self-interpretation itself.

General problems of self-construction, self-objectivation (logic of desire), self-repair, self-observation at the conscious and unconscious level, and so on are of paramount importance for the erection of a bio- and psycho-logical system of classification of abnormal behavior. Indeed the abnormality of behavior construction cannot be evaluated if the underlying logic of normal behavior construction is not understood.

To give an example: The concept of system "protection" is an essential objective of general systems theory. Kohout and Gaines (1976, p. 3) show that "protection structures present necessary constraints on sub-systems in order to maintain the basic functions of the system as a whole and prevent them being impaired by the independent and uncoordinated activities of its individual parts". Do different moods use different protection structures? (Pritz, 1983) Or, have sexual differences in symptomatology something to do with different ideals of protection operations? (Pritz and Mitterauer, 1980)

FINAL REMARK

At the end I like to endorse Royce (1975) that the various schools of psychiatry need a constructive effort towards sophisticated theoretical frames. Such a theoretic approach is viable at present and it will not contradict Royce's paradigmatic title: "Psychology is Multi-: Methodological, Variate, Epistemic, World View, Systemic, Paradigmatic, Theoretic, and Disciplinary". The 'autolinguistic' viewpoint underscores only "that nothing is more practical than good theory" (p. 58) To maintain that such a theory is not possible means to prolong the distorting influences of psychiatric discontinuity in diagnosis.

REFERENCES

Conant, R. C., and Ashby, W. R., 1970, Every good regulator of a
    system must be a model of that system, Int. J. Systems
    Sciences,1:89.
Getzels, J. W., 1979, Problem finding: a theoretical note, Cogn.
    Science,3:167.
Goodwin, B. C., 1972, Biology and meaning, in: "Towards a Theore-
    tical Biology 4: Essays," C. H. Waddington, ed., Edinburgh
Guenther, G., 1976, 1979, 1980, "Beiträge zu einer operationsfähigen
    Dialektik, Bd. I, II, III," Meiner, Hamburg.
Kohout, L. J., and Gaines, B. R., 1976, Protection as a general
    systems problem, Int. J. Genral Systems, 3:3.
Loefgren, L., 1977, Complexity of descriptions of systems: a foun-
    dational study, Int. J. General Systems, 3: 197.
Loefgren, L., 1981, Life as an autolinguistic phenomenon, in: "Auto-
    poiesis," M. Zeleny, ed., North Holland, New York.
Maturana, H. R., 1970, "Biology of Cognition," BCL report No. 9.0,
    University of Illinois, Urbana.
Owens, H., and Maxmen, J. S., 1979, Mood and affect: a semantic
    confusion, Am. J. Psychiatry, 136:97.
Pask, G., 1981, Organizational closure of potentially conscious
    systems, in: "Autopoiesis", M. Zeleny, ed., North Holland,
    New York.
Pattee, H. H., 1972, Physical problems of decision-making con-
    straints, Int. J. Neuroscience, 3:99.
Pattee, H. H., 1982, Cell psychology: an evolutionary approach to
    the symbol-matter problem, Cogn. Brain Theory, 5: 325.
Peterson, L. J., 1975,"The Recursive Nature of Descriptions: A
    Fixed Point," BCL 252, University of Illinois, Urbana.
Pritz, W. F., 1983, Mood congruent/incongruent dichotomy: the need
    for an advanced mood concept, Psychiatria Clin., 16: i.p.
Pritz, W. F., and Mitterauer, B., 1980, Bisexuality and the logic
    of narcissism, World J. Psychosynthesis, 12:31/2.9.
Rosen, R., 1979, Sixth annual Ludwig von Bertalanffy memorial
    lecture, Behav. Science, 24:283.
Royce, J. R., 1975, Psychology is multi-: methodological, variate,
    epistemic, world view, systemic, paradigmatic, theoretic,
    and disciplinary, in: "Nebraska Symposium on Motivation,"
    University of Nebraska Press, Lincoln.
Von Foerster, H., 1982, "Observing Systems", collected papers,
    Intersystems Publications, Seaside.
Weston, P. E., and Von Foerster, H., 1974, Artificial intelligence
    and machines that understand, Ann. Rev. Physical Chemistry,
    24:1.

ARE THERE PLUS AND MINUS SYMPTOMS "SPECIFIC" FOR SCHIZOPHRENIA?

P. Berner, B. Küfferle and H. Schanda

Psychiatric University Clinic
Vienna
Austria

During the last decade research on schizophrenia has brought about a disillusionment with Schneider's first rank symptoms. The main reason for this lies in the increasing evidence that first rank symptoms frequently occur in affective disorders as well. Consequently, and in accordance with Kraepelin's hypothesis of schizophrenia as a disease progressing to a deficiency state, attention has become focused on Bleuler's basic disturbances, symptoms which may be regarded as the expression of a functional deficit. With regard to Jackson's hierarchic brain model (1) and Birkmayer's concept of plus and minus symptomatology (2) these basic disturbances have been called 'negative' or 'minus' symtoms as opposed to florid 'positive' or 'plus' symptoms. On the basis of this distinction several researches, leaving aside the problem of differential diagnosis between manic-depressive and schizophrenic disorders, proposed to divide the latter into those with a predominantly negative and those with a predominantly positive symptomatology (3, 4). They hypothesized that these two groups may differ in many respects, such as course, outcome, response to neuroleptic treatment and underlying pathologic processes. Recent attempts to test his hypothesis suggest indeed that 'negative schizophrenia' may have an underlying pathologic process involving cerebral atrophy, whilst in 'positive schizophrenia' the underlying process may well be predominantly neurochemical (5).

Andreasen (6) underlines the congruency of Bleuler's basic disturbances with her negative symptoms, but with the exception of blocking, ranges formal thought disorders among her positive symptoms. This may be based on the experience that formal thought disorders occur frequently during florid psychotic episodes. Furthermore, in the criteria of Andreasen and Olsen (4) formal thought disorders

427

represent only one of four optional including elements for positive schizophrenia. The Vienna Research Criteria (7), called the 'endo-genomorphic schizophrenic axial syndrome' don't differentiate between negative and positive schizophrenia.

TABLE 1

Endogenomorphic-Schizophrenic AS

A) Formal Thought Disorders

1. blocking 2. derailment 3. pathologically 'muddled speech'

B) Affective Blunting

      Definite: A present   Probable: only B present

They require the presence of operationally defined formal thought disorders for diagnostic assignment to schizophrenia, whereas the presence of affective blunting alone makes the diagnosis only probable. Our research criteria were so conceived in order to filter out the endogenous schizophrenic from the whole of functional psychoses. For this purpose the following assumption is taken into account: Although formal thought disorders and affective blunting may occur in both endogenous schizophrenia and organic brain disorders, the latter are generally of a coarse nature when giving rise to formal thought disorders and thus easy to detect, whereas somatic blunting may be insidous and therefore often difficult to detect. Basing the diagnosis of endogenous schizophrenia on the grounds of the affective blunting alone would thus encompass a whole range of organic disturbances of brain function evading discovery and thereby blur investigations. On the other hand, since formal thought disorders are frequently present only during transient stages of schizophrenic disorders, this approach contains a major disadvantage: If used for cross-sectional diagnosis, the Viennese criteria identify for sure only a portion of those patients who would be otherwise identified when the whole illness course is taken into account. Furthermore, patients in no instance exhibiting formal thought disorders will never be accredited with certainty to the research diagnosis of endogenous schizophrenia, although they may quite well belong to this group. It is not our intention to discuss the pros and cons of Andreasen's and Olsen's approach on the one side and ours on the other; both serve different purposes. Our only aim here is to demonstrate, in view of results of two longitudinal studies, that formal thought disorders are predictors of an evolution towards deficiency and thus may be related to negative symptoms.

A catamnestic study covering a mean observational period of 12 years was carried out on 68 patients who met the ICD - 9 criteria for schizoaffective psychoses on first admission (8). This study was

428

based on the assumption that schizoaffective disorders represented a heterogenous group encompassing both affective disorders and true schizophrenia and set out to investigate whether schizoaffective disorders were involved in the development of deficiency states, and if so, to what extent. The appearance, at any time during the entire observational period, of symptomatology or from Bleuler's basic disturbances, of first rank symptoms or of catatonic symptoms was registered and related to the presence or absence of a deficiency state, defined as affective blunting, at the moment of re-examination. (Affective blunting was most frequently accompanied by avolition/ apathy). These correlations are presented in Table 2.

TABLE 2

SCHIZOAFFECTIVE PATIENTS (N : 68)

Vienna Research Criteria for Schizophrenia

	yes	no
No deficiency	2	42
Development of deficiency	17	7

$$x^2 = 33.89 \ (p < 0.001)$$

Bleuler's Basic Disturbances

	at least 2 of all		Assoc. Disturb.		Affect. Disturb.	
	yes	no	yes	no	yes	no
No deficiency	11	33	2	42	14	30
Development of deficiency	16	8	13	11	16	8
	$x^2 = 11.26$ $(p < 0.001)$		$x^2 = 22.24$ $(p < 0.001)$		$x^2 = 7.65$ $(p < 0.01)$	

429

	at least 1 of all		Imperat. Voices		Thought Insert.		one of all Hall.	
	yes	no	yes	no	yes	no	yes	no
No deficiency	31	13	4	40	3	41	7	37
Development of deficiency	19	5	8	16	6	18	9	15
	n.s.		$x^2 = 6.28$ $(p < 0.05)$		$x^2 = 4.47$ $(p < 0.05)$		$x^2 = 4.02$ $(p < 0.05)$	

The Vienna Research Criteria for Schizophrenia show the highest correlation with the development of a deficiency state. If at least two of the six Bleurlerian basic disturbances (disturbances of association, of effectivity, of volition and acting, of the subjective experience of the self, autism, and ambivalence) are present, the correlation with deficiency is still highly significant; this correlation becomes even stronger when the associational disturbances are taken alone. The significance drops on the other hand to a lower level when disturbances of affectivity alone are compared with deficiency. The presence of at least one first rank symptom (as required in many diagnostic criteria) has no significant relation with the development of a deficiency state. If the first rank symptoms are taken individually, only imperative voices and thought insertion reach a slight significance on the 5% level; the same correlation prevails when at least any one of the hallucinations specified with the first rank symptoms is brought into relation with deficiency. No significant correlation appeared between deficiency and catatonic symptoms.

These findings were corroborated by a prospective study embracing 90 delusional patients (9). Eighty-four of whom had been followed for a period ranging from 6 to 9 years.

TABLE 3

DELUSIONAL PATIENTS (N : 84)

Vienna Research Criteria for Schizophrenia

	yes	no
No deficiency	0	65
Development of deficiency	7	12

$$x^2 = 26.12 \ (p < 0.01)$$

All seven cases which met at least once the Vienna Research Criteria for Schizophrenia during the observational period subsequently developed a deficiency state. However, the state also appeared in 12 other cases for which the obligatory symptoms of the Viennese criteria were never reported. The reason might be that in 'negative schizophrenia' formal thought disorders either do not occur at all or are so insidious and transitory that they could not be grasped by the follow-up examinations. Such predominantly 'negative' cases are less likely to be found among schizoaffective psychoses which by definition have an affective component than among a cohort of patients sampled in view of presence of delusions. This may explain why correlation between the Vienna Research Criteria for Schizophrenia and the development of a deficiency state reaches a significance of 0·1% in the first study and only 1% in the second. Anyhow, both studies demonstrate that the appearance of formal thought disorders is a strong indicator for an evolution towards deficiency. The second study also investigated the relation between psychopathological findings and illness course, the result being that formal thought disorders showed a highly significant correlation with a chronic evolution. These findings are reported in detail in the symposium on the polydiagnostic approach (10).

The results of our research suggest that formal thought disorders are strong indicators for a chronic illness course leading to deficiency. Why, then, should they not be regarded as 'negative' symptoms? As already mentioned, formal thought disorders seem to occur mainly during florid episodes characterized by 'psychotic' features, such as first and second rank symptoms, and emotional turmoil. If psychotic features appear without formal thought disorders the illness usually takes an episodic course with a restitutio ad integrum; when they appear together with formal thought disorders the illness usually takes a chronic course leading to deficiency. We therefore hypothesize that an underlying process characterized by an impairment in information processing already exists in the latter situation. The emotional turmoil here unmasks the impairement, whereby formal thought disorders become clinically manifest. In our opinion the same also applies to blocking, which many authors, such as C. Schneider (11) and Fish (12) include under formal thought disorders. This is apparently why Andreasen (4) found blocking to show the lowest correlation with her alogia complex. This complex is a component of the clinical picture of negative schizophrenia, whose symptoms, such as poverty (of content) of speech, affective flattening etc., may on the contrary be masked by the emotional turmoil.

In conclusion we hypothesize that endogenous schizophrenia is the expression of a neurochemical disturbance which leads to an impairment of information processing. Psychotic episodes with emotional turmoil frequently, but not obligatorily, mark its course, unamsking the 'loss of function' that mainifests as formal thought disorders. The neurochemical disturbance in endogenous schizophrenia may possibly be accompanied by or result in structural changes of the brain correlating with atrophy. Other organic brain disorders may also be hallmarked by an impairment of information processing, display or lead to atrophy and produce a deficiency state characterized by negative symptoms; here, states of emotional turmoil occur rarely if at all, so that formal thought disorders are seldom seen. Affective psychoses don't lead to an impairment of information processing; emotional turmoil occuring in these disorders therefore may release only 'psychotic features'. Thus formal thought disorders, hypothetically considered to be unmasked negative symptoms, seem to be very characteristic, albeit unspecific, for endogenous schizophrenia.

REFERENCES

1. J. Hughlings-Jackson, Selected Writings. Taylor (ed.)
    Hoddler and Stoughton, London 1931
2. W. Birkmayer, Die Vegetative Dystonie, eine Funktions-störung
    der Retiklu ren Formation. Mediz. Welt 27/28, 1-16, 1960
3. J. Strauss, W. Carpenter and J. Barkto, The Diagnosis and
    Understanding of Schizophrenia: II. Speculations on the
    Process that underlie Schizophrenic Symptoms and Signs.
    Schizophr. Bull. 11: 61-76, 1974
4. N. Andreasen and S. Olsen, Negative and Positive Schizophrenia.
    Definition and Validation. Arch. Gen. Psych. 39:789-794, 1982
5. T. Crow, Molecular Pathology of Schizophrenia: More than one
    Disease Process? Brit. Med. J. 280: 1 - 9, 1980
6. N. Andreasen, Negative Symptoms in Schizophrenia. Definition
    and Reliability. Arch Gen. Psych. 39: 784-788, 1982

7. P. Berner, E. Gabriel, H. Katschnig, W. Kieffer, K. Koehler, G. Lenz and Chr. Simhandl, Diagnostic Criteria for Schizophrenic and Affective Psychoses. Amer. Pscyh. Press Inc., 1983

8. B. Küfferele and G. Lenz, Classification and Course of Schizoaffective Psychoses. Pscyhopathology, in press.

9. P. Berner, E. Gabriel, M. L. Kronberger, B. Küfferle, H. Schanda and R. Trappl, Course and Outcome of Delusional Pscyhoses. Psychopathology 17: 28-36, 1984

10. H. Schanda, K Thau, B. Küfferle and P. Berner, The Polydiagnostic Approach in Delusional Syndromes. Proceedings of the 7th World Congress of Psychiatry, Vienna

11. C. Schneider, Die Pscyhologie der Schizophrenen. Thieme, Leipzig 1930

12. F. Fish, Schizophrenia. Bristol, John Wright, 1976

LATERAL IMBALANCE AND POSITIVE AND NEGATIVE SYMPTOMS

John Gruzelier

Department of Psychiatry
Charing Cross Hospital Medical School
University of London, U.K

While substantial evidence exists for a lateralised anomaly of the left hemisphere in schizophrenia (Gruzelier & Flor-Henry, 1979; Flor-Henry and Gruzelier, 1983; Reynolds, 1983) recent research in our laboratory suggests that the consequence of this for hemispheric function may depend on the syndrome (Gruzelier, 1983a). Using a left or rightward psychophysiological asymmetry as the independent variable Gruzelier and Manchanda (1982) found that the two groups so defined, comprising a sample of 48 recent hospital admissions with a diagnosis of schizophrenia, differed in syndromes described by the Present State Examination with the CATEGO system of classification (Wing, Cooper and Sartorius, 1974) and by the Brief Psychatric Rating Scale (Overall and Gorham, 1962). These are shown in abbreviated form in Table I and define a syndrome of positive symptoms in one group and a syndrome of negative symptoms in the other.

The psychophysiological measure was the bilateral asymmetry in the electrodermal orienting response to tones. Frontal-limbic systems have important modulatory influences on this brainstem autonomic response such that lesions of the amygdala generally abolish the response while lesions of the hippocampus delay its habituation (Pribram and McGuinness, 1975).

An arousal dimension is in many respects central to the behaviour described in the syndromes which encompass self concepts, affect, cognition and motor functions. Quite apart from the fact that a lateral asymmetry is the method by which the syndromes are classified, their character is also consistent with an imbalance of activity between the hemispheres. The hemispheres have been shown to differ in their emotional polarities, the most straight-

435

forward interpretation of which associates euphoria with the left hemisphere and sadness with the right hemisphere (Tucker, 1981).

Table 1. Features of the Positive (L > R Asymmetry) and Negative (R > L Asymmetry) Syndromes.

Positive (L > R)

Heightened self consciousness (simple ideas of reference).
Exaggerated self opinion and conviction of unusual ability (grandiosity).
Exaggerated concern about bodily welfare(hypocondriasis).
Euphoria (hypomania).
Situational anxiety; avoids situations: phobias.
Pressure of speech.
Flight of ideas.

Negative (R > L)

Lack of self confidence.
Social withdrawal.
Uncooperative (resistance, resentment, unfriendliness).
Irritable to hostile.
Emotional withdrawal.
Reduced emotional tone (blunted affect).
Depressed mood.
Motor underactivity.
Slow speech.
Muteness, restricted quantity of speech.
Inefficient thinking (muddled, slow, not goal directed).

On these grounds the euphoria of the florid syndrome reflects left hemispheric overactivity. The accompanying flight of ideas, pressur of speech and exaggerated self concepts are also parsimoniously explained by an overactivation of left hemisphere cognitive processes.

Conversely the negative syndrome with its emotional valence of depressed mood and blunted affect is in keeping with an over-activation of the right hemisphere reflected in restricted quantity of speech and retarded, sluggish thinking. A reciprocal relation between the hemispheres in dynamic systems is consistent with theoretical views of Kinsbourne (1973) and evidence from electro-dermal recording where fast and slow habituation of orienting responses were associated with opposite electrodermal asymmetries (Gruzelier, Eves and Connolly, 1981). The direction of imbalance in hemispheric activity is also consistent with a model of hemis-pheric influences on the electrodermal system in which larger

436

left than right hand responses reflect a left hemisphere polarity and the opposite response asymmetry a right hemisphere polarity (Gruzelier et al, 1981).

The validity of the model of hemispheric functions underpinning two syndromes in schizophrenia found support from a review of the literature which revealed asymmetries in opposite directions in different forms of schizophrenia having an affinity with the syndromes outlined above (Gruzelier, 1983a; 1983b this collection). Validity was confirmed by a spectral analysis of the EEG activity of patients classified by both electrodermal response asymmetries and positive and negative symptoms (Gruzelier, Jutai, Connolly and Hirsh, 1984), results elaborated elsewhere in this collection.

What are the implications of the syndromes for current interests in positive and negative symptomatology in schizophrenia? While a positive syndrome is distinguished from a negative one the symptoms described form only a part of the clinical picture. Positive symptoms such as Schneiderian symptoms of first rank accompanied both syndromes. In this regard it is of interest that in the review of Davison and Bagley (1969) relating schizophrenic symptoms to organic lesions, the majority of schizophrenic symptoms were associated with the left hemisphere, particularly the temporal lobe, with the exception of Schneider's symptoms which had no lateral associations and instead were associated with the brainstem.

The coexistance of Schneiderian symptoms and negative symptoms sets this syndrome apart from the negative symptom, Type II schizophrenia of Crow (1980). Nevertheless it does contain those symptoms thought by Crow (1983) to be essential to the negative syndrome - blunted affect and poverty of speech. In fact blunted affect was the most reliable differentiator (Gruzelier and Manchanda, 1982). Furthermore in clinical practice the negative syndrome in a pure form is rare in schizophrenia in all but burned out, defect states. The most common clinical outcome is a mixture of positive and negative symptoms, and, prior to a patient reaching a state of chronic deterioration where negative symptoms predominate, the question as to the relative weighting to give them is a vexed one. Thus where negative symptoms are masked by positive ones the electrodermal measure may offer an objective method of assigning patients to the appropriate syndrome. This could be important if differential courses of treatment were implicated, as might well be the case if positive and negative symptoms have a bearing on prognosis.

However, it is too soon to say whether the psychophysiological marker provides a means of predicting the form the illness will take and delineating from the outset a group who have a poor prognosis. It is not known to what extent the psychophysiological asymmetry represents a trait of state factor, though it has been shown in some patients that the asymmetry may be reduced or reversed with drug treatment (Gruzelier, Eves, Connolly and Hirsch, 1981). Should this turn out to be a viable marker, at least in some, it is worth noting that the measures in our sample of 48 cases were examined within a few days of hospital admission while patients were unmedicated. None at that time could be categorised as possessing a chronic defect state.

At a neurophysiological level there are a number of implications. The syndromes are underpinned by hemispheric asymmetries in opposite directions and these are depicted by measures that reflect dynamic processes rather than fixed structural ones. Accordingly the syndromes reflect dynamic states of hemispheric imbalance which may be ammenable to modification. As neuroleptics have been shown to have asymmetrical effects (Gruzelier & Flor-Henry, 1979) and neurotransmitter concentrations may be asymmetrical (Reynolds, 1983), the alteration of hemispheric imbalance may be an important component in the efficacy of neuroleptics and a psychophysiological means is thereby provided of monitoring drug change.

Finally, theories of hemispheric specialisation when applied to the syndromes provide a neuropsychological explanation for different forms of schizophrenic behaviour. For example a dependence on right hemisphere processes would account for why the poor prognosis syndrome has negative affect, avoids social encounters and withdraws into fantasy, behaviour all ascribed to the right rather than left hemisphere. That the substrate is an activation imbalance, and hence lies with a dynamic process, allows for the not uncommon shifts between syndromes, in which it would be inferred hemispheric balance alters, and for the observation by M. Bleuler (e.g. 1983) that even patients with long standing chronic illnesses, which give the appearance of chronic deterioration, may recover.

References

Bleuler, M. (1983) Schizophrenic deterioration. Brit. J. Psychiat. 143, 77-84.
Crow, T.J. (1980) Molecular pathology of schizophrenia: More than one disease process? Brit. Med. J. 280, 66-68.
Crow, T.J. (1983) Schizophrenic deterioration. Brit. J. Psychiat. 143, 77-84.
Davison, K., and Bagley, C.R. (1969). Schizophrenia-like psychoses associated with organic disorders of the central nervous system: A review of the literature. In "Current Problems" in Neuropsychiatry" (R.N. Herrington, ed.), pp. 113-184. Headley Bros., Ashford, Kent.
Flor-Henry, P., and Gruzelier, J.H. (1983) eds. Laterality and Psychopathology. Elsevier Science Publishers, Amsterdam.
Gruzelier, J.H. (1983a) A critical assessment and integration of lateral asymmetries in schizophrenia. In M. Myslobodsky (ed) Hemisyndromes: Psychobiology, Neurology, Psychiatry, Academic Press, London, 265-236.

Gruzelier, J.H. (1983b) Dynamic hemispheric imbalance in schizo-phrenia. This collection.

Gruzelier, J.H. and Flor-Henry, P. (1979) Hemisphere Asymmetries of Function in Psychopathology, Elsevier Biomedical Press, Amsterdam.

Gruzelier, J.H., and Manchanda, R. (1982) The syndrome of schizo-phrenia: Relations between electrodermal response, lateral asymmetries and clinical ratings. Brit. J. Psychiat. 141, 488-495.

Gruzelier, J.H., Eves, F.F., and Connolly, J.F. (1981). Habituation and phasic reactivity in the electrodermal system: reciprocal hemispheric influences. Physiol. Psychol. 9, 313-317.

Gruzelier, J.H., Eves, F.F. Connolly, J.F. and Hirsch, S.R. (1981) Orienting, habituation, sensitisation and dishabituation in the electrodermal system of consecutive, drug free, admissions for schizophrenia. Biological Psychology, 12, 187-209.

Gruzelier, J.H., Jutai, J., Connolly, J., and Hirsch, S.R. (1984) Cerebral asymmetries in unmedicated schizophrenic patients in EEG spectra and their relation to clinical and autonomic parameters. To be published in Advances in Biological Psychiatry.

Kinsbourne, M. (1973) The mechanisms of hemispheric control of the lateral gradient of attention. In S.   (ed) Attention and Performance IV, London, Academic Press.

Overall, J.E., and Gorham, D.R. (1962) The Brief Psychiatric Rating Scale. Psychol. Rep. 10, 799-812.

Pribram, K.H., and McGuinness,D. (1975) Arousal, activation and effort in the control of attention. Psychol. Rev. 82, 116-147.

Reynolds, G.P. (1983) Increased concentrations and lateral asymmetry of amygdala dopamine in schizophrenia. Nature, in press.

Tucker, D. (1981) Lateral brain function, emotion and conceptual-isation. Psychol. Bull. 89, 19-46.

Wing, J.K., Cooper, J.E., and Sartorius, N. (1974). "The Measurement and Classification of Psychiatric Symptoms". Cambridge University Press, London.

BIOCHEMICAL AND CLINICAL INVESTIGATIONS WITH REGARD TO PLUS AND MINUS SYMPTOMATOLOGY IN SCHIZOPHRENIA

Margot Albus

Psychiatric Hospital-University of Munich

Nussbaumstr. 7, D 8000 Munich, GFR

There is no doubt about the antipsychotic efficacy of neuroleptics, which act mainly over blockade of the dopamine receptor and thus secondarily increase dopamine turnover. The so-called dopamine-hypothesis (CARLSSON & LINDQVIST, 1963) has won wide support and an antagonism of dopamine receptors is most probably the critical element in diminishing productive schizophrenic symptoms such as delusions, hallucinations and thought disorders. On the other hand, neuroleptics are of limited value in many chronic patients, where the so-called negative symptoms like flattening of affect, lack of speech, loss of impetus are - contrary to the positive symptoms - much less affected (JOHNSTONE et al., 1978). Therefore, CROW (1982) proposed the differentiation between the "Type I"-syndrome, approximating "acute schizophrenia", characterized by the positive symptoms and in some way associated with a change in dopaminergic transmission. The "Type II"-syndrome, however is characterized by negative symptoms and is unrelated to dopaminergic transmission. During the last years more and more investigations support an involvement of the noradrenergic system in the etiology of schizophrenia and the mode of action of neuroleptics. LAKE et al. (1980) reported elevated NE-levels in the cerebrospinal fluid (CSF) of acute schizophrenic patients, who had been drug free for at least 2 weeks. STERNBERG et al. (1979) found a significant decrease in NE CSF levels after application of pimozide. This decrease correlated significantly with a decrease in the

patients' psychopathology, similar to the decrease in
CSF MHPG after clorpromazine, found by SEDVALL (1978),
which also correlated with a decrease in psychosis.
Furthermore, receptor binding studies showed an effect
of neuroleptics (NL) on the dopaminergic as well as on
the noradrenergic system (PEROUTKA et al., 1977; GROSS
& SCHUMANN, 1980; REISINE, 1981). Besides this possible
involvement of the noradrenergic system i would like to
discuss, if different conditions of the dopaminergic
system could account for productive and negative respec
tively plus and minus symptoms, as proposed by
LECRUBIER et al.,(1980), who postulated an overactivity
of dopaminergic functions in productive patients and an
hypoactivity in defective patients. KING et al.(1982)
proposed, that psychotic individuals exhibit an instability in dopaminergic function. This instability again
could be caused by other systems, e. g. the peptide
system, which acts as neuromodulator (ZETTLER, 1981) i.
e. as part of a inhibitory feed-back system. Taking in
account all these possible explanations for the develop
ment of minus symptoms we investigated the effects of
drugs, which act mainly on the noradrenergic system,
one alpha-adrenergic, the other an alpha-adrenolytic
one, on plus and minus symptoms in chronic schizophrenics. As well as this, the influence of an additional
application of a peptide was expected to induce amelio-
rations of negative symptoms in schizophrenics.

METHODS

Study I:Blood samples for the estimation of NE were
taken from 53 male chronic schizophrenics at two
successive days during rest and after cold pressor test
(CP) under NLs (day 1). From the sample 24 patients
were selected, 12 with the highest, 12 with the lowest
NE-levels. After 12 days drug withdrawal (day 2) blood
was collected again during rest and after CP for the
estimation of NE, E, prolactin, cortisol and psycho
pathology was rated by BPRS. Following this, the patients received the alpha-adrenergic Sulpiride-analogue
(CGP 11109) for 15 days (day 3) and the same biochemical investigations were carried out as well as after
the following 15 days application of the identical NL
medication as at day 1 (day 4).

Study II:From 20 male chronic schizophrenics under
neuroleptics (day 1) blood samples for the estimation
of NE, Cortisol, HGH, ß-Endorphin were taken in rest,
after CP and after 0.075 mg Clonidin intravenuosly,
psychopathology was rated by BPRS and AMDP. The neuroleptic treatment was discontinued and no verum medication was given for a period of 12 days . These patients

days, and the same biochemical and clinical ratings as under neuroleptics were carried out after 12 days withdrawal (day 2), 15 (day 3) and 30 (day 4) days Nicergoline application.

Study III: Again 20 male chronic schizophrenics were investigated(double-blind-design, 10 patients receiving ceruletide,10 placebo under unchanged neuroleptic therapy). Blood samples for estimation of NE, Prolactin, Cortisol and ß-Endorphin were taken under neuroleptics (day -14) in rest, then at 3 successive weeks in rest and after intramuscular injection of 0.3 ug/kg ceruletide (day 0, 7, 14). Clinical ratings (AMDP, BPRS, NOSIE, GAS) were carried out at day -14, 0. 7, 14, 21, 28.

RESULTS

Study I: 1. Biochemical data: Prolactin secretion decreased significantly between day 1 (NL) and day 2 (withdrawal) in both groups (day 1: high level: $x = 5.41$ ng/ml, standard deviation (SD) = 3,38; low level: $x = 8,42$, SD = 8.03; day 2: high level: $x = 4,7$, SD = 3,71; low level: $x = 3,21$, SD = 4.43). On the other hand, cortisol secretion increased significantly between day 1 and 2 (day 1: high level: $x = 20.25$ ug/%, SD = 5.87; low level: $x = 17.59$, SD = 2.37; day 2: high level: $x = 25.07$, SD = 5.1; low level: $x = 22.12$, SD = 5.59) and decreased significantly between day 3 and 4 in both groups without any differences between the groups (day 3:high level: $x = 28,5$, SD = 26.4; low level: $x = 25,13$, SD = 7,87; day 4: high level: $x = 21.15$, SD = 4.96; low level: $x = 19,29$, SD = 3,62).In the high level group, NE decreased highly significantly between day 1 ($x = 948.75$ pg/ml, SD = 447.15) and day 2 ($x = 318.29$, SD = 111.85), where the values were lower than in the initial low level group (day 1: $x = 404.25$, SD = 250.46; day 2: $x = 406.33$, SD = 193.63) and increased significantly between day 2 and 3($x = 623.17$, SD = 177.98), whereas no significant changes ere found in the low level group (day 3: $x = 458.33$, SD = 196.54). There were significant group differences at day 1,3 and 4 (high level: $x = 611.33$, SD = 172.53; low level: $x = 374$, SD = 169.16), but no clear differences at day 2 (placebo).

2. Psychopathology: BPRS: The BPRS total score differed already significantly at day 1 and was worse for the high level group (high level: $x = 48.17$, SD = 11.81; low level: $x = 39$, SD = 8.66). The high level group

showed a significant deterioration between day 2 (x = 44.92, SD = 11.89) and day 3 (x = 49.83, SD = 12.61), whereas the low level group showed no significant differences. A decrease in the subscore "ANERGIA" between day 1 (high level: x = 14.25, SD = 6.08; low level: x = 14.83, SD = 4.61) and day 2 (high level: x = 12.25, SD = 6.47; low level: x = 12.67, SD = 5.53) occurred in both groups without group differences. No significant changes occured in the subscores "Thought Disturbances" (THOT) and "Hostility" (HOST), but in THOT a significant group difference at day 4 (high level: x = 10.67, SD = 4.36; low level: x = 6.67, SD = 2.64)was seen in that the high level group had worsened. The subscore "Anxiety-Depression "(ANDP) showed a clear worsening (p .05) between day 1 (x = 9.83, SD = 5.02) and day 2 (x = 7.75, SD = 4.37) in the high level, but not in the low level group (day 1: x = 7.67, DF = 3.31; day 2: x = 9.33, SD = 4.09). Moreover, the high level group showed a significant elevation of the subscore "Activity" (ACTV) between day 2 (x = 7.83, SD = 3.09) and day 3 (x = 75, SD = 3.41) and is not so in the low level group.

Study II: 1. Biochemical data: CP induced an increase of plasma NE, whereas clonidine, due to the presynaptic a-2-stimulation showed a decrease of plasma NE in every period.(day 1: rest: NE = 452 pg/ml, SD = 227; CP: x = 591, SD = 256; 30 min. after Clonidin: NE: x = 292, SD = 205). Drug withdrawal induced a decrease (p. 05) in plasma NE (day 2: rest: NE: x = 343, SD = 147; CP: x = 455, SD = 199; 30 min. after Clonidin: x = 235, SD = 135), this decrease continued (p.01) after 15 days Nicergoline application (day 3: rest: x = 304, SD = 106; CP: x = 370, SD 159 ;30 min. after Clonidin: x = 171, SD = 67), whereas under 30 days an increase which lead to no significant differences to the NE levels under neuroleptics occured (rest: x = 465, SD = 374; CP: x = 509, SD 216, 30 min. after Clonidin: x = 253, SD = 189)

2. Psychopathology: in "THOT" there was an deterioration under withdrawal, an amelioration similar to the level under NL after 15 days Nicergoline (p.05) and a slight deterioration after 30 days Nicergoline (day 1: x = 12.75, SD 4.29; day 2: x = 14, SD 4.72; day 3: x = 13, SD = 4.5; day 4: x = 13.3, SD 4.18)In ACTV we found an deterioration under withdrawal (p.05), a slight amelioration after 15 days and again a deterioration (p.05)to a slight higher level than after withdrawal under 30 days Nicergolin day 1: x = 7.6, SD = 2.1; day 2: x = 8.9;, SD = 3.39; day 3: x = 8.47, SD = 2.93; day 4: x = 9.05, SD = 2.75)

Study III: I. Biochemical data:Prolactin showed no significant changes over the time nor between the groups. In cortisol, too, no significant changes occured under ceruletide treatment nor in comparison of groups. The ceruletide group showed a significant (p.05) decrease in Cortisol-level 60 min. after Ceruletide between day 0 and 14 (day 0: x = 14.66 mg%, SD 6.34; day 14: x = 10.1, SD = 2.5), the placebo group between day 7 and 14 (day 7: x = 11.03, SD = 3.7); day 14: x = 9.81, SD = 3.17, p .01). No significant differences between the groups occurred in NE, but in the ceruletide group significant decreases in NE-base level and after Ceruletide-application are to be shown in the sense, that at day 14 all levels were lower than at day 7. The Ceruletide group showed wider variance than the placebo group, this already before ceruletide application (day 7, Ceruletide:-10 min: NE: x =712.8, SD = 388.37; +20 min: x = 674.6, SD = 344.2; +40 min: x = 612.8, SD = 378.6; day 14: -10 min: x = 533.5, SD = 284.97; +20 min: x = 511.5, SD = 236.47; +40 min: x = 507.1, SD = 268, 92.

II. Psychopathology:
The Ceruletide group showed a significant amelioration between day 0 and 7 (p.05) and 0 and 21 (p.01) in BPRS total score (day 0: x = 47.9, SD = 11.52; day 7:x = 44.5,SD = 10.34; day 21: x = 42, SD = 10.83).The placebo-group, too, showed a significant amelioration at day 21 and 28 compared with day 0 (day 0: Placebo: x = 45.2, SD = 14; day 21: x = 36.1, SD =7.61, p .01; day 28: x = 37.4, SD = 8.54, p .01), but without significant differences between the groups. In ANER no significant changes occured, but the ceruletide group was worse (p.05) at day 7 and 14 than the placebo group (day 7: ceruletide: x = 16.7, SD = 4; placebo: x = 13. SD = 3.56; day 14: Ceruletide: x = 15.7, SD = 4.16, Placebo: x = 12. 1, SD = 3.51). In HOST and THOT no significant changes occured neither between the days nor between the groups. In ACTV the ceruletide group showed a significant (p.05) amelioration between day 0 and 7 (day 0: x = 6.2, SD = 3.1; day 7: x = 4.9, SD = 3.1), the placebo group between day 7 and 14 (day 7: x = 7.4, SD = 1.8; day 14: x = 6.2, SD = 1.8, p = .05) but without significant differences between the groups. In ANDP the ceruletide group showed a significant (p .01) deterioration between day 21 and 28 (day 21: x= 7.7, SD = 3.6; day 28: x = 8.7, SD = 4.1)

DISCUSSION

Comparing the effects of the two drugs, influencing the

noradrenergic system on biochemical and clinical parameters different profiles are evaluable: whereas the
alpha-adrenergic Sulpirid-analogue induced only in the
initial high-level group a similar increase as under
neuroleptics without inducing alternations in the NE-
levels of the initial low-level-group, Nicergoline
leads initially (after 15 days) to an even further
decrease of NE-levels, followed by a decrease up to NE-
levels found under neuroleptic treatment. For this a
delayed effect of Nicergoline is to discuss, as alpha-
adrenolytics due to their feedback regulation should
increase NE. The sulpiride-analogue shows a similar
influence on Cortisol and prolactin secretion as do
neuroleptics. Ceruletide, which is supposed to act
mainly on the dopaminergic system leads to no changes
in prolactin and Cortisol secretion and only weak
changes in NE-levels, where only after twice application NE-levels were found to be significantly lower.
The alpha-adrenergic Sulpirid-analogue lead to an deterioration in the initial NE-high-level group, this
mainly because of the worsening in productive symptoms
In the subscore"ANER" both groups showed a significant
amelioration i. g. application of an alpha-adrenergic
substance leads to an unspecific activation , especially in patients with high NE-levels under classical
neurolep- tics, but is eventually inducing a deterioration of productive symptoms. For a short time (15 days)
the alpha-adrenolytic Nicergoline was able to amelio-
rate the withdrawalinduced deterioration in productive
symptoms (THOT), as well as "ACTV", but it seems to be
not effective enough for protecting for developing
acute "productive" symptoms for an longer intervall.
The additional administration of the Dekapeptide
Ceruletide to the unchanged neuroleptic therapy leads
to an amelioration in BPRS-total Score - but for the
Ceruletide as well as for the placebo-group,only in the
subscore ACTV to an amelioration, whereas productive
symptoms (THOT) as well as HOST were not influenced As
no significant differences between the groups exist the
amelioration is probably mainly effect of the more
intensive care patients received during the investigation and not related to a specific drug effect. Summarizing we have to conclude, that neither drugs influencing the adrenergic system nor a drug which is said to
act as neuromodulator on the dopaminergic system are
capable to improve valid and specifically minus symptoms in chronic schizophrenic patients. The initial
amelioration in "ACTV" under Nicergoline-treatment and
the more pronounced amelioration in this BPRS-Subscore
under Ceruletide treatment may reflect psychotropic
effects of these substances.

446

References

CARLSSON,A. & LINDQUIST, M.: Effect of chlorpromazine and haloperidol on formation of 3-methoxytyra-tyramine and normetanephrine in mouse brain. Acta Pharmacol. Toxicol.,20, pp 140-144, 1963.

CROW, T. J.: Two Dimensions of Pathology in Schizophrenia.Dopaminergic and Non-Dopaminergic. Psychopharmacology Bulletin,Vol. 18, No. 3, pp 22-29, 1982

GROSS, G. & SCHUMANN, H. J.: Enhancement of Noradrenaline Release from Rat cerebral Cortex by Neuroleptic Drugs. Arch. Pharmacol.315, pp 103-109, 1980.

JOHNSTONE, E. C.; CROW, T. J.; FRITH, C. D.; CARNEY, M. W. P. & PRICE, J.S.: Mechanism of the antipsychotic effect in the treatment of acute schizophrenia. Lancet, i: pp 848-851, 1978.

KING, R. J.; RAESE, J. D.; HUBERMAN, B. A. & BARCHAS, J. D.:Dopamine Neuronal Instability: A Model for the Schizophreniform Psychoses. Psychopharmacology Bulletin, Vol. 18, No. 3, pp 70-72 1982

LAKE, C. R.; STERNBERG, D. E.; VAN KAMMEN, D.P.; BALLENGER, J.C.; ZIEGLER, M. G.; POST, R.M.; KOPIN, I.J. & BUNNEY, W. E.:Schizophrenia: Elevated Cerebrospinal Fluid Norepinephrine. Science, 207, pp 331-333, 1980.

LECRUBIER, Y.; PUECH, A.; SIMON, P. & WIDLOCHER, D.: Schizophrenie: hyper ou hypofonctionnement du systeme dopaminergique? Une hypothese bipolaire. Psychologie Medicale,12,11, pp 2431-2441, 1980.

PEROUTKA, S.J.; U'PRICHARD, D.C.; GREENBERG, D. A.; SNYDER, S.H.:Neuroleptic drug interactions with norepinephrine alpha-receptor binding sites in rat brain. Neuropharmacol. 16, pp 549-556, 1977.

REISINE, T.: Adaptive changes in catecholamine receptors in the central nervous system. Neuroscience, 6, No. 8, pp 1471-1502,1981.

SEDVALL, G.: Relationships among biochemical, clinical and pharmacokinetic variables in neuroleptic-treated schizophrenic patients. In: F. Cattabeni et al. (eds).: Adv. Biochem. Psychopharmacol., 24, pp 521-528, 1978.

ZETTLER, G.: Central depressant effects of caerulein and cholecystokinin octapeptide (CCK-8) differ from those of diazepam and haloperidol. Neuropharmacology, 20, pp 277-283, 1981.

POSITIVE <u>VERSUS</u> NEGATIVE SCHIZOPHRENIA:

CRITERIA AND VALIDATION

Nancy C. Andreasen

Department of Psychiatry, University of Iowa

Iowa City, Iowa 52242

The distinction between positive and negative symptoms was originally proposed by Hughlings-Jackson, who conceptualized these symptoms in terms of an evolutionary and hierarchical theory of brain structure. Interest in this distinction smoldered quietly for many years, but recently enthusiasm for conceptualizing the psychopathology of schizophrenia in terms of positive and negative symptoms has rekindled vigorously. The reawakening of interest in this distinction has occurred largely because many investigators believe that it may lead to improved methods of classification, assist in predicting response to treatment and outcome, and ultimately improve our understanding of the underlying brain pathology in this illness.

The application of the concept of positive <u>vs</u>. negative symptoms to research has been handicapped, however, by the lack of reliable and valid instruments for measuring these symptoms, particularly negative symptoms. Many investigators have been concerned that negative symptoms are relatively "soft," and that therefore they cannot be defined reliably. This paper reports on a set of instruments designed to remedy this problem. One of them, the Scale for the Assessment of Negative Symptoms (SANS), provides definitions and a rating scale for five important negative symptoms: alogia, affective flattening, anhedonia-asociality, avolition-apathy, and attentional impairment. In addition, a complementary scale for evaluating positive symptoms is also under development and will provide similar definitions and ratings for delusions, hallucinations, bizarre behavior, and positive formal thought disorder. These rating scales should assist future investigators, particularly those who undertake psychopharmacological research.

449

This paper also reports on the development of diagnostic criteria for subtyping schizophrenic patients as positive, negative, or mixed. These criteria should be useful to those investigators who wish to explore new approaches to classification or subtyping. The criteria were written a priori, based on the author's clinical experience in working with schizophrenic patients over the last 15 years. The selection and weighting of criteria were based primarily on clinical intuition, with the goal of defining relatively homogeneous groups that would differ on important validating correlates. The test of these criteria is their predictive validity. In a study of 52 schizophrenic patients described in this paper, evidence of CT scan abnormalities, poor premorbid functioning, and cognitive impairment were treated as the major validating variables. It was predicted a priori that patients meeting criteria for negative schizophrenia would show more evidence of CT scan abnormality, more cognitive impairment, and poorer premorbid functioning than would the positive or mixed patients.

The criteria for positive, negative, and mixed schizophrenia are as follows:

Positive Schizophrenia

1. At least one of the following is a prominent part of the illness.
   (a) Severe hallucinations that dominate the clinical picture (auditory, haptic, or olfactory). (The judgment of severity should be based on various factors such as persistence, frequency, and effect on lifestyle.)
   (b) Severe delusions (may be persecutory, jealous, somatic, religious, grandiose, or fantastic). (The judgment of severity should be made as described for hallucinations.)
   (c) Marked positive formal thought disorder (manifested by marked incoherence, derailment, tangentiality, or illogicality).
   (d) Repeated instances of bizarre or disorganized behavior.

2. None of the following is present to a marked degree.
   (a) Alogia, (b) affective flattening, (c) avolition-apathy, (d) anhedonia-asociality, (e) attentional impairment.

Negative Schizophrenia

1. At least two of the following are present to a marked degree.
   (a) Alogia (e.g., marked poverty of speech, poverty of content of speech), (b) affective flattening, (c) anhedonia-asociality (e.g., inability to experience pleasure or to feel intimacy, few social contacts), (d) avolition-apathy (e.g., anergia, impersistence at work or school), and (e) attentional impairment.

2. None of the following dominates the clinical picture or is present to a marked degree.
   (a) Hallucinations, (b) delusions, (c) positive formal thought disorder, (d) bizarre behavior.

Mixed Schizophrenia

This category includes those patients that do not meet criteria for either positive or negative schizophrenia, or meet criteria for both.

The application of these criteria must be based on the use of a systematic structured interview that evaluates the various positive or negative symptoms in terms of frequency, persistence, severity, and impact on the patient's lifestyle. Using the SANS and our rating scale for positive symptoms, we allocated each patient a score ranging from 0 to 5 for the various criterion symptoms. These symptoms were considered to be present to a prominent or marked degree (and therefore to reach criterion level) when a rating of at least 4 was given. Since most schizophrenics have some mixture of positive and negative symptoms to a mild degree, the distinction between the positive and negative subtypes turns on the severity of individual symptoms.

When these criteria were applied to 52 schizophrenic patients, 16 were classified as negative, 18 as mixed, and 18 as positive. The sociodemographic characteristics of these three groups are summarized in Table 1.

The three subtypes do not differ significantly from one another in age, sex ratio, or marital status. They do show highly significant differences in the expected direction in educational level,

TABLE 1

Negative vs. Positive Schizophrenia

Sociodemographic Characteristics

Variable	Negative (n = 16) Mean	s.d.	Mixed (n = 18) Mean	s.d.	Positive (n = 18) Mean	s.d.	Pr > F	Duncan (α = 0.05) Follow-up
Age	34.37	14.49	27.28	7.73	28.72	8.09	.1241	–
Years education	11.06	1.48	12.05	2.44	13.55	2.04	.0032	P > M,N
Premorbid adjustment (Phillips Scale)	8.40	3.58	5.50	3.20	5.05	1.95	.0047	N > M,P
% Female	50		44		50		.9336*	–
% Never married	63		67		78		.6175*	–
% Employed	6		41		55		.0066*	P,M > N

* F statistics result from a normal approximation to the binomial distribution.

premorbid adjustment, and ability to hold a job. The negative schizophrenics are consistently more impaired in these areas.

Other major validating variables examined in this study are summarized in Table 2.

Nearly all the hypothesized differences between the three groups were found to be present. The negative schizophrenics had a significantly larger mean ventricular/brain ratio than did the mixed or positive schizophrenics, suggesting that the negative patients as a group have some evidence of structural brain abnormality. The mean VBR among the negative patients is 8.48, which is significantly different from the VBR of 4.5 found among normals in our previous work. These results are further supported through the Mini Mental Status data. The Mini Mental Status provides a thirty-point rating of cognitive function. The negative schizophrenics have a mean score of only 20.6, which is significantly lower than either the mixed or positive schizophrenics. Finally, the negative patients also have a significantly higher rate of left-handedness, providing further evidence for some type of brain injury occurring early in life that has driven dominant processing from the left to the right hemisphere.

We also assessed the interrater reliability and internal consistency of the various items on the SANS that were used in order to make clinical ratings to apply the above diagnostic criteria. These results are summarized in Table 3, which also indicates the various items used to rate the five negative symptoms, included on the SANS.

As that table indicates, interrater reliability (measured by intraclass R) was consistently high for both individual items and

TABLE 2

Negative vs. Positive Schizophrenia

Indices of Cognitive Dysfunction and Outcome

Variable*	Negative (n = 16)		Mixed (n = 18)		Positive (n = 18)		Pr > F	Duncan (α = 0.05) Followup
	Mean	SD	Mean	SD	Mean	SD		
VBR	8.48	4.55	5.20	2.93	4.59	3.24	.0063	N > M,P
Mini mental status	20.60	8.96	26.47	3.00	28.67	1.88	.0011	P,M > N
GAS admission	20.31	6.04	27.25	6.04	26.61	5.68	.0026	P,M > N
GAS discharge	28.00	10.62	37.50	12.30	33.33	7.30	.0381	M > N
Handedness (% right-handed)**	67		83		100		.0403	P > N

*Some missing observations in some variable cells; **F statistics result from a normal approximation to the binomial distribution.

TABLE 3

Interrater Reliability of Negative Symptoms

Item	Intraclass Reliability
Affective Flattening or Blunting	
Unchanging facial expression	.895
Decreased spontaneous movements	.910
Paucity of expressive gestures	.873
Poor eye contact	.872
Affective nonresponsivity	.858
Inappropriate affect	.765
Lack of vocal inflections	.702
Subjective rating of affective flattening	.858
Global rating of affective flattening	.696
Subscale score	.925
Alogia	
Poverty of speech	.876
Poverty of content of speech	.748
Blocking	.704
Increased latency of response	.914
Subjective rating of alogia	.845
Global rating of alogia	.877
Subscale score	.903
Avolition-Apathy	
Grooming and hygiene	.918
Impersistence at work or school	.832
Physical anergia	.834
Subjective complaints of avolition-apathy	.701
Global rating of avolition-apathy	.763
Subscale score	.864
Anhedonia-Asociality	
Recreational interests and activities	.853
Sexual interest and activity	.853
Ability to feel intimacy and closeness	.898
Relationships with friends and peers	.798
Subjective awareness of anhedonia-asociality	.820
Global rating of anhedonia-asociality	.731
Subscale score	.860
Attentional impairment	
Work inattentiveness	.867
Inattentiveness during mental status testing	.918
Subjective complaints of inattentiveness	.926
Global rating of inattentiveness	.749
Subscale score	.924
Summary score (global ratings)	.838
Composite score	.920

for global rating. In addition, we also assessed the internal consistency of each symptom complex using Cronbach's alpha, a coefficient that is essentially a mean of all the split-half reliabilities for each subscale. Thus, this coefficient provides an index of the extent to which all items in a given subscale measure the same symptom complex: the higher the coefficient alpha, the greater the likelihood that all the items measure the same symptom complex. Coefficient alpha is very high for each of the five negative symptom complexes: affective flattening (.814), alogia (.834), avolition-apathy (.799), anhedonia-asociality (.632) and attentional

impairment (.844). In addition, the overall scale has an alpha of
.740. These results suggest that, not only is the scale reliable
in the sense of yielding consistent ratings between clinicians,
but it is also reliable in the sense that it is internally consistent.

In summary, several new tools have been developed in order to
measure the positive vs. negative distinction in schizophrenia.
One of these, the SANS, provides clinicians and researchers with a
useful instrument for collecting symptom measurements for research
on diagnosis, response to treatment, and outcome. In contrast to
previous clinical lore, the SANS indicates that negative symptoms
can be evaluated reliably. In addition, diagnostic criteria for
classifying patients a priori as positive, negative, and mixed
have also been developed. In a pilot study involving 52 schizophrenic patients, these diagnostic criteria have been found to
have significant predictive validity. They were useful in defining
and identifying patient groups that differed significantly on measures of brain structure and function.

REFERENCES

Andreasen, N. C., and Olsen, S. A., 1982, Negative v positive schizo-
    phrenia: Definition and validation, Archs. Gen. Psychiatry,
    39:784.
Angrist, B., Rotrosen, J., and Gershon, S., 1980, Differential ef-
    fects of neuroleptics on negative versus positive symptoms
    in schizophrenia, Psychopharmacology, 72:17.
Bleuler, E., 1950, Dementia Praecox or the Group of Schizophrenias,
    trans. J. Zinkin, International Universities Press, New York.
Crow, T. J., 1980, Molecular pathology of schizophrenia: More than
    one disease process? Br. Med. J., 280:1.
Folstein, M. F., and McHugh, P. R., 1975, Mini Mental State, J.
    Psychiat. Res., 12:189.
Harris, J. G., 1975, An abbreviated form of the Phillips rating
    scale of premorbid adjustment in schizophrenia, J. Abnorm.
    Psychol., 84:129.
Hughlings-Jackson, J., 1931, Selected Writings, ed. J. Taylor,
    Hodder & Stoughton, London.
Kraepelin, E., 1950, Dementia Praecox and Paraphrenia, trans. J.
    Zinkin, International Universities Press, New York.

SYMPTOM PATTERNS IN SCHIZOPHRENIA

A FACTOR-ANALYTIC STUDY

Hamilton, M., Hughes J. and Hill M.

Storthes Hall Hosital

Kirkburton, West Yorks, England

The number of symptoms to be found in schizophrenia is not
only greater than that found in any one patient, but indeed very
much greater. One of the reasons for this is that some symptoms
are incompatible, e.g. a mute patient cannot show disturbances of
speech. All this was of very minor interest until the
introduction of modern neuroleptics in many varieties made it
imperative to evaluate them in proper clinical trials.

An important difficulty soon appeared. It is well known
that when a total score on a multi-item rating scale is used, the
rationale for using such a sum depends on the existence of
positive correlations between all the items. Hamilton et al.
(1960) pointed out that this did not occur in chronic
schizophrenia, where the items fell into two groups. Within the
groups the inter-correlations were positive, but between them the
correlations were negative. There were three ways of dealing with
this situation: the first was to sum the scores on the items,
weighted positively or negatively according to which group they
they belong. The second was to treat the two groups of symptoms
as separate criteria. The third was to ignore the correlations
and to add all the scores, on the basis that they were all
symptoms of schizophrenia. This is the most common practice.
Although this is not a satisfactory method, it is not entirely
meaningless, as symptoms are either absent or present to some
degree, whereas correlations are calculated with the scores
treated as deviations from the mean score.

In general, when a matrix of correlations is factor

analysed by the centroid or similar method, the first factor is a general factor with all the loadings positive. Subsequent factors are bipolar, with positive and negative loadings. The reason for this is that when the first factor is removed, the matrix of residuals, from which the next factor is derived, fall into a pattern in which there are two groups where within the groups the inter-correlations are positive and the cross correlations are negative - exactly the same as is found with data derived from a sample of chronic schizophrenics.

With chronic schizophrenics, the first factor obtained from the matrix of correlations is, strictly speaking a second and therefore a bipolar factor. Defining the type of patients narrowly has more or less eliminated the variance of the first factor. If the sample had included all types of schizophrenia and all grades of severity from the most severe to the mildest, the correlations would have all been positive, the first factor would have been a general factor with positive loadings, and the second would have been bipolar.

This type of factor analysis produces a classification of the variables, in this case, of symptoms. When the nature of the factor is examined it is clear that at one end the symptoms are the 'positive' symptoms of schizophrenia and at the other end they are the 'negative ones'.

The correlations are obtained from data which consists of a set of persons who have scores on a set of symptoms. The usual method of analysis produced inter-correlations between the symptoms, but it is equally possible to calculate the correlations between persons and to analyse these, a method sometimes referred to as inverse factor analysis. Without going into the details and simplifying somewhat, the matrix of correlations obtained in this way shows a 'bipolar' pattern, i.e. there is no general factor, only bipolar factors, which classify the persons. When this is done with chronic schizophrenics, it will be seen that the first factor classifies the patients into those who have predominantly positive symptoms and those who have predominantly negative ones. Both methods of analysis yield the same results and it is therefore convenient to talk of two patterns of symptoms or syndromes in schizophrenia: Type P and Type N. (In the 1960 paper the P and N referred to the sign of the loadings of items on the factor).

The results of factor analysis therefore correspond to some extent with the clinical classification. However, it is inadvisable to rely strongly on the results of factor analysis, as the correlations are calculated from items in a scale the scores of which have some peculiar properties. Even within a group of chronic schizophrenics the appropriate items have a high proportion of zero scores. In consequence, the value of the

456

correlations will depend very much on the presence or absence of a few high values in the scores. In fact, in the original scale used (consisting of items selected from the Lorr scale), some of the items had such few scores that it made them unsuitable for inclusion.

In a recent trial carried out with my colleagues, the scale was modified to include only those items which had scores above zero in at least ten per cent of the records. This reduced the scale from 18 to 10 items. As the scores in all the items showed an asymmetrical distribution, the values were changed so as to normalise the distribution. On recalculating the correlations, it was found that the new values differed only slightly from those correlations calculated with the original crude scores. This showed that the the selection of items had been adequate for the purpose of calculating correlations. It was therefore considered that for that sample of 57 patients, the further analysis would yield confirmable results. The matrix was factorised by the method of principal components and yielded four factors using the Kaiser criterion for the number of factors. However, it is unlikely that the third and fourth factors would show sufficient stability to reappear exactly the same in another sample.

The results conformed to expectation. On the first component, the three items Mannerisms, Poverty of Thought and Conversation and Affective Blunting showed high negative loadings and the rest showed high positive loadings. The other factors split the items of the two halves into further subgroups. A Varimax rotation of the loadings gave results which were much clearer to interpret. It yielded four Varimax factors of course, the second of which showed high loadings on the three negative symptoms mentioned above. If loadings below 0.4 are disregarded (as is customary) there were no other symptoms on this factor, and the negative symptoms did not appear in any other factor, i.e. they formed a very coherent group.

This did not apply to the positive symptoms which split into three groups almost completely non-overlapping. The fourth factor contained the items Delusions of Influence and Auditory Hallucinations. The first factor contained the items Other Delusions, Thought Disorder and Incongruity of Affect, overlapping slightly with the third, which contained Incongruity of Affect, Delusions of Persecution and Hostility.

Clinicians have long been aware that the therapeutic value of neuroleptics is much greater in acute than in chronic schizophrenia. In fact, it could be said that the chief value of these drugs in chronic schizophrenia is to diminish the risk of relapse. The work of Crow and his colleagues has proved that the therapeutic effect of neuroleptics lies almost entirely in their control of positive symptoms.

This has important implications on the conduct of clinical trials. It indicates that to carry out such trials using scales which bring together all symptoms in one total score entails the risk that changes in the drug-responsive symptoms may be obscured by the non-responsive symptoms, which show little response and much random variation. The present results indicate that one should go further and not regard the positive symptoms as a homogeneous group. Further work needs to be carried out to determine if the present subdivision of positive symptoms is stable. It would then be better to examine the results of treatment in terms of these subgroups.

In the past, many trials have been analysed in terms of the changes produced in individual symptoms, but this has usually been a post hoc procedure. Given an adequate basis, the specific effects of different neuroleptics could be ascertained and thus improve considerably the choice of drug for individual patients, as well as indicating appropriate directions for the introduction of new drugs.

References

Hamilton, M., Smith, A. L. G., Lapidus, H. E., and Cadogan, E. P. 1960
> A controlled trial of Thiopropazate dihydrochloride, (Dartalan), Chlorpromazine and occupational therapy in chronic schizophrenics, J. ment. Sci. 106:40

NEWER CONCEPTS OF BASIC DISORDERS AND BASIC SYMPTOMS

IN ENDOGENOUS PSYCHOSES: INTRODUCTION

Gerd Huber

Psychiatric Clinic of the University of Bonn
D-5300 Bonn 1

Newer concepts of basic disorders and basic symptoms developed by SÜLLWOLD and our group have much in common with researchers like ZUBIN who conceptualized schizophrenia in terms of vulnerability due to faulty information processing (4,5). According to our concept a neurochemical disturbance results in the transphenomenological area in a disorder of processing of information, levelling of experience hierarchies and a few basic disorders. These constitute with different shares the manifold substrate-close basic symptoms that are experienced in the basic stages ("Basisstadien") by the patients and likewise the typical schizophrenic end- and superstructure-phenomena which result from the amalgamation of the basic symptoms with the "anthropological matrix". The majority of the schizophrenics in consideration of the whole course of the disease is able to perceive the basic deficiencies, to view them with critical detachment and to develop strategies of coping and compensation. Therefore, it was possible with the help of the subjective experience of the patients to confirm findings of the American and Russian experimental-psychological research (BUSS, LANG 1965; BROEN, STORMS 1966; POLJAKOV 1973; s. in 5; REY, OLDIGS 1982, s. in 3) and develop training programs which take into consideration the cognitive basic deficiencies. The subjective experience of the basic deficiencies which can be elicited with the descriptive-phenomenological method of JASPERS and SCHNEIDER, and the findings of psychological research offer a chance to clear up what so-called schizophrenic symptomatology truly is. These basic phenomena from their noncharacteristic first (Stufe 1-Basissymptome) over their characteristic second (Stufe 2-Basissymptome)

to the schizophrenia-typical third stage, i.e. the schizophrenic end-phenomena, are conceptualized as existing on a
psychopathological continuum. Thus the third stage to which
the stage 1- and stage 2-basic symptoms in one and the same
patient may progress also includes such symptoms as those
of the first rank of K. SCHNEIDER.

The psychopathological picture of basic stages is determined by dynamic and cognitive basic deficiencies which
are perceived and communicated by the patients themselves
and can be registered with the "Frankfurter Beschwerde-
fragebogen" by L. SÜLLWOLD. We have described the phenomenological aspects of pure defect and of the other four
types of basic stages as "substrate-close basic symptoms"
1966 and 1968 (s. 2,5,6). Because the phenomenological
aspects of the pure defect syndromes, the postpsychotic
basic stages, the prodromes and outpost syndromes and the
intrapsychotic basic stages, too, intersect each other,
these five non-psychotic manifestations of schizophrenic
diseases can be summarized as "basic stages more widely
taken". We could point out in basic stages in psychological tests a decrease of performance that is correlated
with the symptoms which were found in the "complaint
questionnaire" in the same patients.

Some features common to all basic symptoms are: they
are not accessible to observation of behaviour but have to
be found out by psychopathological exploration using the
patient's remaining ability for self-perception of deficiencies; they often occur in a rather characteristic
psychopathological quality, i.e. as stage 2-symptoms, and
at the same time with a higher degree of process activity
only transitory-intermittent and fluctuating,and that's
why they can be observed only by follow up studies. The
fluctuation is not only endogenous but largely dependent
on the situation, on non-specific stress, f.i. on emotional
or optic or acoustic relative overstimulation. Furthermore, it is often difficult to separate basic symptoms
from secondary efforts of coping, managing and compensation. For this reason and to get more knowledge about the
relation between basic deficiencies and psychotic final
symptoms, it is necessary to extend the analysis to the
early and prodromal phases, too, in which the disorders
most likely can be elicited in the original form, not yet
modified by secondary processes of working up. But, the
basic symptoms are not only initial symptoms but they
also are present in the later stages and especially in the
residues in the sense of pure defect. The "pure defect",
too, is strictly spoken no defect but a basic phase which
shows generally no or a very low degree of "process activity".

The basic symptoms are, though more rarely, also observed phenomenal identically in definable diseases of the brain. However, they do not occur in stage 2 and 3 at healthy persons or patients with psycho-reactive disorders and neuroses. The stage 2-basic symptoms are not characteristic for schizophrenia in the sense of the conventional concepts. But with growing experience it becomes possible to identify the peculiar quality of the phenomena, f.i. of cognitive thinking disorders or cenesthesias of stage 2. It is a task of the current research to detect the "characteristic in the non-characteristic" (s. in 3; 5) of the basic symptoms also with the help of special experimental arrangements.

It is important to see that the patients in basic stages notice their deficiencies as deficiencies, that they are able to describe the deficiencies and to develop coping reactions, mechanisms of defence and compensation. They learn from personal experiences f.i. that they are not allowed to overstrain their forces without paying for it, e.g. in the form of excitation, troubled sleep or psychotic relapses. As a reaction to the increased impressionability by stimulation result kinds of behaviour understandable as mechanisms of shielding, avoiding and coping. This is a root of the "secondary autism" (s. in 5).

The attempts of management are more or less intentional: the patients try to avoid everything that could evoke their disturbances and try to bring about conditions that help them to keep control. Therefore, the severity of the disease and its course and outcome also depend on the interindividual differences in the reactions on the basic symptoms and in this connection also on the level of premorbid intelligence (s. 7).

In order to try to correlate certain somatical data with psychopathological syndromes, those concepts as true or nuclear schizophrenia or atypical, schizophreniform, schizoaffective or cycloid psychoses are in our opinion not yet sufficient. In the search for highly fluctuating neurochemical or neurophysiological changes it seems necessary to define by means of the descriptive-phenomenological method of JASPERS and SCHNEIDER syndromes as homogenous as possible characterized by basic symptoms which have to be assessed as to the degree of "process activity" (see above), corresponding exactly to the time of biological investigation. That is to say that longitudinal studies with simultaneous psychopathological and somatical investigations in intervals as short as possible are indispensable. The degree of process activity

461

can be determined on the base of the clinical-psychopathological state. Hints of process-active basic phases that
can be correlated with neurochemical or certain findings
in EEG are f.i. cenesthetic or perceptual or thinking
phenomena of stage 2, or already yet more characteristic
schizophrenic basic symptoms as the vague delusional mood,
i.e. delusional perception of stage 1 and 2 in the sense
of CONRAD and HUBER and GROSS (s. in 5). In process-active
basic stages we could point out f.i. abnormal rhythmicity
in EEG (theta-, alpha- or delta-parenrhythmias), attribut-
able presumably to disturbed functions of limbic system
(s. 6; s. PENIN, GROSS, HUBER in 3).

The basic symptoms and basic stages reveal a marked
intraindividual fluctuation that may indicate on its part
fluctuating neurochemical and/or neurophysiological disturbances. But the fluctuation of the supposed disturbance
of processing of information and its equivalence in the
phenomenological area depend on the situation, too. Basic
symptoms and underlying basic disorders are the primary
phenomena which are according to our hypothesis nearer
to a supposed biological substrate than the most typically,
highly complex schizophrenic end-phenomena.

Whereas the cited changes in EEG can be found in
reversible transitory process-active basic stages, changes
ascertainable with static-morphological methods as CT
have to be related with irreversible psychosyndromes in
the sense of pure defect. Only schizophrenics with marked
signs of pure deficiency, persisting continuously at least
three years, reveal in their majority pathological deviations in CT concerning preferably the third ventricle
(s. in 3). Against it, persisting deformations of personality structure and full remitted schizophrenic psychoses have in the whole no pathological CT findings.

The changes in EEG and CT and the phenomenological
quality of basic symptoms can point at limbic system as
the location of the pathological altered cerebral function.
On the base of our results we assume that disturbances of
interpretation of information, of selective filtration
and of aimed utilization of stored experiences underlie
the basic deficiencies in schizophrenia.

To explore the fundamental disturbances in schizophrenias we must abandon some conventional ideas about
schizophrenia, e.g. that a reduction of capacity in the
field of perception and memory could not occur on principle; that always the whole personality would be af-

fected; that the schizophrenic would always be ruled by his disease, and, in contrary to a patient with a definable, well-known disorder of the brain, would not be able to self-perception, critical distance, insight of deficiencies, coping, adaption, compensation and self-organizing. The schizophrenic patients in basic stages show less a change of personality than a failure of efficiency. The ability for work and social contact, mainly in the sense of secondary autism, are impaired, whereas the capabilities of being responsible and guilty, of acting and contracting are maintained. This is of considerable importance for treatment, for psycho- and social therapy, the rehabilitation and the social appreciation of the phenomenon "schizophrenia" at all.

References

1. Huber, G., 1957, Die coenästhetische Schizophrenie, Fortschr. Neurol. Psychiat. 25: 491-520
2. Huber, G., 1966, Reine Defektsyndrome und Basis-stadien endogener Psychosen, Fortschr. Neurol. Psychiat. 34: 409-426
3. Huber, G., ed., 1982, "Endogene Psychosen: Diagnostik, Basissymptome und biologische Parameter," Schat-tauer, Stuttgart New York
4. Huber, G., 1983, Das Konzept substratnaher Basis-symptome und seine Bedeutung für Theorie und Therapie schizophrener Erkrankungen, Nervenarzt 54: 23-32
5. Huber, G., Gross, G., and Schüttler, R., 1979, "Schizophrenie. Eine verlaufs- und sozialpsych-iatrische Langzeitstudie," Springer, Berlin Heidelberg New York
6. Huber, G., and Penin, H., 1968 , Klinisch-elektro-encephalographische Korrelationsuntersuchungen bei Schizophrenen, Fortschr. Neurol. Psychiat. 36: 641-659
7. Süllwold, L., 1977, "Symptome schizophrener Erkran-kungen. Uncharakteristische Basisstörungen," Springer, Berlin Heidelberg New York

THE NEWER CONCEPTS OF BASIC DISORDERS

AND THE ORIGINAL CONCEPT OF SCHIZOPHRENIA

J. Klosterkötter

Universitäts-Nervenklinik
Köln, Josef-Stelzmann-Str. 9

1. STATEMENT OF THE PROBLEM

The fact that this symposium is dedicated expressly to the newer concepts of basic disorders immediately raises the question of their relationship to older concepts of basic disorders. In the following, the attempt is therefore made to compare the basic disorder concept by HUBER and SÜLLWOLD with the original concept of schizophrenia by KRAEPELIN and E. BLEULER (4).

2. SIMILARITIES

The necessary points of departure for such a comparison can be found in the three categories which the basic disorder concept lays down for the derivation of schizophrenic symptoms. In the most recent summary of the concept, in January of this year, HUBER differentiates between:

- one or more fundamental disorders in the processing of information
- completely uncharacteristic or more or less characteristic basic symptoms, and,
- typically schizophrenic end phenomena (3).

These terms refer to the corresponding importance in the derivation context which the basic disorder concept determines. One can therefore speak of structural similarities only if a functional correspondence for each of these categories can actually be shown. First of all, what about the transphenomenal level, where the attempt is made to link the basic symptoms to the prephenomenal data of brain research by means of the fundamental disorder hypothesis? HULL's construct of a "conditioned hierarchy of goal reaction tendencies", whose deterioration can be characterized equally well psychopathologically as well as somatopathologically, today serves this purpose (2). From the viewpoint of modern experimental psychology such a deterioration allows an instrusion of irrelevant aspects of stimuli and competing reaction tendencies. From the neurophysiological and neurochemical aspect this information processing disorder is equated with a defect in the limbic integration system. The "Loss of habit hierarchies" as a thoroughly effective deranging mechanism can be imputed to the various basic symptoms in such a way that their linkage to organic brain diagnostic evidence appear plausible. It would seem apparent that also the original theory of schizophrenic symptoms already has in its "hypothesis of the loosening of association" a similar substruction, which correlates phenomenal and pre-phenomenal given facts. This loss of hierarchies of association is interpreted physiologically as deficiency of a kind of diffuse cortical energy and at the same time used psychologically in the derivation of cognitive symptoms. The partial deterioration in the storing of associative experience reduces the control of the purposive ideas in the cognitive process. "If", however, according to E. BLEULER, "in thinking, the purposive ideas are missing, there arises confusion of every kind; the ill person loses himself in side associations, he is distracted by externals in cases where he would not otherwise be so, and reversely, pays no attention to external events which under given circumstances would be noticed (1, p.291).

In this manner, a kind of phenomena is already being treated in which direct reference is made to cognitive interferences and disorders of selective attention, exactly as in the case of basic symptoms. Although it of course appears in the original concept of schizophrenia under the category of secondary symptoms, stemming from the fact that the term primary symptom has already misleadingly been used for the transphenomenal loosening of association itself. Within this category, however, E. BLEULER unmistakeably differentiates confusion – along with less distinct displacements, symbolizations, and condensations of thought as direct and therefore substrate-close results of the fundamental disorder – from the remaining secondary symptomatology. Should one ask what basic symptoms are thus already anticipated here, the most likely to be considered would be the relatively characteristic "loss of control of the thought processes". This sub-category includes only subjectively experienced disturbances in the cognitive capacity, which can be specified by cognitive blocks, cognitive gliding, or disturbances of receptive and expressive language. Here the loss of cognitive-linguistic control is derived stringently from the loosening of the habit hierarchies just as traditionally "concept splitting" is derived from the construct of "loosening associations". The point to be emphasized here is that also the second category of the newer concept of schizophrenia can be shown to correspond to a surprisingly large extent, at least in the case of the cognitive basic symptoms in a more narrow sense with the original symptom theory.

How does the comparison bear out concerning the typical schizophrenic end phenomena? If the fundamental disorder constructs have succeeded in deriving only a portion of deficiencies from neurochemical functional disorder, a further mode of derivation must be given for the remaining phenomena. In the basic disorder concept experiential reactions take over this function and link, for example, elaborated delusional perceptions, ego disturbances, and acustic and bodily hallucinations indirectly, as it were, to the fundamental cognitive disorder. Concerning this HUBER remarks: "According to our concept [...] the typical schizophrenic end phenomena are to be conceived of as the 'superstructure of the human Psyche' arising from changes in the primary basic functions, as the reaction of the individual to the experiencing of the cognitive basic symptoms, i.e. as the result of a secondary process of working it out and forming changes" (3, p.26). According to this the forming of the superstructure is not motivated by arbitrary experiences, but rather is set in motion by coping with the immediate results of the fundamental disorder. This is also linked, although of course not in a causal sense, back to the cognitive fundamental disorder, in such a way that this reaction is understood as the mediation of highly complex experience symptoms with the process of the disease. Such a mediating function bears very exact similarity indeed to that provided in E. BLEULER's derivation of delusive phenomena, hallucinations and catatonic symptoms. Also according to him the somatic hypothesis only then becomes plausible if the psychotic experience change can be linked back to processing mechanisms in which the psyche reacts on a secondary level to the process of the disease. Such products do not represent, therefore, direct, but rather indirect results of the psycho-physiological fundamental disorder. In this way the category of the schizophrenic end phenomena is also to be found in the original concept of schizophrenia. It comprises exactly these indirect secondary symptoms so that now a functional correspondence can actually be demonstrated for each of the three categories in the basic disorder concept.

3. DIFFERENCES

Concerning the differences attention must first be drawn to the precise characteristic of the psycho-reactive mediation which, as outlined above, both theories posit between the "cognitive defect" and "psychotic otherness". At present the formulation of the "amalgamation" of basic symptoms with an "anthropological matrix" keeps the question open for various possible solutions. The schizophrenic voices could, following the learning theory arise from self commentaries, which at first serve to cope with the loss of cognitive control, with increasing interference, however, they cannot be discriminated from external auditory perceptions (5). No matter what explanation be offered for these secondary processes, one principle of the basic disorder concept remains unaffected: the way to be elaborated end phenomena does not follow a psychodynamic regression, but rather represents a compensatory struggle against cognitive disturbances within the frame of life-history and personality. In contrast to this, the original concept of schizophrenia used the complex theory of C.G. JUNG for the interpretation of the productive reaction. According to it the transphenomenal loosening of associative influences in experience disinhibit "emotionally charged idiational complexes" and thus confine the processing of information to the autistic perspective of wishes and fears. Any psychodynamically meaningful "life-event" affecting such a "split personality" is sufficient to trigger, for example, paranoid-hallucinatory "falsification of reality".

E. BLEULER, however, classified the phenomena of "personality splitting" as typical and those of "concept splitting" as specific signs of schizophrenia. Thus the psychoreactive mediation leads to a reduction of the diagnostic validity, but on the other hand, the validity progresses from the more uncharacteristic basic symptoms of the first level to the less uncharacteristic basic symptoms of the second level and further to the typical end phenomena. This second difference is especially important, because it affects the derivation plausibility in the basic disorder concept. The indifference of more or less uncharacteristic basic symptoms as opposed to clearly brain organic psychosyndromes provides only superficial support for the somatic hypothesis. The question arises, namely, as to whether one can derive typical phenomena from phenomena which are at best more or less characteristic. At least the same diagnostic validity, however, must be assured for both the cognitive basic symptoms and the end phenomena, if the disease process is to determine the superstructure psychoreactively. The two concepts of schizophrenia are in the meantime, however, no longer as different from each other as it first seemed under the influence of the "purity" of prodomal, outpostlike, postpsychotic and residual basic stages. Also for E. BLEULER, namely, the specifity of the direct results of basic disorders presupposed a "certain degree of development" which is possibly by no means reached by far the majority of cases from the beginning up to the final stage. "Concept splitting" remains then below the objectively measureable degree of confusion and allows only the assumption of a "latent schizophrenia", just as in the case of the "more subjective-experential given" loss of control of the thought processes. Conversely, at present, the gradation of validity requires in itself that one seeks the characteristic signs even for basic processes with a minimal degree of intensity. Should this search prove successful, the different grades of validity between the psychoreactive superstructure and the psychophysiological substructure would be equalized as in the older specifity hypothesis, but not only as a postulate, but moreover, as a clinically given fact. Thus the further development of the basic disorder concept at present attempts to prove the plausibility of that which the original concept of schizophrenia apparently prematurely attempted to demonstrate.

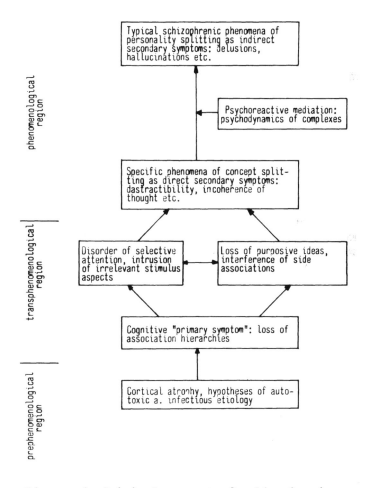

Diagram 1 Original concept of schizophrenia

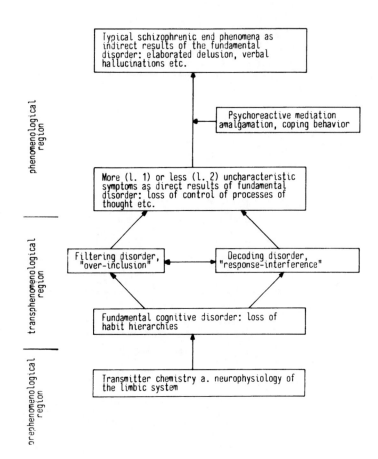

Diagram 2 Basic disorder concept

4. RESULTS

In summary: the "loss of associative hierarchies" corresponds on the transphenomenal level to the "loss of habit hierarchies". For the phenomenal sphere, this accordance in the psycho-physiological model of derivation entails two further points of correspondence: that of the cognitive basic symptoms with the secondary symptoms of "concept splitting" and that of the end – and superstructural phenomena with the indirect secondary phenomena of "personality splitting". The differences, along with the hypothesis of a pre-phenomenal somatic sphere remain limited to two problems: the question of specifity – the basic symptoms of level 1 or 2 as opposed to the characteristic phenomena of "concept splitting" and the concept of psychoreactive derivation – amalgamation, for example, as a coping reaction, as opposed to the complex theory. We can therefore conclude, in answer to our question concerning the older concepts of basic disorders, that the original theory of schizophrenia can indeed be regarded as a far-sighted and instructive precursor of the newer basic disorder concept (see diagrams 1 and 2).

REFERENCES

1. BLEULER, E.: Dementia praecox oder Gruppe der Schizophrenien. In: HdB der Psychiatrie, Teil 4. Hrsg. Aschaffenburg, G., Deuticke: Leipzig, Wien (1911).

2. BROEN, W.E.: Schizophrenia. Research and Theory. Academic Press: New York, London (1968).

3. HUBER, G.: Das Konzept substratnaher Basissymptome und seine Bedeutung für Theorie und Therapie schizophrener Erkrankungen. Nervenarzt 54:23-32 (1983).

4. KLOSTERKÖTTER, J.: Assoziationspsychologische versus lernpsychologische Schizophrenietheorie. Fortschr. Neurol. Psychiat. 50:165-170 (1982).

5. SÜLLWOLD, L.: Symptome schizophrener Erkrankungen. Uncharakteristische Basisstörungen. Monographien aus dem Gesamtgebiete der Psychiatrie. Bd.13. Springer: Berlin, Heidelberg, New York (1977).

SCHIZOPHRENIC BASIC DISTURBANCES: PSYCHOLOGICAL ASPECTS

THE TYPE OF "PSYCHOLOGICAL DEFICIENCY"

Lilo Süllwold

Zentrum der Psychiatrie
Klinische Psychiatrie II
Universität Frankfurt a.M

As the case research of Huber et al. (1) could
establish, uncharacteristic disturbances in the overall
development of disease are present more extensively than
the acute syndromes. These discrete disturbances are often
an obstacle to rehabilitation because they lead to
overstrain and thus provoke the risk of a renewed decompen-
sation.

From experimental schizophrenia research, which is
only gradually becoming integrated into psychopathology
(L. Süllwold (2)), it can be derived as generalizable
result that the intellectual capacity is apparently
retained but all psychic functions become susceptable to
disturbance and instability. The overall behaviour is thus
difficult to predict. A hypothetical basic disturbance,
from which all observable phenomena can be deduced, is
most likely to be assumed where it is a question of the
integration of incoming information with stored up memory
material. This higher, assessing and integrating phase of
information processing does not appear to function
continuously. This has the consequence that the consciousness is flooded with unselected, irrelevant internal and
external stimuli. The extent of the disintegration
fluctuates spontaneously but it can be provoked by certain
conditions such as a too manifold and too unstructured
stimulation. This applies to many social situations which
therefore give rise to difficulties for the sick person.
Blockages and false reactions, such as have been described,
for instance, as "formal thought disturbances", can be
observed in all areas of behaviour. Efforts to solve

473

problems and take action are interrupted by such interferences. This applies in the same manner for emotional
reactions which indeed presuppose a cognitive assessing
activity.

THE SUBJECTIVE SIDE

Many sick persons describe more discrete disturbances
which were previously neglected by the clinical diagnosis.
as also reported by Chapman (3), Freedman (4) and Huber
(1), these self-perceived deficiencies are frequent. On
the basis of descriptions collected by us which originated
from the patient themselves, we constructed a questionnaire which required only a simple recognition and therefore did not overtax the patients. (L.Süllwold (5))
(Example from 103 items: I often cannot differentiate
correctly between noises and hear everything as if mixed
together.) In an initial study, this was presented to
200 clinical patients diagnosed as schizophrenic and to
200 healthy persons as control group. The questionnaire
fulfilled the statistical quality criteria which are
required for such prodecures and separated with a high
degree of significance between the patient and the
healthy control group. These results were confirmed in
a replication study with 263 cases and the statistical
characteristics obtained were almost identical. The fact
that such self-perceived disturbances with schizophrenia
patients represent a regularly distributed feature was
confirmed by further follow-up investigations. The
descriptions were immediately understood in this clinical
group but they were easily misinterpreted by those not
suffering from schizophrenia.

Classified according to phenomenal features, the
deficiencies concern thought processes, speech, memory,
perception and motoric processes. The sick persons attempt
to reduce the disturbances by intensified self-monitoring
of their own behaviour. Even simple routine activities
therefore require high concentrative strain. The observed
losses produce anxiety in many patients which leads to
avoidance actions. Activities are consciously restricted.
A factor analysis led 4 dimensions well capable of
interpretation and clarified over 70 % of the variance:

  1. The loss of automated processes concerns apart
     from the motoricity also simple thought and speech
     acts, these must be controlled consciously.

2. Optical, acoustic and proprioceptive perceptions are impaired by irritating disturbance phenomena.

3. Emotional reactions are each time negatively shaded and dedifferentiated. (Anhedonia)

4. The patients experience a no longer controllable profusion of ideas and stimulations.

Patients with formal thought disturbances and patients who are clinically still unimproved indicate more subjective disturbances.

If the patients can recognize with the aid of these disturbances that functional disturbances occur with overstrain, the uncanniness of this psychosis is alleviated since the observed phenomena represent only deviations in degree from healthy persons. The insight that possible self protection methods exist for critical situations, however, imparts a certain amount of control. The "small disturbances" are therefore a useful basis for communication with the patient.

References

1. G. Huber: Reine Defektsyndrome und Basis-Stadien endogener Psychosen. In: Fortschr. Neurol.Psychiat. 34:409 Stuttgart (1966)

2. L. Süllwold: Schizophrenie Verlag Kohlhammer Stuttgart (1983)

3. J. Chapman: The early symptoms of schizophrenia Brit. J. of Psychiat. 112: 225 (1966)

4. G.J. Freedman: The subjective expierence of perceptual and cognitive disturbances in schizophrenia. Arch.Gen.Psychiat. 30: 333 (1974)

5. L. Süllwold: Symptome schizophrener Erkrankungen Verlag Springer Heidelberg (1977)

THE VIENNESE CONCEPT

OF ENDOGENOMORPHIC AXIAL SYNDROMES

P.Berner, E.Gabriel, H.Katschnig,

B.Küfferle, and G.Lenz

Psychiatric University Clinic, Vienna, Austria

The development of the Vienna endogenomorphic
schizophrenic and cyclothymic axial syndromes as research criteria for endogenous psychoses is based on
the results of a follow-up study on paranoiac patients
by Berner (1). He was able to demonstrate that part of
these patients were suffering from a clear schizophrenic
or manic-depressive disorder at the time of reexamination. Further catamnestic studies on paranoiac patients
as part of the Lausanne Survey (2) gave rise to the
formulation of criteria enabling an attribution to these two diagnoses. The term 'axial syndromes' for these
criteria was derived from the term 'axial symptoms'
coined by Hoche (3). They were called 'endogenomorphic'
(the adjective used formerly, 'endomorphic' was abandoned to avoid confusion with Sheldon's physical types), to emphasize their use as research criteria
and not as nosological classifications. The criteria
were defined in 1969 and underwent several modifications
as a result of experience gained in their use.

What were the reasons behind the creation of this
research instrument, and which hypotheses were taken
into account for their formulation? The reasons were
twofold: firstly, the systems of the Bleulerian and
Schneiderian schools, until then generally used in
German-speaking countries, left some dissatisfaction
concerning their modalities of diagnostic attribution
and lack of clearly and systematically definable criteria. Secondly, the Vienna criteria were to investigate the hypothesis that both the aforementioned schools

often attribute cases to schizophrenia which really
may belong to cyclothymia (used synonymously for major
affective disorders) or other illnesses.

As to the hypotheses, the first one is founded on
the theoretical concept of 'basic disturbances' of the
Bleulerian school, whereby on the one hand associational disturbances, manifesting themselves as formal thought
disorders, and on the other hand affective blunting are
considered to be central symptoms for schizophrenia.
The second one takes into account Janzarik's (4) concept of basic dynamic constellations in endogenous
psychoses. This concept has provided a theoretical
explanation for the unspecificity of atleast part of
the 'classic' schizophrenic symptoms.

Janzarik designated as 'dynamic' a fundamental
realm embracing affectivity and drive, which is contrasted with the 'psychic structure' containing behaviour patterns and representations (cognitive notions),
both inborn and acquired largely throughout the developmental period. Parts of this structure become 'dynamically invested' meaning that they are connected
with positive, negative, or ambivalent feelings. Those
markedly invested or 'dynamically loaded' parts of the
structure are called 'values' and comprise the 'value
structure'.

'Dynamics', however, are not entirely tied to
structural elements. Everybody has at his disposal a
certain amount of 'free floating dynamics', subject to
alterations called basic dynamic constellations. When
attaining a level of morbidity, these modifications
correspond either to 'dynamic depletion', seen clinically as affective blunting, or to 'dynamic derailments'.
There are three types of derailments: dynamic 'expansion', as in mania, 'restriction', as in depression,
and 'instability', characterized by rapid fluctuations
or 'swings' between the first two states.

Dynamic derailments effect an actualization of
specific values: in states of expansion, for example,
the positive elements of the structure are actualized,
while in states of restriction the negative ones prevail, since positive values find no actualization.

In states of dynamic instability, rapid changes
in actualization of differently 'invested' parts of
the structure occur, whereby 'ambivalently' invested
elements of the value structure also become conscious.

Higher levels of instability lead to 'delusional impressions', delusional perceptions, illusions and hallucinations. The rapid swings in drive, emotional resonance and affectivity are overpowering, making one feel to be at their mercy; this may explain how feelings of will-deprivation, alien influence, depersonalization and ambivalence arise.

In the light of this theory, dynamic instability appears to be the source of Schneider's first rank symptoms and a part of Bleuler's basic symptoms. Janzarik's assumption that the dynamic instability may arise in abnormal mental conditions, stemming from various origins, creates doubts as to the specifity of the phenomena.

Nosological unspecifity can also be claimed for formal thought disorder and affective blunting. These symptoms seem not to occur in manic depressive disease, so that the problem of differential diagnosis they pose may be limited to schizophrenia and illnesses of organic origin.

The third hypothesis is derived from the work of Bürger-Prinz (5) and Mentzos (6) on manic-depressive mixed states and Specht's (7) opinion that dysphoric states could constitute a special form of affective psychosis: endogenous cyclothymic disorders manifest themselves not only in the form of typical mania or depression, they can also appear in the form of dysphoria, 'unstable mixed states' (rapidly alternating changes in affectivity, emotional resonance, and drive), or stable mixed states. Whilst the latter occur rarely, unstable mixed states manifest rather frequently in the course of manic-depressive disease. The dynamic derailments lying behind these various expressions of cyclothymia are stable ones as far as mania, depression, dysphoria, and stable mixed states are concerned; unstable mixed states are labile derailments corresponding to 'dynamic instability'.

Biorhythmic disturbances hypothetically constitute a fundamental aspect of endogenous cyclothymia. Since the dynamic derailments mentioned above are nosologically unspecific, attribution to cyclothymia may only be justified when they are coupled with biorhythmic disturbances.

We will now mention the axial syndromes in detail.

Table 1
ENDOGENOMORPHIC-SCHIZOPHRENIC AXIAL SYNDROME
(Definitive: A and /or B present
Probably: only C present)

A) Incoherence (without marked pressure or retardation of thinking or marked autonomous anxiety; at least one of the following symptoms is required)

1. Blocking: Sudden cessation in the train of thought; after a gap the previous thought may be taken up again or may be replaced by a different thought.
2. Derailment: Gradual or sudden deviation from the train of thought without gap.
3. Pathologically 'muddled speech': Fluent speech, for the most part syntactically correct, but the elements of different thoughts (which, for the patient, may belong to a common idea) get muddled together.

B) Cryptic neologism (the patient does not explain their private meaning spontaneously)

C) Affective blunting (without evidence of marked depression, tiredness, or drug effect). This term includes flatness of affect, emotional indifference and apathy; essentially, the symptom involves a diminution of emotional response.

ENDOGENOMORPHIC-CYCLOTHYMIC AXIAL SYNDROME
A and B obligatory

A) Appearance of marked changes in affectivity, emotional resonance, or drive following a period of habitual functioning.
B) Appearance of biorhythmic disturbances
1. diurnal variations of mood or drive
2. sleep disturbances (interrupted sleep, early awakening, prolonged or shortened sleep)

The endogenomorphic-schizophrenic axial syndrome consists exclusively of symptomatological criteria dealing primarely with disturbances of expression. The presence of formal thought disorders is obligatory, more specifically: at least one of the symptoms of incoherence and/or cryptic neologisms. Incoherence can not be accurately evaluated when thought tempo is markedly accelerated or retarded, or if marked autonomous anxiety is present. For us, affective blunting is restricted to the sense of a global impoverishment in emotional resonance and thus in contrast to the opinion of other authors does not embrace parathymia (inappropriate affect).

Affective blunting is difficult to evaluate in the presence of psychic drug effects or of marked depression or tiredness. It may also appear in (unrecognized) somatic illnesses so that its presence alone can make the diagnosis only probable. When any of the above symptoms cannot be accurately evaluated for the reasons mentioned, their use for diagnosis must be disregarded.

On the grounds of the hypotheses mentioned above, symptoms judged to be expressions of a dynamic instability, such as first rank symptoms and some of Bleuler's basic symptoms, were excluded from the axial syndrome.

The endogenomorphic cyclothymic axial syndrome is also based exclusively on symptomatological criteria.

Obligatory are both A, the appearance of marked changes in affectivity, emotional resonance, or drive following a period of habitual functioning, and B, the appearance of biorhythmic disturbances. Of the symptoms in group A, only one is required for diagnosis. This means that the presence of mood abnormalities is not obligatory for diagnosis. On the basis of the various aforementioned affective expressions of cyclothymia, 5 cyclothymic axial syndromes have been established: a manic, depressive, and dysphoric axial syndrome and the axial syndromes of the unstable and stable mixed states.

The biorhythmic disturbances concern on the one hand diurnal variations of mood or drive and on the other hand sleep disturbances in the form of interrupted sleep, early awakening, prolonged sleep or shortened sleep. Prolonged sleep was included because it does occasionally occur in depressive phases. Difficulty in falling asleep was not included because it occurs frequently in mental disturbances of various origins.

In the simultaneous presence of the endogenomorphic cyclothymic and the schizophrenic axial syndromes, a schizoaffective syndrome is diagnosed. A hierarchical priority of either illness is thus avoided. However it can be said that a hierarchical principle concerning both functional endogenous psychoses does exist:

the presence of organicity exclude either one.

The axial syndromes for the functional psychoses were formulated for the purpose of cross-sectional diagnosis and carry no nosological connotations. A nosological weight can only be given through additional validating criteria such as illness course or genetic loading.

As a tool of research the endogenomorphic axial syndromes have proved to be of value in several investigations into the nature of psychoses in general. Some of these investigations will be dealt with in detail in other congress symposia.

References
1. P.Berner, "Das paranoische Syndrom". Monograhien aus dem Gesamtgebiete der Neurologie und Psychiatrie, 11o, Springer, Berlin-Heidelberg-New York, (1965)
2. C.Müller, "Psychische Erkrankungen und ihr Verlauf sowie ihre Beeinflussung durch das Alter." Hans Huber, Bern-Stuttgart-Wien, (1981)
3. A.Hoche, "Die Bedeutung der Symptomkomplexe in der Psychiatrie." Zbl.ges.Neurol.Psychiat. 12: 54o-551, (1912)
4. W.Janzarik, "Dynamische Grundkonstellationen in endogenen Psychosen." Springer, Berlin-Göttingen-Heidelberg, (1959)
5. H.Bürger-Prinz, "Probleme der phasischen Psychosen." Enke, Stuttgart, (1961)
6. S.Mentzos, "Mischzustände und mischbildhafte phasische Psychosen." Enke, Stuttgart, (1967)
7. W.Specht, "Über den pathologischen Affekt in der chronischen Paranoia". Festschrift der Erlanger Universität, (19o1)

PHENOMENOLOGICAL ASPECTS OF PURE DEFICIENCY SYNDROMES IN SCHIZOPHRENIA

Reinhold Schüttler

Bezirkskrankenhaus Günzburg/Abteilung Psychiatrie II der Universität Ulm
D-8870 Günzburg

The psychopathological picture of basic stages (incl.
pure residual syndromes) is determined by dynamic and
cognitive deficiencies which are experienced and communicated by the patients themselves (3).They can be
registered with the "Bonner Beschwerden- und Symptom-
liste zur Dokumentation der Basissymptome und Basisstadien" (4).Following I shall enumerate those items,
which include especially the dynamic deficiencies, the
disturbances of the general well-being; lack of energy,
resilience, vitality, persistence and patience; increased excitability and impressionability, a category which
corresponds to the lowering of the threshold of tolerance for non-specific stress.

Item 124 (I 1 a): Increased physical and psychical fatigability

The complaints are also concerned with manual, purely bodily actions and everyday - performances: "I get tired faster, I need more
rest than before." - "I am no longer as good at work as I used to
be. In between I have to rest to be able to continue. It is like a
constant psychical "to-pull-oneself-together". - "Everything strains
me in particular, much more than before, physical work wears me out,
so that I cannot keep a thought in my mind." - "Even after walking
just 100 meters, I am completely exhausted. It is even difficult
for me to put my clothes on."

Item 125 (I 1 b): Increased need for sleep

"I have to fight constantly against the desire to sleep.Even if I have been sleeping through for 8 hours, I hang around in the morning like a wet bag, and I get only alert after I have reached my usual routine." - "I have such an outstanding need for sleep, that I can rather do without food than without sleep." - "I can only stay awake till 8 o´clock, for I depend on sleep, since I am so tired."

Item 128 (I 2 a): Loss of vigour, energy, vitality, endurance, patience to learn, creative power; need to rest; listlessness

Appearing noticeably perplexed the patients try to express their loss of activity, briskness, liveliness, drive, spirit of enterprise, their general "listlessness", their decline in "creative power": "In the past I´ve had more endurance and drive than today. Staying power and energy are no longer with me". - "For the past years I have lost energy and activity. I get slower and slower." - "When I had difficult temporary work, I could not stay longer than a few hours in the morning, in the afternoon strength was gone. Drive and energy ... like I see it in others, I don´t have it any more." - "To play cards with my son is too much for me. I still have the will to do something, but my body cannot cope with it."

Item 131 (I 2 d): Intolerance of - generally present and non-specific - stress and conflicts; feeling of effort in social surroundings; inability to work under time pressure

Possibly also secondary defense and coping mechanisms as well as secondary autistic behavioral patterns are included here, like in other categories of disorders of pure deficiency: "I´d like to be in company, but this affects me and stirs me up." - "I can no longer care so much about things like to go shopping, or to go to the savings bank. That strains me too much." - "Whenever there is some sort of stress coming upon me, I am even more labile. After excitements I have always a bad phase." - "I don´t like guests, that makes me nervous and fidgety. That strains me too much, the noise, the whole fuss." - "I am disturbed by many people. I feel much better when I am alone. I am afraid of people, it just irritates me."

Item 134 (I 3 b): Lack of naivety and unaffectedness; compulsion to reflect

By this is meant a compulsion-like tendency to reflect and to ponder fruitlessly, a lack of unaffectedness often paralleling a tendency towards anancastic-phobic phenomena of derealisation or depersonalisation: "Since I am sick I need a very long time to get over something. I am forced to ponder over it again and again. Before I get to sleep or when I wake up at night,the thought ist present again instantaneously and I cannot go back to sleep." - "All times, all events turn around in the centre of my brain. I am forced to think it." - "Whenever I write a letter, and I am writing for a while and in doing so I am thinking, I have to think now, because I have to put the phrases correctly, then I am writing a bit and then there is a moment like 'turned off'. Then I say to myself, I cannot make it."

Item 136 (I 3 d): Inability to enjoy

Utterances like: "Everything is so dark", "always depressed" return frequently: "My mood is depressed. I can in no way be gay any more." - "I cannot be so glad any more, I am not capable to be glad like before. Formerly I enjoyed nature, that is no longer there, only a faint reflection. It is like something burst that was there before."

Item 137 (I 3 e): Experience of decrease of impulse; lack of inner drive; lack of spirit of enterprise

"I have to bring myself to do my work." - "The creative power is missing." - "I cannot make up my mind to do something." - "I can do everything only with disgust." - "Agility, spirit of enterprise, "esprit" are missing".

Item 138 (I 3 f): Experience of loss of feeling; sense of lack of feeling; lack of interest

"I can simply not feel the emotions, not even for my family." - "Joy does not come from the roots any more. This is no real joy. Not the way that I can laugh heartily from within." - "I have no proper feelings, I cannot cry any more and not be glad any more properly."

Item 139 (I 4 a): Disorders of general well-being and lack of performance. Tendency towards laying down; general weakness and tiredness; sense of not being allowed to exert oneself; sense of powerlessness

"I cannot do anything, I am lying in bed. I have to bring myself to care for my body". - "I get tired easily. Part of the time it works quite well, then I have no strength any more, I am exhausted." - "For the recent time I lay down mostly. After having coffee I have to lay down again till noon ... completely run down and exhausted. It goes up and down, but it is never enough to work." - "There is no comparison to previously, there is an unbelieveable tiredness, also physical tiredness."

Item 140 (I 4 b): Tendency towards coenesthetic symptoms in connection with loss of potential

"After working for a longer period of time my arms get numb. Then everything gets cramped, like dead and died off, somehow cramped. Sometimes I have a pressure in my head, then again a pressure over my ear, over the forehead and over the eyes. This sense of pressure travels throughout the body." - "While working I keep feeling a sudden pain shooting into my left side, as if someone were pushing a knife through. Then I cannot catch my breath and I think that I have to die. My heart starts beating extremely rapidly then. I feel so shaky and weak then, and this happens all of a sudden. When I lay down it passes away."

Item 142 (I 4 b): Phasic subdepressive, hypergic or hypomanic moods

"I have bouts of no desire for anything, I have to cry terribly then." - "I have often to do with melancholy, and then I have difficulty to get up in the morning. I have to force myself to get breakfast ready for my children."

Item 143 (I 4 c): Sleeping disorders

"My sleep is often poor.When I have to get up very early because of the children, I lay down again afterwards as I cannot sleep well at night. Whenever I don´t sleep through well for several nights in a row, then I get quite nervous." - "Sleep could be better. I cannot understand that, always so weak in the morning, like beaten down in the morning. I have never known this before." - "Whenever I get upset because of the children I cannot sleep and I lie awake half of the night, even if I have to exert myself too much in my plant, poor sleep, therefore I don´t do piecework any more ... cannot get to sleep immediately, lie in my bed awake for an hour... take sleeping pills only very rarely."

Item 144 (I 4 d); Central-vegetative disorders

Under this item there are 47 different vegetative single phenomena described by the patients with sufficient accuracy. Among the vegetative cardiovascular disorders paroxysmal tachycardia and brady-cardia, sensations of dizziness and disturbance of equilibrium are the most frequent ones. In vegetative disorders of the digestive tract nausea, vomiting and constipation are the most prominent ones. In disorders of single vital urges there is loss of appetite and libido. Palmar and plantar hyperhydrosis occurs frequently: "I can´t even look into a newspaper, for I get dizzy,this constant dizziness never disappears. Sometimes my pulse is running like a sewing machine, it goes on like this for hours, I have to lie completely still and cannot move then." - "I perspire frequently at night, dizziness, so that I have to sit down, no real headaches, such a pressure on the forehead mainly. First of all my eyes hurt. Appetite is missing, too." - "Enormous heat, sweats and chills. While running I am perspiring so much, shortness of breath, cardiac troubles, cannot sleep at all."

Item 146 (I 4 f): Intolerance against certain foods or stimulants

"My troubles come from food, I only tolerate special food like carrots or green beans, rice and noodles; I cannot tolerate at all cucumbers, cabbage and potatoes, then I get the difficulties, I like to eat everything, I just cannot tolerate it; I also cannot tolerate coffee or coffee-substitute, I get sick to my stomach from it, I drink only pure water." - "Since getting sick I quit smoking completely, I also drink no wine, no alcohol and no coffee any more, I live like a monk, formerly I smoked a lot." - "Whenever I cannot refuse to have alcohol or coffee, with visitors for instance, then my pains also extend to the left side ... For breakfast I have only malted coffee, if possible no ground coffee, because it is not pure any more." - "I have to be on my guard against spicy food. I cannot tolerate black tea, nor hawthorn tea nor warm lemon, real coffee only very little und with much milk ... I have also to be careful with alcohol, I cannot tolerate beer, wine a little better ..." The difficulties are said to be quite variable, according to the presumed cause, either the weather or the stimulants listed.

Item 147 (I 5 a): Loss of self-confidence; sense of insufficiency; to be ashamed in front of people

"In first place my self-confidence has decreased. The disease made that I lost the feeling to be also capable to do something. Whenever others come to me who want to know something from me, then I feel insecure." - "I see negative aspects more than the positive ones in everything." - "Whenever I plan something, I think it must go wrong." - "I have less self-confidence, less self-assertiveness. Formerly I was able to assert myself much more in everything."

Item 148 (I 5 b): Sense of being sick; consciousness of being sick

"I have had a disease that has to do with nerves, and my troubles are an expression of this disease". - "Because of the disease something has stayed with me despite all efforts. Something that one cannot overcome. The surrounding don't sense that." - "I don't feel healthy yet, cannot work yet as in former times. For complete recovery I have no confidence.

Item 149 (I 5 c): Experience of change of personality or
potential reduction

"I am just worn out, I cannot manage like before the disease." -
"I cannot work any more like before. I think the disease made me
harder and firmer." - "It has never improved 100 %. Outsiders don't
notice it. I am frequenty desperate myself, though." - "When I was
well, I was much more self-confident. Before I behaved as I was ...
Today I watch myself too much. I watch not to do this and that the
wrong way."

Item 150 (I 5 d): Defense not to occupy oneself with the
disease

"To recall the past into the presence after so many years, that is
trying, that does not help me any further." - "I dislike to think
of that time, I get sick whenever I think of it, I do not like
that." - "These are things that one does not like to be reminded of,
one does not want to touch them any more, too; bad enough if one
has had something like that. Because I am reminded of everything
today, I am so upset and nervous." - "Actually this case is over
for me, I don't want to talk about it. I have taken that out of my
head, I don't want to talk about it any more now."

The pure residues in the majority of schizophrenics
which develop pure or mixed residues, namely in 75 %,
become manifest already in the 3 years after the first
psychotic manifestation.

The pure defect develops independently of psychopharmacological treatment. In 52 % the pure residues of the
Bonn-Study had already developed before 1953. Other evi-
dences for morbogenic and not pharmacogenic or psychogenic charakter of pure defect were listed in our monograph (1;2). It can, however, be assumed that the
psychopharmacological drugs and especially the long-term
medication have supported a disease-immanent tendency to
reduce the psychosis to nonlong-characteristic residues
and basic stages; especially the long-term medication has
accelerated in individual case this tendency.

Noncharacteristic prodromes, which lead to initial psychotic episodes after an average course of 3.2 years,
occur in 37 % of the sample. Phenomenologically, these
prodromes are nearly identical to the pure residues and
the reversible postpsychotic asthenic basic stages and
the free-standing outpost syndromes that precede the prodromes or the initial psychotic manifestations by an

average of 10.2 years. Outpost syndromes, which were observed in 15 % of cases, are likewise noncharacteristic
episodes that completely remit after duration of 3 days
to 4 years, in average of 5 months.

The postpsychotic reversible basic stages appear immediately after the remission of the productive-psychotic
schizophrenic manifestation and can in the cross section
picture not be differentiated by psychopathological and
psychological methods from irreversible pure residues;at
this time it is not possible to judge whether the state
is reversible or not. Only if such basic stages, which
can look more asthenic or depressive, persist contio-
nously more than 3 years, we speak of irreversible pure
residues.

The pure residuum shows during the course very different
degrees of process activtiy (3) with all transitions
form noncharacteristic to more or less characteristic
phenomena. It is no fixed permanent state, shows fluctuations, f.i. depressive and coenaesthetic phases.

It is probably no true residuum but rather a "basic process in latency" (3). Moreover, the visible syndromes
of pure residues and basic stages are codetermined by
interindividual variable mechanism of compensation and
overcoming, by manifold coping reactions.

Basic disorders (5) were also found in outpost syndromes and prodromes and reversible postpsychotic basic
stages which are phenomenological, as we have seen,almost
identical with pure residues; at least, the symptoms overlap largely.

In many courses the development goes from noncharacteristic prodromes through the characteristic schizophrenic
productive-psychotic phases to a noncharacteristic syndrome again, i.e. to pure residuum.

The noncharacteristic periods were a short time ago
either not seen and taken into consideration by the
scientific psychiatry. Really,in the majority of courses
the in the sense of traditional concepts noncharacteristic periods predominate against to the typical ones.

Just in these more or less noncharacteristic stages the
chance to find basic symptoms, which are relatively close
to the biological substrate and not modified by secondary working over, is better than in chronic psychoses
with fixed structural deformation or in florid psychoses

without the possibility of self-perception and description of the disorders by the patients themselves.

REFERENCES

1. G. Huber, G. Gross and R. Schüttler, "Schizophrenie," Monographien aus dem Gesamtgebiete der Psychiatrie, Bd. 21. Springer, Berlin-Heidelberg-New York (1979.
2. G. Huber, G. Gross, R. Schüttler and M. Linz, "Longitudinal Studies of Schizophrenic Patients," Schizophrenia Bulletin, Vol. 6, Nr. 4:592 (1980).
3. G. Huber, G. Gross, R. Schüttler and L. Süllwold, "The concept of substrate-close basic disorders and basic stages," in: "Concepts of Schizophrenia," Ed. by U.H.Peters, in press.
4. R. Schüttler, G. Gross and G. Huber, "Zum Problem der operationalisierten Dokumentation der Potentialeinbuße bei reinen Defizienzsyndromen," in: "Endogene Psychosen: Diagnostik, Basissymptome und biologische Parameter," Schattauer, Stuttgart-New York (1982).
5. L. Süllwold, "Symptome schizophrener Erkrankungen. Uncharakteristische Basisstörungen", Monographien aus dem Gesamtgebiete der Psychiatrie, Bd. 13. Springer, Berlin-Heidelberg-New York (1979).

COGNITIVE DISORDERS IN SCHIZOPHRENIC DISEASES

Gisela Gross

Psychiatric Clinic of the University of Bonn
D-5300 Bonn 1

Since the early fifties, G. HUBER had tried to find
an answer to the question which kind of disturbances of
psychic functions constitute the symptomatology of schizophrenic psychoses or precede it. Since 1957, he had developed a typology of prodromal and residual syndromes
of schizophrenic diseases based on long-term investigations of schizophrenic in- and out-patients of the
Psychiatric University Clinic of Heidelberg. A new aspect
of this typology was the emphasis of more or less noncharacteristic types of remission in the sense of "asthenic defect" or "pure defect". The psychopathological
picture of noncharacteristic stages, which prevail in
the long-term course of schizophrenic diseases compared
to typical schizophrenic periods, is characterized by
manifold dynamic and cognitive deficiencies, experienced
and communicated by the patients themselves. HUBER called
these pre- or postpsychotic noncharacteristic deficiency
syndromes, that often have a depressive, asthenic, pseudoneurasthenic or cenesthetic symptomatology, "basic stages"
and described the phenomenological aspects of these reversible or irreversible basic stages as "substrate-close
basic symptoms" (1,2; see also in 5).

Regarding the descriptions of 350 schizophrenic patients of the Bonn study with pure (202 cases) and mixed
residues (83 cases) and postpsychotic basic stages (65
cases), we ranked the frequency of occurrence of complaints and disorders in the reversible and irreversible
basic stages. In the following we describe cognitive disorders of schizophrenic diseases and want to adjust our

491

main interest to (1.) the "loss of ability to direct the thinking processes" and (2.) to the "sensorial disturbances on optic, acoustic, gustatoric and sensible field".

(1.) The cognitive disorders in a stricter sense, i.e. the noncharacteristic thinking disorders, which are not yet characteristic for schizophrenia, described by HUBER 1966 (2) as "lack of control of processes of thought" are one of the most frequent basic symptoms in reversible and irreversible basic stages. These disorders usually are registered by the patients, e.g. as impairment of thinking and attention, as loss of thoughts, forced thinking, interferences of concentration, easy distractability or disturbances of memory in the sense of forgetfulness. Contrary to typically schizophrenic thinking disorders (incoherence of thoughts and thought blocking) these disorders are only subjectively.

Patients with cognitive thinking disturbances show disorders of immediate memory, ultra-short- and short-term-memory or disturbances of remote memory and of selective recalling of experiences from the long-term store. Patients complain e.g. to be inable to remember more complicated procedures, to be more forgetful than earlier, to be incapable to learn new things or to renew their knowledges, f.i. of foreign languages. Other patients report of an incapacity to understand the meaning of words or longer sentences or numerical series by reading or listening. Or they have to write down exactly the ingredients of usual meals and have to concentrate strongly during cooking to avoid burning or wrong spices; before the disease they never had such problems. Weakness of comprehension, disturbances of receptive or expressive speech are also among these categories of cognitive disorders. The patients tell that they don't understand the meaning of more complicated sequences of words either listening to them or reading them, and therefore they are not able to follow television films with many actors or books with complicated stories.

Patient often report, that the disturbances of memory occur or worsen especially in stress-situations or in times of deteriorations in the sense of dysthymic or hypergic shallow-waves ("Flachwellen"). The interferences paraphrased by the patients as disorders of capacity to register or memorize ("forgetfulness") corresponding to disorders, described by HUBER and SÜLLWOLD as "cognitive gliding" with permanent penetration of side associations and inability of focussing the attention which is determined by accidental stimuli of the surrounding. Disturbances in the sense of interference of thoughts can be linked with a lack of actualization of experiences (4). The (compensatory) derangement of task set with a too limited spectrum of attention and rigidity belongs to disturbances of selective attention.

These disorders quite often are connected to a weakness of discrimination, e.g. an uncertainty in discriminating imaginations and perceptions, reveal in the phenomenon of ideas of obsession in mental or optic field. The patients complain f.i. to have to brood especially in early morning whether something could happen during the work or to their relatives; trivial thoughts are stuck in their head, unimportant problems occupy them for weeks and they can't think of anything else. Sometimes they tell that they are unable to control or stop these ideas. This compulsion to reflection and the incapability to stop to think these thoughts is often amalgamated with increased impressionability and lowering of the threshold of tolerance for external influences and conflicts. These symptoms occur especially in subdepressive"shallow-waves" of irreversible basic stages.

Furthermore, our patients complain that intellectual work is too exhausting. Reading or other intellectual tasks cause excitement. Especially in connection with increased efforts or stress and during impairment in the sense of dysthymic-cenesthetic depressions the ability to concentrate is deteriorated compared to the premorbid one. Others notify an increased distraction by external impressions or interferences of own thoughts. They are unable to suppress competitive tendencies or reactions or are incapable to ignore irrelevant data. An impairment of concentration power during physical or intellectual work is often connected with an abnormal physical and psychic exhaustibility and fatigability in general, a lack of stress capacity and with sensorial disturbances on optic field.

Often our patients complain of thought rushing, forced thinking or loss of thoughts. According the latter symptom, patients sometimes report that their thoughts are just as cut off. This phenomenon corresponds to the symptom - emphasized by the traditional psychiatry - of thought break off or thought blocking, the "escaping" and "blending of the thoughts" (s. in 3). Similar to it is also a blockade with suddenly pausing of thinking and unability to react, especially appearing after overstimulation and overcharging, i.e. in the sense of "impotence of impulse of motion", analogous to states of being spell-bound ("Bannungszustand" - s. in 5). Moreover, patients have an <u>impediment or retardation of thinking</u> with interference of thinking energy, thinking initiative or thinking impulse. They are unable to deal with them as fast as before the disease; exact thinking or changing over from one task to another are far more difficult. Sometimes they cannot work or decide under shortage of time.

It is most important to state that patients with reversible and irreversible basic stages perceive their own losses, suffer from them and develop <u>coping-reactions, mechanisms of defence and compensation</u>. Results of the increased sensitivity against stimuli are patterns of behaviour understandable as mechanisms of shielding, avoiding and coping; the "<u>secondary autism</u>" ("sekundärer Autismus" - s. in 5) has to be classified here, too. Autistic behaviour patterns are secondary phenomena originated by learning processes: the patients learn to what extent they may exert and charge themselves regarding working performance and social contacts and how to avoid situations with the risk of stimulation that could aggravate their symptoms, e.g. new, unaccustomed and complicated situations that are difficult to survey, are estimated to be dangerous from the patients' own experience. They retire from reality, from the contact to other people. "Secondary autism" and other coping reactions are frequent and often hard to separate from the primary basic symptoms.

<u>Decrease of psychomotoric speed and rigidity</u> can also be interpreted as mechanisms to compensate the cognitive disorders, e.g. the disorders of selective attention. The patients try to avoid everything that could evoke their disturbances and try to arrange conditions that help them to keep control. Like interference of thoughts the <u>interference of motor reactions</u> also can be seen under the common aspect of an inability to suppress rivaling tendencies to react. The lack of self-acting abilities belongs to the loss of directing processes of acting, a "loss of the way of acting" ("Verlust des Handlungsfadens"). The disturbance of interpretation of information becomes also effective in the psychomotor level. There are disabilities in motor processes, f.i. by <u>sudden blockings</u> or <u>unvoluntary movements and actions</u>. Patients who describe this, tell that they have to stop during a movement and think about its continuation or that their face doesn't show the intended expression. Trivial actions, normally done automatically, f.i. walking, clothing, phoning, intend strain adjustment of attention.

The inability to distinct between positive and negative emotional qualities, the "feeling of loss of emotion" and the "inability to be pleased", are also frequent in the asthenic basic stages. The mentioned uncertainty in discriminating imaginations and perceptions,
often in connection with no longer dirigible "inside
speaking" and transitions to thought hearing ("Gedankenlautwerden") can be related to the "loss of hierarchies
of habituation".

(2.) Like other basic symptoms as cenesthesias and
central-vegetative disturbances the disorders of perception, i.e. sensorial disturbances, also have a neurological-psychopathological transition character ("somato-
psychischer Übergangscharakter" - s. in 1). The sensorial
disturbances were observed in the first year of the schizophrenic disease in 15 % of the patients. In an even
higher degree than other basic symptoms the sensorial
disorders occur paroxysmally or phasically in transitoric
phases with a duration of seconds, hours, days or weeks
(s. in 1,2,5). Most frequent are sensorial disturbances
on optic field, special types for example are hazy, cloudy
and coloured seeing, oversensitivity to light, feeling of
beeing dazzled, micro- and macropsy, changes of perceptions on face and shape of other people or of the own
face or body (so-called mirror sign), uncertainty in estimation of distances, experiences of pseudomovements, alterations of intensity and quality of colours, metamorph-
opsy, porropsy or photopsia (photisms). A disturbance of
selection of optical perception focussed only on details
and not on the whole of an object ("Herauslösung von Wahr-
nehmungsdetails"), f.i. on a face or a house, belong here,
too ("partial seeing").

More rarely are perceptional disorders on acoustic
field with alterations of intensity or quality of noises,
e.g. hypersensitivity to sounds and noises or an augmentation of the intensity of acoustic stimuli. The patients
suffer seriously from their difficulty to tolerate noises
which irritate them and cause physical trouble; motor
hooping or running engines may produce tachycardia, even
the slamming of doors they can hardly bear. On olfactoric
or gustatoric field we see either an augmentation or diminution of the intensity of perception or an alteration
of its quality. Patients report about a hyperosmia or an
alteration of the quality of smells and tastes. Perceptional alterations on sensible field often lead to a
hypersensitivity to touches of certain regions of the
body and to disturbances of the perception of the structures of surfaces of touched objects. The patients e.g.

sometimes report that they can't tolerate hair-cutting, because it causes pains and leaves them exhausted for a whole day or more. A woman told us that the surface of her knitting-needles felt strangely altered, entirely sticky and curious.

Sensorial disturbances can be released by physical or intellectual defatigation or sleeping deficit and often occur in connection with paroxysmal or phasic dysthymic-cenesthetic depressions, central-vegetative disturbances and intolerance to some food or beverages. Alterations of perception on face or shape of other people are already phenomena leading to delusional mis-identifications of persons and perceptual founded forms of delusional perceptions (s. in 5).

Basic symptoms, as cognitive, sensorial or cen-esthetic disturbances, are explained as consequences of a disturbance of selective filtration and of re-calling of experiences from the long-term store of the limbic system. The experimental research assumes a "more diffi-cult application of stored experiences" and a "levelling of probability of occurrence of certain reactions". The basic stages reveal a marked intraindividual fluctuation that may indicate on its part fluctuating neurobiochemi-cal and/or neurophysiological disturbances. These find-ings must be followed by consequences for therapy and re-habilitation of schizophrenic patients. Treatment con-cepts based on psychological methods can help the patient to compensate distinct basic deficiencies and to re-aquire lost abilities.

References

1. Huber, G., 1961, "Chronische Schizophrenie," Hüthig, Heidelberg Frankfurt
2. Huber, G., 1966, Reine Defektsyndrome und Basisstadien endogener Psychosen, Fortschr. Neurol. Psychiat. 34: 409-426
3. Huber, G., ed., 1982, "Endogene Psychosen: Diagnostik, Basissymptome und biologische Parameter," Schat-tauer, Stuttgart New York
4. Huber, G., 1983, Das Konzept substratnaher Basissym-ptome und seine Bedeutung für Theorie und Therapie schizophrener Erkrankungen, Nervenarzt 54: 23-32
5. Huber, G., Gross, G., and Schüttler, R., 1979, "Schizophrenie. Eine verlaufs- und sozialpsych-iatrische Langzeitstudie," Springer, Berlin Hei-delberg New York

TEXT ANALYSES IN SCHIZOPHRENIC BASIC DISORDERS

Uwe Henrik Peters

Professor and Chairmann
Dpt. of Psychiatry and Neurology
University of Cologne, W.Germany

I would like to begin my contribution with a remark concerning a small observation I made at a congress. A few years ago I listened to a speech by SCHÜTTLER about uncharacteristic schizophrenic basic disorders. While listening I had the following impressions: Yes, the models he uses for his descriptions are taken from schizophrenics. This impression - although it is correct and shared by others - more or less goes against the theory of basic disorders, since the theory clearly states that basic disorders are uncharacteristic. They are disorders that schizophrenics suffer from but they are a) no symptoms of schizophrenia and b) apart from schizophrenics other people can tell about very similar experiences.

This small observation already justifies some conclusions. Apparently the "competent psychiatrist" knows rules that are typical for schizophrenia, but, however, he is only able to apply them implicitly. Indeed this signifies his experience, his competence, that he could unknowingly apply rules that he learned in his clinical experience with schizophrenics. This could not be done by a non-psychiatrist or a psychiatrist who is not yet competent.

Because this reflection is so simple yet so unusual I would like to stay with it for a moment. One of the reasons why basic disorders have been neglected is the fact that they are not considered as symptoms of th usual type. Kurt SCHNEIDER, whose reputation is based mainly on his labelling and valuation of symptoms of schizophrenia like no other, is also the one who rarely ever misses the opportunity of referring to the diagnosis of schizophrenia as having elements that cannot be expressed in words:

But outside of these symptoms (the 1st rank symptoms
of schizophrenia) a lot more else can also be regarded
as schizophrenia.

By mentioning the second rank symptoms of schizophrenia he states:

If one only has these second rank symptoms, then the
diagnosis is dependent entirely on the clinical context.

But what does the "clinical context" mean other than the application of implicit rules that the psychiatrist can not make explicit.

It is not a coincidence that I chose the term "competent psychiatrist" to correspond to Chomsky's concept of "competent speaker" which
is commonly applied to linguistics. The competent psychiatrist is
namely in the same situation as the user of a primary language. He
uses its complex system of rules without knowing them in detail and
without being able to make them explicit. The scientific task, however, consists in rendering these implicit rules in an explicit way.

Text analysis has proved to be an apt method for the solution of
this problem. Here the texts of schizophrenics are analysed according to their particularities in form and in content and naturally
also for schizophrenic symptoms. Although we have analysed and published numerous cases, it is not possible to present them in detail
here because of the shortage of available time. Only the results can
be summarized here.

1) On the whole it can be established that only very little of
what has changed and is prevalent within schizophrenics can be used
for diagnostic purposes as signs, symptoms. If the theory of basic
disorders had only this one result, namely to have shown us the wide
spectrum of schizophrenic disorders that are only irrelevant when
used within the clinical theory of symptoms, but usually constitute
the most important elements for the schizophrenics themselves, then
its practical meaning would already be extraordinary.

2) According to the text analysis none of the described basic
disorders are continually present with an individual schizophrenic.
A given disorder does not even have to be present for a very short
time - since even in a short text of the size of a manuscript page
- from a formal point of view - the disorder changes from being
present to being absent a number of times.

Although this does not correspondend to the self-perception of
the schizophrenic, it indirectly becomes clear in their statements.
For this purpose I had a look at the questionaire of SÜLLWOLD. Of
the 103 pre-formulated questions concerning basic disorders there
were 70 times formulations concerning special occasions or a reference to a temporary limitation: for example, sometimes (20 questions),
occasionally (5), often, repeatedly, repeated, frequent (14),

whenever (4), from time to time (6). With the remaining 30 formulations the schizophrenic abstracts his mental and physical state in a meta-language more or less according to the pattern, "Whenever I am thinking, I am constantly being diverted by inappropriate ideas" (sentence 13). Only with generalizations like that in the meta-language do the words "always" or "constantly" appear.

3) The fact that basic disorders only occur at particular times and certain occasions presents a serious argument against the notion of a "system disorder", or demands at least the addition of other hypotheses that may be very risky.

But according to which rules do disorders occur in the normal flow of thinking and action of the schizophrenic? Schizophrenics themselves, however, can give very little information about this. Most of these things are so far back in the past that when we speak to them about it, they are unable to recall any of the facts with the exactness we require. Or the disorder is presently acute. In this case they cannot have the disorder and at the same time speak about it coherently. Therefore the texts in which these disorders show unnoticeably are the best material for research.

Hence it follows that the formal changes are closely connected to what the speech is about, to the theme; or to express it more linguistically: That the surface-structure of the language (thinking) is disturbed in the semantic deep structure (figure 1). There are always particular themes - touched in a specific way - that lead to these changes.

Whichever these themes are has already been formulated with a striking clarity by Eugen BLEULER in 1907 when he spoke of "several thousands of individual symptoms" and stated:

that we normally find sexual roots in the symptoms of dementia praecox and only very rarely find other aspects as more or less unimportant factors...

The same theme always reoccurs with one and the same patient and is connected to specific events of life in the beginning of the psychosis, which again keeps on generating schizophrenic symptoms and basic disorders.

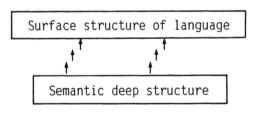

figure 1:

Instead of presenting a textual example which is not possible here, I will deal shortly with HÖLDERLIN. This famous German poet, who had so perfectly mastered the German language in his special way, was inflicted round about 1806 when he was 36 with a language schizophrenia, a schizophasia, which I think I have proved recently in a book. After that HÖLDERLIN lived another 36 years. During these decades he continued writing poetry although very little of his writing survived. This poetry gave his contempories and also the psychiatrists of his century the impression that he was schizophrenic, although there is nothing in his poetry that could be classified as schizophrenia even with the aid of a list of symptoms or a psychiatric textbook. If one uses these so-called latest poems of HÖLDERLIN for text analysis, then it shows that over the many years they contain an abundance of unusual language rules that I would call "avoidance rules". The following was to be avoided:

0 All information that concerns the inner state of the author, but also the lyrical I (ego). The word "heart" disappears completely by 1832;
0 any mentioning of the relationship between the two sexes;
0 but also love between people in the widest sense, between mother and child, between siblings, between women and men, and even love to God;
0 interpersonal relationships, for example friendship, but also hate;
0 intellectual brooding, (...) veiled symbolism (Häussermann) all hints (that can hence be misinterpreted) that might be associated with the above mentioned themes;
0 everything individual;
0 everything sacred, religious, Christian, or connected with God;
0 heroic existence;
0 beauty; female, male but also beauty in the wider sense, for example classical Greek (Bernhard Böschenstein was the first to notice this fact);
0 all words whose meaning refers to the above mentioned things in a figurative way.

All of these themes are very frequent in the earlier poems of HÖLDERLIN, as in poetry in general. But, to add this viewpoint too, the rest of HÖLDERLIN's earlier poetry themes reoccur in his so-called latest poems.

As we have have shown, these are themes that could not be mentioned or touched at all. Their absence goes hand in hand with certain formal changes. To be avoided are:

0 all imperfect rhymes;
0 all masculine rhymes;
0 all antique syllabic metres.

It is not difficult to see that these complicated rules cannot be demonstrated as an individual symptom but can only be worked out after a troublesome study of the whole corpus is accomplished. The "competent psychiatrist" - and thus we return to our initial question - nevertheless learns these rules and some others more intuitively and this is what enables him to sense the praecox feeling. Here I can only hint at the thematic background: It has to do with HÖLDERLIN's complicated attitude to homosexuality and heterosexuality which he tried to combine on a high ideal plain. At the time of the outbreak of the disease these were personified in his female friend Susette GONTARD and his male friend SINCLAIR. One may add that over the years even the most subtle hints concerning the themes he tried to avoid already led to formal contextual changes.

After all this preparation I would like to quote two lines of one of HÖLDERLIN's poems even at the risk of being misunderstood. In one of the latest poems entitled "Winter" the second stanza begins as follows:

> Just as a day of rest, thus is the ending year,
> Like a question's tone.........................

The comparison of the ending year, the beginning of winter, with a day of rest presents a "good" image. The second line increases the impression, because it begins with an image of extraordinary poetic strength. The slightly rising tone of a question arouses expectations. What could the lyrical I or ego enquire for at the end of the day, the year, in winter, and the already announced start of a new year?

Could he mean death? Life after death? Birth? Conception? At any rate it could mean something deep and emotional. But HÖLDERLIN's continuation is merely banal:

> ....
> .... and thus may be perfected.

Here we find a break in the train of thought, an incoherence that was also noticed by linguists, therefore an uncharacteristic basic disorder. This means: knowing the rules, we can discover basic disorders even in two lines of a poem from HÖLDERLIN.

Sentence 102 in SÜLLWOLD reads as follows:

> I should avoid everything that touches my feelings.

And sentence 100 reads as follows:

> I must by all means learn to shield myself better,
> otherwise I will go mad.

This touches a fear that is apparently quite justified with schizophrenics, at least according to a central European conception.

So what can be learned about basic disorders from text analyses?
They reveal that these schizophrenics elaborate a complicated strategy to avoid certain themes. Of course they do this unconsciously -
hence what they complain about (the basic disorders) is not a primary
symptom but already the result of an intrapsychic (avoiding-) process
which has escaped their self-perception. By means of interpretation
it can be shown that each concrete disturbance is a specific one,
although it cannot be used in a symptom list. And that is where the
competence of the competent psychiatrist is derived from.

References

Huber, G., G. Gross, R. Schüttler: Schizophrenie. Eine verlaufs-
und sozialpsychiatrische Langzeitstudie.
Springer-Verlag: Berlin/Heidelberg/New York 1979

Peters, U.H.: Hölderlin. Wider die These vom edlen Simulanten.
Rowohlt: Reinbek bei Hamburg 1982 (English and French translation
to be prepared)

Süllwold, L.: Symptome schizophrener Erkrankungen.
Springer-Verlag: Berlin/Heidelberg/New York 1977

NEUROLOGICAL-PSYCHOPATHOLOGICAL TRANSITION SYMPTOMS

IN SCHIZOPHRENIC DISEASES

Bärbel Armbruster

Psychiatric Clinic of the University of Bonn
D-5300 Bonn 1

INTRODUCTION

The concept of basic disorders in schizophrenia has been developed on the basis of phenomenological observation and detailed description of the experiences described by the patients and regularly occuring in postpsychotic basic stages, in prodromes, and outpost syndromes. These symptoms are noncharacteristic in the sense of the traditional schizophrenia concepts. Our concept is founded on the hypothesis that these basic symptoms are substrate-close, i.e. that they are evoked by disorders which are caused by the disease. This hypothesis is supported a.o. by the phenomenological relationship of the described symptoms and syndromes with corresponding features in defined, known brain diseases. In the following we shall describe phenomenologically the relationship of certain neurological-psychopathological transition phenomena with symptoms of defined brain diseases. In this way we refer to the descriptions of the self-perception of 202 patients of the Bonn study with postpsychotic persistent basic stages, i.e. so-called pure deficiency syndromes. With the neurological-psychopathological transition symptoms, G. HUBER (1957) has ranked disorders of body sensations, i.e. cenesthesias, motor symptoms and central-vegetative disturbances. The linkage of these symptoms is frequent and typical in the mentioned stages.

CENESTHESIAS

With cenesthesias we mean different types of disorders of body sensations which can vary rapidly in time, often occuring paroxysmally or phasically depending on physiological rhythms and periodicity. Frequently the patients describe their perceptions in comparisons and pictures. G. HUBER has distinguished three stages of body sensations: 1. Simple "hypochondrisms" as the noncharacteristic degree of intensity can hardly be differentiated from hypochondric features of neurotic disorders. 2. Cenesthesias strictly speaking experienced as abnormal, strange, and of another kind show a phenomenological relationship to thalamic sensations and are already "roughly characteristic". 3. Experiences of body sensations with the "criterion of the made" are already typical schizophrenic symptoms and caused by interpretation of the experienced basic symptom. As to development and regression of the cenesthetic phenomena, continuous transitions from stage 1 via stage 2 to stage 3 and down can be observed. Therefore, it is phenomenologically a question of flowing devolution, i.e. quantitative and/or qualitative different phenomena of the same substrate-close basic disorder. Only the step from the quantitative to the qualitative character which we can notice by the strangeness transfers to the psychopathologically characteristic and finally typical schizophrenic end-phenomena. In the following we will demonstrate by some examples the transition sequence of these phenomena and their phenomenological relationship to neurological disorders.

According to G. HUBER, type 1 of cenesthesias are "sensations of numbness, stiffness and strangeness of the own body and with the feeling of non-existence of organs and limbs" (somato-psychic depersonalization). The patients often complain that an arm or a leg is numb or it feels stiff. These sensations occur paroxysmally, partially released by physical or psychic strain, often in connection with dysthymic mood, and can persist for seconds, minutes or even longer. Daily fluctuations can be observed, too. - "Especially in the morning I used to have a permanent drawing in the neck region combined with dizziness in my head." - The feeling of the non-existence of parts of the body could be interpreted as aschematia, as it were the opposite of phantom-limb pains. - "I have the feeling as if my head would be filled and the other limbs would be not existent at all." - Also the circumscript sensations of single organs seem to be similar to thalamic caused phantom-limb sensations: "I feel my heart quite isolated like a muscle, the heart works his own way as if it would be separated from my body." - If these sensations are referring to the head, the transition to the disorders of ego-experience will be understandable, and from the quality of the sensation combined with the resulting process of explanation and interpretation dynamically derivable. This interpretation is especially obvious if the cenesthetic sensation occurs combined with a cognitive disorder which is experienced as a disorder of concentration.

The relationship of cenesthesias to thalamic spontaneous sensations is still more evident in the "circumscript pain" and "migrating sensations" (type 3 and 4) and in the "sensory, affective or sensorial released sensations" (type 12). - "In the region of the ribs there is a tension, nearly handbreadth enlarged and often occuring." "There is a traction in the shoulder running through the whole body, a feeling that something is moving from the neck to the hips." - Similar transitions from the noncharacteristic to the characteristic and typical stage can be demonstrated in all other types of cenesthetic symptoms, too.

"Sensations of becoming smaller, diminution and shrinking respectively of enlargement and dilatation" (type 9) are phenomenologically and in the experience related to the neurological symptom of aschematia: "I often have the feeling as if both parts of the body would be shifted one against the other; often the feeling as if the right leg would be shorter than the left one." - Aschematias which are perceived as swelling or diminishing of one half of the body, as shortening of one limb or as shrinking of the trunk can be observed in circumscript lesions of the thalamus. They are phenomenologically not discernible from cenesthetic disorders in basic stages of schizophrenic psychoses.

"Kinesthetic sensations" (type 10) show the transition to vestibular symptoms in which complaints about vertigo combined with the feeling of dizziness predominate: "When I am lying, I have the feeling as if I would be swinging."

The "sensation of motor weakness" (type 2) is described as a feeling of paralysis or a lame feeling and can increase to the inability to carry out an intended movement: "When I am running, my legs are lame, a kind of lame feeling, a kind of stopping." - This type of cenesthesia leads over to the motor phenomena, the impotence of impuls of motion. These phenomena, described by G.HUBER as spell-bounded states ("Bannungszustand"), are observed as sleep paralysis in narcolepsy and argue for a disturb-

ance in the area of the diencephalon. Symptomatic narco-
lepsias have been registered mainly in the train of ence-
phalitis epidemica, of malaria and of carbon disulphide
poisoning. A similar experience also is reported by patients with beginning Parkinson's disease as JACOB has
described.

MOTOR SYMPTOMS

According to L. SÜLLWOLD, G. HUBER has termed these
phenomena "interference of reactions on motor fields" and
has included them in the basic symptoms. Phenomenologically we can find similarities and correspondences of the
extrapyramidal system. In these phenomena, too, we can
follow up quantitatively different steps from the noncharacteristic over the nearly characteristic to the typical
stages.

The "loss of automated abilities" requires an increased level of attention to carry out properly every-
days motions and actions, normally done automatically. -
One patient respected as good secretary reported that she
often would make mistakes in typing since she had suffered
from the schizophrenic psychosis; that she could not type
as automatically as in former times; nowadays she would
need more attention to manage her secretary function as
well as previously. This patient experienced that the described disorder increased as soon as she had forgotten
to take her drugs.

In the case of "motor interference symptoms" intended
movements will be interrupted by suddenly occuring, not
controllable, competitive impulses of motion: "I am not
sure at all where my legs will going to, f.i. when I wish
to go to the street exit, I move in spite of that to another direction, or if I want to walk to a certain goal,
I always deviate to the right or to the left side."

Suddenly occuring, unvoluntary movements, as in
Huntington's disease, athetotic-like movements or jerky,
ballistic-like rotary motions of the limbs, a paroxysmally
occuring grimacing or perioral hyperkineses, a hoarse and
monotonous voice combined with a general bradykinesia, an
increased tonus, a post-encephalitic-like seborrhea remind
of corresponding disorders of the extrapyramidal system.
Such as in defined brain diseases, the patients percept
the impuls of motion without being able to influence it.

Visual spasms, also existing in extrapyramidal disorders, are characterized by a self-percepted and voli-

tionally not or hardly interruptable deviation of the bulbs upward like a dystonic movement. A fine nystagmus on deviation and a tic of an eyelid occur often in addition. This disturbance partially starts with forced thinking, and can be combined with productive-psychotic phenomena. In our opinion this disturbance therefore is a phenomenon of stage 2 changing to stage 3 and argues in favour of a high degree of process activity. - "At the beginning my thoughts get all mixed up, so that I am not able to form an idea. This state can last some hours. Then my eyes rise automatically and then the hearing of voices starts off." - In this case we could observe that the patient's eyes deviated up to the right and he seemed to be extraordinary anxious. Phenomenologically similar visual spasms can be observed in lesions of the diencephalon just as in extrapyramidal syndromes as extrapyramidal paroxysms often lasting for minutes or hours.

Tic-like hyperkineses, complete coordinated movements and trembling attacks are subsumed phenomenologically to the catatonic hyper-symptoms, i.e. to the expression symptoms in a wider sense according to K. SCHNEIDER, and are therefore already likely characteristic phenomena.

All these motor phenomena are characteristic as to the expectation that they are based on a symptomatic or endogenous psychosis, but they are not specific. This phenomenological relationship or identity can be observed as one evidence that these basic symptoms are substrate-close. Therefore, they are real symptoms, that means hints at a pathological process, a pathological change of brain function.

CENTRAL-VEGETATIVE DISORDERS

Central-vegetative disorders can be registered during active psychotic manifestations as well as in outpost syndromes, prodromes and postpsychotic basic stages as far as these stages show a sufficient degree of process activity. The episodic, often paroxysmal occurrence and a swing between hyper- and hypofunction is characteristic. These disturbances, too, indicate an involvement of the diencephalon. Paroxysmal tachycardia, bradycardia or tachypnoe, juvenile hypertension, hyper- and hyposalivation, nausea and vomiting, disorders of the day-and-night-rhythm, of thermoregulation, and of single vital drives have to be mentioned here. The different types of central-vegetative disorders occur phenomenologically identical in defined brain diseases as well as in endogenous psychoses: Analogous symptoms can be released by stimulation of corresponding areas in the diencephalon, as has been demonstrated already 1925 by W.R. HESS (s. G. HUBER 1957). The central-vegetative symptoms are substrate-close basic symptoms, too, and furthermore an evidence for the presumption that schizophrenia are caused by disorders of brain function. We suppose that these disorders are localized in the limbic system in a wider sense, particularly because central-vegetative disorders occur together with other basic symptoms.

CONCLUSION

These neurological-psychopathological transition symptoms are all unspecific regarding to the diagnosis and are during the psychotic manifestations covered up by the amalgamation with the "anthropological matrix", that means they result in typical schizophrenic superstructure and end-phenomena. Therefore, it must be our future task to examine patients in postpsychotic basic stages especially with regard to these symptoms and to follow up patients with prepsychotic prodromes and outpost syndromes. These symptoms have been neglected by the different concepts because they are relatively noncharacteristic, and not usuable for the diagnosis in the traditional sense. But they do indicate on the basis of their substrate-closeness more distinctly to the disorder in the prephenomenal-somatic field than it is done in a clearly marked, acute or chronic schizophrenia. Therefore, it is our opinion that certain somatic investigations in the more or less characteristic phases with stage 2-symptoms are more promising and can be carried out more successfully than in typically psychotic manifestations. Relations to neurochemical and EEG parameters can be expected most likely in basic stages with marked process activity. In our team we try to make possible the survey of these more or less characteristic basic symptoms and to prove them in a rating scale.

References

Huber, G., 1957,"Pneumencephalographische und psychopathologische Bilder bei endogenen Psychosen," Springer, Berlin Göttingen Heidelberg
Huber, G., 1983, Das Konzept substratnaher Basissymptome und seine Bedeutung für Theorie und Therapie schizophrener Erkrankungen, Nervenarzt 54: 23-32
Huber, G., Gross, G., and Schüttler, R., 1979, "Schizophrenie. Eine verlaufs- und sozialpsychiatrische Langzeitstudie," Springer, Berlin Heidelberg New York

DISTURBANCES OF AWARENESS AND "BASIC SYMPTOMS" OF A SENSORY KIND

Karl Koehler and Heinrich Sauer

Psychiatric University Clinic
Voss Strasse 4
6900 Heidelberg
West Germany

In a large-scale investigation, carried out in 1972, Gross and Huber[1] systematically studied certain perceptual -or sensory, as they called them- abnormalities found in 757 schizophrenic patients admitted to the Schneider-oriented University Clinic in Bonn, West Germany. At some time in the course of their illness, usually at the beginning, 106 (14%) experienced unusual visual, auditory, olfactory, or gustatory phenomena. Symptoms in the visual area occurred most often, being reported by 82 (77%) of the 106 probands. Since there was difficulty in satisfactorily classifying all the visual sensory disturbances found, Gross and Huber for the most part restricted them-selves to presenting a few dramatic "Prägnanztypen" of the phenomena at issue. For example, these included: micropsia, macropsia, meta-morphopsia, porropsia, increased intensity of color vision, blurred vision, the perception of facial changes in looking in a mirror or at others and so on. In other words, Gross and Huber's concept of "basic symptoms" of a sensory kind were almost exclusively refer-ble to Jaspers'[2,3] chapter dealing with disorders of the awareness of objects as outlined in his "General Psychopathology."

Most recently, Huber[4] pointed out that the uncertainty or in-ability of differentiating between memory and phantasy imagery might also be regarded as a "basic symptom"; this disturbance had not be-longed to those "basic symptoms" of a sensory type investigated ear-lier[1]. As for Jaspers[2,3], he definitely considered experiences invol-ving abnormal imagery and false memory as disorders of the awareness of objects. Furthermore, although not formally classified in terms of a "basic symptom" of a sensory kind, the vague delusional mood (vage Wahnstimmung) also appears to be seen by Huber[4] as yet another characteristic type of disorder from this group of phenomena. This is of no little importance in the context of the present discussion since the delusional mood clearly has close psychopathological ties to Jaspers'[2,3,5] concept of delusional awareness (Wahnbewußtheit). And delusional awareness is in turn certainly related to the issue of the confusing psychopathological status of the "leibhaftige Bewußtheit" or the sense of presence, one of the Jasperian central disturbances of the awareness of objects[2,3]. The classification, however, of this latter phenomenon is by no means resolved.

In Jaspers' writings the word "leibhaftig" was unfortunately used differently in different places[6]. For example, Jaspers stated that the general quality of truly perceiving something with the five exteroceptive senses -the very quality he meant by "leibhaftig"- was, paradoxically, lacking in the case of the "leibhaftige Bewußtheit." In this context, then, the "Leibhaftigkeit" he was referring to was really only of a "pseudo" sort. In addition, the quality of being really "close by", that is, the proximate nature of that which the patient is falsely aware of or actually has an awareness of without there being any true perceptual basis was another most important feature of the "leibhaftige Bewußtheit" emphasized by Jaspers. Yet this essential aspect is usually either not recognized or, when recognized, not given more prominence in most definitions. Thus, the "leibhaftige Bewußtheit" or the sense of presence should more precisely be referred to as a deception involving the non-perceptual awareness of a proximate presence, or, in shorter form one might speak of a deceptive or false proximate awareness.

The major psychopathological differential described by Jaspers with respect to the "leibhaftige Bewußtheit"[2,3,5] seemed to involve the phenomenon of the delusional awareness (Wahnbewußtheit) mentioned earlier. This distinction primarily hinged on the separation of the features of proximity and non-proximity, which are associated with false awareness experiences, from one another. Thus, his definition of the delusional awareness stressed the awareness of someone not close by, that is, not in the immediate proximity. One could refer to this experience as the non-perceptual and non-imagined awareness or sense of a non-proximate presence. Most clinicians, however, would probably simply speak of a delusion in such instances due to this very quality of non-proximity, especially if the content should also be "non-understandable"[2,3]. However, even an awareness phenomenon in the previously defined sense of the false proximate awareness or "leibhaftige Bewußtheit" would also be simply and globally sized up as a delusion by most. In other words, the false awareness and the "leibhaftige Bewußtheit" are not focused upon, much less are any further phenomenological distinctions between the two seriously considered, by the majority of clinicians.

In addition, Jaspers[5] warned against interpreting the false proximate awareness in terms of an illusion. Although based on remembered earlier sensations and perceptions in a so-called primary manner, he

speculated that the phenomenon did not involve sensations or perceptions capable of being misperceived or misidentified. Jaspers, in this
connection, spoke of the so-called "pure form" of the false proximate
awareness (reine leibhaftige Bewußtheit). Yet he also admitted that
a phenomenon of this kind at times could occur on the basis of some
meager sensory material (leibhaftige Bewußtheit mit spärlicher sinn-
licher Repräsentation). Thus, Jaspers appeared to view the false
proximate awareness more in terms of a group of phenomena that could
be hypothesized as being located at different points on a continuum.
And on this continuum there would be transitions in one direction
to pseudo-hallucinations, in another to illusions and true hallucinations, and lastly, transitions could also be found to false non-
proximate awareness as well as to other delusional phenomena.

It would appear reasonable, then, if one accepts what has been
said thus far, to conceptualize most false proximate awareness phenomena in terms of a sensory or perceptual disorder. That is, the experience of the pure form of false proximate awareness, as hypothesized by Jaspers[5], probably occurs much more infrequently -if it ever
truly occurs- than the similar awareness phenomenon Jaspers had assumed to be grounded in so-called unnoticed sensation. It most likely
would be difficult if not impossible to test hypotheses regarding
the genesis of different assumed types of false proximate -as well
as non-proximate- awareness phenomena. For clinical descriptive
purposes, however, such considerations are not really important.
Yet of practical worth might be the act of arbitrarily classifying
the experience of false proximate awareness among the "basic symptoms" of a sensory kind in Huber's[4] sense. Perhaps in so doing more
interest might be finally focused on and more effort expended towards
detecting all phenomena demonstrating an awareness quality of some
type, sharpening their operational criteria, and determining their
frequencies.

REFERENCES

1. G. Gross and G, Huber, Sensorische Störungen bei Schizophrenien,
   Arch. Psychiat. Nervenkr. 216:119 (1972).
2. K. Jaspers, "Allgemeine Psychopathologie," Springer, Berlin-Heidelberg-New York (1965)
3. K. Jaspers, "General Psychopathology," J. Hoenig and M. Hamilton,
   translators, Manchester University, Manchester (1963).
4. G. Huber, Das Konzept substratnaher Basissymptome und seine Bedeutung für Theorie und Therapie schizophrener Erkrankungen,
   Nervenarzt 54:23 (1983).
5. K. Jaspers, Über leibhaftige Bewußtheit (Bewußtheitstäuschungen),
   ein psychopathologisches Elementarsymptom, Zschr. Pathopsych-
   olog. 2:157 (1913).
6. F. Kräupl-Taylor, On pseudo-hallucinations, Psychol. Med. 11:
   265 (1981).

ANXIETY STATE AND DEPRESSIVE DISORDERS: SEPARATION IN TERMS OF

SYMPTOM-CLUSTER, PATIENT-GROUPS AND PERSONALITY FEATURES

D. Caetano, M. Roth, and C. Mountjoy

Department of Psychiatry, Clinical Medical School
Cambridge University
Cambridge CB2 2QQ - U.K

INTRODUCTION

Since the recognition of anxiety as a syndrome in 1871 by Da-Costa[1] there have been disagreements about the relationship between anxiety state and depressive illness. These disagreements are concerned with two viewpoints: one that brings anxiety along the same continuum with depression[2-4], and another that states that there is a relevant difference between depressive and anxiety states[5-7]. The former approach represents a unitarian view[8,9], while the latter one postulates a categorical model[10]. With the development of computer technology sophisticated statistical techniques became feasible and have been applied to tackle the problem of classification of affective disorders. Although some of these investigations[11-13] favor the unitarian view, the great majority, however, have consistently shown that anxiety and depressive state, despite some overlap, constitute two distinct syndromes[10,14-20]. However, there is still some confusion in the nomenclature used to nominate the affective disorder where anxiety and depressive symptoms are combined. This is exemplified by the current concept of "anxious depression" used by many psychiatrists.

The separation of groups of patients exhibiting the syndromes of anxiety state and depressive disorder, rather than the separation of these syndromes themselves, is of great practical importance for the study of psychophysiological measures and personality factors that may contribute to the development of these disorders. Attempts at separating groups of patients have previously been made by Prusoff and Klerman[21], Roth and co-workers[10,22,23] and more recently by Mountjoy and Roth[20]. Roth and colleagues obtained a good separation between anxiety and depressive states by means of discriminant func-

tions. However, in neither study was the patients' overall discriminant score distribution formally tested, which might raise the question as to whether these two groups only represent extremes of a single normal distribution (unitarian view).

Bearing that in mind, the present enquiry was undertaken with
the purpose of investigating whether within the clinical material of
affective disorders dominated by anxious or depressive features or
exhibiting a blend of both forms of mood disturbance, anxiety and
depression are separable in terms of: I) symptom-clusters; II) patient-groups; III) personality measures. Accordingly, three hypotheses were put forward: I) that within this clinical material there
are two distinct syndromes corresponding to anxiety and depression
respectively; II) that the patients exhibiting the syndromes under
enquiry (I) fall into two clear-cut separated groups; III) that any
discrimination between groups of patients achieved with the aid of
the enquiries under I) and II) would be independently validated by
self-rating personality measures.

Patient-sample and Data acquisition

The sample comprised 150 acute in-patients of either sex suffering from a primary mood change to depression and/or anxiety. The pa-
tient-sample ranged in age from 30 to 80 years, with a mean of 46.7
(SD+16);36.2% of the patients were below 40 years, 47.2% between 40
and 64, and 16.4% equal or above 65 years. The patients' age distribution was normal and women outnumbered men by a ratio of approximately 2:1.

The patients' mental state was assessed within the first week
of admission to hospital by means of the Present State Examination
(PSE)[24] and their personality was independently assessed by means of
the Maudsley Personality Inventory (MPI) and the Cattell 16PF (form
C), after recovery from illness.

Clinical Diagnostic Groups

At the end of the clinical enquiries and before the analysis of
the patients' personality profiles, each patient was allocated to
one of the three clinical diagnostic groups tentatively defined as
follows: 1) Depressive disorders (N=105). Patients were assigned to
this group if they had been depressed during the past month and/or
at interview, i.e. if they had a positive score on item 23 and/or
121 of the PSE. It comprised endogenous and neurotic depressives.
2) Anxiety state (N=41). This group was tentatively defined by a, b
and c: a) anxious mood (i.e. a positive score on PSE item 120);
b) at least two out of the six features: 1. free-floating autonomic
anxiety; 2. panic attacks; 3. situational autonomic anxiety;
4. autonomic anxiety on meeting people; 5. specific phobias, 6. anxiety avoidance. c) absence of marked and persistent depression

during the past month and/or at interview (i.e. the patient should not have a score of 2 on PSE item 23 and/or 121). 3) Doubtful group (N=4). This group comprised patients who failed to fit into one the above groups. It was mainly constituted by anxious patients who failed to satisfy criterion "b" of the group Anxiety state. The validity or otherwise of these hypothetical groupings were investigated with the aid of multivariate statistical techniques.

Results

A principal component analysis performed on the intercorrelation matrix of the PSE 42 items yielded two main components. The first one accouting for 15.4% of the total variance was bipolar and contrasted anxiety and phobic symptoms at the positive pole with depressive symptoms at the negative one. The highest positive loadings were for Anxiety avoidance (.72). Observed anxiety (.71), Autonomic anxiety on meeting people (.68), Situational autonomic anxiety (.62), Free-floating autonomic anxiety (.59), Panic attacks (.59), Specific phobias (.58), Tension pain (.55), and Muscular tension (.54). Obsessive symptoms (.36). Irritability (.30), Depersonalization (.28) and Derealization (.24) also had highly significant loadings. High negative loadings were for: Observed depression (-.59), Depressed mood (-.56), Subjective retardation (-.43), Morning depression (-.37), Retardation (-.34), and Early waking (-.33). Pathological guilt (-.20) and Agitation (-.20) also had significant loadings. Component I clearly corresponded to an anxiety versus depression dimension.

Component I was rotated to Varimax, Quartimax and Equimax criteria. The factor pattern remained practically unchanged. Standardized factor-score with mean 0 and standard deviation 1 were computed for each case and plotted along unrotated and rotated component I. Neither of the overall patients' factor-score distributions departed appreciably from normality.

Fig. 1 shows the factor-score distribution of the clinical diagnostic groups along unrotated component I (anxiety-depression). The depressed patients tended to concentrate at the negative (depressive) end of the continuum, while the anxious ones were on the positive (anxiety) end of the same continuum; the four uncertain cases are also represented. Patients with anxiety state were thus broadly separated from those with depressive disorders. However, the overall patients' factor-score distribution when checked by Least Squares Fit failed to indicate any bimodality. Nevertheless, the exam of this distribution shows that there is a reasonable degree of separation between the tentative clinical diagnostic groups, which justifies the use of these groups in the attempt to improve further the discrimination between subjects with anxiety state and depressive disorders. That was accomplished with the aid of discriminant function analysis.

Table 1 - Discriminant Function Analysis I: standardized discriminant function coefficients and group means scores

Symptom	Coefficient
Observed anxiety	.64
Anxiety avoidance	.40
Muscular tension	.30
Situational autonomic anxiety	.28
Aut. anxiety on meeting people	.25
Obsessive symptoms	.21
Free-floating aut. anxiety	.19
Observed depression	−.47
Tension pain	−.34
Morning depression	−.26
Self-depreciation	−.23
Hysterical symptoms	−.17
Agitation	−.17
Guilty ideas of reference	−.13
Diagnostic group	Group mean score
Depressive disorders	−1.50
Anxiety state	3.55

Discriminant Function Analysis

Before the discriminant function analysis was actually performed, the dimension (anxiety-depression created by component I (Fig. 1) was used as a criterion of the accuracy of the clinical assignment of patients to the groups of anxiety state or depressive dirsorders. Accordingly, a cut-off point was placed where the groups overlapped least (0.5); (Fig. 1), thus defining two exclusive regions of anxiety and depresssion. Eight cases of depressive disorders fell within the anxiety region and four cases of anxiety state fell within the depression region. These 12 cases were considered "misclassified" and together with the four cases for which a clinical diagnosis could not be made were omitted in the first step of the discriminant function analysis. That left 134 definitive cases, of which 39 suffered from anxiety state and 95 from a depressive disorder.

Table 1 presents the 14 variables selected by the stepwise procedure and their standardized coefficients which correspond to the relative contribution of each variable to the discriminant function. Negative weights are associated with depressive disorders and positive ones with anxiety state. The two group means on the discriminant function are shown in the lower part of the Table. The mean of the group of depressive disorders is about 1.5 standard deviations away from zero point (the grand mean) of the function while that of anxiety state is 3.5 standard deviations away the same point but in the opposite direction, and the two group means are 5 standard deviations away from each other.

516

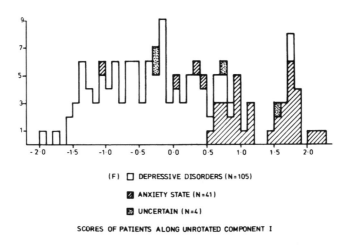

(F) ☐ DEPRESSIVE DISORDERS (N=105)

▨ ANXIETY STATE (N=41)

▧ UNCERTAIN (N=4)

SCORES OF PATIENTS ALONG UNROTATED COMPONENT I

Fig. 1

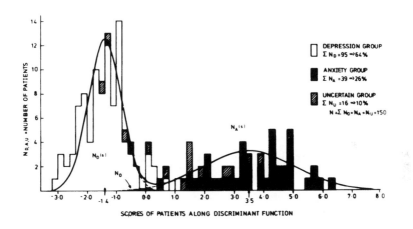

Fig. 2 Discriminant Function Analysis I: Frequent distribution of patients' scores with the "best fit" superimposed on it (dashed curves). This is composed of two normal curves with means of −1.4 and 3.5, respectively.

The group separation is more clearly shown in Fig. 2, where the overall patients' discriminant function scores, including the 16 doubtful cases omitted in the first step of the analysis, is displayed. Superimposed on the sample distribution are frequency curves of the "best" fitting normal distribution. The fit of the theoretical to the actual data distribution was tested by means of X^2, "goodness of fit". The small expected frequencies at the tails of the distribution were combined. The integration of the expected frequency was 149.6 which corresponds well with the 150 observed cases. Altogether there were 22 cells giving 19 degrees of freedom. $X^2 = 27.13$; $20 > p > .10$.

Thus the difference between expected and observed frequencies is small and non-significant at the 10% level. That lends statistical support to the hypothesis that the theoretical distribution, which is indeed composed of two Gaussian curves (one with mean of -1.4 and standard deviation of .57, and the other with mean of 3.5 and standard deviation of 1.55), describes well the sample distribution. It shows that patients suffering from anxiety state come from one population and those suffering from depressive disorders from another.

Personality Measures

Personality inventories were included in the enquiry later on. The present data refer to 89 subjects with a definitive diagnosis of Anxiety state (N=30) or Depressive disorders (N=59) who completed both the MPI and the 16PF after recovery from illness. A discriminant function analysis carried out on the patients' self-ratings on these tests showed that the patients' overall discriminant score distribution did not depart appreciably from normality; however, the two groups of anxiety state and depressive disorders tended to occupy opposite parts of distribution. A cut-off point placed where the groups overlapped least defined two exclusive regions of anxiety state and depressive disorders. Accordingly, out of the 59 cases of depressive disorders, 8 (13.6%) fell within the anxiety region; and 6 out of the 30 cases of anxiety state (20%) fell within the depression region. The overall classification rate was 84.3% (75 out of 89).

That means that 84.3% of the patients assigned to the groups of Anxiety state or Depressive disorders, on the basis of their current symptoms, were also assigned to these same groups on the basis of independent personality measures.

Discussion

In this paper the clinical material has been examined only in terms of two broad groups of anxiety state and depressive disorders. Further sub-divisions within these two groups have been examined with aid of cluster analytic techniques and the findings will be reported later.

A principal component analysis both before and after rotation to Varimax, Quartimax and Equimax criteria, yielded a bipolar component which contrasted two clusters of symptoms corresponding to anxiety state and depressive disorders, respectively. A similar anxiety-depression factor has been consistently identified in various samples with different sex ratios and making use of a number of different techniques for ratings of the symptoms[10,14-20]. The present study, thus does not stand alone when showing that anxiety state and depressive states, despite some overlap, constitute two distinct syndromes.

Owing to similarities in the kind of patients and symptom-items utilised, the findings from Roth et al.[10] and Mountjoy and Roth[20]'s studies are of special interest for comparison with the present one. Despite some methodological differences, the clusters of symptoms corresponding to anxiety state and depressive disorders depicted by these studies were very similar. Thus, Panic attacks, Autonomic manifestations of anxiety, Phobias, Muscular tension, Depersonalization. Derealization, Obsessive symptoms, and Irritability, all emerged in the three studies as heavily loaded on the phobic-anxiety syndrome, while Depressed mood, Persistent depression, Morning depression, Retardation and Early waking, were at the core of the depressive syndrome. In Roth et al.'s study, Delusion was also among the depressive symptoms, whereas in the present one, perhaps owing to the relative rarity of this symptom, it did not have a significant loading; Pathological guilt and Agitation emerged instead. The symptom "Anxiety avoidance" had in the present study the largest loading on the phobic-anxiety syndrome which is in good agreement with findings reported by Fleiss et al.[25] and Derogatis et al.[19]. Roth et al.[10] and Mountjoy and Roth[20] did not include this item in their studies.

These symptoms could be used as clinical criteria for the assignment of patients to either group of anxiety or depressive state. A clearer delineation between these syndromes would provide better guides for further refinement of the classification of affective disorders as well as for biological markers, drug prescription and other forms of scientific enquiries.

A reasonable separation of patients with anxiety state and depressive illnesses was obtained by Roth et al.[10], and Mountjoy and Roth[20]. However, the patients' discriminant function score distributions were not formally tested. In the present study the overall patients' score distribution was fitted with two Gaussian curves and the fit was actually checked by means of X^2, afterwards. The result showed that patients suffering form anxiety state come from one population while those suffering from depressive disorders come from another.

The separation of the affective population into groups of subjects with anxiety state and depressive disorders was submitted to further validation by means of independent personality measures. A discriminant analysis on the patients' self-ratings on the MPI and 16PF showed that 84% of the subjects assigned to the groups of Anxiety state or Depressive disorders on the basis of their current symptomatology were also assigned to these same groups on the basis of their personality features.

Although procedures such as i) reasonable subject variable ratio, ii) accurate assignment of the subjects to the groups before the discriminant function was actually carried out, and iii) minimization of bias and halo-effect; were taken in order to make a replication of the present findings possible, these procedures, however, should not rule out completely the necessity of cross-validation on a second set of data, preferably collected by an independent investigator.

Notwithstanding this, the independent personality data here reported together with genetic and family studies, response to treatment, course and outcome, already give support for the clinical differentiation between the categories of anxiety state and depressive disorders. Hence, genetic and family studies indicate that there is a genetic factor in determining the predisposition to anxiety state, while neurotic depression seems to lack such a factor. Moreover, this genetic factor is more or less specific to anxiety state and unrelated to depressive disorder[26-32]. Further support for this differentiation is given by therapeutic response presented by these two groups. Thus, depressive disorders as a whole respond well to electroconvulsive therapy (ECT)[33] or tricyclic compounds[33-44], while anxiety state responds less favourably[42, 45-47] and may even get worse after ECT[48]. On the other hand, anxiety state responds favourably to MAOI and/or benzodiazepines[47,49-55], whereas depressive disorders show a feeble response to these drugs[39,43,57-60].

Investigation of the course and outcome of affective disorders provides other independent criteria for the validation of the phenomenological distinction between anxiety state and depressive disorders. Follow-up investigations suggest that anxiety state has a poorer outcome than depressive disorders[61-73], that the diagnosis of anxiety state is stable over time[66], and that diagnostic crossover between the two illnesses is exceptional[73].

In conclusion, althought it is desirable to have a cross-validation before definitive conclusions may be drawn, the phenomelogical differentiation between anxiety state and depressive disorders achieved in this study with the aid of multivariate statistical tecniques has already been validated by independent genetic and family studies, response to treatment, course and outcome.

Acnowledgements

One of the author (D.CAETANO) would like to thank the Conselho Nacional de Desenvolvimento Cientifico e Tecnológico (CNPq) (Brasil) for its financial support of this research.

REFERENCES

1. J.C.Nemiah, Anxiety Neurosis, in: "Comprehensive Textbook of Psychiatry, "A.M. Friedman, H.I. Kaplan, B.J. Sadock, eds., Williams
   & Wilkins Company, USA (1976).
2. S. Freud, Inhibitions, Symptoms and Anxiety, in: "Complete Psychological Works, Vol. XX, Hogarth Press, London (1959).
3. H. Harris, Anxiety: its nature and treatment, J. Ment. Sci 80:482
   (1934).
4. M.E.P. Seligman, "Helplessness on Depression, Development, and
   Death". W.H. Freeman and Company, San Francisco (1975).
5. E. F. Buzzard, Discussion on manic-depressive psychosis, Brit.
   Med. J: 2:877 (1926)
6. T. A. Ross, The Cassel Hospital Seventh Annual Report. Cited in
   C. H. Rogerson, The differentiation of neuroses and psychoses
   with special reference to status of depression and anxiety, J.
   Ment. Sci: 86:632 (1940)
7. G. Germany, "Anxiety states", Brit. Med. J. 1:943 (1956).
8. E. Mapother, Opening paper of discussion of manic-depressive psychosis, Brit. Med. J. 2:872 (1926).
9. A. J. Lewis, Melancholia: a clinical survey of depressive states,
   J. Ment. Sci 82:488 (1934).
10. M. Roth, C. Gurney, R. F. Garside, and T.A. Kerr, Studies in the
    classification of affective disorders: the relationship between
    anxiety states and depressive illnesses, Brit. J. Psychiat. 121:
    147 (1972).
11. H. J. Eysenck, Classification and the problem of diagnosis, in:
    "Handbook of Abnormal Psychology" H. J. Eysenck, ed., Pitman
    Medical Publishing Co., Ltd., London (1960).
12. J. Mendels, N. Weinstein, and C. Cochrane, The relationship be-
    tween depression and anxiety, Arch. Gen. Psychiat. 27:649
    (1972).
13. R. C. Benfari, M. Beiser, A. H. Leighton, and C. Mertens, Some
    dimensions of psychoneurotic behavior in an urban sample, J.
    Nerv. Ment. Dis. 155:79 (1972).
14. M. Hamilton, A rating scale for depression, J. Neurol. Neuros.
    Psychiat. 23:56 (1960).
15. M. Lorr, and R.M. Hamlin, A multimethod factor analysis of behav-
    ioral and objective measures of psychopathology, J. Consult.
    Clin. Psychol. 36:136 (1972)
16. E. S. Paykel, Classification of depressed patients: a cluster
    analysis derived grouping, Brit. J. Psychiat. 118: 275 (1971).
17. E. S. Paykel, Predictions of treatment response, in: "Psycho-
    pharmacology of Affective Disorders", E.S. Paykel, H. Coppen,
    eds., Oxford University Press, Oxford (1979).
18. R. M. Mowbray, The Hamilton Rating Scale for Depression: a factor
    analysis, Psychol. Med. 2:272 (1972).
19. L. R. Derogatis, R.S. Lipman, L. Covi, and K. Rickels, Factorial
    invariance of symptom dimensions in anxious and depressive neu-
    roses, Arch. Gen. Psychiat. 27:659 (1972).

20. C.Q. Mountjoy, M. Roth, Studies in the relationship between depressive disorders and anxiety states, Part 2 (Clinical items), J.Affect. Dis. 4:149 (1982).

21. B. Prusoff, G. L. Klerman, Differentiating depressed from anxious neurotic out-patients, Arch. Gen. Psychiat. 30:302 (1974).

22. M. Roth, The phobic anxiety-depersonalization syndrome, Proc. Roy. Soc. Med. 52:587 (1959)

23. C. Gurney, M. Roth, R. F. Garside, T.A. Kerr, K. Schapira, Studies in the classification of affective disorders: the relationship between anxiety states and depressive illnesses-II, Brit. J. Psychiat. 121:162 (1972).

24. J. K. Wing, J. E. Cooper, N. Sartorius, "The Measurement and Classification of Psychiatric Symptoms", Cambridge University Press, Cambridge (1974).

25. J. L. Fleiss, B. J. Gurland, J. E. Cooper, Some contribution to the measurement of psychopathology, Brit. J. Psychiat. 119:647 (1971)

26. R. G. McInnes, Observations on heredity on neurosis, Proc. Roy. Soc. Med. 30:895 (1937).

27. F. W. Brown, Heredity in the psychoneuroses, Proc. Roy. Soc. Med. 35:785 (1942).

28. M. E. Cohen, D. M. Badal, A. Kilpratick, W. Reed, P.D. White, The high familial prevalence of neurocirculatory asthenia (Anxiety neurosis, Effort syndrome), Amer. J. Hum. Gen. 3:126 (1951).

29. P.L. Broadhurst, The biometrical analysis of behavioural inheritance, Sci. Prog. Oxf. 55:123 (1967).

30. E. Staler, V. Cowie, "The Genetics of Mental Disorders", Oxford University Press, London (1971).

31. R. Jr. Noyes, J. Clancy, Anxiety neurosis: a 5-year follow-up. J. Nerv. Ment. Dis. 162:200 (1976).

32. R. R. Crowe, D. L. Pauls, D. J. Slymen, R. Noyes, A family study of anxiety neurosis. Morbidity risk in families with and without mitral valve prolapse, Arch. Gen. Psychiat. 27:659 (1980).

33. C. Gurney, M. Roth, T.A. Kerr, K. Schapira, The bearing of treatment on the classification of the affective disorders, Brit. J. Psychiat. 117:251 (1970).

34. R. Kuhn, The treatment of depressive states with G 22355 (imipramine hydrochloride), Am. J. Psychiatry 115:459 (1958).

35. J. R. B. Ball, L.J. Kiloh, A controlled trial of imipramine in treatment of depressive states, Brit. J. Psychiat. 2:1052 (1959).

36. L. J. Kiloh, J. R. B. Ball, Depression treated with imipramine: a follow-up study, Brit. Med. J. 1:168 (1961).

37. C.G. Burt, W. F. Gordon, N.F. Holt, A. Hordern, Amitriptyline in depressive states: a controlled trial, J. Ment. Sci: 108:711 (1962).

38. R. S. Master, Amitriptyline in depressive states, Brit. J. Psychiat. 109:826 (1963)

39. M. E. Martin, A comparative trial of imipramine and phenelzine in the treatment of depression, Brit J. Psychiat. 109:279 (1963).

40. A. Hordern, C. J. Burt, W. F. Gordon, N.F. Holt, Amitriptyline in depressive states: six-month treatment results, Brit. J. Psychiat. 110:641 (1964).
41. Medical Research Council, Clinical trial of the treatment of depressive illness, Brit. J. Psychiat. 1:881 (1965).
42. J. E. Overall, L. E. Hollister, M. Johnson, V. Pennington, Nosology of depresssion and differential response to drugs, J. Am. Med. Assoc. 195:946 (1966).
43. D. W. K. Kay, R.F. Garside, T. J. Fahy, A double-blind trial of phenelzine and amitriptyline in depressed out-patients. A possible differential effect of the drug on symptoms, Brit. J. Psychiat. 123:63 (1973).
44. L. Covi, R.S. Lipman, L.R. Derogatis, J. E. Smith, J.H. Pattison, Drugs and groups psychotherapy in neurotic depression, Am. J. Psychiatry 131:191 (1974).
45. E. S. Paykel,Depressive typologies and response to amitriptyline, Brit. J. Psychiat. 120:147 (1972).
46. E. S. Paykel, D. Haskell, H. Dimascio, Clinical response to amitriptyline among depressed women, J. Nerv. Ment. Dis. 156:149 (1973).
47. D. V. Sheehan, J. Ballenger, G. Jacobsen, Treatment of endogenous anxiety with phobic, hysterical, and hypochondriacal symptoms, Arch. Gen. Psychiat. 37:51 (1980).
48. E. D. West, P. J. Dally, Effects of iproniazid in depressive syndromes, Brit. J. Psychiat. 1:1491 (1959).
49. W. Sargant, P. Dally, Treatment of anxiety states by antidepressant drugs, Brit. Med. J. 1:6 (1962).
50. D. Kelly, W. Guirguis, E. Frommer, N. Mitchel-Heggs, W. Sargant, Treatment of phobic states with antidepressants: a retrospective study of 246 patients, Brit. J. Psychiat. 116:387 (1970
51. L.E. Hollister, J.E. Overall, A.D. Pokorny, J.Shelton, Acetophenazine and diazepam in anxious depressions, Arch. Gen. Psychiat. 24:273 (1971).
52. D.S. Robinson, A. Nies, L. Ravaris, K.R. Lamborn, The mono-amino oxidase inhibitor, phenelzine in the treatment of depression- -anxiety states, Arch. Gen. Psychiat. 29:407 (1973).
53. L. Solyom, G.F.D. Heseltine, D.J. McClure, C. Solyom, B.Ledwidge, G. Steinberg, Behaviour therapy versus drug therapy in the treatment of phobic neurosis, Can. Psychiat. Ass. J.: 18 (1973).
54. P. Typer, J. Candy, D. Kelly, Phenelzine in phobic anxiety: a controlled trial, Psychol. Med. 3:120 (1973).
55. A. Raskin, J.G. Schulterbrandt, N. Reating, T.H. Crook, D.O. Rockville, Depresssion subtypes and response to phenelzine, diazepam, and a placebo: results of a nine hospital collaborative study, Arch. Gen. Psychiat. 30:66 (1974).
56. J. A. Harris, A.A. Robin, A controlled trial of phenelzine in depressive reactions, J.Ment. Sci: 106:1432 (1960).
57. J.T. Hutchinson, D. Smedberg, Phenelzine (Nardil) in treatment of endogenous depression, J.Ment. Sci: 106:704 (1960).
58. E.H. Hare, J. Dominian, L. Sharpe, Phenelzine and dexamphetamine

in depressive illness: a comparative trial, <u>Brit. Med. J.</u> 1:9 (1962).

59. C. Mountjoy, M. Roth, A controlled trial of phenelzine in anxiety, depressive and phobic neuroses, in: "Excerpta Medica International Congress Series", J. R. Boissier, H. Hippius, P.Pichot, eds. (1974).

60. A.F. Schatzberg, J.O. Cole, Benzodiazepines in depressive disorders, <u>Arch. Gen. Psychiat.</u> 35:1359 (1978).

61. W.L. Neustatter, The results of fifty cases treated by psychotherapy, <u>The Lancet</u> 1:796 (1935).

62. J.A. Harris, The prognosis of anxiety states, <u>Brit. Med. J.</u> 2:649 (1938).

63. E. O. Wheeler, P.D. White, E.W.Reed, M.E. Cohen, Neurocirculatory asthenia (Anxiety neurosis, Effort Syndrome, Neurasthenia). A twenty-year follow-up study of one hundred and seventy-three patients, <u>J. Am. Med. Assoc.</u> 142:878 (1950).

64. R.Blair, J.M. Gilroy, F. Pilkington, Some observations on out--patient psychoterapy with a follow-up of 235 cases, <u>Brit. Med. J.</u> 1:318 (1957).

65. H.H.W. Miles, E.L. Barrabee, J. E. Finesinger, "Evaluation of psychotherapy with a follow-up of 62 cases of anxiety neurosis", <u>Psychos. Med.</u> 13:83 (1951)

66. L. Eitenger, "Studies in neuroses", <u>Acta Psychiat. Scand.</u> Suppl. 101 (1955).

67. K. Ernst, "Die prognose der neurosen "Cited in Greer (1969) The prognosis of anxiety states, <u>in</u> "Studies of Anxiety", M.H.Lader, ed., <u>Brit. J. Psychiat.</u> Special Publication N⁰ 3 (1969).

68. H.S. Greer, The prognosis of anxiety states, in: "Studies of Anxiety" M.H. Lader ed., Brit. J. Psychiat., Special Publication N⁰ 3 (1969).

69. H.S. Greer, R.H. Cawley, "Some observations on the natural history of neurotic illness", Australian Medical Publishing company, Sydney (1966).

70. M. Raskin, J.W. Rondestuedt, G.Johnson, Anxiety in young adults: a prognostic study, <u>J. Nerv. Ment. Dis.</u> 154:229 (1972).

71. T.H. Kerr, M. Roth, K. Schapira, C. Gurney, The assessment and prediction of outcome in affective disorders, <u>Brit. J. Psychiat.</u> 121:167 (1972).

72. R. Jr. Noyes, J. Clancy, Anxiety neurosis: a 5-year follow-up. <u>J. Nerv. Ment. Dis.</u> 162:200 (1976).

73. K. Schapira, M. Roth, T.A. Kerr, C. Gurney, The prognosis of affective disorders: the differentiation of anxiety states from depressive illnesses, <u>Brit. J. Psychiat.</u> 121:175 (1972)

ANTHROPOLOGICAL ASPECTS AT JEALOUSLY

Kalle Achté and Taina Schakir

Department of Psychiatry
University of Helsinki
SF-00180 Helsinki 18, Finland

Considered on the individual level, jealousy is often based on feelings of insufficiency and inferiority. A predisposition to it generally develops as a result of childhood conflicts, associated either with the oedipal triangle situation or sibling rivalry. Jealousy may also reflect the individual's own infidelity wishes, in such a way that these are denied and the partner is blamed for them (1). Sometimes, latent homosexual trends or an unconscious wish to get rid of the beloved one may form its background. In these cases, wishes that the individual does not dare to admit even to himself have been transformed into jealous suspicions and fears.

Not only individual-level factors but also social factors bear on the experiencing of jealousy. A threat to the individual's self-esteem gives rise to jealousy, but the situations forming such a threat differ, depending on the individual's environment. Values and ideals, and people's possibilities of living up to them vary greatly from one culture to another. The attainment of a good social position, for example, may prerequire the acquisition of wealth, its display and its distribution or use in the pursuit of other values (4).

In the sexual area the reputation of a male may depend on his number of sexual partners or, as among the Manus, on the number of temptations he has successfully resisted. Micronesian males proudly compare the scars caused to them by reluctant women with their shark-tooth knives. As for women, chastity is appreciated in many cultures, but, in some cases, women are expected to show activity in pre-marital relations. For instance, the ancient Natchez Indians thought that a very chaste virgin would not find a firm foot-hold on the bridge leading to the spirit world. The accomplishments that the norms of a community may demand of an individual in order to gain the apprediation of other people may vary indefinitely. Yet, whatever they demand, an individual's self-esteem is in jeopardy unless he is able to behave in the way they require (4).

Jealousy that has its origin in the narrowness of the norms dictating the ideals of a culture can be regarded as purely culture-determined. On the east coast of Africa, for instance, where girls of marrigeable age have to live, according to the local custom, in the "Fatting House" for months, a girl who remains lean will be in a socially unfavourable position and is likely to experience herself as failure. The same applies to a Bush Negro in Ghana who doesn't know how to carve: girls will sneer at him and the rest of the community will accept him only grudgingly. Some individuals always depart from the norms set, and in most cases just they are prone to jealousy (4).

The social causes of jealousy may also be associated with membership of some particular group of people. How easily the members of a community are likely to meet situations liable to shake their self-esteem depends in a large measure on the social system of the community. A system where there are inequalities in social position based, say, on radical, economic or religious differences between groups of people is conductive to insults and jealousy. Likewise, a society in which social and family life unavoidably leads to conflicts of interests is favourable soil for them. The practice, for instance, that the daughters of the family have to get married in order of age will often cause jealousy which can very directly be traced to social factors (4).

Since a negative value is attributed to jealousy, there is reason, when various cultures are compared, to stress, with Mead (4), the difference between jealousy and positively valued zeal. She employs the word 'zeal' to refer to a live interest in the pursuit of some personal or social goal and in its maintenance on it has been attained. On the other hand, an effort to defer one's own position fearfully and angrily amounts to jealousy. What is involved thereby does not mean protection of the individual's natural rights but, instead, a worried fight against breach of rights sanctioned by society. In some cultures, the male shows laudable zeal by taking several wives in order to increase this prestige.

But an impotent owner of a harem who devotes himself to watching over his wives, instead of allowing them to keep lovers, is simply jealous. Jealousy is always an unpleasurably tinged emotion apt to cause pain. In a love relationship it is not an indication of the depth of affection but, mostly, an indication of the insecurity of one or the other of the parties.

JEALOUSY IN POLYGAMOUS SOCIETIES

In various communities, the members' right to own their spouses have been violated and altered in numerous ways. We may well assume that polygamy and other practices with simply sexual relationships of the members of the community with more than one partner are apt to arouse jealousy. The observations made by researchers of communities where such social arrangements are part of everyday reality suggest, however, that people's attitude toward them is often quite calm. These observations demonstrate, on their part, how complex a phenomenon jealousy is and how it is intertwined with the totality of the community's mores, beliefs and values.

The data collected in trans-cultural studies definitely supports the view that there is a connection between jealousy and self-esteem. In cases where the sharing of the sexual partner with others amounts to an injury to the individual's self-esteem - as a result of, e.g., the liberties taken by the partner himself - it easily gives rise to jealousy. But insofar as it adds, according to the views held in the community, to the person's social prestige and his self-confidence, such problems will not necessarily arise.

Only some 16 per cent of the world's population lives in communities which are purely monogamous. Both pogyny and, though more rarely, polyandry are met with in various cultures (5). Under exceptional conditions a group of men may live together with a number of women, in group marriage. Even where polygyny is permissible, it need not necessarily be generally practised. In primitive cultures, where it chiefly occurs, only few men are in a position to maintain more than one woman. In a polygynous society, a man's social prestige is related to his number of wives. An Eskimo man, for example, usually has one wife, but men who are more well-to-do than others or aspire for prestige may marry several wives. The Bushmen the Kalahari typically have one wife, but a man who is particularly well-off may also marry another. In Australia too, an aboriginal male who is more influential than others can be recognized by his having two wives (3).

In communities where men of influence generally have several wives, women may also be, in conformity with local views, for polygamy (4). A woman might even feel very humiliated if she were her husband's sole spouse, since such a state of affairs would not be good for the family's social prestige. When polygamy is an accustomed practice, it need not insult the first wife, and in many instances the decision to marry a second wife is taken jointly by the married couple (3). It not infrequently happens that the wife, urges her husband to marry other wives, because this would increase her own self-esteem by offering her the rank of chief wife. At the same time, it would provide the household with labourers and child beaers. A case has been recorded where a woman hailed her husband into court because she had been married to him for three years and borne him two children, and he had not yet taken another wife. The native court obliged the husband to rectify the situation within six months (4).

In polygamous families, wives are usually said to be on good terms with one another. Among the Wabenoes, in Tanganyka, wives may even get allied against their husband and unanimously keep their love affairs secret to him (3). It doesn't seem self-evident, however, that harmony is always safeguarded, particularly not if all the family members live together, as a so-called joint family. The wives may feel that they have to compete for their husband's attention and affection and their interrelationships are characterized by at least potential conflicts and rivalry (2). According to Westermarck, the fact that the wives live peacefully together is often simply a consequence of the husband's strict discipline, a long-standing custom and the advantages that polygyny brings to them (6).

It is known, for example, that, among certain India tribes and the aborigines of Ghana, the wife sometimes commits suicide when her husband takes another wife (6). In communities where people believe in witchcraf wives easily accuse one another of practising black magic. Such accusations may lead to homicide and suicide. The word for concubine in the language of the Central African Ruanda people actually means jealousy (2). It has been said that a Charruas woman will leave her husband if she finds another man who will take her as his wife (6).

As a matter of fact, the instability of a polygynous family unit has been allowed for institutionally in most cultures where polygyny occurs. The husband is supposed to show attention evenly to his wives. There is usually a clear-cut hierarchy among the wives, so that the status of each considerably differs from that of all others, which prevents them from being sufficiently equal to compete with one another (2). In order to preserve peace in the family, all the wives may be taken from the same series of sisters. Attempts are often made to avoid discord by placing the wives to live separately from one another (6).

Comparable means of control are connected with polyandry which has been found to occur in Tibet and in some parts of India, and occasionally, everywhere on the sides of the Himalayan Mountains facing to India. If a woman has several husbands, they are usually brothers of one another. Detailed rules regulate the husbands' rights to approach their common wife (3). Moreover, in a polyandrous household, more than one man is infrequently simultaneously at home. For instance, the husbands of a Nairs woman, who may number even twelve, are known to get well along with one another, since each of them will in turn cohabit with the wife (6).

The custom prevailing in some cultures that another man has firsti access to a man's wife may or may not give rise to feelings of jealusy. The man will revolt against this practice if it humiliates him. During the ancient régime, the French peasant had reason to resent it, since his seigneur's jus primae noctis underscored the peasant's social impotence, and he did not have any soothing philosophy to console himself. On the other hand, if such a custom is one accepted by the community, the young husband may be less concerned with the girl's ordeal than with the possibility of her not being a virgin.

In a society where wife lending is considered natural and a husband who wants to possess his wife alone is regarded as stingy, a man expects his wife to willingly meet the quest's demands (4). It has been supposed that wife lending and prostitution indicate the absence of jealousy, but, in their own contexts, such customs do not imply the absence of jealousy more than other ways of showing hospitality imply the absence of proprietary feelings ( ). In some cultures, the married couple's common interests simply requires infringement of their mutual proprietary rights - in the form of wife lending, for example, or as a part of a religious ceremony (4). However, adultery has to be under the husband's control. Among the aborigines of New South Wales, a man was frequent ready to give one of his wives to a friend but was likely to be very jealous and to resent any freedom taken by other men with their wives (6).

It seems that, as a rule, the husband will permit sexual relations between his wife and other men only as an act of hospitality or friendship or in order to gain some advantage. Negro husbands have used their wives for entrapping other men and making them pay a heavy fine. The Cree Indians have not regarded adultery as a crime, provided that the husband has received sufficient consideration for his wife's prostitution; and, in Nukahiva, men sometimes offered their wives to foreigners in order to get iron or other European article (6). Men have usually been unwilling to haggle about the exchange value of women. For example, in North-East Siberia a group of men, numbering twelve at most, might contract an exchange marriage, which meant an agreement on reciprocal rights to the wives of one another; however, unmarried men and men differing greatly in age from other members were not welcomed to join the group (3).

Man is inclined to feel jealous more or less exclusively of his equals. The jealous individual compares himself with other people. In order for such a comparison to have significance for his self-esteem, the other individuals in question have to resemple him sufficiently. The aborigine of Australia, for instance are more jealous of the members of their own tribe than of white men and will more commonly prostitute their wives to strangers than to their own people. The Negroes of Benin were very jealous of their own country men but not in the least of European foreigners, and the same has been stated to hold true of the Sandwich Islanders (6). A dark coloured native will undoubtedly experience an European as quite distant and, therefore, a situation or rivalry will seem impossible to him. Jealousy will also be avoided if the rival is considered to come out the loser in the comparison. A British upper-class woman was not jealous if her husband had a relation with a woman representing a lower social class, whereas a mistress belonging to the same class as herself made her feel jealous.

REFERENCES

1. Achté, K.A., Alanen, Y.O. and Tienari, P., 1981, Psykiatria. 4th edit. WSOY, Porvoo-Helsinki-Juva.
2. Beattie, J., 1976, Other Cultures. Routledge & Kegan Paul Ltd., London.
3. Davies, A., 1948, Mating and marriage customs, in: Man and His Life the World Over. Ohhams Press, Long Acre-London.
4. Mead, M., 1931, Jealousy: Primitive and civilized, in: Woman's Coming of Age, S.D. Schmalhausen & V.F. Calverton, eds., Horace Liveright, Inc., New York.
5. Sarmela, M., 1979, Johdatus yleiseen kulttuuriantropologiaan. Ihminen ja yhteisöt cross-cultural -tutkimuksen valossa. Suomen Antropologisen Seuran monisteita 2. Helsinki.
6. Westermarck, E., 1891, The History of Human Marriage. MacMillan and Col., London.

PARANOID-HALLUCINATORY FUNCTIONAL PSYCHOSES IN LATER MIDDLE AGE

Vilho Mattila

Psychiatric Policlinic of the Turku University
Central Hospital
Kiinamyllynkatu 4-8, 20500 Turku 50, Finland

INTRODUCTION

The findings presented here are based on a broader study,[1] in which the etiology of functional psychoses in individuals of middle age was investigated from a social-psychiatric and psychodynamic point of view. The purpose of the present paper is to draw comparisons between paranoid-hallucinatory and affective psychoses of later middle age and between paranoid-hallucinatory patients and the general population of the same age.

Recent research on narcissism has opened up new possibilities for the understanding of psychoses and for integrating psychodynamic insights which previously were relatively unorganized. Kohut[2] and Kernberg[3,4] described the so-called narcissistic personality disorder, which is more severe than ordinary neurosis but milder than psychosis; this personality disorder is characterized by emotional constriction and grandiose fantasies associated with a greater-than-average vulnerability of self-esteem. Kernberg has in fact suggested that it is precisely narcissistically disturbed individuals who are particularly susceptible to severe mental disturbance in later life, since they need continuous external support to their self-esteem.

SUBJECTS

The patient body studied consisted of 74 consecutive

Turku cases aged 45 to 64 who had been admitted to the mental hospital during the study period for the first time for functional psychosis. For the purposes of this report two groups were formed out of these patients: one with paranoid-hallucinatory (N=28) and one with affective (N=29) psychosis, excluding from consideration the 'mixed' or atypical cases.

For each patient, a control born in the same year and of the same sex was randomly selected from the population register. Of these 74 controls, however, twelve refused the interview. The research method consisted of an extensive semistructured psychiatric interview. In the case of the patients, interviews were also carried out with family members, primarily spouses and children.

The consideration of the prepsychotic development of the patients and their somatic and psychosocial predisposition is confined to the period beginning at the age of 15 years and ending five years prior to entry into the study, which is equivalent to the hospital admission. In the case of the controls this period is better called the 'period of adolescence and adulthood', and is defined as ending five years before the hospitalization of the corresponding patient. The precipitating factors playing a part in the illness were studied for the five-year period preceding hospitalization.

RESULTS

The role of somatic predisposing and precipitating factors cannot be dealt with here.

Psychosocial Predisposition

The marital-status distribution of the patients did not clearly differ from that of the controls. The proportion of single persons was only slightly higher in the paranoid-hallucinatory group than in that with affective psychosis and in the control group. The same held also for the social class distribution: differences between the study groups were quite small.

The interviews, however, showed that the marriages of the patients were clearly less often successful than those of the controls. Likewise it turned out that patients had had fewer friends and leisure activities and that they had shown less sexual activity than controls. Both the social and the psychic total development had been clearly poorer in the patients than in the controls already during the period of adolescence and adulthood.

The prepsychotic personality disorder of the patients had been clearly more severe than the personality disorder of the controls during the corresponding period. Only slightly under one third of the patients but over two thirds of the controls had been clinically healthy during the period of adolescence and adulthood.

The occurrence of a history of a narcissistic personality disorder in subjects is shown in Table 1. A clear difference was found between patients and controls. The diagnostic groups did not differ in this respect. It thus seems that narcissistic problems play a fundamental role in all functional psychoses of later middle age.

Table 1. Occurrence of narcissistic disorders in subjects in period of adolescence and adulthood (%)

	Patients		Controls
	Paranoid-hallucinatory psychosis N 28	Affective psychosis N 29	N 62
No pathological narcissistic traits	-	-	37
Mild/suspected narcissistic disorder	32	31	44
Evident narcissistic disorder	68	69	19

A narcissistic disorder usually implies two things: (1) The psychic equilibrium of the narcissistically disturbed individual usually rests on a very narrow basis, his psychologic defence system is fragile, and he is therefore in danger of being overwhelmed by uncontrolled inner conflicts. (2) Such an individual therefore needs other persons or other objects, to replace what might be called the gaps in his psychic structure. Both these aspects are evident in the following case history.

Case A, a widow, had been an illegitimate child and had early formed a highly symbiotic relationship with her mother. After leaving home in adolescence she gradually drifted into promiscuity and at 23 into marriage with an alcoholic.
The patient's marriage was throughout chaotic,

due to her husband's drinking and to her continuous marital infidelity and attempts at illegal abortion. A daughter and then a son were born in the marriage. The patient developed a very close relationship with her daughter. In the interview, the latter felt that her mother had tried to delegate to her her own failed and unrealistically grandiose ambitions. The mother told her daughter about her sexual adventures and attempted abortions trying to make her into accomplice.

In some cases the narcissistic disorder took the form of a cold and dominating attitude toward other family members and toward other people in general. Features found more commonly than these, however, were massive dependency problems and an obsessive need to work and sacrifice oneself for others in order to gain a sense of personal worth. The following case is an example of this.

Case B, a housewife with five children, had experienced her childhood home as insecure and hostile. She was therefore married as early as 18, with unrealistic hopes. Her husband turned out a severely disturbed, dominating and jealous alcoholic.

The patient described having been extremely fond of her children; she said she particularly liked young children and taking care of them. She was sterilized 13 years prior to hospitalization. After this she long dreamt of adopting a child, but gave it up due to her husband. She did not in any way try to keep her children from becoming independent, although she felt it to be hard for herself. The family was chaotically schismatic. The mother and the children allied themselves against the frightening father. In this sense too the children were important to the mother's psychic equilibrium.

Potential Psychosocial Precipitating Factors

Since the operationalization of psychosocial precipitating factors is very difficult, they were classified on the one hand as exactly definable factors occurring in general independently of the subject, i.e. 'objective' factors, and on the other hand as more diffuse, i.e. 'subjective' factors, the recall and encoding of which were in considerable measure dependent on the subject's memory, or which were provoked by the subject. The occurrence of potential precipitants is shown in Table 2.

Table 2. Psychosocial precipitants as cumulative percentages

	Patients		Controls
	Paranoid-hallucinatory psychosis N 28	Affective psychosis N 29	N 62
Objective psychosocial precipitant			
During last yr	21	41	19
During last 5 yrs	46	79	63
Subjective psychosocial precipitant			
During last yr	57	83	13
During last 5 yrs	93	100	53

The potential precipitating factors generally did not involve exceptional adversity; rather these events presented a new developmental challenge for the patient. They nevertheless turned out to be crucial due to the fact that the patients were exceptionally vulnerable to such new experiences. Due to the age in question, these factors fairly often consisted of losses. The precipitants were often specifically narcissistic traumas, through which they thus lost the support on which their psychic equilibrium had rested.

The following examples shed further light on the nature of narcissistic traumas and the dynamics of illness onset.

Case A, described above, began to display paranoid symptoms for the first time after her husband's death. A few years after that she retired from work due to her somatic diseases. The most important precipitant preceding the hospitalization, however, was the effort made by her daughter toward greater independence in connection with her own divorce, when she refused any longer to act as a support for her mother.

Case B was admitted to the mental hospital due to paranoid schizophrenia when the last child was leaving home. The patient was left unoccupied and isolated, and increasingly dependent on her frightening husband. Now that she no longer had her children to wait on, she lost the safeguard of her self-esteem and the allies she had had against her husband.

The dynamics of the illness onset was of this type in many of the cases of paranoid-hallucinatory psychosis and in almost all the cases of affective psychosis; in the former, however, the dynamics relatively often were not quite clear. The crucial psychic trauma could also be a somatic illness.

DISCUSSION

In the light of this study, narcissistic problems seem to form the main basis for susceptibility to psychoses of later middle age. The role of heredity, on the other hand, seemed relatively limited and nonspecific.[1]

In both diagnostic groups, most precipitating events were losses in character. Losses have generally been considered to be associated with the onset of depression. On the basis of the present study, it may be concluded that in later middle age losses and the consequent depressive mechanism play a crucial role in the dynamics of paranoid psychoses as well. The question why some developed a psychotic depression and others a paranoid-hallucinatory psychosis could not be answered.

REFERENCES

1. V. Mattila, "Onset of Functional Psychoses in Later Middle Age," doctoral dissertation, manuscript, Turku University (1983).
2. H. Kohut, "The Analysis of the Self," Int. Univ. Press, New York (1971).
3. O. F. Kernberg, A psychoanalytic classification of character pathology, J. Am. Psychoanal. Ass. 18: 800-822 (1970).
4. O. F. Kernberg, Further contributions to the treatment of narcissistic personalities, Int. J. Psychoanal. 55: 215-240 (1974).

PSYCHOSOCIAL CONSTELLATIONS IN DEVELOPING PARANOID PSYCHOSES

Christoph Mundt

Psychiatrische Universitätsklinik
Voßstraße 4
D-69oo Heidelberg

The discussion of the pathogenesis of delusion has been controversial even polemical in psychiatry since Karl Jaspers. In the tradition of the Heidelberg School of psychopathology the claim of the non-understandability of the delusional perception made by Jaspers and Gruhle was connected with the process-hypothesis of schizophrenia. Thus following their lead, Kurt Schneider[1] distinquished real delusional experiences from ideas of reference which have a sufficient emotional basis to make them understandable. According to him this meant that there was an absolute cut-off point between a schizophrenic psychosis and an abnormal reaction. It is well known that this postulate of non-understandability led to much controversy with - among others - the Tübingen School as represented by Gaupp and Kretschmer. They had described paranoid developments by trying to reveal their inner logic and to make them psychologically understandable. If we analyse the empirical findings and hypotheses regarding psychosocial influences on the pathogenesis of delusional syndromes we have to overcome this postulate of non-understandability. We have to assume a position that views the entanglement of autonomous and reactive psychic processes not as a contradiction in itself but as a challenge for posing further questions. Observations with respect to the influence of psychosocial constellations in the development of the delusion can obviously more easily be made in diseases, which display at least a reactive aspect in addition to the endogenous one. In this sense then, in the following, diagnostic considerations which have in the past drawn so much attention shall deliberately be disregarded in favour of the following question: whether and if so which psychosocial variables facilitate the development of delusion without any consideration of the syndrome in which it might be embedded.

537

Three areas of research will be chosen for our purpose out of the multitude of different methodological approaches and then questioned as to the psychosocial constellation they posit for the development of delusion: first, experiences and personality structure, second, social isolation, and third, symbiontic psychoses.

1. Experiences as an element of psychosocial constellations important in the development of delusion can not be viewed apart from personality structure. The effort to determine those experiences precipitating the delusion stretches from the last century with Heinroth, Griesinger, Hecker and others, who thought "protuberant emotions" were responsible for setting off the development of delusion, up to the life-event-research of our day, which has found an increase of stressful experiences which were not self-induced in a time span before the onset of psychotic episodes. The question of the specifity of these experiences has shifted more and more to the question of the specifity of a certain personality structure, which might be vulnerable for the precipitating experiences. The most subtle descriptions of the entanglement of personality and situation stem from the Tübingen School and from v.Baeyer's[2] investigations in the psychoses of the persecuted. Kretschmer[2] focused on the importance of the precipitating experience in a certain social environment in the case of the sensitive delusion of reference yet the vital role is played by the personality structure in which a particular conflict occurs and whose content expresses itself in the precipitating experience. The sensitive structure, according to Kretschmer, is determined by a mixture of asthenic and sthenic-expansive features. Janzarik[3] also spoke of a structurally bound tendency in the personality against itself which becomes predominant before the onset of delusion. Thus, he defines situation as well as experience in terms of "lived out structure"[4].

The sthenic-expansive element in the character of late-onset-schizophrenics whose main symptomatology consisted of delusion also was described by Bostroem, Klages, Lange and others[5]. They found that their premorbid personalities contained much ambition and oddness whereby they trapped themselves in a particular life-situation. M. Singer and L. Wynne[6] have distinguished an amorphous from a fragmented type of schizophrenia, the latter with an affinity toward developing paranoid symptomatology. In our own study[5] on the affective make-up of the premorbid personality of late schizophrenic patients we found that lasting paranoid features developed in those dynamic characters demonstrating clear cut conflicts, comparatively mature in their development, but conflict-laden; whereas paranoid symptoms were less often found in amorphous, naive-open characters showing little structure at all. Wulff[7] demonstrated in a cross-cultural study comparing Vietnamese and German schizophrenics that a clearly structured and developed personality is necessary for the development of a delusional psychosis. This hypothesis is also sustained by the experience that

schizophrenic psychoses in children remain unspecific in their
symptomatoloy as long as a clear-cut personality structure has
not yet developed.

In v. Baeyer's[8] investigation of patients who suffered from
persecution, their extreme experience has a double impact: first,
as a damaging influence on the personality structure which
v. Baeyer has called "annihilation" and second, as a pervasive theme
which remains effective after the initiating situation has ceased.
Moreover, it tinges later experiences with the same emotional colouring, which v. Baeyer refers to as a gliding transposition of
delusions, if f.e. a delusion of persecution should ensue. In such
a case the original mode of working over a terrifying experience in
a delusional fashion is maintained, also the basic topic, but the
content of experiences changes and is permanently assimilated by
the delusion. Stierlin[9], as other psychoanalysts, stresses the element of alienation of feelings in families where delusion occurs
in one member. However, this alienation of feelings created a cognitive deficit for them and thereby made effective projection
possible.

Thus, all the investigations focusing on experiences which may
precipitate the development of delusion in the end refer to the
premorbid personality structure, which is described as strong in
its frailty and coupled with expansive features and a tendency for
alienation. Although this alienating tension in premorbid characters of late paranoid schizophrenics has often been worked out, the
description does not reach a high degree of specifity. Fritsch and
v. Zeersen[10] demonstrated that Kretschmer's concept of the schizoid
character was the most successful one in blindly allotting premorbid characters to the schizophrenic patients, yet a quantitative
factor plays a role as well, since neurotics and the psychosomati-
cally ill display signs of schizoidism as well.

2. Isolation and loneliness before the development of delusion has often been described. Kraepelin mentioned the risk of the
deaf, who not only suffer a partial sensory deprivation, but above
all a social separation which required an increased striving for
social contacts in order to overcome it. In experimental research
on sensory deprivation, hallucinations and inconstant delusions
have been observed[11]. Usually the delusions occured with the abnormal perceptions and they also disappeared with them. J. Gross et
al.[11] have collected some case reports from the literature, in
which, for example, the prison psychosis is mentioned as well as
the delusion of a single sailor, who produced a catathymic delusional elaboration of his main psychic theme at that time, the attempt
to prove a certain scientific hypothesis by means of his travels
around the world. Social isolation due to the language barrier was
also mentioned by Frost[12]. But in methodologically careful studies
such as the one by Ödegaard[13] on Norwegian immigrants in the USA,

the premorbid personality was once again more decisive for developing a psychosis than the situation of being in a foreign country. Janzarik described a special syndrome of paranoid states due to lack of social contact in late-onset-paranoid - developments of a schizophrenic or paranoid kind, as did Berner, Klages, Peters et al.[14]. Especially premorbidly not autistic, but extraverted, gregarious patients suffered from the social restriction of growing old. An expansive feature in their personality was also considered equally responsible for the fact that they removed healthyly until an advanced age as well as for the paranoid character of the eventually arising psychosis. Social isolation also became important with respect to the delusional content. Often the delusion was concerned with the boundaries of their appartment or house and then proceeded to invade the body. They imagined society, which became less accessible, to have a hostile and aggressive attitude towards them. In contrast to the self inflicted autism of young schizophrenics, the unexpected, undesired segregation in this instance made them feel ostracized by society.

It can be concluded from these observations on the topic of social isolation and delusion, that isolation can precipitate the development of delusion in a two-fold way: first as a theme and content of experience; as such it is hardly distinguished from other biographical catastrophes, except if it occurs at an early stage of personality development; and second, as an interruption of the dialectic relationship with society, the world, and with oneself, whose proper functionning is apt to bring about a feeling for a common sense reality shared and joined in by others. If the emotionally correcting feed-back of the social surroundings is reduced, it becomes increasingly difficult to prevent strong rebellious feelings from projectively filling in the cognitive defects. Thus, in predisposed patients delusional ideas may occur which - without any special constellations-disappear when the isolation subsides.

3. Following the French late 19th century authors Laségue and Falret, Regis and Maradon de Montyel, who presented a rich description of collective delusional psychoses, v. Baeyer, Mechler, and Scharfetter have focused on the psychology and psychodynamics of "shared delusion" or "symbiontic psychoses" as they called the folie a deux[15]. V. Baeyer [16] stressed the pathologic union between the two patients, which inflicts autism and social withdrawal - a well known feature in the schizophrenic individual - on the couple. Mechler[17] and v. Baeyer emphasized the importance of a delusional theme, which matches the demands of the partner and helps him to express an existential conflict which was about to express itself in some way. In other words, the delusional theme which is offered by the inducer must be usable by the induced. These were usually those delusions with more general themes,which give way to the development of a deviant existence by both part-

ners, for example, as v. Baeyer put it, the "persecutory self relation". Scharfetter[18] sees a gain from the illness in terms of maintaining the relationship with at least one human being by giving up
the obligatory contact to reality; and Mechler spoke of a communicative function of the delusion in the deluded couple. Our own case
study[15] demonstrated a schizoid mistrustful inducer, who could only in symbiosis with his manic-depressive wife receive the affective dynamism needed to produce a full delusion, which in turn was
adopted by his wife, a case in which Janzarik's concept of struc-
tural-dynamic-coherence proved to be useful. Both v. Baeyer and
Scharfetter pointed out, that among inducers and induced there are
many abnormal personalities whose pathology already dovetailed in
the relationship before the onset of the shared psychosis. Indeed
it may even have been the reason for choosing that particular mate.

If we consider the pathologic union of a deluded couple as a
model of the deluded Ego in one particular individual we may draw
some conclusions out of the reported findings: There seems to be a
latent readiness for becoming deluded in the induced; a suitable
content has to be offered at a suitable time with the necessary
affective dynamism in the relationship, an aspect referred to by
E. Bleuler as a readiness for delusion governed by affects[19]. There
may be a sort of shutting off the outside world in favour of a stabilizing effect and harmonious state of the inner world of the two.
The delusion arising out of a confusion of feelings and perceptions
exerts the function of making sense again, whereby the couple is
then able to experience itself wholly and fully again, reality
being split off but not the system in itself. At any rate, the
communicative function of delusion becomes obvious, as Stierlin[9]
pointed out, since it contains a part of the emotional reality. As
an experienced counter-reality it represents the autistic withdrawal as well as its defeat in one.

Summing up our remarks we can say that findings and their
interpretations with respect to the psychosocial constellations in
developing delusional syndromes remain vague. Stressful precipitating experiences are unspecific and must always be first referred
to the vulnerability of the experiencing structure. This is usually described in terms of beeing clearly figured, affectively tense,
conflict-laden and prone to alienation. Social isolation, no matter if self-inflicted or not, interrupts the dialectic relationship to the world, which is necessary for establishing a feeling
for common sense reality; moreover, social isolation can also
arouse fear for one's safety and a loss of the feeling of being
protected. Thus, the induced delusion in symbiontic couples clarifies some intrapsychic processes found in the individual such as
the necessity of demarcation against the outside world in favour of
innerpsychic coherence and stability, the reintroduction of purpose in previously confused affects and thoughts as well as the
function of the communicated delusion to overcome autism.

Blankenburg[20] differentiates two paths leading into delusion:
the psychotic impairment of psychic functioning - the formal pole -
and the insidious increase in the autonomy of a theme, the pole representing content. Psychosocial constellations which become relevant for the generation and perpetuation of delusion refer to the
latter pole, while the axial-syndromes formulated by Berner and
Gabriel - following Hoche - refer to the psychotic pole with its
constellations of perpetuating psychotic or organic dysfunctioning.

Thus, psychotic dysfunctioning on one side, the growingly
autonomous nature of a theme on the other, with their particular
constellations of perpetuation represent two different objectives
for research. Their complicated interdependence creates the
inexhaustible clinical variety of delusional syndromes.

References

1. K. Schneider, "Klinische Psychopathologie", Thieme, Stuttgart(1976).
2. E. Kretschmer, "Der sensitive Beziehungswahn", Springer,
   Heidelberg (1950).
3. W. Janzarik, Die produktive Psychose im Spannungsfeld pathogener
   Situationen, Nervenarzt 36: 238-244 (1965).
4. W. Janzarik, Situation, Struktur, Reaktion und Psychose,
   Nervenarzt 52: 396-400 (1981).
5. Ch.Mundt, Die schizophrene Primärpersönlichkeit im Lichte psychopathologischer und tiefenpsychologischer Ansätze, in:
   "Psychopathologische Konzepte der Gegenwart", W. Janzarik,
   ed., Enke, Stuttgart (1982).
6. M. Singer and L. Wynne, Thought disorder and family relations
   of schizophrenics. IV. Results and implications,
   Arch. Gen. Psychiat. 12: 201-212 (1965).
7. E. Wulff, Psychiatrischer Beitrag aus Vietnam, in: "Beiträge
   vergleichender Psychiatrie", N. Petrilowitsch, ed.,
   Akt. Fragen, Psychiatr. Neurol. /Vol. 5: 1-84 (1967).
8. W. v. Baeyer, "Endomorphe Psychosen bei Verfolgten",
   Springer, Stuttgart (1982).
9. H. Stierlin, Die Gestaltung und Übermittlung des Wahns in der
   Familie, Stud. gen. 20: 693-700 (1967).
10. W. Fritsch, Die prämorbide Persönlichkeit der Schizophrenen in
    der Literatur der letzten hundert Jahre, Fortschr. Neurol.
    Psychiat. 44: 323-372 (1976).
11. J. Gross, P. Kempe und C. Reimer, Wahn bei sensorischer Depri-
    vation und Isolierung, in: "Wahn", W. Schulte, R. Tölle,
    ed., Thieme, Stuttgart (1972).
12. L. Frost, Home sickness and Immigrant Psychoses, J. Ment.
    Sci. 84: 801 (1938).
13. O. Ödegaard, "Emigration and insanity", Acta psychiat.
    scand. (Suppl. 4) (1932).
14. W. Janzarik, Über das Kontaktmangelparanoid des höheren Alters
    und den Syndromcharakter schizophrenen Krankseins,
    Nervenarzt 44: 515-526 (1973).

15. Ch.Mundt, Psychopathologische Überlegungen an Hand einer symbiontischen Psychose, Nervenarzt 49: 235-239 (1978).
16. W. v. Baeyer, Über konformen Wahn, Z. Ges. Neurol. Psychiat. 140: 398-438 (1932).
17. A. Mechler, Über konformen Wahn, Nervenarzt 32: 49-57 (1961).
18. C. Scharfetter, "Symbiontische Psychosen", Huber, Bern (1970).
19. P. Berner, "Das paranoische Syndrom", Springer, Heidelberg (1965).
20. W. Blankenburg, Anthropologische Probleme des Wahns, in: "Wahn", W. Schulte and R. Tölle, ed., Thieme, Stuttgart (1972).

COMPARING FRENCH AND INTERNATIONAL CLASSIFICATION SCHEMES :

III PARANOIA AND OTHER PARANOID STATES

C. B. Pull, M. C. Pull, and P. Pichot

Centre Hospitalier, 1210 Luxembourg and
Clinique des Maladies Mentales et de l'Encéphale
75014 Paris

INTRODUCTION

The adjective "paranoid" is one of those psychiatric terms which has have become polysemantic in the course of time. The concept is used with vastly different connotations from country to country and, in a given country, from textbook to textbook. Its meaning has changed considerably from DSM I to DSM II and again from DSM II to DSM III [1,2]. The DSM III diagnosis paranoid disorders is, at least partially, irreconcilable with the ICD-9 diagnosis paranoid states, which in turn cannot be equated with the Scandinavian diagnosis paranoid psychosis.[3]

In France, the adjective paranoid is used exclusively in connection with "schizophrenie paranoïde", to specify a type of schizophrenia characterized by -in addition to Bleulerian fundamental symptoms - mood-incongruent delusions with or without persecutory content.

Reference of the present report is on the classification and descriptions provided in the ICD-9 [4] glossary. Starting from the ICD-9 definitions, an attempt is made to explain the present French position on paranoia and possible equivalents of other categories listed under ICD-9 class 297.

FRENCH EQUIVALENTS OF ICD-9 PARANOID STATES

In a comprehensive review [5] on French nomenclature and comparison with other nomenclatures, one of the present authors has provided the background and current views on possible French equivalents to ICD-9 paranoid states. The conditions known in France as chronic delusional states correspond roughly to ICD-9 paranoid states, in so far as the disorders belonging to the latter are viewed as chronic conditions. Chronic delusional states are subdivided into three groups : (1) chronic interpretative psychosis, (2) chronic hallucinatory psychosis and (3) chronic imaginative psychosis. The two first are at least partially equivalent to one or several ICD-9 paranoid states.

The same author expressed the view that French psychiatric concepts are highly amenable to both empirical and comparative studies and has, in fact, instigated a nation-wide investigation with the aim to elucidate diagnostic criteria emerging from French diagnostic practices. Based on a survey [6] carried out in a sample group representative of experienced French clinicians, the co-authors of the present report have developed empirical diagnostic criteria for a number of categories included in the French classification of mental diseases [7] . The instrument used in this investigation was a List of Integrated Criteria for the Evaluation of Taxonomy in the field of non-affective disorders (LICET-S) [8] . The methodology has been exposed in detail elsewhere .

In what concerned chronic interpretative psychosis and chronic hallucinatory psychosis, the description of cases provided through LICET-S was of a quite remarquable homogeneity. The results were highly consistent in what concerned age of onset, duration, symptom pattern and exclusions. Moreover, the data relevant to a definition of the two concepts consisted of objective observable behaviours and reported feelings for which there is no need for inference. As a consequence, the major elements required to operationalize diagnostic concepts could be elucidated, which in turn permitted to construct the corresponding algorithms.

CHRONIC INTERPRETIVE PSYCHOSIS

As stated by one of the authors [5] , various methods have been suggested for organizing the disorders included under chronic interpretive psychosis, but the distinctions usually made are trivial. The present report does not consider these subtle subdivisions of French nosology for which there is no general consensus anyway and for which it would be difficult to establish rigorous diagnostic criteria.

1. French empirical diagnostic criteria for
   chronic interpretive psychosis

   A. Age of onset : between 25 and 50

   B. Onset : acute or (as a rule) progressive

   C. Chronicity : acute phases are followed by a residual
      phase characterized by the presence of at least some
      signs of the illness

   D. Characteristic symptoms : all of the following

      1. Delusional interpretations
      2. Delusional references
      3. Persistent delusional ideas of either persecution,
         prejudice, grandeur or love or delusional jealousy
      4. Delusions are coherent and form a delusional system

   E. No formal thought disorder

   F. Not due to any organic mental disorder

2. Comparisons with ICD-9

   Cases meeting the criteria for paranoia (ICD-9 297.1)
would all be diagnosed in France as chronic interpretive psychosis, as would, in addition, most cases meeting the diagnostic criteria for paranoid state, simple (ICD-9 297.0). Induced
psychosis (ICD-9 297.3) is perceived in France merely as a
special aspect of chronic interpretive psychosis.

3. Comparisons with DSM III

   Cases meeting the criteria for paranoia (DSM III-297.10)
would all be diagnosed in France as chronic interpretive psychosis. Shared paranoid disorder (DSM III-297.30) would be
considered as a special case of chronic interpretive psychosis.
Acute paranoid disorder (DSM III-298.30) corresponds, to a
certain degree, to reactive bouffée délirante.

   The general diagnostic criteria provided in DSM III for
paranoid disorder correspond to the French usage of paranoid =
paranoïaque. In the French edition of DSM III, paranoid
disorders could thus be translated accurately as "troubles pa-
ranoïaques".

CHRONIC HALLUCINATORY PSYCHOSIS

1. French empirical diagnostic criteria

    A. Age at onset : between 30 and 55

    B. Onset : acute or progressive

    C. Chronicity : active phases are followed by a residual
       phase with at least some signs of the illness

    D. Characteristic symptoms : all of the following

        1. Auditory hallucinations
        2. Persecutory delusions
        3. Delusions of being controlled, thought broadcasting,
           thought insertion, thought withdrawal
        4. Formal thought disorder, if present, does not
           dominate the clinical picture
        5. Delusions tend to develop into a delusional system

    E. Not due to any organic mental disorder

2. Comparison with ICD-9

    Chronic hallucinatory psychosis corresponds closely to
the description provided in the ICD-9 glossary for paraphrenia.
There is, however, no comment in ICD-9 for age at onset.

3. Comparison with DSM III

    There is no category in DSM III which corresponds directly
to chronic hallucinatory psychosis. Chronic hallucinatory psychosis with onset before age 45 meet the DSM III criteria for
schizophrenic disorder. For chronic hallucinatory psychosis
with onset after age 45, the only possible DSM III category
would be atypical psychosis. This is however a residual category encompassing in addition a number of other disturbances
that do not meet the criteria for any specific mental disorder.

    The diagnosis of chronic hallucinatory psychosis implies
the presence of "automatic mental activity" (automatisme mental). This specific French syndrome corresponds basically to
a constellation of Schneiderian first rank symptoms, and, in
DSM III, to symptom criteria 1 and 4 for schizophrenic
disorder.

DISCUSSION

The French position on paranoia and other paranoid states is in fact more complex as presented here. Theoretical considerations and subtle subdivisions have been lost in the operationalization process. Our definition of chronic hallucinatory psychosis does not, for instance, render all of the highly complex implications of "automatic mental activity". In the same way, the definition provided for chronic delusional psychosis omits time-honored references to spreading or non-spreading delusions, and a bewildering number of additional subdivisions. On the other hand, it would make little sense to analyse the finer distinctions of French nosology at a time when French positions on diagnosis and classification are, on the whole, viewed as unique and impossible to understand outside of France.

The present report is in fact part of a more global attempt initiated by the authors to transpose essential elements of French nosology into internationally recognizable criteria. The striking outcome of this endeavour, which is based on actual French diagnostic practices, is that :

1. Basic French diagnostic concepts are amenable to translation into operational diagnostic criteria and terminology, that raise no obstacle to international understanding. In particular, the traditional French categories chronic interpretive psychosis and chronic hallucinatory psychosis may be defined by criteria as rigorous as those in DSM III.

2. French diagnostic concepts defined in this way are directly comparable to concepts defined in other nomenclatures. Chronic hallucinatory psychosis is close to paraphrenia as described in ICD-9 and chronic delusional psychosis to paranoid disorder as defined in DSM III.

3. Traditional French positions, such as the exclusion from schizophrenia of specific chronic delusional and/or hallucinatory disorders may be related to similar trends in recent classifications, as shown by the addition of paraphrenia to paranoid states in ICD-9 and the exclusion from schizophrenic disorders of cases with onset after age 45 in DSM III.

REFERENCES

1. American Psychiatric Association, Diagnostic and
   Statistical Manual of Mental Disorders (3rd edn,
   DSM III), A.P.A., Washington D.C. (1980)
2. J. I. Walker, H. K. H. Brodic, Paranoid disorders,
   in : "Comprehensive textbook of Psychiatry/III",
   H. I. Kaplan, A. M. Freedman, B. J. Sadock, eds,
   Williams and Wilkins, Baltimore/London (1980)
3. N. Retterstøl, The course of paranoid psychoses in
   relation to diagnostic grouping, in : "Proceedings
   of the VII World Congress of Psychiatry", P. Berner,
   ed, the VII World Congress of Psychiatry (1982)
4. World Health Organization, Mental Disorders, Glossary
   and Guide to Their Classification in Accordance
   with the Ninth Revision of the International
   Classification of Diseases, W.H.O., Geneva (1978)
5. P. Pichot, The diagnosis and classification of mental
   disorders in French-speaking countries : background, current views and comparison with other
   nomenclatures, Psychol. Med., 12, 475 (1982)
6. C. B. Pull, M. C. Pull, P. Pichot, Etude Nationale
   sur les Critères de Diagnostic des Psychiatres
   Français dans les Psychoses Non-Affectives :
   Premiers Résultats, Comptes rendus du Congrès des
   Psychiatres et Neurologues de langue Française,
   P. Sizaret, ed, Masson, Paris (1981)
7. Institut National de la Santé et de la Recherche
   Médicale, ed, Classification française des troubles mentaux, Bull de l'INSERM, 24, Suppl. to N° 2
   (1969)
8. C. B. Pull, M. C. Pull, P. Pichot, LICET-S : Une
   Liste Intégrée de Critères d'Evaluation Taxinomi-
   ques pour les Psychoses Non-Affectives, J. Psych.
   Biol. Thérapeut., 1, 33 (1981)

THE COURSE OF PARANOID PSYCHOSES IN

RELATION TO DIAGNOSTIC GROUPING

Nils Retterstøl

Professor of Psychiatry University of Oslo

Gaustad Hospital, Oslo, Norway

INTRODUCTION

In this lecture I shall give an overview on my own research on the course of paranoid psychoses, based on the diagnostic system used in Scandinavia between 1945 and 1963. The course is evaluated in relation to the diagnostic system then used. As the case material is kept in detail, we are now in the process of rediagnosing every case according to the ICD-9 system, the DSM-III system and the RDC-system, and a new follow-up is running. I had hoped to be able to present the preliminary report on this new investigation to this congress, but this has not been possible. Reinvestigation with personal home visits is a time-consuming process, and another year will pass before the final results can be presented.

DIAGNOSTIC CONCEPTS USED IN THE PRESENT INVESTIGATION

Three diagnostic concepts were crucial in the present investigation, which is based on the Scandinavian terminology.

1. Reactive Psychosis

Although the World Health Organization has approved of the term, and the diagnosis is also accepted in the DSM-III system, the Scandinavian concept is broader and more widely used. A reactive psychosis is defined as a psychosis in which the development of a psychosis seems understandable in terms of the affected person's constitutional background and personality development within a life situation which facilitated a mental disturbance in that specific

551

person at that particular time in the individual's life.

2. Schizophreniform Psychosis

The term is coined by the Norwegian psychiatrist Langfeldt (1939), and his concept (which is different from the present DSM-III concept) has been used in the present study. It is a symptomatological and not a nosological entity.

Symptoms are acute or episodic rather than chronic, often developing in previously well-adjusted persons, and are often precipitated by problems in the life situation or by organic factors or a combination of both. Consciousness is often mildly clouded, and the patient often presents affective symptoms in addition to paranoid symptoms. Recovery from the episodes is usual, though relapses may appear, and the illness may take a more schizophrenic course.

3. Schizophrenia

Contrary to the schizophreniform psychosis, the concept of schizophrenia as used in this study is a strict one (Langfeldt, 1937), which may be defined as nuclear schizophrenia or process schizophrenia, where the schizophrenic splitting symptoms are present in a clear sensorium, and the development often is insidious.

4. Paranoid Psychoses

Paranoid symptoms or features occur in many psychiatric disorders, while paranoid disorders do not constitute a diagnostic entity. In the material I am going to present in paranoid psychoses are counted psychoses accompanied by delusions. The clinical group will thus include reactive psychoses, schizophreniform psychoses and schizophrenia of paranoid type. The DSM-III concept (Spitzer and Williams, 1980) includes the concept of reactive psychosis under the group of psychotic disorders not elsewhere classified, a group which also includes schizophreniform psychoses, schizo-affective disorders and atypical psychoses, so the group will include a great part of what we in Scandinavia label reactive psychoses. If the group paranoid disorders (297) in DSM-III is included, most of the psychoses in Scandinavia labelled as reactive psychoses will be traced.   In the material I am going to present, schizophrenia of paranoid type is also included.

MATERIAL

In the material I am going to present, all patients with a paranoid psychosis, as defined above, consecutively admitted to the University Psychiatric Clinic of Oslo during two defined time periods, were included (Retterstøl, 1966). The defined periods were 1946-1948 and 1958-1961. Paranoid psychoses were found to constitute about the same percentage of the consecutively admitted patients in the two periods (12.5 and 11.8% respectively). In both periods about 30 per cent of the patients had a diagnosis of psychosis. The hospital admitted patients for only a relatively short stay, up to 3-4 months, and had no long-stay patients. The patients were all systematically diagnosed according to the diagnostic traditions already introduced. What I here want to present, is the course of the psychoses in relation to the diagnostic grouping. The course is systematically evaluated by personal follow-up investigations by myself, mostly in the patients' home, giving me a travelling distance of more than 10.000 miles. The home visits gave me a unique experience in seeing the patients in their home and environment, interviewing the patients as well as their family members and often also the family doctor. All the patients from the last time period, more than half of all the patients in the total material, I knew personally from their hospital stay. The time spent in the homes varied from an hour to a whole day. All data were also checked in our national central bureau of statistics, our national register of psychoses as well as the national social insurance company and the national suicide register.

Out of a total of 334 such patients, five only refused contact, and 28 had died during the observation period. Thus, the sample under discussion consists of 301 living, personally contacted patients, i.e. 98 per cent of the living patients selected for follow-up. Of these 132 were in the long-term group (15-18 years of observation), and 169 were in the short-term group (2-6 years of observation). 55 per cent were males, 60 per cent were in the age group 30-49 years, 27 per cent in the group under 30 and 13 per cent only in the age group over 50 years.

Table 1 shows the hospital diagnosis on discharge. The group labelled psychosis e genere incerto is the group coined schizophreniform psychosis by Langfeldt (1937) and just defined. It has, therefore, a special interest to study the course of this group. The group of other psychoses includes 9 patients with organic brain disorders and 1 patient with an alcoholic psychosis. These are the only patients in the material not belonging to the major group of functional psychosis.

On basis of the course of illness and all data verified and brought to light on follow-up, a final diagnosis was made. The

Table 1. Hospital Diagnosis on Discharge

Reactive Psychosis	Psychosis e Genere Incerto	Schizophrenia	Other Psychoses	Total
167	76	52	10	301

group of "psychosis e genere incerto" has been avoided, and the patient has been placed in another group in the final diagnostic system.

The reactive psychoses, which made up the bulk of the material, were divided into: cured reactive psychoses without relapse, cured reactive psychoses with subsequent relapse, recovered again, and chronic reactive psychoses.

As chronic reactive psychoses were counted reactive psychoses that did not take a schizophrenic course, but which presented psychotic symptoms during the entire or main part of the observation period. These were mainly those with systematic paranoiac delusions.

The schizophrenias were divided into "cured" and "non-cured" according to outcome. The "cured" group included those patients in whom the illness left no definite trace of deterioration, and where the patient's future life had not been noticeably affected by the past illness.

In Table 2 the findings are concentrated in a simple way. It is clearly seen that the bulk of the "psychosis e genere incerto" or schizofreniform group in the long run turn out to be

Table 2. Changes from Discharge Diagnosis to Final Diagnosis

			N	%
Schizophrenia	to	Reactive psychosis	7	14
Reactive psychosis	to	Schizophrenia	16	10
Psychosis e genere incerto	to	Reactive psychosis	48	63
Psychosis e genere incerto	to	Schizophrenia	23	30

Table 3. Recovered on Follow-up, in Percentage,
in Relation to Discharge Diagnosis

Discharge Diagnosis	Percentage Recovered	Basis
Reactive psychosis	81	167
Psychosis e genere incerto	61	76
Schizophrenia	23	52

relatively benign reactive psychoses, as can be more accurately seen from Table 3. The group of schizophreniform psychosis thus is clearly inbetween schizophrenia and reactive psychosis as to course, but closer to the reactive group.

For the social course the group of schizophreniform psychosis was also inbetween, and still closer to the reactive group, as can be seen from Table 4.

Also in other respects the group was inbetween. More of the patients with a discharge diagnosis of schizophreniform psychosis than those with a diagnosis of schizophrenia had stayed out of mental hospitals during the observation period, while still more of those with the discharge diagnosis of reactive psychosis did so.

It is striking to notice the continuum as to course from the reactive psychoses via the schizophreniform psychoses to the schizophrenias.

SECOND FOLLOW-UP

For the short term material the patients were personally

Table 4. Social Course in Relation to Discharge Diagnosis

Discharge Diagnosis	Self-supporting	Basis
Reactive psychosis	79	167
Psychosis e genere incerto	67	76
Schizophrenia	30	52

followed up again 3 years after the first follow-up, thus bringing the observation period up to 5 to 8 years for this group (Retterstøl, 1970). There were no diagnostic changes.

In the long-term as well as in the first and second short-term investigation, the diagnosis on discharge is of highly statistical prognistic importance. Clinical course and work status have proved to be favourable for the patients discharged under the diagnosis of reactive psychosis. In the total material, the difference is statistically significant in relation to every one of the other diagnostic categories.

CONCLUSION

It seems possible to make a distinction between 2 main groups of functional paranoid psychoses, schizophrenia and reactive psychoses, and also between a nuclear group of schizophrenia and a different group with a much better prognosis: the schizophreniform psychoses. There is a strong correlation between diagnostic grouping and clinical and social course.

ADDITIONAL REMARKS

A new personal follow-up, undertaken by Dr. Opjordsmoen, is now on the way, giving an observation period varying from 18 to 36 years. The material will be rediagnosed according to ICD-9, DSM-III and Winokur's system DD and SDD (Kendler 1980,a-b).

REFERENCES

Kendler, K. S., 1980a, Are there delusions specific for paranoid disorders vs. schizophrenia, Schizophr Bull, 6:1.
Kendler, K. S., 1980b, The nosological validity of paranoia (simple delusional disorder), Arch Gen Psychiatry, 87:699.
Langfeldt, G., 1937, The prognosis in schizophrenia and the factors influencing the course of the disease, Acta Psychiatr Scand, Suppl 13.
Langfeldt, G., 1939, "The Schizophreniform States", Munksgaard, Copenhagen.
Retterstøl, N., 1966, "Paranoid and Paranoiac Psychoses", Thomas, Springfield.
Retterstøl, N., 1970, " Prognosis in Paranoid Psychoses", Thomas, Springfield.
Spitzer, R. L., and Williams, J. B. W., 1980, Classification of mental disorders and DSM-III, in: "Diagnostic and Statistical Manual of Mental Disorders", 3rd edit., Am Psychiatric Ass, ed., Washington.

BIOLOGIC MOTHERS IN THE FINNISH ADOPTIVE FAMILY STUDY;

ALTERNATIVE DEFINITIONS OF SCHIZOPHRENIA

Pekka Tienari, Ilpo Lahti, Mikko Naarala, Anneli Sorri,
Jukka Pohjola, Merja Kaleva and Karl-Erik Wahlberg

Department of Psychiatry
University of Oulu
90210 Oulu 21, Finland

Our study was started in 1967, after the International Symposium on Transmission of Schizophrenia organized by David Rosenthal, Ph.D. and Seymour Kety, M.D. (1968). All the participants were highly impressed by the new strategy for separating heredity and environment. Still some problems remained in Rosenthal's Danish study on adopted-away offspring of schizophrenics (Rosenthal 1971, Lidz 1981). Their series was rather small. The diagnoses of the index parents were based on hospital records, not on psychiatric interviews. The family environment was not investigated directly, although some historical information was obtained through individual interviews of the offspring, of whom 80 % participated. There was also the chance of omitting cases of early onset of schizophrenia in biological parents, because the regulations in Denmark discouraged known schizophrenics from giving their offspring up for adoption. Finally, the diagnostic concepts have changed considerably since the late 50's, when their study was planned. Because of these problems, we considered it justifiable to replicate the study, including direct family measurements of the rearing environment and personal diagnostic interviews of the biological index parents, too.

A total of 19447 schizophrenic women have been identified from the resident hospital population and consecutive admissions. The sample covers the whole of Finland. Only women were collected because they could be checked through registers if they had given their children up for adoption. Also, we knew more surely that they were the biologic parent than if the index parent would have been the father.

557

Through parish and civil population registers, it was found that 287 children of 267 schizophrenic mothers have been given away for adoption, 192 of them during their first five years of life. Cases were excluded for field study for several reasons, especially because adoption occurred after age 5, took place abroad or with a relative, or because the adoptee was still young (born in 1968 or later). A total of 161 children of 149 biologic index mothers remained in the sample and were eligible for study. These children were the adopted-away offspring of schizophrenic mothers who had been placed in a non-relative, Finnish adoptive family during their first five years of life. The control cases were picked up from the files of a private national adoption organization, which handles 80 % of adoption cases in Finland,and from the files of community social boards.

The matching was done outside the Department of Psychiatry by persons who were given the criteria and who carried out the matching case-by-case procedure quite independently. The criteria for matching the controls case by case with the index groups were as follows: the age difference between index and control adoptee is $\leq$ 1 year; the age of the adoptive parents versus control parents $\leq$ 10 years; index and control adoptees are matched for sex; the age of placement in the family in 9 groups (< 6 months, 6-12 months, 12-18 months, 18-24 months, 24-30 months, 30-36 months, 36-42 months, 42-48 months and 48-60 months). The two series were further matched with regard to social class, family residence (town, country), and family structure (mother and father versus only father or only mother). Only if some of the biologic control parents have been treated because of psychosis have they been excluded from the control series. Hence, some of the biologic parents in the control series have needed psychiatric help for reasons other than psychosis. The research and control series are numbered randomly in such a way that the psychiatrist conducting the examination is blind as to whether this is an index or a control family.

Adoptive families have been investigated intensively with procedures that usually take two days (14-16 hours). Family relations are studied through family and spouse interviews, as well as Consensus Rorschach and the Interpersonal Perception Method. Both the adoptive parents and the offspring are interviewed personally and the individual Rorschach is given after the Consensus Rorschach is given. The MMPI is only given to the adopted offspring.

All the interviews and most of the experimental examinations are tape-recorded. This makes it possible to carry out comparable blind ratings and re-classifications later on. The examination procedures and classification principles are described in more detail elsewhere (Tienari 1981, 1983).

By March 1983 we had contacted about 230 families of which 215 have been preliminarily scored. In this phase, only some tentative trends can be presented.

The total family interview material has been used for rating the overall mental health of the families as units. The most common characteristics of the families with the different ratings have been described elsewhere (Tienari 1983). We consider the following factors to contribute most significantly to our ratings: anxiety and its level, boundary functions, quality of interaction, flexibility of homeostasis, "transactional defences", conflicts, empathy, power relations, reality testing and basic trust.

Each adoptive offspring has been rated on a degree of disturbance scale from 1 to 6, where 1 and 2 signify healthy in the clinical sense and 3-6 refer to clinical cases. 113 (53 %) have been rated as healthy and 101 (47 %) as disturbed. Altogether 38 (17,8 %) have been considered more severely ill than neurotic.

Table 1.   The Mental Health Ratings of the Adoptive Children
(82 index cases and their matched controls.

Ratings of the Offspring	Offspring of Schizophrenics	Offspring of Controls
1. Healthy	2	9
2. Mild disturbance	38	36
3. Neurotic	22	28
4. Character disorder	7	5
5. Borderline	7	4
6. Psychotic	6	-
Total	82	82
"Mean"	2.96	2.50

If we look at the first 82 index cases and their matched controls, which have already been investigated (Table 1), we can see that 24 % (20/82) of the index offspring are rated more severely ill than neurosis as compared with only 11 % (9/82) of the controls. All the subjects with psychosis have had a schizophrenic mother.

The two groups of offspring have not very different ratings in normal and neurotic families, whereas in the more seriously disturbed families (rigidly syntonic and severely disturbed) there is a clear-cut difference between the index group and the control group (Tienari 1983). This might mean that the offspring of schizophrenic mothers are more vulnerable when they have been reared in disturbed families.

Table 2. The Mental Health Ratings of the Offspring in
Relation to the Ratings of the Adoptive Families
(in percentages)

Ratings of the Index Offspring (N=92)	Ratings of the Adoptive Family		
	"Healthy"	Neurotic	"Severe Disturbance"
"Healthy"	85	39	6
Neurotic	$12\frac{1}{2}$	50	32
"Severe disturbance"	$2\frac{1}{2}$	11	62

Ratings of the Control Offspring (N=122)	Ratings of the Adoptive Family		
	"Healthy"	Neurotic	"Severe Disturbance"
"Healthy"	86	50	29
Neurotic	14	41	40
"Severe disturbance"	0	9	31

In Table 2 the ratings of all 214 offspring investigated so far (92 index offspring and 122 control offspring) have been presented. If we look at the distribution of offspring diagnoses according to the degree of disturbance of the rearing environment, we can see that when the index offspring (offspring of a schizophrenic mother) have been reared in severely disturbed adoptive families, only 6 % of them have been rated as healthy and 62 % have had a severe diagnosis (psychosis, borderline or character disorder). The control offspring are distributed evenly even when they have been reared in severely disturbed adoptive families. Because the interviewing psychiatrists did not know who was a control and who was an index case, their subjective bias cannot have any influence on this result. It seems to me that genetic vulnerability has interacted with a disordered rearing environment.

If we consider the rates of severe diagnoses in the index offspring (Table 3), we can see that 8 % of the index cases have had a diagnosis of psychosis, 16 % are psychotic or borderline patients, and 26 % have psychosis, a borderline condition or a character dis-

order. Among those 34 index offspring who had been reared in severely disturbed adoptive families, 18 % appear to have been psychotic,
and 38 % psychotic or borderline, and a total of 62 % have had
either psychosis, a borderline condition or a character disorder.
This again supports the hypothesis of interaction between heredity
and family environment.

Table 3. Index Offspring with a Severe Diagnosis
          (psychosis, borderline or character disorder)

Diagnosis of the Offspring	All Cases (N=92)	Cases Whose Rearing Environment Has Been Severely Disturbed (N=34)
Psychotic	(7/92) 8 %	(6/34) 18 %
Psychotic + borderline	(15/92) 16 %	(13/34) 38 %
Psychotic + borderline + character disorder	(24/92) 26 %	(21/34) 62 %

The patient records of the biological mothers have been obtained
an copied. Their diagnoses have been checked by several psychiatrists
performing the classifications independently of each other (87 biologic mothers of 92 index offspring). In May 1982 we initiated the
personal interviews of the biologic parents. In their interview
schedule we use Present State Examination added items, which give
the DSM III and Research Diagnostic Criteria-diagnoses.

Two raters have applied the Research Diagnostic Criteria to the
hospital records of the biologic mothers (Table 4). Of the 85 cases
reviewed so far they were able to confirm the diagnosis of schizophrenia in 57 cases, whereas in 21 cases hospital record data were
insufficient. Their reliability in this tentative phase is not
high, 74 % (50/66 cases which both have reviewed). All the nine
offspring with a borderline diagnosis have had a mother whose
symptoms had met RDC criteria of schizophrenia, as have also four
of the six psychotic cases. On the other hand, we must be careful at this stage before the biologic fathers have also been
diagnosed. Assortative mating might be much more important than
the diagnoses of the mothers only. We had expected that chronicity
or severity in the biologic mothers would be correlated with serious
diagnoses in the adopted-away offspring. Instead, we found that
certain characteristic symptoms of schizophrenic mothers were
correlated with serious disorders of the biologic offspring.

Table 4. Research Diagnostic Criteria in Biologic Mothers
in Relation to Ratings of Their Offspring

Ratings of the Offspring	RDC-Diagnosis of the Biologic Mother (based on hospital records)			
	Schizo-phrenia	Major depressive disorder	Unspecified functional psychosis	Other psychiatric disorder
1. Healthy	1	1	1	–
2. Mild disturbance	26	3	8	2
3. Neurotic	13	3	4	2
4. Character disorder	4	–	2	–
5. Borderline	9	–	–	–
6. Psychotic	4	–	–	2
Total	57	7	15	6
"Mean"	3.10	2.29	2.46	3.67

REFERENCES

Lidz, T., Blatt, S. and Cook, B., 1981, Critique of the Danish-
American Studies of the Adopted-Away Offspring of
Schizophrenic Parents, Am. J. Psychiat., 138:8:
1063-1068.
Rosenthal, D., and Kety, S. S., eds., 1968, "The Transmission
of Schizophrenia", Pergamon Press, London.
Rosenthal, D., Wender, P. H., Kety, S. S., Welner, J. and
Schulsinger, F., 1971, The Adopted-Away Offspring of
Schizophrenics, Am. J. Psychiat., 128:3:307-311.
Tienari, P., Sorri, A., Naarala, M., Lahti, I., Boström, C.,
and Wahlberg, K-E., 1981, The Finnish Adoptive Family
Study: Family-Dynamic Approach on Psychosomatics. A
Preliminary Report, Psychiat. and Soc. Sci., 1:107-115.
Tienari, P., Sorri, A., Naarala, M., Lahti, I., Pohjola, J.,
Boström, C., and Wahlberg, K-E., 1983, The Finnish
Adoptive Family Study: Adopted-Away Offspring of Schizo-
phrenic Mothers, in "Psychosocial Intervention in
Schizophrenia", H. Stierlin, L. C. Wynne, and M. Wirsching
eds., Springer-Verlag, Berlin Heidelberg New York Tokyo.

[3]H-SPIPERONE BINDING TO POST MORTEM HUMAN PUTAMEN

IN PARANOID AND NONPARANOID SCHIZOPHRENICS

Peter Riederer, Kurt Jellinger and Eberhard Gabriel[*]

Ludwig Boltzmann-Institute of Clinical Neurobiology,Lainz-Hospital, and *)Psychiatric
Hospital, Baumgartner Höhe, Vienna, Austria

The dopamine hypothesis is widely believed to be an attractive explanation for a variety of symptoms of schizophrenic patients. Paranoid behavior and tardive dyskinesia are the most prominent symptoms which have been related to dopaminergic overactivity. While pre-synaptic activity with increased synthesis or release of dopamine (DA) might contribute to this functional state of the DA-neuron, measurement of postsynaptic receptor function by radiolabelled neuroleptic drugs has been used to define more precisely the functional significance of sub- and supersensitive receptors. Positive symptoms defined as hallucinations, delusions and formal thought disorder were positively correlated with increased spiperone binding sites in post mortem human putamen of schizophrenics while there was no significance to negative symptoms (Owen et al,1981). Although neuroleptic drug treatment might have contri-buted to an increase in binding number as shown in animal studies and human post mortem analysis (Seeman, 1980) in a certain subgroup of schizophrenics an endo-genous overstimulation of postsynaptic receptors as pathogenic cause of specific symptoms might occur. It is, however, very unlikely to assume that a single and localized disturbance contributes to such a hetero-genous complex of symptoms (or diseases) like schizo-phrenia. Therefore, we have tried to characterize the human post mortem brain tissue with regard to clinical and biochemical criteria.

CLINICAL CLASSIFICATION AND ASSOCIATED SYMPTOMS

For biochemical analysis of brain tissue was obtained from 40 patients where clinical histories fulfilled both Feighner's Research Diagnostic Criteria (RDC) and International Classification of Disease (ICD-8th version) criteria for schizophrenia and its subgroups. For clinical research purpose also other rating scales have been used (e.g. Bleuler, Schneider and Berner) and compared to the RDC and ICD-8 diagnostic criteria in these patients (see Gabriel, *)). We have decided to define the last clinical rating prior to death (ICD-8) as that, which probably correlates most with eventually observed biochemical measurements. Tab. 1a shows, how often shifts in the diagnostic evaluation occur. It seems to be noteable that the <u>first</u> number of diagnosis might be predictive for the interpretation of results obtained according to the <u>last</u> number because of possible differences in the development of symptom complexes. As an enormous amount of brain tissue would be necessary to account for significant results in a group of patients like that of table 1a more closer results could be obtained with groups of patients without disease fluctuations (shown by single number) or at least with groups changing from ICD-8 295.3 (the paranoid state) to 295.6 (the defect stage).

Moreover, according to the ICD-classification, a number of paranoid states cannot be thought as to be "schizophrenia" and in such an unselected material as shown in tables 1a and 1b only about 59% fulfill the RDC criteria of schizophrenia. Furthermore, the patients condition is stable in 85% the last three months prior death, while behavioral changes were noteable in 10%. No exact information can be given for 5% of the patients according to the case histories. Organic psychosyndrome was seen in 56% and extrapyramidal symptoms were noted in 49% occurring at any time and in 28% three months prior to death. Furthermore, 59% of the patients received neuroleptic treatment within the last three months and 38% within the last three days before death (table 1b).

It seems to be an important information to biochemists to have such data available especially for evaluation of subgroups of patients.

---

*) this volume

Table 1a.   Changes in Diagnosis Depending on the Progression of "Schizophrenia" (ICD-8) in an Unselected Material of a Psychiatric Hospital

	n		n			n
295.6	(2)	295.2 295.3 295.6	(1)	296.2	297.1 290.0	(1)
295.3	(4)	311 297.9	(1)	297.1 293.0	295.7	(1)
295.6	(6)	297.9	(3)	295.8 297.0 290.0	295.3 297.9	(1)
297.1	(1)	295.7 294.3	(1)	295.6 / 290.0	295.6 / 290.1 / 290.0	(1)
295.3	(4)	297.1	(3)	290.0	295.9 / 315.4	(4)
297.9	(1)	296.3	(1)	297.1 295.3	296.2 / 295.6 / 311.9	(1)
311						

Table 1b.   Patients Status Prior to Death

n	M/F	age (yrs)	duration of disease (yrs)	RDC/ SCHIZO %	condition 3 mo prior to death %	O P S %	E P S ever %	prior to death — E P S 3 mo %	prior to death — neuroleptic medication 3 mo %	prior to death — neuroleptic medication 3 d %
40	10/30	71,7 ± 1,32	27,7 ± 2,5	59+ / 41–	85 stable / 5 ? / 10 instable	56 + / 10 ? / 34 –	49 + / 51 –	28 + / 15 ? / 57 –	59 + / 41 –	38 + / 62 –

means ± sem;

RDC = Research Diagnostic Criteria (Feighner)
OPS = organic psychosyndrome
EPS = extrapyramidal symptoms

+ with   }
– without } symptoms or treatment
? not known

STRUCTURAL BRAIN DEFICITS

Another criteria to select brain tissue is the confirmation of the clinical diagnosis by pathological and neuropathological examination. Weinberger and Wyatt (1981) by CT-studies found that schizophrenics have significantly larger lateral cerebral ventricles. They showed a higher prevalence for dilated cortical fissures and sulci, an apparent atrophy of the anterior cerebellar vermis and a greater frequency of reversed occipital lobe asymmetry. Sometimes, the ventricles are clearly larger than the upper limit of the normal range. Another CT-study showed 55% abnormalities of mild degree in series of patients including 50% hebephrenia, 19% catatonia and 16% paranoia(Takahashi et al.,1981).

However, the morphological substrate of major psychoses is still controversial (Stevens,1982; Riederer and Jellinger,1982). Structural changes are often present in dementias and a variety of neurological disorders. If morphological changes would account for "schizophrenia" significant associations between morphology and clinical parameters should exist. Unfortunately, cortical atrophies do not correlate with severity of illness, time course of disease processes, present episodes, age or EEG findings (reviewed by Takahashi et al.,1981). In our material neuropathology in an unselected group of 90 patients with the clinical diagnosis of schizophrenia revealed nothing abnormal in only 53,4%, while the others showed pathological changes either due to lesions superimposed on the basic process (10%) or other brain diseases including senile and presenile atrophy of Alzheimer type, inflammatory and vascular lesions, or brain tumors (25,6%) (table 2).

The fact that structural changes occur in almost half of the patients with a clinical diagnosis of major psychoses explain some of the discrepancies in recently published data in human post mortem brain pathobiochemistry (Seeman,1980; Owen et al.,1981; Reynolds et al.,1981).

DOPAMINE RECEPTOR DENSITY AND SCHIZOPHRENIC ILLNESS

In accordance with the clinical criteria and neuropathologic findings described above, data obtained from neuroleptic drug binding have been subdivided as shown in table 3. In addition to our initial reports (Reynolds et al.1981; Reynolds et al.1980) this closer study confirms that neuroleptic drug treatment increases spiro-

Table 2. Neuropathology Findings in Autopsy Series of Patients With Clinical Diagnosis of Schizophrenia (Vienna Psychiat. Hospital, 1978–1982)

Diagnosis (ICD-NR) Neuropath.	Paranoid Schizoph. (295.3)	Acute/other Schizoph. (295.0/4)	Schizophr. Defect (295.6)	Schizo-Aff.Psych. (295.7)	Paranoid Psychos. (297.1)	Senile Paranoid (293.0, 290.1)	Unclassified	TOTAL N	TOTAL %	Median Age at Death
Normal	13	3	16	5	8	1	2	48	53,4	63,6
S.D.A.T.	–	–	9	–	–	–	–	9	10,0	79,2
Anoxia,	2	–	–	–	–	–	1	3	3,3	58,0
Hemorrhage	1	–	1	–	–	–	–	2	2,2	62,5
Metastases	–	–	3	–	–	–	–	3	3,3	52,0
Hep.enc.	–	1	–	–	–	–	–	1	1,1	50,0
CNS leukemia	–	1	–	–	–	–	–	1	1,1	65,0
Cerebellar atrophy	–	–	–	–	–	–	–	–	–	–
Normal/Super imposed les.	16	5	29	5	8	1	3	67	74,4	
S.D.A.T.	1	–	–	–	5	2	–	8	9,0	81,0
Alzheimer dis.	1	–	–	–	1	1	–	3	3,3	67,0
Sen.vasc.enc.	–	–	1	–	–	1	–	2	3,3	81,7
Vasc.enceph.	–	–	2	–	1	–	–	3	3,3	70,3
Alcohol.enc.	–	–	1	–	–	–	–	1	1,1	65,0
Meningioma	1	–	–	1	–	–	–	2	2,2	61,0
Mult.scler.	1	–	–	–	–	–	–	1	1,1	74,0
Fahr's dis.	1	–	1	–	1	–	–	3	3,3	70,0
Other process	5	0	5	1	8	4	0	23	25,6	
T O T A L	21	5	34	6	16	5	3	90	100,0	
Median Age	62,3	57,0	67,1	56,5	76,1	77,0	48,0			

Table 3.   ^{3}H-Sprioperidol Binding in Post Mortem Putamen

	n	B_{max} (pmol/g)	K_D (nM)
Controls	22	$21,9 \pm 2,0$	$0,15 \pm 0,03$
Schizophrenia			
ICD 295.3 + NL	5	$28,8 \pm 5,6$	$1,05 \pm 0,53$**
ICD 295.3+297+NL	11	$24,4 \pm 2,9$	$0,69 \pm 0,25$**
ICD 295.6 + NL	8	$24,0 \pm 5,2$	$0,46 \pm 0,23$**
ICD 295.6 - NL	10	$25,6 \pm 1,4$*	$0,16 \pm 0,017$
Tardive Dyskinesia			
ICD 295.6 (1), 295.3 (1)			
297.1 (1) + NL	3	$26,8 \pm 6,7$	$0,44 \pm 0,15$
ICD 295.6(6),295,7(1)-NL	7	$16,2 \pm 1,5$	$0,22 \pm 0,07$

* p< 0,01 vs controls and ICD 295.6 + NL
** p< 0,01 vs controls
+ with neuroleptics (1 day - 7 months prior to death)
- without   "   (drug free for at least 3 months)
age (yrs): $72,5 \pm 3,1$; schizophrenics: $69,7 \pm 2,7$
post mortem time: 1 to 10 hours for schizophrenics and
                  3 - 15 hours for controls

Table 4.   Lisuride Binding in Human Putamen

Group	n	NL	B_{max} (nmol/g)	K_D (nM)
ICD-8 295.3	4	+	$0,268 \pm 0,056$	$6,5 \pm 0,42$
295.6	7	+	$0,183 \pm 0,03$	$3,58 \pm 0,73$
295.6	4	-	$0,163 \pm 0,01$	$3,96 \pm 1,42$
295.1(1), 290,0(1) 295.7(2), 296.1(1)	5	-	$0,136 \pm 0,03$	$3,25 \pm 0,91$
Controls	15	-	$0,173 \pm 0,018$	$2,48 \pm 0,047$

means $\pm$ sem; NL = neuroleptic drugs; + with, - without neuroleptics;
correlations between lisuride and spiroperidol binding (B_{max}):
controls: r = 0,789, t = 4,06, n = 15, p< 0,005
all other: r = 0,716, t = 4,35, n = 20, p< 0,0005

peridol binding sites. This is evident for schizophrenics with a defect stage (ICD-8 - 295.6) while all our patients with paranoid behavior were on neuroleptic drug treatment. Therefore the increase above normal observed in this group seems to be related to neuroleptics. The major difference between our reports and that of others (Owen et al.,1981; Seeman for review,1980) seem to be the fact that all our non neuroleptic patients belong to a subgroup characterized by negative symptoms of the defect stage.

Tardive dyskinesia in patients on neuroleptic showed spiroperidol binding number comparable to that of patients on drugs but without dyskinesias. Furthermore, patients with tardive dyskinesias but without neuroleptic drug treatment have spiroperidol binding sites similar to non treated patients of the defect stage, but show lower affinity (table 3). Therefore,our data do not show an association of tardive dyskinesia with increased numbers of dopamine receptors in the putamen. This finding agrees well with recent data by Cross et al. (1983), although in the latter study both schizophrenics with and without movement disorders had significantly higher D-2 receptor numbers than controls. This finding compared to our data again shows that differences in patient selection seem to account for these divergencies. In another trial lisuride binding has been measured in some of the brains from which spiperone data were available. The results shown in table 4 indicate that neuroleptic drugs lead to an increase in binding number and change in affinity in patients on long term drug treatment. No substantial changes have been measured in paranoid psychosis and patients meeting ICD-8 criteria of 295.6 without neuroleptics, although a slight decrease is noteable. It might be of some interest to mention that there are clear correlations between changes in spiroperidol and lisuride binding numbers (table 4) indicating binding of both ligands to a similar group of membrane binding sites. In the human putamen these may be associated with a preferentially dopaminergic function.

REFERENCES

Cross,A.J., Crow, T.J., Ferrier,I.N., Johnstone,E.C., Mc Creadie,R.M., Owen,F., Owens,D.G.C., and Poulter,M., 1983, Dopamine receptor changes in schizophrenia in relation to the disease process and movement disorder, J.Neural Transm. Suppl.18:265-272

Owen,F., Cross,A.J., Crow,T.J., Poulter,M., and
    Waddington,J.L., 1981, Increased dopamine receptor
    in schizophrenia: specificity and relationship to
    drugs and symptomatology, in: Biological Psychiatry
    1981, C.Perris,G.Struwe, B.Jansson eds, Elsevier,
    North Holland, Amsterdam pp 699-706
Reynolds, G.P., Reynolds,L.M., Riederer,P., Jellinger,K.,
    and Gabriel, E., 1980, Dopamine receptors and
    schizophrenia: Drug effect or illness, Lancet,Dec.6:
    1251
Reynolds,G.P., Riederer,P., Jellinger, K.,and Gabriel E,1981,
    Dopamine receptors and schizophrenia: the influence
    of neuroleptic drug treatment and disease symptoms,
    in: Biological Psychiatry 1981, C.Perris, G.Struwe,
    B.Jansson eds, Elsevier, North Holland,Amsterdam,
    pp 715-718
Riederer,P., and Jellinger,K., 1982,Biochemie und
    morphologische Aspekte der Schizophrenie, Schwer-
    punktmed. 5:32-40
Seeman,P.,1980, Brain dopamine receptors, Pharmacol.
    Rev. 32:230-313
Stevens, J.R., 1982, Neuropathology of schizophrenia,
    Arch.Gen.Psychiat. 39:1131-1139
Takahashi,R., Inaba,Y., Inanaga,K., Kato,N., Kumashiro,
    H., Nishimura,T., Okuma,T., Otsuki,S., Sakai,T.,
    Sato,T., and Shimazono,Y., 1981, CT scanning and
    the investigation of schizophrenia, in: Biological
    Psychiatry 1981, C.Perris, G.Struwe, B.Jansson eds,
    Elsevier,North Holland,Amsterdam pp 259-258
Weinberger,D.R., and Wyatt,R.J., 1981, Computed
    tomography (CT) findings in schizophrenia: clinical
    and biological implications, in: Biological
    Psychiatry 1981, C.Perris, G.Struwe, B.Jansson,eds.
    Elsevier, North Holland, Amsterdam, pp 255-258

ON THE SENSE OF STRESSING PARANOID PSYCHOSES

Eberhard Gabriel

Medical Direction
Psychiatric Hospital
A-Vienna 1140, Baumgartner Höhe 1

1. For a long time nosology dominated psychiatric classification.
In this way descriptive psychopathology has been neglected. For example schizophrenia has been understood as a nosological group of pathological states characterized by the although unknown endogenic
etiology and its grouping together seemed more important than its
differentiation. A still effective example for this decision about
the classificatory importance of different aspects which even has
grown in interest is K. Schneider (1959), who gave with his first
rank symptoms regulations for a typological classification of what
he called schizophrenia but postulating at the same time a special
etiology, the endogenous and stressing the sharp distinction of organic, endogenous and reactive disorders. Thus the instruments of classification relate to different areas of characteristics, to the descriptive psychopathological area on the one hand to the area of non
psychopathological so called external criteria on the other hand.
Only states containing these criteria and which can not be interpreted as of organic origin are schizophrenic. Though in K. Schneider's teaching organic, endogenous and psycho-/sociogenic factors
are not of the same order because he assumes a hierarchical row
from organic to endogenous and furthermore psych-/sociogenic. In
a tradition of general pathology causes only have been imaginable
as organic causes. The word endogenous alluded to unknown factors
which have been presumed organic. Detectable psychogenic or socio-
genic factors did not respond to this view and thus have been pushed
away from this system of genetic factors. That the genetic factors
which have been expected to be the important remained unknown and
detectable by means of descriptive psychopathology only from the
phenomenological periphery was seen as a dramatic deficiency. The
distinction of different conditioning factors for the existence
(Da-Sein) and the special form (So-Sein) of schizophrenic psychoses

in the sense of K. Schneider was an attempt to focuse on the psychological and sociological factors which had so much grown in interest
from a social and political view point (remind the psychoses of persecuted and displaced persons) and a therapeutic view point as well.
But the hierarchic position of these factors was a subordinated one
and remained underestimated. The withdrawal of the concept of basically genetic or causal factors and the attempt to stress on multiple conditions interelated one with the others created the fundamental
equivalence of genetic factors in different phenemonological areas
at least in the interpretation of the so called functional psychoses.

Diagnostic systems like the International Classification of
Diseases (ICD) reflect this situation of our science and its evolution. In its 8th revision paranoid psychoses are found within the
schizophrenic psychoses (295.3, .7) and with a very poor phenomenological and conceptual spectrum in 297 (.0 paranoia, .1 involutional
paranoid psychosis, .9 other paranoid syndromes) and as acute paranoid reaction (298.3). No organic psychoses except the well differentiated group of psychoses basing on alcool addiction (291.2 hallucinosis, .3 paranoia of jealousy) can be differentiated syndromatolo-
gically. The 9th revision changed the situation highly. The syndromatological differentiation of schizophrenia and alcoolic psychoses
remained the same. But in contrast to the 8th revision it is now
possible to stress paranoid psychoses in the group of organic psychoses within the senile dementia (290.1) and within the drug induced
psychotic states (292.1). And there are now more possibilities to
diagnose paranoid syndromes outside of schizophrenia (297.0 simple
paranoid psychosis, .1 paranoia, .2 paraphrenia, .8 other paranoid
syndromes, .9 paranoid syndromes not specified and 298.3 acute paranoid reaction, .4 psychogenic psychosis with paranoid symptomatology).

2. What are the motives for changing the classificatory attitudes and wheigts in this way?

2.1 I begin with Kraepelin (1913). His attemp to create a system
of functional psychoses survives mainly in the grouping of different
forms of disorders as different types of one entity denominated dementia praecox and the dichotomy of functional psychoses in dementia/
schizophrenia and manic depressive illness. But it is not so known
that even in the 8th edition of his textbook of psychiatry he grouped
the paraphrenias together with dementia praecox under the heading
of 'endogeneous dementias' (endogene Verblödungen) and that he quoted
paranoid psychoses on the first place in the series of disorders
which he did not feel able to affiliate to dementia praecox. (Berner
et al., 1983) With respect to the paraphrenias Kraepelin's pupil
Mayer (1921), often is called as a witness that paraphrenias are
schizophrenic psychoses basing this testimony on his catamnestic
examination of Kraepelin's own cases of paraphrenia. In fact this
study is not conclusive. Mayer only stressed the similarities of
these cases with schizophrenia more than their particularities. Thus

572

he did not find new facts but proposed only another interpretation
of the same or similar facts. (Gabriel, 1976) The problem was not
solved but only had found a ficticious solution desactualising it
for some time. But in different connexions the rigid dichotomy was
not efficient enough, mainly in the phenomenological analysis of
syndromes, prognostics and in the interpretation of findings of the
basic sciences. Therefore a peculiar position of paranoid psychoses
even within schizophrenia was proposed repeatedly.

2.2 An other motive is a renewed interest in pathogenetic analysis of symptoms and syndromes. Examinating paranoiac patients in
a retrospective catamnestic design Berner (1965), found that the
course of the paranoiac syndromes was determinated by phenomena which
he felt able to evalute in a reliable manner and to group easily.
From this study the attempts of the Viennese research group on paranoid psychoses started. I like to remind you only of three other
studies of this group which I consieder to be the most important with
respect to their special topic and their methodological connexion
(generation of hypotheses, testing within a retrospective design,
reconsideration of hypotheses, testing within a prospective design:
Berner et al. (1966), Berner et al. (1984). It seems to me important
to point out that this interest in the pathogenetic analysis of
symptoms and syndromes goes back to Eugen Bleuler (1911), and his
distinction between primary symptoms indicating an illness process
and secondary symptoms which are reactions to the primary ones.

The findings of the Viennese group coincided with the theory of
Janzarik (1959), on fundamental dynamic constellations in psychoses
and their bearing on actualization and fixation of certain contents
representative for a personality (coherence of structure and dynamics)
as a theory valid for the pathogenetic interpretation of productive
phenomena.

I only mention that this row of motives unevoidably leads to
the problems of schizoaffective psychoses. (Gabriel, 1983)

2.3 A third motive relates to changing views of the etiopathogenesis of psychic disorders in general. In a rigid threefold system
of organic, endogenous and psychogenic/reactive disturbances genetic
research only can meet limited topics/problems. Examples are the genetic research restricted for a long time on endogenous psychoses
and the psychological research in functional psychoses which for an
important period of time did not lead to meaningful accumulations
of knowledge but to a game changing pots and the neglection of the
respectively other important facts. Genetic factors were pushed away
in the interpretation of psychogenic disorders (paranoid psychoses
may be) and psycho-/sociogenetic factors were pushed away in the
interpretation of endogenous disorders (paranoid psychoses may be
too).

573

Two concepts seem to be very important, both basing much more differentiated views.

2.3.1 The one relates to methodology. There is no search of 'causes' but of conditions and their constellations which are variable over time. In the German speaking countries for instance this concept was introduced in important study of Helmchen (1968), on constellations of conditions in paranoid hallucinatory syndromes which is a study mainly on neurophysiological conditions of such psychoses. This concept led to a differentiation of the questions to the non psychopathological basic sciences and to much more modesty but also to much more precision in these questions.

Our group contributed to the research on biological conditions of paranoid psychoses mainly with two studies on genetics (Berner and Gabriel, 1973, Schanda et al., 1983) and a study of Lange (1981), on serological genetic markers.

2.3.2 It was a great merit of Danisch and Norwegian psychiatry to stress on psychogenesis of paranoid psychoses. The concept of psychogenic psychoses breaks through the rigid threefold diagnostic system, which was in fact psychopathological but postulated an etiological order. With regard to paranoid psychoses important studies of the last decades emerged from this tradition (Retterstøl, 1966, 1970). The effect was twofold: on the one hand psychogenic factors in paranoid psychoses have been pointed out - and this led to a better basis for therapeutic concepts, and on the other hand it led to etiological relativation of the concept of psychosis. The growing interest in multiaxial classification systems seems to be an indicator of this evolution of concepts.

2.4 To summarize: The uncertainty of the position of paranoid psychoses in the traditional system of functional psychoses, the bearing in mind of pathogenetic analysis of psychopathological symptoms and syndromes and their theoretical interpretation and the consideration of multidimensional genetic concepts seem to be important motives for the growing interest exemplified in the ICD evolution with respect to paranoid psychoses. They occur frequently, they are frequent in therapeutic institutions where in principle clinical research is done and in general they can be examined easily. Therefore paranoid psychoses form not only a peculiar field of interesting and fascinating phenomena but they are suitable as a natural model of psychic disorders and their genesis in general.

References

Berner, P., 1965, "Das paranoische Syndrom", Springer, Berlin.

Berner, P., Kryspin-Exner, C., and Panagiotopoulos, P., 1966, Themenwahl und Wahnfixierung bei der alkoholischen Eifersuchtsparanoia, Wien.Z.Nervenheilk., 24:204-218.

Berner, P., and Gabriel E., 1973, Beziehungen zwischen Psychopathologie und Genetik sogenannter Spätschizophrenien, Wien.Z.Nervenheilk., 31:1-11.

Berner, P., Gabriel, E., Lenz, G., Katschnig, H., Simhandl, C., and Wallner, W., 1983, Diagnostic Criteria for Schizophrenia and Affective Psychosis, American Psychiatric Press, Washington.

Berner, P., Gabriel, E., Kronberger, M. L., Küfferle, B., Schanda, H., and Trappl, R., 1984, Course and Outcome of Paranoid Psychoses, Psychopathology, 17:28-36.

Bleuler, E., 1911, "Dementia praecox oder Gruppe der Schizophrenien", Deuticke, Leipzig. Reprint: 1978, Minerva Publikation, München.

Gabriel, E., 1976, Spätschizophrenie und ihre Prognose, Vortrag, Universität Oslo.

Gabriel, E., 1978, "Die langfristige Entwicklung von Spätschizophrenien", Karger, Basel.

Gabriel, E., (Ed.), 1983, Problems of Schizoaffective Psychoses, Psychiat.Clin., 16:69-304

Helmchen, H., 1968, "Bedinungskonstellationen paranoid-halluzinatorischer Syndrome", Springer, Berlin.

ICD 8th Rev., 1968, (1965 revision), "WHO Manual of the International Statistical Classification of Diseases", V, WHO, Geneva.

ICD 9th Rev., 1978, "Mental disorders: Glossary and Guide to their Classification in accordance with the 9th Revision of the International Classification of Diseases", WHO, Geneva.

Janzarik, W., 1959, "Dynamische Grundkonstellationen in endogenen Psychosen", Springer, Berlin.

Kraepelin,E., 1913, "Psychiatrie", 8th ed., vol.III, Barth, Leipzig.

Lange, V., 1981, Genetische Markierungsbefunde bei Wahnkrankheiten der Lebensmitte, Psychiat.Clin., 14:23-34.

Mayer, W., 1921, Über paraphrene Psychosen, Z.ges.Neurol.Psychiat., 71:187-206.

Retterstøl, N., 1966, "Paranoid and paranoiac psychoses", Universitetsforlaget, Oslo.

Retterstøl, N., 1970, "Prognosis in paranoid psychoses", Universitetsforlaget, Oslo.

Schanda, H., Berner, P., Gabriel, E., Kronberger, M. L., and Küfferle, B., 1983, in press, Familienbilduntersuchungen an Patienten mit paranoiden Psychosen, Psychiat.Clin., 16.

Schneider, K., 1980, "Klinische Psychopatholgie", 12th ed., Thieme, Stuttgart.

Specht, G., 1901, Über den pathologischen Affekt in der chronischen Paranoia, Festschrift der Erlanger Universität.

DEPRESSION IN SCHIZOPHRENIA:

CRUCIAL ISSUES AND FURTHER EVIDENCE

Steven R Hirsch   Julian Leff

Dept of Psychiatry   MRC Social Psychiatry Unit
Charing Cross Hospital   Friern Barnet Hospital
London W6   London N11

The concurrence of depressive symptoms and schizophrenia is not disputed but the nature of the depressive syndrome in schizophrenia, its natural history, whether it is separate from depressive illness, its aetiological relationship to schizophrenia, and its treatment, all remain open questions. However this symposium is directed at aetiological issues. To date, the question of prevalence and incidence have only been explored in selected samples. In the absence of a proper epidemiologically based sample involving a follow up of a previously untreated schizophrenia from its start, we must rely on piecing together the puzzle from isolated samples to build up a picture of the relationship of depressive syndromes to the epoch of the illness in relation to onset, chronicity, and relapse and the effect of intervening variables such as life events, social environment, and treatment.

The International Pilot Study of Schizophrenia which includes 1202 patients from 9 centres throughout the world is the most ambitious study to date. Newly admitted patients with less than 5 years previous illness were drawn as a continuous sample of 100 or more at each centre. Table 1 shows the prevalence of the PSE affective syndromes HM (Hypomania), DD (depressive delusions), ED (special features of depression), OD (other symptoms of depression) and SD (simple depression) in schizophrenia, mania, psychotic depression and 50 neurotic depressive states respectively.

Table 1

AFFECTIVE SYNDROMES IN FOUR DIAGNOSTIC GROUPS

WHO, IPPS - 1973

ICD	N	% Syndrome Present				
Categories		(HM) N = 355	(DD) N = 167	(ED) N = 409	(OD) N= 942	(SD) N= 950
Schizophrenias 295.1, 3, 4, 7	588	30	15	39	78	81
Mania 296.1, 296.3 298.1	79	90	8	19	76	52
Psychotic Depressive 296.2	73	9	34	59	96	97
Neurotic Depressive 300.4	70	4	10	42	94	99

Note the high incidence of depressive symptoms in those diagnosed as schizophrenics - not dissimilar to the results reported by Knights and myself[2], but far greater than most psychiatrists would expect. The diagnosis schizo-affective psychosis (295.7) was used by 4 of the 9 IPSS centres. Although there was a greater qualitative loading of affective syndromes in the profiles of schizo-affectives in these centres, it was still not possible to separate individuals with this condition from those with paranoid schizophrenia, 295.3. Thus depressive syndromes are extremely prevalent in acutely ill schizophrenic patients throughout the world.

From an epidemiological perspective the aetiological relationship of affective syndromes to schizophrenia can be simplified into three main hypotheses with subsidiary hypotheses. Are affective symptoms in schizophrenia due to neuroleptic treatment? Are they an inherent part of the disease itself, or are they purely a psychogenic reactive condition? Although Dr Roy has presented evidence that they are related to social environment and life events, there is nothing to suggest that these are not merely provocation factors in otherwise predisposed individuals.[3] Drs Van Putten[4], Johnson[5], and Galdi[6], have each published evidence which suggests that an extra-pyramidal mechanism involving akinesis, presumably arising as part of the drug induced extra-pyramidal syndrome, is the basis for most of the dysphoric affective reactions seen in schizophrenia. At the same time Möller and von Zerssen[7], and Knights and I[2], have shown that affective syndromes are most prevalent on admission in the acute phase, and become less common as recovery proceeeds - this is the opposite of which one would expect if affective symptoms wwere mainly drug induced or were psychological reactions which occurred when insight was regained during the recovery phase. Johnson's data[5] from a small cohort of previously untreated patients supports this, but most reports unfortunately confound the factor of drug treatment with the epoch of the illness because a large proportion of acutely admitted patients have been put under treatment prior to admission.

The two competing hypotheses - that affective syndromes are drug related, hypothesis DR, and illness related, IR, lead to opposite but testable predictions. Hypothesis DR predicts a decrease in the prevalence of depressive syndromes, DS, if drugs are discontinued. Strictly speaking under the DR hypothesis the prevalence of affective syndromes should not vary according to the state of the illness whether the patient is in an acute phase or in remission:

$$\text{If DR, then Scz} + R_x \longrightarrow DS \uparrow \text{(increase or the same)}$$
$$\text{but Scz} - R_x \longrightarrow DS \downarrow \text{(decrease)}$$

As reported elsewhere[2,8], the illness related hypothesis leads to an opposite prediction: Affective syndromes, DS, should increase with an exacerbation of schizophrenia, decrease as schizophrenia improves, but otherwise not be related to drug treatment.

Two cohorts of patients were examined to test these predictions,[9,8]. The first consists of 28 patients discharged from hospital after an acute episode of schizophrenia who were switched under randomized double blind conditions to treatment with either placebo, chlorpromazine 100-300 mgm, or Stelazine 5-15 mgm daily for one year.[9] The second consisted of 73 chronic outpatients on depot fluphenazine decanoate blindly and randomly switched to placebo or to continue active medication for 9 months.[9] Assessments were repeated at the end of the trial period or when the patient relapsed. Twenty six of 28 patients in the acute cohort had a depressive affective syndrome. This could mean that there was as little as one affective symptom, simple depression, present on the PSE; it is not equivalent to a diagnosis of depression. Because almost all patients in the acute cohort were dysphoric when entering the study we could not see if relapse resulted in an increased incidence of depression as predicted by the illness related hypothesis, IR, but of 12 patients who remained on drugs without relapse, 6 lost their depression and none developed it ($p < 0.02$ binomial) see table 2. In fact there was a strong tendency for all patients to lose their depressive syndromes regardless of whether they were switched to placebo or not. Both these findings tend to disconfirm the drug related hypothesis, DR. A decrease in depressive syndromes when neuroleptics are discontinued and placebo substituted would be expected if the drug related hypothesis is correct. This could not be tested in the non-relapsing placebo group because the numbers were too small,

Table 2

NUMBER OF PATIENTS WITH AFFECTIVE SYNDROMES

LEFF & WING'S SERIES - 1971

Schizophrenics	N	First Interview	Second Interview	decrease in dsyphoria
Patients not relapsing				
on drug	12	11	5	6 (p<.02,binomial)
on placebo	2	2	0	2 against DR
Patients who relapsed				
on drug	6	6	4	2
on placebo	8	7	7	0 against DR&IR
All patients	28	26	16	10 p=.006 (binomial) against DR

but in the relapsing placebo group a decrease in the number of those with affective syndromes did not occur, again disconfirming the DR hypothesis. It was not possible to test the opposite prediction of the increase in the number with affective syndromes with an exacerbation of schizophrenia which would be expected from the Illness Related hypothesis. Almost all patients in this subgroup had an affective syndrome from the start and the numbers are too small to test for a change in affective syndromes among those who relapsed on drugs.

In the second series, of 13 patients remaining well on placebo 4 lost their affective syndrome. This is predicted by the Drug Related Hypothesis, DR (p = 0.0625 binomial) and aginst Hypothesis IR. There was no change in the proportion of patients affected by dysphoria among those who did not relapse but continued with drug treatment; one-third at the beginning and end of the trial, but this is as predicted by both hypotheses. However of patients switched to placebo who then relapsed, the prediction of an increase in the number with depressive syndrome, as expected with the IR hypothesis, did not occur. Eleven patients did not have an affective syndrome when they entered the trial (1st interview) of whom 3 showed an affective syndrome at relapse. Conversely, of 13 patients with affective syndrome at the 1st interview, 4 lost it by the second, as would be predicted by the DR hypothesis. The overall change in affective syndrome among those who relapsed on placebo, reflects minimal overall change with nearly equal numbers developing and losing their affective syndrome. If, as we hoped, either hypothesis IR or DR is correct, we would have expected an overall increase or decrease in depressive syndrome respectively in this crucial subgroup. Unfortunately there was no

580

Table 3

NUMBER OF PATIENTS WITH AFFECTIVE SYNDROMES

HIRSCH ET AL. SERIES − 1973[10]

Schizophrenics	N	First Interview	Second Interview	decrease in dysphoria
Patients not relapsing				
on drug	33	11	11	0
on placebo	13	9	5	4 p=.06 against IR favouring DR
Patients who relapsed				
on drug	3	2	3	1
on placebo	24	13	12	1 against DR & IR
All patients	73	35	31	4 NS

significant change in either direction so we are unable to find
support for either hypothesis in this crucial test. Patients
relapsing on drug treatment could not be considered because the
number was too small.

Conclusion

A recently discharged acute sample and a sample of chronic out-
patients on long term medication were observed under conditions
of maintenance, neuroleptic or placebo treatment. The results
tended to disconfirm the hypothesis that depression is drug
related, but did not show a net increase in depressive dysphorias
when relapse occurred, as predicted by the illness related
hypothesis. A tendency for depressive syndrome to decrease over
time, whether on drug or placebo was observed. The results are
not conclusive. A prospective study beginning before treatment
is instituted is necessary to properly document the natural
history of the affective syndromes in schizophrenia.

References

1. World Health Organisation. Internation Pilot Study of Schizophrenia. Volume I, Basel (1981).

2. Knights,A. and Hirsch,S.R. 'Revealed' depression and drug treatment for schizophrenia. Archives of General Psychiatry, 38, 806-11 (1981).

3. Hirsch, S.R. Depression 'revealed' in schizophrenia. 'Comments' British Journal of Psychiatry, 140, 421-424 (1982).

4. Van Putten, T. and May, P.R.A. 'Akinetic depression' in schizophrenia. Archives of General Psychiary, 35, 1101-7 (1978).

5. Johnson, D.A.W. Studies of depressive symptoms in schizophrenia. British Journal of Psychiatry, 139, 89-101 (1981).

6. Galdi,J., Rieder, R.O., Silber, D. and Bonato,R.R. Genetic factors in response to neuroleptics in schizophrenia. A psychopharmagenic study. Psychological Medicine, 11, 713-728 (1981).

7. Möller, H.J. and von Zerssen,D. Depressive symptomatik in stationären Behandlungsverlauf von 280 schizophrenen Patienten. Pharmacopsychiatria, 14, 172-9 (1981).

8. Leff, J. and Wing, J. Trial of maintenance therapy in schizophrenia. British Journal of Psychiatry, 3, 599-604 (1971).

9. Hirsch,S.R. Gaind, R., Rohde, P., Stevens, B. and Wing, J. Outpatient maintenance of chronic schizophrenic patients with long acting fluphenazine: Double-blind placebo trial. British Medical Journal, 1, 633-637 (1973).

THE NATURE OF THE DEPRESSIVE SYNDROME IN SCHIZOPHRENIA AND ITS RELATIONSHIP TO PROGNOSIS

Hans-Jürgen Möller, Detlev von Zerssen

Max-Planck-Institute of Psychiatry
Kraepelinstr. 10
D-8000 Munich 40, F.R.G

The growing literature on depression in schizophrenia not attributed to the schizo-affective psychosis indicates that this is an important clinical phenomenon. But the constructs (Hirsch, 1982) used to describe them - pharmacogenic depression, akinetic depression or akinesia, postpsychotic depression, schizophrenic depression - are not well defined, and their empirical basis seems weak. That is especially true for depressive states occuring during the acute neuroleptic treatment of schizophrenic psychoses.

Also the knowledge about the prognostic meaning of such depressive states in schizophrenia (we are not talking about the typical depressions of the schizo-affective disorders!) is unconclusive. While they were regarded as a sign for a good long-term outcome by some authors, other authors described them as a sign of an unfavourable prognosis (McGlashan and Carpenter, 1979; Mandel, 1982; McGlashan, 1982).

To broaden the knowledge about depressive states that occur during neuroleptic therapy of acute schizophrenic psychoses we used data from our clinical documentation system (Möller et al., 1983) for a group of 280 schizophrenic inpatients (ICD 295, schizo-affective psychoses were excluded). We were interested in the following problems:

[a] symptomatology of the schizophrenic psychosis in comparison to endogenous depressions
[b] frequency and course pattern of depressive states
[c] predictors of depressive states at discharge
[d] prognostic value of depressive states concerning long-term outcome.

In this paper we will briefly report the results of different analyses without going into the details.

Syndrome Pattern of Acute Schizophrenic Psychoses

The analysis of the IMPS-profile (Lorr, 1974) of acute schizophrenic patients at admission leads to the result, that this profile is not only characterized by the typical schizophrenic syndromes (e.g. "Paranoid Projection", "Perceptual Distortion", "Hostile Belligerence", "Conceptual Disorganization", "Motor Disturbances" etc.), but also by a high intensity of the IMPS-factors "Anxious Depression", "Retardation and Apathy" and "Impaired Functioning", which are typical for depressive states (Möller et al., 1981; 1983). Thus, we can conclude, that acute schizophrenic psychoses are not only described by the spectrum of the so-called productive schizophrenic symptoms, but also by a broad spectrum of depressive-apathetic symptoms, a result, which was also reported by other authors (Mombour, 1974; Knights and Hirsch, 1981). The comparison with the IMPS profile of a group of inpatients suffering from an acute endogenous depression shows that the schizophrenic patients have almost similarly high scores on the factors "Anxious Depression", "Retardation and Apathy", and "Impaired Functioning" at admission. This result is very interesting especially under the aspect that schizo-affective psychoses were excluded from the analysis. Thus we can conclude, that the depressive spectrum symptoms were considered by the doctors as an integral part of the schizophrenic psychosis, not as a part of a schizo-affective one.

What has been described as a syndrome pattern at admission, is also true for discharge. The three IMPS-factors describing depressive ("Anxious Depression"), apathetic ("Retardation and Apathy") and neurasthenic ("Impaired Functioning") symptoms have almost the similar intensity in schizophrenic patients as in endogenous depressives.

We also can notice that there is a significant decrease of the intensities of the three syndrome scores in the two diagnostic groups between admission and discharge. That is remarkable under the aspect that the two groups were treated in a different way: the endogenous depressives were treated with antidepressive drugs, the schizophrenic patients were treated with neuroleptic drugs. Thus, we have to conclude, that neuroleptic drugs are able to reduce depressive symptoms of acute schizophrenic patients - symptoms, which seem to be an integral part of the acute schizophrenic psychosis - as well as do antidepressives in patients suffering from an endogenous depression.

Frequency and Course Pattern of Depressive States

If neuroleptics do induce depression one might expect the levels of depression to increase during the hospitalization when the dosages of neuroleptics are generally higher than before admission (if there was any neuroleptic medication before admission). In opposite to this hypothesis the level of depression is lower at discharge than on admission (Möller and von Zerssen, 1982b). Psychiatrists' ratings were in good agreement with the patients' self-ratings (von Zerssen, 1976b) concerning this fact. Such a decrease was also observed by other investigators.

In order to collect more detailed informations we counted the frequency of marked intensity (more than 20% of the maximum score) of the different depression scores at admission and discharge. 48% of the patients had a marked "Depressive-Apathetic Syndrome" (this superfactor contains the three IMPS-factors mentioned above; von Zerssen and Cording, 1978) at admission, 17% at discharge. The analysis of the original IMPS-factors and of the self-rating factors gave similar results: The frequency of marked depressive syndromes is decreased at discharge as compared to admission. Most patients who had a marked depressive syndrome at discharge suffered from a marked depressive syndrome of the same or greater intensity on admission (Möller and von Zerssen, 1982b). Only from 5 to 10% of the patients - the percentage depends on the syndrome in question - were more depressed at discharge than on admission, a finding which does not provide strong support for the concept of pharmacogenic depression. Nevertheless, there is a rather high frequency (17%) of depression at discharge, which coincides with the clinical observation concerning "pharmacogenic" or "post-psychotic" depressions.

Analyses of the self-rating data on actual mood - the Actual Mood Scale (von Zerssen, 1976c) was given every other day - provides additional insight into the course of depressive disturbances of schizophrenic inpatients. 56% of the patients had a "depressive period" defined as a sequence of at least three abnormal scores higher than 21. Only 14% of all patients developed such a "depressive period" during hospitalization without also having had abnormal mood scores on admission. Depressive periods were overrepresented in those patients with an abnormal mood score on admission (Möller and von Zerssen, 1982b). The self-rating data on actual mood were plotted for each patient of a subgroup of 81 patients. A classification of these curves, made by visual analysis, proved similar results: Only 17% of the patients developed a depression without having been depressed at admission (Möller and von Zerssen, 1982a).

A small group of acute schizophrenic inpatients (N = 30), who were treated with a standard dose of Haloperidol, was rated repetitiously using the IMPS (Möller et al., 1982c). The analysis of original IMPS-factors and the analysis of the superfactor "Depressive-Apathetic Syndrome" shows in a very impressive way, what was called "revealed depression" by Knights and Hirsch (1981): The depressive symptoms remain hidden behind the florid feature of psychosis and are revealed during the remission phase (Fig. 1). There is no evidence in this group-statistical analysis for an increase of depressive-apathetic syndromatology. That is also true for the three original IMPS-factors ("Anxious Depression", "Retardation and Apathy", "Impaired Functioning") describing different aspects of depression. Analysing the courses of the single cases we found, that mostly a persistance or decrease of depressive symptomatology happens whereas an increase of the syndrome "Anxious Depression" was only observed in four cases, an increase of the syndrome "Retardation and Apathy" only in one case.

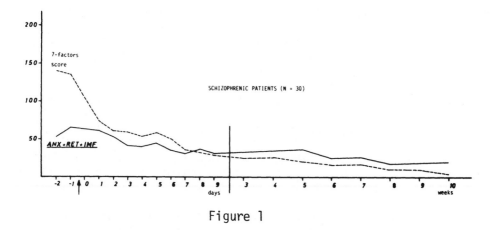

Figure 1

Prediction of Depressive States at Discharge

Depressive states at discharge of schizophrenic patients seem to be a more important phenomenon for clinicians than the depressive states at admission, when the florid psychotic symptoms are apparently of greater interest. To get some more ideas on factors correlated to these depressive states at discharge, we tested a large set of potential predictor variables, among others, data on premorbid personality dimensions (von Zerssen, 1980), data on premorbid psychosocial adjustment, socio-demographic data and data on the course of illness. Taking into account only the superfactor "Depressive-Apathetic Syndrome" as outcome-criterion, we found the following variables significantly ($p < 0.05$) correlated to a depressive state at discharge: poor premorbid adjustment (measured on the Gittelman-Klein-Scale, on the Goldstein-Scale and on the Phillips-Scale), schizoid traits (rated by relatives, not self-rated) and neurotic traits (self-rated) of premorbid personality, insiduous onset of first and index manifestation, duration of continuous neuroleptic treatment before index hospitalization and depressive symptoms at index admission. The IMPS-superfactor "Depressive-Apathetic Syndrome" at admission proved the highest correlation to the "Depressive-Apathetic Syndrome" at discharge (Möller et al., in prep.). None of these or the other variables tested were correlated to an deterioration of depressive-apathetic symptomatology between admission and discharge. Some of the predictors of the "Depressive-Apathetic Syndrome" at discharge were also predictive for the original IMPS-factors of depression: e.g. poor premorbid adjustment (measured by the Phillips Scale) for "Retardation and Apathy" and "Impaired Functioning", neurotic traits of premorbid personality (self-rated) for "Anxious Depression", duration of neuroleptic treatment for "Retardation and Apathy". Most of the predictors of the "Depressive-Apathetic Syndrome" are also predictive for the depression self-rating factor at discharge. In summarizing these results, we have to conclude that,among other variables, schizoid and neurotic traits of premorbid personality and poor premorbid adjustment are to the same extent related to depressive states at discharge as duration of neuroleptic treatment before admission. This gives some evidence for the hypothesis that depressive states at discharge cannot be explained only by one factor, e.g. the neuroleptic treatment or pre-treatment respectively, but that also other factors must be taken into consideration. It should be tested in multivariate regression analyses, whether and if so, how these factors are interrelated within the frame of a multiconditional model.

Depressive States in Schizophrenia as Predictors of Long-Term-Outcome

The subsample of 81 schizophrenics was reexamined five years after discharge. By this we had the opportunity to test the predictive value of depressive symptomatology at admission and discharge for the long-term outcome. There was no relationship between depression at admission and outcome-criteria, neither between the three IMPS-syndromes, nor for the depression self-rating factor and outcome criteria. In opposite to this the syndrome "Retardation and Apathy" at discharge was significantly ($p < 0.05$) correlated with some outcome criteria tested, among others, to the Global Assessment Scale. Higher scores of the IMPS-syndrome "Retardation and Apathy" were related to a poor outcome. The other IMPS-factors ("Anxious Depression", "Impaired Functioning") and the depression self-rating factor did not prove to be of prognostic value. Also there was no significant difference in the GAS-score between those patients who had higher depression scores at discharge than at admission compared to the other patients. To interprete these findings we would like to say that only depressive symptoms in the sense of "Retardation and Apathy" at discharge are of prognostical importance for long-term outcome, possibly because they are indicators of personality change.

REFERENCES

Knights, A., Hirsch, S.R., 1981, Revealed depression and drug treatment for schizophrenia. Arch. Gen. Psychiat. 38:806-811
Kokes, R.F., Strauss, J.S. and Klorman, R., 1977, Measuring premorbid adjustment: the instruments and their development. Schizophrenia Bull. 3:186-213

Lorr, M., 1974, Assessing psychotic behavior by the IMPS. In: Psychological measurements in psychopharmacology. Modern problems in pharmacopsychiatry, Vol. 7, Pichot, P., Olivier, R., eds., Karger, Basel

Mandel, M.R., Severe, J.B., Schooler, N.R., Gelenberg, A.J., Mieske, M., 1982, Development and prediction of postpsychotic depression in neuroleptic-treated schizophrenics. Arch. Gen. Psychiat. 39:197-203

McGlashan, T.A., 1982, Aphanisia: the syndrome of pseudo-depression in chronic schizophrenia. Schizophrenia Bull. 8:118-134

McGlashan, T.H., Carpenter, W.T., 1976, Postpsychotic depression in schizophrenia. Arch. Gen. Psychiat. 33:231-239

McGlashan, T.H., Carpenter, W.T., 1979, Affective symptoms and the diagnosis of schizophrenia. Schizophrenia Bull. 5:547-553

Möller, H.J., Zerssen, D.v., Werner-Eilert, K. and Wüschner-Stockheim M., 1981, Psychopathometrische Verlaufsuntersuchungen an Patienten mit Schizophrenien und verwandten Psychosen. Arch. Psychiat. Nervenkr. 230:275-292

Möller, H.J. and Zerssen, D.v., 1982a, Depressive states occuring during the neuroleptic treatment of schizophrenia. Schizophrenia Bull. 8:109-117

Möller, H.J. and Zerssen, D.v., 1982b, Depressive Symptomatik im stationären Behandlungsverlauf von 280 schizophrenen Patienten. Pharmacopsychiat. 14:172-179

Möller, H.J., Kissling, W., Lang, C., Doerr, P., Pirke, K.M. and Zerssen, D.v., 1982c, Efficacy and side effects of haloperidol in psychotic patients: oral versus intravenous administation. Am. J. Psychiat. 139:1571-1575

Möller, H.J., Barthelmes, H. and Zerssen, D.v., 1983a, Forschungsmöglichkeiten auf der Grundlage einer routinemäßig durchgeführten psychiatrischen Basis- und Befunddokumentation. Psychiatria clin. 16:45-61

Mombour,W., 1974, Syndrome bei psychiatrischen Erkrankungen.Eine vergleichende Untersuchung mit zwei Schätzskalen (IMPS und AMDP-Skala). Arch. Psychiat. Nervenkr. 219:331-350

Spitzer,J., Endicott, R.L., Fleiss, L., 1976, The Global Assessment Scale. A procedure for measuring overall severity of psychiatric disturbances. Arch. Gen. Psychiat. 33:766-771

Zerssen,D.v. , 1976, Klinische Selbstbeurteilungsskalen (KSB-S) aus dem Münchner Psychiatrischen Informationssystem (PSYCHIS München). Manuale. a) allgemeiner Teil; b) Paranoid-Depressivitäts-Skala; c) Befindlichkeits-Skala; d) Beschwerden-Liste. Beltz, Weinheim

Zerssen,D.v., Cording, C., 1978, The measurement of change in endogenous affective disorders. Arch. Psychiat. Nervenkr. 226: 95-112

Zerssen,D.v., 1980, Persönlichkeitsforschung bei Depressionen. In: Neue Perspektiven in der Depressionsforschung. Heimann, H., Giedke, H., eds., Huber, Bern, Stuttgart, Wien

SOME OBSERVATIONS ON THE FREQUENCY OF DEPRESSION IN SCHIZOPHRENIA

D.A.W. Johnson

Consultant Psychiatrist
University Hospital of South Manchester
West Didsbury,   Manchester   M20 8LR

The aim of the studies reported is to investigate the frequency of depression in the schizophrenic patient and to provide some information that is relevant to the present controversy on aetiology.

Depression was only identified if consistently present for more than a week, and under normal clinical conditions would provoke considerations for treatment. The definition used would meet all the requirments of the D.S.M.-111. The severity of depression had to rate a minimum of 15 on either the Hamilton Rating Scale for Depression or the Beck Depression Inventory.

Seven separate evaluations were carried out (Johnson, 1981).

(a) First illness schizophrenic patients who had not been prescribed neuroleptic medication prior to examination.

(b) Chronic schizophrenic patients who were currently not on neuroleptic drugs and were admitted to hospital in acute relapse. Patients had to be free from oral medication for two months or received no depot injection within the preceding three months (mean period = 9 months).

(c) Chronic schizophrenic patients in acute relapse on regular depot medication by injection.

Assessment of groups (b) and (c) were made blind to the current prescription of medication.

(d) Three groups of chronic schizophrenic patients maintained on regular depot injections and free from acute schizophrenic symptoms.

(i) Two month prevalence rate evaluated by prospective monitoring.

(ii) Patients prescribed antidepressant medication during a 15 month prospective assessment of extrapyramidal symptoms. (Johnson, 1973).

(iii) Random selection of patients attending the depot injection clinic and evaluated by nurses and a self-rating scale.

(e) A small group of chronic schizophrenic patients randomly selected at the time of relapse and followed-up prospectively for two years. All patients were on a single neuroleptic by a long-acting injection.

RESULTS

The mean age of patients with a first illness (21.7 years) was younger than the mean ages of the other groups (27-31 years). In all groups there were an excess of female patients (51-64 per cent).

Only two depot preparations were used for the patients on regular medication (fluphenazine decanoate N=176; flupenthixol decanoate N=112). No other medication was used apart from anti-Parkinsonian agents in 23 per cent of patients.

The prevalence of derpession for each group is shown in Table 1.

These results indicate that depression is a frequent symptom in both drug-free and drug treated patients. However, the particularly high prevalence of depression in first illness patients who have never received neuroleptics (37 per cent with a history of recent depression and 19 per cent with depression at the time of examination), and in drug-free relapsed chronic schizophrenic patients (30 per cent) clearly indicates that drugs are not the only cause of depression, nor is it likely that they are responsible for the majority of depressive episodes. The patients in remission, stabilised on maintenance depot therapy, and free from schizophrenic symptoms for some months consistently had the lowest prevalence of depressive symptoms (15-25 per cent). This result is consistent with the conclusions of Knights and Hirsch (1981) that depressive symptoms decrease rather than increase with adequate treatment.

A more detailed analysis of the results in the drug treated patients does provide some indication that at least some contribution may come from drugs, albeit a minority contribution, since both a higher dose regimen and the presence of extrapyramidal symptoms correlate at a level of significance with the presence of depression.

Table 1

Prevalence of depression in schizophrenia

	Sample N	Depression present	B.D.I.			H.R.S.		
			15–19	20–24	>25	15–19	20–25	>25
(a) First illness schizophrenia. No previous drugs:								
Depression present on admission	37	7	4	1	0	4	2	1
History of depression in the previous two months	30	11						
Total depression	37	18						
(b) Chronic schizophrenia: Relapse NOT on drugs:	79	24	2	2	1	14	8	2
(c) Chronic schizophrenia: Relapse ON depot medication	89	34	14	9	4	16	14	4
(d) Patients in remission on depot medication:								
2 month prospective study	41	10	3	7	0	4	6	0
15 month survey of prescribed antidepressants	140	21						
Nurses survey	100	26						
(e) Two year survey:								
Depressed at onset relapse	30	18	7	9	2	6	9	3
Depressed during follow-up	30	21	5	11	5	9	8	4

The full extent of the morbidity from depression is shown in the patients who were followed-up prospectively from the time of relapse (Group (e)). At the time of relapse 60 per cent of patients had depression present and during the next two years 70 per cent of patients experience at least one episode of depression. A comparison of the morbidity from depressive and more specific schizophrenic symptoms is shown in Tables 2 and 3. These results clearly indicate that a schizophrenic relapse is more serious in both a change of social function and treatment consequences, but nevertheless the morbidity from a depressive mood change is considerable.

A detailed analysis of the results failed to show any constant correlation with life events, drug dose change, extrapyramidal side-effects or relapse. On occasions when an association appeared clear the patient had subsequent depressions without the apparent precipitant being present. This illustrates how misleading it can be to identify causal associations from a single episode rather than a longitudinal study. The apparent lack of precipitating factors coupled with different associations being identified with different episodes of depression in the same patient strongly suggests that none of the factors studied were causative in the majority of depressions, and raised the strong possibility that depression is an intrinsic part of a schizophrenic illness.

'Depression' would appear to be more universally present and frequent in appearance than previously believed. Mood disorder in the total treatment of schizophrenia requires more careful evaluation, and in particular its modification needs urgent research. The present studies suggest only a minority contribution from drugs, with the best prognosis for depression being amongst the patients adequately stabilised on regular depot maintenance medication.

Table 2

Symptoms responsible for morbidity

| | Morbidity | |
Symptom	%	Weeks
Depression	70	356
Schizophrenia	20	104
Mixture	10	64

Table 3

Change of social function with depression and

schizophrenic relapse

	Depression %	Schizophrenia %
In employment - stopped work	69	100
No employment - work pattern deteriorated	71	100
Environment change	86	100
Mental Health Act admission	0	33
Relatives report substantial deterioration	52	100

REFERENCES

Johnson, D.A.W. (1973). The side-effects of fluphenazine decanoate. British Journal of Psychiatry, 132, 27-30.
Johnson, D.A.W. (1981). Studies of depressive symptoms in schizophrenia. British Journal of Psychiatry, 139, 89-101.
Knights, A. and Hirsch, S.R. (1981). 'Revealed' Depression and drug treatment for schizophrenia. Archives of General Psychiatry 135, 515-23.

THE DYSPHORIA SYNDROME

AND ITS RELATION TO EPS

Theodore Van Putten and
Stephen R. Marder

Veterans Administration Medical Center
Brentwood
Los Angeles, CA   90073

The measurement of extrapyramidal side effects (EPS) is in a primitive state. Groves and Mandel,[1] for example, in a survey of the long-acting fluphenazine studies, found the reported incidence of EPS with the enanthate ester to range from 0% to 100%, and with the decanoate ester the reported incidence of EPS ranged from 10% to 83%. Since the dosages in these studies were conventional, these marked differences in the reporting of EPS indicate that physicians differ greatly in their ability to detect the EPS of akinesia and akathisia: presumably everybody would record such readily observed EPS as tremor, dyskinesia, or dystonia.

Another reason for the underdiagnosis of akathisia and akinesia is that they have not been thought of as all that important. Generally, EPS have been regarded as a small price, a small discomfort that the patient should tolerate. Freyhan[2] even believed that akinesia is "a regular effect of neuroleptic drugs, part and parcel of their therapeutic action, which in many instances makes it seem arbitrary to define borderlines between therapeutic quanta of hypomotility and early signs of Parkinsonism."

Everyone would agree that severe akathisia or akinesia can cause dysphoria. The question is whether more moderate, or even subtle, EPS are all that important.

Dosage Comparison Studies

If subtler EPS cause dysphoria, then schizophrenic outpatients maintained on very low doses should feel better provided they do not relapse (Inpatient dose comparison studies were performed primarily in chronically hospitalized treatment refractory schizophrenics.(3,4) We do not believe that these results generalize to the more usual schizophrenic patient).

In a six week after care study Goldstein et al[5] compared 1 vs ¼cc (25 vs 6½mg) of fluphenazine enanthate in young, predominantly first-admission schizophrenics. Men (but not women) on the low dose experienced less anxious-depressive symptoms, but at the price of a somewhat higher tendency to relapse. EPS were not systematically recorded.

Kane and coworkers[6] tested the limits of a low-dose strategy by comparing standard dose fluphenazine decanoate - 12.5 to 50 mg every two weeks--to a 10% dilution--1.25 to 5.0 mg every two weeks--in stabilized schizophrenic outpatients. Even though low-dose patients relapsed more (the one-year relapse rate was 56% cumulatively for the low dose group and only 7% for the regular dose group) low-dose patients did better on measures of patient and family satisfaction, even with relapsing low-dose patients included. Nonrelapsing low-dose patients were also judged by the "blind" social adjustment raters to be doing significantly better than regular dose patients in social leisure activities and general adjustment. Marder and coworkers[7] similarly compared fluphenazine decanoate 25 vs 5 mg every two weeks in stabilized, rather chronic schizophrenic outpatients. On the SCL-90,[8] a self-report measure of subjective feeling states, patients on the higher dose experienced elevation in all nine SCL-90 factor scores. First year survival curves for the two doses show no differences in relapse rates (35% on 5 mg vs 42% on 25 mg).

These studies examine a complex risk-benefit area. They indicate, on balance, that patients on doses often regarded as homeopathic feel better at the price of a modest increase in relapse rate. The reasons why patients feel better on these very low maintenance doses is less certain.

In both the Marder[7] and Kane[6] studies, there was no difference in manifest EPS between the standard and low dose. This, however, does not invalidate our belief that differences in EPS account for the differences in outcome; rather, the measurement of EPS is so inexact given today's crude rating instruments that only gross differences can be detected.

For example, it can be impossible to distinguish between akinetic apathy and the negative symptoms of schizophrenia; between complaints of tension and anxiety and a mild treatment-resistant akathisia.

An "Exact" Incidence of Akathisia

Akathisia refers not to any type or pattern of movement but, rather, to a subjective need or desire to move. It is generally considered to occur within a few days or weeks of starting antipsychotic medication, but not within the first several hours. Actually, little is known about the incidence of akathisia, for no one has systematically attempted to measure it.

Following a test dose of haloperidol 5 mg, p.o., a substantial percentage of schizophrenic patients experienced akathisia: a few experienced akathisia already 2 hours after taking the tablet, and some 6 hours later, 40% of patients experienced akathisia! This akathisia was not mild or inconsequential: 28% experienced moderate, 17% severe and 22% experienced very severe akathisia.[9]

Treatment-resistant Akathisia with Haloperidol

If akathisia were promptly diagnosed (which, in our experience, it is not), it would still not pose a problem if it responded to treatment with antiparkinson drugs.

Of the 32 patients who developed akathisia during their first week of treatment with haloperidol 10 mg daily, akathisia was completely suppressed in 14 (44%). In the remaining 18 it was not possible to suppress the akathisia in spite of the maximal allowable (by the manufacturer) doses of antiparkinson drugs (either benztropine, 8 mg daily or trihexyphenidyl, 15 mg daily).[9]

Correlations between akathisia ratings (at 4 weeks) and BPRS [10] anxiety-depression scores ranged from $r=.35 - .42$; $p<.025 - .005$. On the SCI-90, a self-rating form attuned to subjective feeling states, akathisia is experienced by the patient as anxiety ($r=.512$) and depression ($r=.56$).

These correlations indicate a modest relationship between akathisia and anxiety-depression. They, however, do not reflect the anguish that akathisia often causes: one complained of "never having any comfort or rest," another of "exploding inside," of a "hurry-up feeling," "impatience," that "awful feeling," or "the worst misery."

Akinesia and Depression

Akinesia is defined by Rifkin, Quitken and Klein, as a "behavioral state of diminished spontaneity characterized by few gestures, unspontaneous speech and, particularly, apathy and difficulty with initiating usual activities."[11] So defined, this side effect of antipsychotic drugs often goes unrecognized.

Schizophrenic patients with post-psychotic depression have been described as "wooden" in appearance, motorically "inactive or retarded," lacking initiative to perform routine tasks, experiencing overwhelming fatigue and neuroasthenic symptoms, "hypersomnic" and "emotionally withdrawn". Nearly all reports comment on the patient's disinclination to speak.[3] All of these symptoms, however, can be manifestations of antipsychotic drug-induced akinesia.

In our own work,[3] out of a total of 94 schizophrenic inpatients, 28 developed a mild akinesia and 32 never developed extrapyramidal symptoms. Those who developed akinesia became less psychotic, but they also experienced a significant, although modest, increase in depression ratings. Vigorous treatment of the akinesia with trihexyphenidyl resulted in significant improvements in depression, somatic concern, anxiety, emotional withdrawal, blunted affect and motor retardation on both physician's and nurses' ratings. The 32 non-akinetic patients also became less psychotic, but not more depressed.

In our sample, only half of the akinetic patients experienced an increase in depression ratings and the increase, although statistically significant, was modest. Further, the half who became depressed were different pre-treatment; they were significantly more grandiose, lively, less blunted and in more active contact with their environment. This suggests a super-imposed affective component, although none of these patients, in our opinion, would warrant the diagnosis of schizoaffective disorder and none had histories of cyclic or naturally occurring depressions.

Rifkin and associates(12,13) compared fluphenazine decanoate and oral fluphenazine with a placebo in remitted schizophrenics in an aftercare clinic. 35% of the patients assigned to fluphenazine decanoate (but none of the patients on oral fluphenazine) developed disabling akinesia. The akinetic patients became significantly (although modestly) more depressed and withdrawn when compared to their own baseline and to the survivors who did not develop akinesia.

Mandel, Severe, Schooler et al[14] compared oral fluphenazine with fluphenazine decanoate in 211 schizophrenic patients being maintained in the community. Three to five months after discharge about one fourth of the patients became depressed. There were no significant differences in incidence of depression between the two preparations. There was also no difference in side effects (rigidity, tremor, akathisia, increased motor activity, decreased motor activity) between the depressed and non-depressed patients. Although akinesia was certainly not measured with the same sensitivity as by Rifkin et al[12,13], it is unlikely that akinesia has much to do with these depressions. One would not expect akinesia to develop 3-5 months after discharge nor to improve over time on the same dosage, as was the case in some of these "depressions".

598

Johnson,[15] in a naturalistic study of schizophrenic outpatients, also found the presence of extrapyramidal symptoms (type not specified) to be significantly (p<.001) related to depression. There was also a trend, not reaching statistical significance, for more severe extrapyramidal symptoms to correlate with more severe depression. It is important to note, however, that those patients successfully maintained in remission by depot injections had the lowest prevalence of depression.

Galdi et al[16] studied drug response in two large samples (total n=251) of schizophrenic inpatients treated with a variety of neuroleptics. In both samples schizophrenics with depressed relatives experienced more depression and more pseudoparkinsonism post-treatment. In the second sample, schizophrenics with depressed relatives experienced significantly more severe EPS (muscle rigidity, loss of associated movements, akathisia); correlations between EPS and anxious-depressive symptoms ranged from 0.48 to 0.79, but the paper does not specify which EPS correlated the most. Hogarty et al[17] similarly found depressive heredity in neuroleptic treated outpatients who relapsed with depressive symptoms. This group did not appear to have more side effects, but there was not a "precise assessment of akinesia."

These studies, on balance, indicate a definite association between EPS and depression. One gets the impression that the increase in depression was clinically modest and that the EPS may have been severe.

Conclusions

The findings of a link between EPS and depression should not be taken to mean that neuroleptics greatly increase the risk of depression in schizophrenics. After all, depression occurs frequently in the course of schizophrenic illness--whether patients receive antipsychotic medications or not.[18] In fact, in our own work,[19] as well as others,[20,21] antipsychotic medications, on the average, exert an antidepressant effect. Thus, in a sample of 91 patients, [19] 29 (32%) remained depressed during the drug-free observation period. When these 29 were treated with antipsychotic medication, 45% improved. Of the 62 patients who were not depressed at the start of drug treatment, only 15% became so. Amongst this 15%, there was a significantly (p<.05) greater number of patients with depressive heredity. The following conclusions appear reasonable:

.EPS, particularly akathisia, is often at bottom of dysphoric feelings and even anguish in medicated schizophrenic patients; [22,23] this anguish is not recorded with the standard rating scales. A schizophrenic patient who can "never find any comfort or rest"(because of akathisia) need not be depressed or anxious; he is, however, miserable.

.It is our belief that a good deal of suffering in schizophrenia
is due to unrecognized EPS. The measurement of EPS is in
primitive state, and, until there is some standardized way of
rating it, such an impression is obviously unverifiable.

.Our work and that of others does support a relationship between
EPS and depression. One gets the impression that the EPS was
severe and the increase in depression modest. It would seem
that much would depend on the patient's understanding of the
EPS and the patient's circumstances; a moderate-severe akinesia
would be one thing for a chronic inpatient, and quite another
for a man who is trying to make it on the outside.

.Although neuroleptics, on the average, do not cause and even
alleviate depression, there are over 30 papers[24] on neurolep-
tic-induced depression. With so much smoke, there has to be a
fire. It may be that schizophrenic patients with depressive
heredity are at special risk of severe depression when treated
with neuroleptics.

REFERENCES

1. Groves JE, Mandel MR: The long acting phenothiazines. Arch
    Gen Psychiatry 32:893-900, 1975.
2. Freyhan FA: Psychomotility and parkinsonism in treatment neuro-
    leptic drugs. Arch Neurol Psychiatry 78:465-471, 1957.
3. Van Putten T, May PRA: "Akinetic depression" in schizophrenia.
    Arch Gen Psychiatry 35:1101-1107, 1978.
4. Cole JO: Psychopharmacology update antipsychotic drugs: Is
    more better? McLean Hospital J 7:61-87, 1982.
5. Goldstein MF, Rodnick EH, Evans JR, May PRA, Steinberg M: Drug
    and family therapy in the aftercare treatment of acute schizo-
    phrenia. Arch Gen Psychiatry 35:1169-1177, 1978.
6. Kane J, Rifkin A, Woerner M, et al: Low-dose neuroleptics in
    outpatient schizophrenics. (Paper presented at the NCDEU
    Annual Meeting, Key Biscayne, Florida, May 26, 1981).
7. Marder SR, Van Putten T: Maintenance therapy in schizophrenia
    with either standard or very low dose fluphenazine decanoate.
    (Paper presented at the ACNP Annual Meeting, Puerto Rico,
    December 15, 1982).
8. Derogatis LR, Lipman RS, Rickets K, et al: The Hopkins symptom
    checklist (HSCL): A self-report symptom inventory. Behav
    Sci 19:1-17, 1974.
9. Van Putten T, Marder SR, May PRA: Akathisia with haloperidol
    and thiothixene. Arch Gen Psychiatry, in press.
10. Overall JE, Gorham DR: The Brief Psychiatric Rating Scale.
    Psychol Rep 10:799-812, 1962.
11. Rifkin A, Quitkin F, Klein DR: Akinesia. Arch Gen Psychiatry
    32:672-674, 1975.

12. Rifkin A, Quitkin F, Rabiner CJ, Klein DF: Fluphenazine decanoate, fluphenazine hydrochloride given orally, and placebo in remitted schizophrenics. I. Relapse rates after one year. Arch Gen Psychiatry 34:43-47, 1977.
13. Rifkin A, Quitkin F, Klein DF: Fluphenazine decanoate, oral fluphenazine, and placebo in treatment of remitted schizophrenics. II. Rating scale data. Arch Gen Psychiatry 34:1215-1219, 1977.
14. Mandel MR, Severe JB, Schooler NR, et al. Development and prediction of postpsychotic depression in neuroleptic-treated schizophrenics. Arch Gen Psychiatry 39:197-203, 1982.
15. Johnson DAW: Studies of depressive symptoms in schizophrenia.
    I. The prevalence of depression and its possible causes.
    II. A two-year logitudinal study of symptoms.
   III. A double-blind trial of orphenadrine against placebo.
    Br J Psychiatry 139:89-101, 1981.
16. Galdi J, Rieder RO, Silber D, Bonato RR: Genetic factors in the response to neuroleptics in schizophrenia: A psychopharmacogenetic study. Psychological Medicine 11:713-728, 1981.
17. Hogarty GE, Schooler NR, Ulrich R, et al: Fluphenazine and social therapy in the aftercare of schizophrenic patients: Relapse analyses of a two-year controlled study of fluphenazine decanoate and fluphenazine hydrochloride. Arch Gen Psychiatry 36:1283-1294, 1979.
18. Hirsch SR, Gaind R, Rohde PD, et al: Outpatient maintenance of chronic schizophrenic patients with long-acting fluphenazine: A double-blind placebo trial. Br Med J 1:633-637, 1973.
19. Van Putten T, Marder SR, May PRA: Neuroleptic induced depression and depressive heredity. Am J Psychiatry, in press.
20. Moller HF, Von Zerssen D: Depressive states occurring during the neuroleptic treatment of schizophrenia. Schizophrenia Bulletin 8:109-117, 1982.
21. Knights A, Hirsch SR: "Revealed" depression and drug treatment for schizophrenia. Arch Gen Psychiatry 38:806-811, 1981.
22. Van Putten T, May PRA, Marder SR: Response to antipsychotic medication: The doctor's and the consumer's view. Am J Psychiatry, in press.
23. Van Putten T, May PRA, Marder SR, et al: Subjective response to antipsychotic drugs. Arch Gen Psychiatry 38:187-190, 1981.
24. Ananth J, Chadirian AM: Drug induced mood disorder. International Pharmacopsychiatry 15:58-73, 1080.

THE ROLE OF GENETIC FACTORS IN THE INDUCTION OF EXTRAPYRAMIDAL
SIDE-EFFECTS IN SCHIZOPHRENIC PATIENTS

Joe Galdi, John T. Kelly, Ronald O. Rieder, and Roland R. Bonato

New Hampshire Hospital, Concord, NH USA; University of Minn-
esota Hospitals, Minneapolis, MN; National Institute of Mental
Health, Bethesda, MD; The Biometric Laboratory, George
Washington University, Washington, DC (respectively)

INTRODUCTION

Extrapyramidal side-effects (EPS) are commonly attributed to
the extraneous dopamine (DA) blocking actions of neuroleptics in the
nigrastriatum.[1] In treating schizophrenia and other disorders, it
is therefore assumed that EPS occur secondarily to the disorder-
related antipsychotic effects of neuroleptics and that the nigrastriatal DA system is not itself implicated in the disorder.

Findings from a recent study by the present authors, however,
have tended to contradict this assumption: some forms of EPS (and
depression) in schizophrenia may not be secondary but may be induced
by the interaction of neuroleptics with a neurogenetic defect in the
nigrastriatum of affected patients.[2] In this study, schizophrenics
who had depressed first-degree relatives exhibited more frequent and
severe expressions of pseudoparkinsonism and akathisia than schizophrenics who had schizophrenic first-degree relatives. Depression,
furthermore, often emerged with EPS in these patients. These findings
not only implied that these side-effects were commonly due to DA-Ach
imbalance in the nigrastriatum,[3-4] but implicated this DA system in
the pathogenetics of the associated disorder. Since they appeared to
characterize the effects of neuroleptics on an extrapyramidal (motor)
component of the disorder, the potential utility of these side-effects
as "pharmacogenetic criteria" by which the disorder may be discriminated was emphasized.

The present study attempted to validate these findings in
another sample of genetically subgrouped schizophrenics.

METHOD

The full sample consisted of 33 recently admitted schizophrenics in whom EPS emerged after being treated with neuroleptics during the normal course of hospitalization.[5] All patients had been diagnosed in routine clinical settings according to DSM-II criteria and lacked signs of organicity, epilepsy, medical disease and true Parkinsonism. In most cases patients were sampled when EPS first emerged which tended to be of milder intensity. Two antiparkinson agents, benztropine mesylate (2-4 mgs/day) and amantadine HCl (200 mgs/day), were randomly assigned and alternately administered in a crossover design while neuroleptics were continued at original dosages. Since few patients entered the crossover phase of the trial, however, only data from the first week outcome were evaluated. Clinical symptoms and drug side-effects were assessed with standard rating scales (see Tables 1 and 2) at pretreatment and after 7 days of therapy. Family history data were obtained using a standard psychiatric history form[6] which assessed the presence of schizophrenia and depression plus alcoholism and "other" disorders in parents and siblings (cf.[2]). Seven patients who had depressed relatives and four patients who had schizophrenic relatives were designated "D" and "S" patients, respectively. One patient who had different relatives diagnosed for schizophrenia and depression was excluded. Among the remaining 21 patients, a few had relatives with alcoholism or other (unspecified) disorders but all lacked a positive family history of schizophrenia or depression. These patients were designated the "0" patients and evaluated for contrast purposes only. Mean dosages of neuroleptics (CPZ equivalents) in use when EPS emerged were nonsignificantly higher in S and 0 patients (1196 and 1219 mgs/day, respectively) than in D patients (850 mgs/day).

Statistical tests applied in the study emphasized a priori t-tests for predictable findings[2] and post hoc tests otherwise.

RESULTS

Rigidity as measured by the Severity of Extrapyramidal Reactions Scale was more severe in D patients than in S patients when EPS emerged, while similar differences in rigidity, posture, and total symptoms score as measured by the Parkinson's Disease Rating Scale approached significance as one-tailed tests (Table 1). Tremor, however, appeared unexpectedly more severe in S patients and akathisia failed to distinguish the subgroups. Tests between these subgroups and the 0 subgroup failed to reveal initial differences in EPS.

Clinical symptoms in these subgroups were also in accord with expected findings (Table 2). BPRS depression and paranoid-hostility levels were significantly higher in D patients than in S patients. Patients in the 0 subgroup also revealed more paranoid-hostility than S patients.

Table 1. Extrapyramidal Side-Effects in Genetic
Subgroups of Schizophrenic Patients

Genetic Subgroups

Side-Effects	n	D 7	S 4	O 21	P-Values[a]
Parkinson's Disease Rating Scale[b]					
Bradykinesia of Hands		1.1	1.0	1.3	
Rigidity		1.9	1.3	1.7	D > S, p < .08, 1-tailed
Posture		1.4	0.8	1.0	D > S, p < .12, 1-tailed
Upper Extremity Swing		1.6	0.8	1.6	
Gait		0.4	0.3	0.8	
Tremor		0.4	1.0	0.8	
Facies		1.1	0.8	1.4	
Seborrhea		0.1	0.0	0.0	
Speech		0.8	1.0	1.0	
Self-Care		0.1	0.0	0.3	
Total Score		9.0	6.8	9.8	D > S, p < .11, 1-tailed
Severity of Extrapyramidal Reactions Scale[c]					
Tremor		0.4	1.5	1.1	S > D, p < .04, 2-tailed
Rigidity		2.6	1.8	2.4	D > S, p < .02, 1-tailed
Akathisia		1.6	2.0	2.2	
Dystonia		1.0	0.0	0.3	
Dyskinesia		1.6	1.3	1.6	
Total Score		7.1	6.5	7.5	

[a] From t-tests for differences between means; shown if $p < .20$.
[b] Scored 0-3 except for Speech, 0-2.   [c] Scored 0-4.

After 7 days of antiparkinson therapy, however, differences between subgroups became nonsignificant. Large reductions of EPS occurred irrespectively of genetic status. Change in total BPRS symptoms including depression at termination or during the first week posttreatment interlude, however, revealed substantial improvement in D and O patients (64 and 63%, respectively) but not in S patients (9%). S patients were also rated as being more severely ill ($p < .005$) and less improved ($p < .05$) than D patients when terminated from the study. Although benztropine induced more overall improvement than amantadine ($p < .05$; cf. [5]), both agents appeared to alleviate EPS in the subgroups (not testable).

Table 2. Clinical Symptoms in Genetic Subgroups of
Schizophrenic Patients With Extrapyramidal Side-Effects

Genetic Subgroups

Symptoms	n	D 7	S 4	O 21	P-Values[a]
Brief Psychiatric Rating Scale (BPRS)					
Anxious Depression		17.0	13.0	14.5	D > S, p < .02, 1-tailed
Withdrawal-Retardation		18.0	15.0	15.4	
Thinking Disturbance		15.9	12.8	14.0	
Hostile-Suspiciousness		11.0	7.3	11.3	D > S, p < .06, 2-tailed
					O > S, p < .003, 2-tailed
Activation		12.7	11.3	11.0	
Clinical Global Impressions Scale (CGI)					
Severity		4.9	4.5	4.8	

[a] From t-tests for differences between means; shown if $p < .20$.

DISCUSSION

These results lend further support to the notion that some forms
of EPS in schizophrenic patients may be pharmacogenetically-induced.
Based on prior findings, these EPS show potential for greater severity and frequently emerge in concert with a depressive syndrome.
Since patients manifesting these side-effects may be suffering from
disorders which are actually genetic variants of affective (bipolar?)
rather than schizophrenic illnesses per se, their potential utility
for discriminating a distinct subgroup (s) of schizophrenia is suggested by these results. To test this proposition further, we compared the (uncorrected) incidences of patients with depressed and
schizophrenic relatives in the 33 EPS-sampled patients with these
incidences in a general sample of 110 recently admitted schizophrenic
patients who had participated in six drug trials at the same hospital. Identical family history and diagnostic criteria had been
applied in both samples. Although patients in the general sample were
older (29 vs 24 yrs, p < .01) and therefore probably had older
relatives who had traversed more age-risk, and although patients
who subsequently exhibited EPS in the general sample could not be
excluded, there was a nonsignificant tendency for more patients in

the EPS sample to have a first-degree relative diagnosed for depression (24.2 vs 12.7%, p > .05 < .10).

Contrasting prior findings, however, in the current study akathisia failed to differentiate the genetic subgroups and tremor appeared relatively more severe in S patients. These discrepancies might have been due to the tendency to sample patients at earlier phases of developing EPS, i.e., before their full severity potential is reached, or they may simply indicate that these EPS are not essential aspects of the pharmacogenetic syndrome. On the other hand, since one sample in the prior study bearing methodologic problems failed to confirm the EPS side of these results altogether, still further replication seems indicated. By the same token, none of the three samples which we have thus far investigated has failed to show higher levels of postdrug depression in schizophrenics with a family history of depression. Unfortunately, lack of symptom ratings at hospital admission in the current sample made it impossible to determine if depression had increased as EPS emerged or whether it was present at admission before the initiation of neuroleptics.

The brevity of this report precludes broader discussion of the pathophysiological aspects of postdrug depressions in schizophrenic patients (q.v. [7-9]). Apart from the contribution of genetic predisposition as suggested by our findings, a critical issue relevant to drug-induction is focused on the presumed nigrastriatal locus[3] and, thus, anticholinergic responsiveness of the depression. If this locus were relevant to induction, then anticholinergic drugs (or DA agonists such as amantadine) would be expected to act on this depression in an ameliorative fashion. To date, however, findings bearing on anticholinergic responsiveness, including our own, are only suggestive. In a controlled study, Johnson[10] recently reported that orphenadrine was mildly, if nonsignificantly superior to placebo in treating these depressions, but low or questionable efficacy[11] may have obscured a clearcut outcome. Several reports of quick remissions following treatment with anticholinergics, while ostensibly convincing, suffer similar shortcomings.[4,12-13] Further controlled studies are obviously required to settle this issue as well as to further clarify competing interpretations of the depression: whether it is a separate, nondrug related syndrome independent from EPS,[7,14] on a severity continuum with EPS,[2] or just a reactive syndrome which occurs secondarily to extrapyramidal motor inhibition.[13,15]

A possibly even more critical issue for future research is suggested by increasing indications that this depression may only be a harbinger of other, more deleterious, iatrogenic effects such as prolonged hospital stay, chronicity, relapse, suicide, and neurologic disorders such as tardive dyskinesia in schizophrenic patients treated with neuroleptics.

REFERENCES

1. C.D. Marsden and P. Jenner, The pathophysiology of extrapyram-side-effects of neuroleptic drugs, Psychol. Med. 10:65 (1980).
2. J. Galdi, R.O. Rieder, D. Silber, and R.R. Bonato, Genetic factors in the response to neuroleptics in schizophrenia: a psychopharmacogenetic study. Psychol. Med. 11:713 (1981).
3. H. Beckmann, Dopaminergic function and depression, q.v. W. Hartmann, J. Kind, J.E. Meyer, P. Muller and H. Steuber, Neuroleptic drugs and the prevention of relapse in schizo-phrenia: a workshop report, Schizo. Bull. 6:536 (1980).
4. F.J. Ayd, The depot fluphenazines: a reappraisal after 10 years' clinical experience, Am. J. Psychiat. 132:491 (1975).
5. J.T. Kelly, R. Zimmerman, F.S. Abuzzahab and B.C. Schiele, A double-blind study of amantadine hydrochloride vs benztropine mesylate in drug-induced parkinsonism, Pharmacol. 12:65 (1974).
6. T.H. McGlashan, The Documentation of Clinical Psychotropic Drug Trials, U.S. Government Printing Office, Washington, DC (1973).
7. S.R. Hirsch, Depression "revealed" in schizophrenia, Brit. J. Psychiat. 140:421 (1982).
8. W. Hartmann, J. Kind, J.E. Meyer, P. Muller and H. Steuber, Neuroleptic drugs and the prevention of relapse in schizo-phrenia: a workshop report, Schizo. Bull. 6:536 (1980).
9. J. Ananth and A.M. Ghadirian, Drug-induced mood disorders, Int. Pharmacopsychiat. 15:59 (1980).
10. D.A.W. Johnson, Studies of depressive symptoms in schizophrenia. Brit. J. Psychiat. 139:89 (1981).
11. R.H.S. Mindham, R. Gaind, B.H. Anstee and L. Rimmer, Comparison of amantadine, orphenadrine, and placebo in the control of phenothiazine-induced parkinsonism, Psychol. Med. 2:406 (1972).
12. T. van Putten and P.R.A. May, "Akinetic" depression in schizo-phrenia, Arch. Gen. Psychiat. 35:1101 (1978).
13. T. van Putten and L.R. Mutalipassi, Fluphenazine enanthate induced decompensations, Psychosom. 14:37 (1979).
14. M.M. Singh and S.R. Kay, Dysphoric response to neuroleptic treatment in schizophrenia: its relationship to autonomic arousal and prognosis, Biol. Psychiat. 14:277 (1979).
15. G.E. Hogarty, N.R. Schooler, R. Ulrich, F. Mussare, P. Ferro and E. Herron, Fluphenazine and social therapy in the after-care of schizophrenic patients, Arch. Gen. Psychiat. 36:1283 (1979).

ACKNOWLEDGEMENTS

The authors gratefully acknowledge Dr. Burtrum C. Schiele, Professor Emeritus, Department of Psychiatry, Univ. of Minnesota Medical School, for contributing data to the study. These data were deposited in the Early Clinical Drug Evaluation Units (ECDEU) data-bank maintained by the Biometric Laboratory of the George Washington University and supported by NIMH contract 5-R01-MH-22019-04 to Dr. Bonato.

DEPRESSION IN CHRONIC SCHIZOPHRENIA

Alec Roy

Clinical Neuroscience Branch
National Institute of Mental Health
Bethesda, Maryland, USA

Other papers in this symposium have highlighted the ubiquitous association of affective symptoms in schizophrenic
inpatients and the high affective morbidity that schizophrenic
patients suffer. Chronic schizophrenic patients also suffer an
increased mortality due to suicide. Follow-up studies demonstrate that 10% of chronic schizophrenics die by suicide
(Miles, 1977). That suicide is associated with affective disorder in chronic schizophrenic patients has been demonstrated
in a recent study (Roy, 1982). Thirty chronic schizophrenic
patients, known to have committed suicide, were matched with
the next presenting chronic schizophrenic patient who did not
commit suicide. Significantly more of those who went on to
commit suicide, than their controls, had been diagnosed in
the past by their psychiatrists as suffering from a major
depressive episode meeting DSM III criteria--over 50%--and
significantly more had been treated in the past with antidepressants or ECT for depression. In the last period of
psychiatric contact, too, significantly more of the chronic
schizophrenic patients who committed suicide in that episode
were diagnosed by their psychiatrist as suffering from a
major depressive episode (DSM III criteria). Thus that study
strongly indicated a link between depression and suicide in
chronic schizophrenia.

To avoid controversy about so-called "postpsychotic
depression," it was decided to study depressed chronic schizo-
prenic patients who had not had an admission within the
previous two months. A consecutive group of 18 chronic
schizophrenic outpatients was collected who, after interview with
the Schedule of Affective Disorders and Schizophrenia (SADS), met

609

DSM III criteria for a major depressive episode (Roy, 1983).
Their mean Hamilton score was 20.3 (range 16 to 26). They
were matched for age, sex and social class with the next chronic
schizophrenic outpatient who was not currently depessed and who
had not had a depressive episode in the previous six months.
There were no significant differences between the two groups for
either the duration of illness, type of schizophrenia or for the
presence in a first-degree relative of depression treated by a
psychiatrist (4 versus 2). Nor were there any significant differences between the groups for mean equivalent daily doses of
chlorpromazine. Sixteen of the 18 depressed schizophrenic
patients were receiving neuroleptics in an equivalent mean daily
dosage of 526.4 mg of chlorpromazine (SD 528.2) as compared to 17
of the 18 nondepressed schizophrenic controls who were receiving
a mean chlorpromazine daily dosage of 303.1 mg (SD 252.8)--no
significant difference.

The statistically significant differences between the
chronic schizophrenics with a current affective syndrome (range
of duration 2 weeks to 7 1/2 months) and the nondepressed chronic
schizophrenic controls are shown in Table 1.

Table 1. Significant Differences between Depressed and
Nondepressed Schizophrenics

	DS* N = 18	NDS** N = 18	Significance
Number of Admissions	6.9	4.1	P<0.02
Past Depressive Episode	15	5	P<0.001
Past Treatment for Depression	13	5	P<0.009
Previous Suicide Attempt	15	7	P<0.007
Early Parental Loss	11	5	P<0.05
Self-esteem	20.9	29.7	P<0.005
Living Alone	11	4	P<0.02
Number of Life Events in Previous Six Months	4.0	1.4	P<0.0005

*DS = Depressed Schizophrenics
**NDS = Nondepressed Schizophrenics

The table shows that the group of depressed chronic schizophrenic patients had had significantly more admissions, more had
had a past episode of depressive disorder and more past treatment

610

with antidepressants or ECT for depression. Significantly more of the depressed schizophrenics had experienced early parental loss and had made an attempt at suicide. The depressed schizophrenics had experienced more life events in the six months before the onset of their depression than their controls. The life events were rated "blindly" by a colleague who did not know the patients or the research hypothesis but who was experienced and reliable with Paykel's life-event methodology. Significantly more of the depressed schizophrenics had experienced undesirable life-events, exits from the social field, work-related, family-related and employment-related life events than their nondepressed schizophrenic controls.

Thus the model proposed by the results of this study is that the chronic schizophrenic outpatient who develops a major depessive episode has risk factors for depression. (In this study these were living alone, early parental loss, and low self-esteem). He encounters adversity (life events) but may not neccessarily relapse with schizophrenia, as Brown and Birley (1968) demonstrated occurs with life events, as he is receiving neuroleptics and thus may be protected from schizophrenic relapse. However, having risk factors for depression he may be liable to relapse with a major affective disorder. Further studies are needed to determine other risk factors for depression in chronic schizophrenic outpatients--i.e., negative symptoms and biological variables. This study highlights the fact that we should pay more attention to the role of precipitating factors and risk factors for depression when studying the aetiology of depression in chronic schizophrenic outpatients.

REFERENCES

Brown, G., and Birley, J., 1968, Crises and life changes and and the onset of schizophrenia, J. Health Soc. Behav., 9:203.
Miles, P., 1977, Conditions predisposing to suicide, J. Nerv. Ment. Dis., 164:231.
Roy, A., 1982, Suicide in chronic schizophrenia, Br. J. Psychiatry, 141:171.
Roy, A., 1983, Depression in chronic schizophrenia. Br. J. Psychiatry, 142:465.

PERSONALITY AND CHRONICITY IN DEPRESSIVE

DISORDERS: INTRODUCTORY REMARKS

Hagop S. Akiskal

Affective Disorders Program
University of Tennessee College of Medicine
Memphis, Tennessee 38163, USA

Current estimates indicate that 15-20% of depressive conditions pursue a chronic course.[1] It was in recognition of such symptomatic chronicity that the DSM-III category of "dysthymic disorder" was created[2]. This term refers to fluctuating depressive symptoms, either continuous or intermittent, over a period of at least 2 years. It is implied that the "typical" course of major depressive episodes is resolution within a time frame considerably shorter than 2 years. Characterologic disturbances are widely believed to contribute significantly to inadequate recovery from depressive episodes. However, the causative role of such disturbances does not rest on firm evidence. Accordingly, while acknowledging the frequent association between dysthymia and personality disorder, DSM-III guidelines are explicit in recommending that personality disorder be coded on a separate axis (II) orthogonal to the phenomenologic axis (I) on which dysthymic disorder is diagnosed.

This position, which considers personality as orthogonal to affective illness, represents the "atheoretical" point of view: Personality and affective disorder may coexist without one necessarily causing the other. This position is in contrast to psychoanalytic, behavioral, cognitive, and Kraepelinian views. Both analytic[3] and cognitive-behavioral[4,6] schools have postulated the existence of maladaptive premorbid personality traits which have formative influence on the development of affective episodes. In neo-Kraepelinian psychiatry, the direction of causation is reversed: Personality disturbances are either considered milder, or subaffective, expressions of the affective disorder[7], or

epiphenomenal to recurrent incapacitating episodes of illness.[8]
In still another theoretical viewpoint, the pathoplasty position,
it is submitted that personality, while not necessarily pathogenic
in affective illness, may nevertheless alter the clinical form of
episodes.[9]

The relationship of personality and affective disorders has
been critically reviewed recently.[10,11] Research in this area,
largely applied to major affective disorders, has been generally
inconclusive in resolving this relationship. Data are sparser,
and direction of causality even less certain, in chronic depressions. This may be due to the heterogeneity of chronic depressions, which represent the final clinical common pathway of
different affective and nonaffective processes. One chronic
depressive pattern, usually late in onset, represents the residuum
of incompletely remitted episodes of unipolar disorder;[12] such
patients are typically free of low-grade depressive manifestations
premorbidly. By contrast, in "double depressions," major episodes
of depression are superimposed on pre-existing low-grade depression;[13] upon recovery from major episodes, return to this premorbid
level is usually the rule. In subaffective dysthymia, tricyclic
antidepressants may bring about brief hypomanic switches, superimposed on the dominant low-grade depressive baseline.[14] Finally,
in secondary chronic dysphorias, fluctuating depression parallels
the course of incapacitating nonaffective psychiatric or disabling
medical disorders.[15]

The relevance of etiologic variables, including putative personality factors, may be different in these subtypes of chronic depression. By way of illustration, incomplete remission from unipolar
episodes[12] seems to be favored by higher genetic loading for affective illness, inadequate therapeutic trials, concurrent rheumatologic
disease, treatment with depressant antihypertensive drugs, multiple
deaths within immediate family, and incapacitating medical or
psychiatric illness of spouse; the relevance of personality factors
could not be established for this subtype in a University of
Tennessee study.[12] Subaffective dsythymia, where personality often
approximates Schneider's depressive type, appears to be an
attenuated genetic form of primary affective disorder.[14] As conceptualized elsewhere,[16] the depressive personality pattern in this
condition may represent a less penetrant form of cyclothymia, where
hypomania is manifest only on pharmacologic challenge.

The concepts embodied in the foregoing paragraph are based on
research findings. In clinical practice, it is often difficult to
determine whether characterologic disturbances are primary or
secondary to the chronic depressive picture. Hence the frequent use
of the clinical concept of "characterologic depression,"[17]
especially in reference to protracted low-grade depressions of
developmental origin. As discussed subsequently in this symposium,

character pathology may be primary in a subtype of such early-onset chronic dysphorias. This symposium will explore the relationship of personality and other relevant variables to chronicity in selected subtypes of affective disorders. Research in this complex interphase of personality and chronic affective disorder is just beginning to yield data of clinical importance. Findings are tentative, often contradictory, but with the new creative and systematic thrust of research in the past few years, this interphase area is emerging as one of the frontiers of research in affective disorders.

References

1. Robins E, Guze SB: Classification of affective disorders: the primary-secondary, the endogenous-reactive and the neurotic-psychotic concepts. In Williams TA, Katz MM, Shields JA (eds): Recent Advances in the Psychobiology of the Depressive Illnesses. Washington, DC, US Government Printing Office (1972)
2. American Psychiatric Association: Diagnostic and Statistical Manual of Mental Disorders, 3rd ed. Washington, DC, APA (1980)
3. Arieti S, Bemporad J: Severe and Mild Depression. New York, Basic Books Inc (1978)
4. Kovacs J, Beck A: Maladaptive cognitive structures in depression. Am J Psychiatry 133:525-533 (1978)
5. Seligman J: Helplessness. San Francisco, WH Freeman and Co (1975)
6. Lewinsohn P: A behavioral approach to depression, in Friedman RJ, Katz MM (eds): The Psychology of Depressions: Contemporary Theory and Research. New York, John Wiley & Sons, pp 97-104 (1974)
7. Akiskal HS, Djenderedjian AH, Rosenthal RH, Khani MK: Cyclothymic disorder: Validating criteria for inclusion in the bipolar affective group. Am J Psychiatry 134:1227-1233 (1977)
8. Cassano GB, Maggini C, Akiskal HS: Short-term subchronic and chronic sequelae of affective disorders. Psychiatr Clin North Am 6:55-67 (1983)
9. Lazare A, Klerman G: Hysteria and depression: The frequency and significance of hysterical personality features in hospitalized depressed women. Am J Psychiatry 124:48-56 (1968)
10. Von Zerssen D: Personality and affective disorders, in Paykel ES (ed): Handbook of Affective Disorders. New York, The Guilford Press, pp 212--28 (1982)
11. Akiskal HS, Hirschfeld RMA, Yerevanian BI: The relationship of personality to affective disorders: A critical review. Arch Gen Psychiatry 40:801-810 (1983)

12. Akiskal HS: Factors associated with incomplete recovery in primary depressive illness. J Clin Psychiatry 43:266-271 (1982)
13. Keller MB, Shapiro RW: "Double depression"; Superimposition of acute depressive episodes on chronic depressive disorders. Am J Psychiatry 139:438-442 (1982)
14. Akiskal HS: Dysthymic disorder: Psychopathology of proposed chronic depressive subtypes. 140:11-20 (1983)
15. Akiskal HS, King D, Rosenthal TL, Robinson D, Scott-Strauss A: Chronic depressions: Part I. Clinical and familial characteristics in 137 probands. J Affective Disorders 3:297-315 (1981)
16. Akiskal HS: Dysthymic and cyclothymic disorders: A paradigm for high-risk research in psychiatry, in Davis JM, Maas JW (eds): The Affective Disorders. American Psychiatric Press, Inc, pp 211-231 (1983)
17. Akiskal HS, Rosenthal TL, Haykal RF, Lemmi H, Rosenthal RH, Scott-Strauss A: Characterological depressions: Clinical and sleep EEG findings separating "subaffective dysthymias" from "character-spectrum" disorders. Arch Gen Psychiatry 37:777-783 (1980)

DYSTHYMIA AND CHRONIC DEPRESSION

Gerald L. Klerman

George Harrington Professor of Psychiatry, Harvard
Medical School and Director, Stanley Cobb Research
Laboratories, Department of Psychiatry
Massachusetts General Hospital
Bulfinch 3
Fruit Street
Boston, MA 02114

The DSM-III included dysthymia as a new diagnostic class within the group of affective disorders. The DSM-III criteria for
dysthymia includes chronic duration, at least two years of
significant mood disturbances, guilt, low self-esteem, and other
symptoms of the depressive syndrome. For the patient to meet the
criteria for dysthymia, depressive symptoms must be present for a
significant proportion of a two year period but not of sufficient
intensity to meet the criteria for major depressive disorder.

In creating this category, the DSM-III highlighted an important clinical phenomena of increasing therapeutic and epidemiologic relevance.

The history of modern understanding of affective disorders began in the late 18 and early 19th century when psychiatry emerged
as a hospital-based on medical specialty. Psychiatrists, then
often called alienists, working in mental institutions described
patients with profound mood disturbance often accompanied by
psychotic features, such as delusions and with severe disability.
The description and classification of these diverse states were
synthesized by Kraepelin in his writings on manic depressive
insanity. His concept has been the foundation for clinical practice and research on the affective disorders well into the 20th
century.

In recent decades, however, the focus of psychiatric practice and clinical interest has shifted from the mental institution to community based programs - in general hospitals, community mental health centers and office practice. The availability of modern somatic treatments, first, ECT in 1940 and later in the late 1950s the MAO inhibitors and tricyclics has revolutionized the treatment of seriously depressed patients. In the 19th century, the clinical issue is, "will this patient get out of the hospital alive?" Currently the issue is, "what will be the long term social and clinical adjustment of the patient discharged into the community?" It is important to recognize that throughout the 19th century and well into the early decades of the 20th century, many hospitalized patients were not discharged before six to 12 months, and a significant portion of patients with affective disorders died of suicide, exhaustion, intercurrent infections, malnutrition or self-inflicted injuries.

One of the significant effects of ECT was the reduction in the death rate and a decrease in duration of hospitalization and disability.

Today the majority of patients with depressive disorders are not hospitalized and if they are hospitalized, the duration of hospitalization is relatively brief, measured in weeks rather than months.

As psychiatry has expanded its therapeutic skill and as the public has become more sophisticated, we are seeing increasing numbers of patients with milder depressive conditions; which in previous decades would have not come to the attention of the psychiatrist, but would have been seen by clergymen or general physicians.

These patients have variously been diagnosed as "neurotic depression," "depressive personality," hypochondriasis," neurasthenia," "masked depression" and "charaterologic depression."

Although the DSM-III criteria for dysthymia are of relatively recent origin, clinical research and epidemiologic studies indicate that it is a wide-spread phenomenon. Early results from the NIMH Epidemiologic Catchment Area (ECA) Project indicate that about 4% of the adult population meet the criteria for dysthymia. Extrapolating to the larger population, this indicates a prevalence of at least five to eight million individuals with this disorder.

Pathways to Dysthymia

There are at least two pathways to dysthymia: -
    One pathway involves the partial resolution of acute
    episodes of Major Depressive Disorder. Since the writings

618

of Kraepelin, clinical psychiatry has emphasized the tendency of affective disorders to remit. Naturalistic follow-up studies indicate that, if death does not occur by suicide or other means, approximately 85% of depressed patients will be symptom free at one year (Klerman, 1978). While this recovery rate is far better than that for schizophrenia, it leaves a moderate percentage of patients with chronic course. Most of these patients are able to function outside of the hospital but at a reduced functioning at work and in the family. Often they are inadequately treated. Others, however, even when treated intensively, are treatment resistant; this group of chronic treatment resistant patients constitute a major challenge to contemporary clinical practice.

The second pathway involves onset of depressive features in adolescence and young adulthood. We are now aware of large numbers of individuals who began to experience feelings of low self-esteem, worthlessness and hopeless- ness in adolescence and young adulthood. These indivi- duals often seek psychiatric and psychological help and are diagnosed as personality disorders. While they often are able to function well in academic and occupational settings, their problems with self-esteem and in the regulation of emotion render them socially impaired. They often feel lonely and isolated, and are unable to gain satisfaction from their social and interpersonal rela- tions. As they proceed into their 30s and 40s, episodes of illness meeting the criteria of Major Depressive Dis- order may occur (Akiskal and Klerman).

Moreover, the NIMH Collaborative Study (Shapiro and Keller) has documented the existence of Double Depression, namely acute episodes of Major Depressive Disorder superimposed on chronic longstanding difficulties of a dysthymic nature.

Differential Diagnosis with Axis II Personality Disorder

In clinical practice, the most difficult diagnostic problems involve the overlap between (Axis I) dysthymia and (Axis II) Personality Disorders. Since these individuals have had longstanding affective symptoms and social difficulties, they are often viewed as having "characterologic depression." The duration of their symptoms seem to have resulted in the depression having become embedded in their personality; many are seen by themselves, friends, and family members as pessimistic, self-depreciating, socially inhibited and withdrawn. Others may focus on their dysfunction and complaints and seek medical attention because of insomnia, backache or headache, where they are labeled hypochrondrical, hysterical or "crocks." Their unrecognized chronic depression creates a heavy burden on the health care

619

system, particularly in primary care. Unnecessary and expensive radiologic and laboratory diagnostic tests are ordered, or they may be treated with viatamins or thyroid supplements.

Since their difficulties are longstanding, dynamic psychiatrists focus upon the character pathology. These patients are often diagnosed as borderline personality disorder, obsessive-compulsive personality disorder or narcissistic personality disorder.

The DSM-III, having created the distinction between Axis I and Axis II disorders, encourage clinicians to make simultaneous diagnoses on both Axes. When this is done, research indicates (Gunderson) (Perry and Soloff) substantial overlap between major depressive disorder and dysthymia (Axis I) and personality disorders (Axis II). The theoretical importance of this overlap is still controversial (Akiskal and Klerman). However, in clinical practice, there are often problems as to which disorder the clinician chooses to emphasize in treatment planning.

In settings where psychoanalytic and psychodynamic theories are emphasized, there is a tendency to focus upon the personality difficulties and to minimize or even ignore the manifest depressive symptomatology and distress. In this view, the "basic" or "underlying" psychopathology is the personality disorder and the depressive symptoms are "just symptoms" "epi phenomenon." Whatever the scientific status of this view, it has the consequences that psychodynamically oriented psychiatrists minimize or ignore the patient's symptomatic distress and delay or withhold use of psychoactive drug treatment, thereby prolonging the period of distress and disability.

On the other hand, psychiatrists who emphasize biological psychiatry and descriptive symptomatology have the opposite tendency, they ignore the longstanding interpersonal and social difficulties and focus exclusively on symptom reduction.

Proposed Treatment Planning

Depression conditions are best viewed as having three components:
1. Symptomatology distress
2. Impairment of social and interpersonal functioning
3. Personality problems

I recommend that treatment planning, particularly for patients with chronic depressions and dysthymia should proceed in these stages:
(1) First, and most important, reduce the level of symptomatology and accompaning distress and disability. This can be done by special focussed psychotherapy such as

620

cognitive behavioral therapy or interpersonal psychotherapy. Often the combination of drugs and psychotherapy is most effective.

(2) As symptom reduction begins to occur, the treatment focus should next turn to the patients current interpersonal difficulties and social impairments. If the depression has been longstanding, as with dysthymia, there will have been adverse consequences in work relations, the marital and child rearing. In many depressions, the interpersonal problems have proceeded the onset of depressive symptoms.

(3) After symptom reduction has occurred and the patient is feeling more comfortable and when interpersonal relations of the patient have been clarified, assessment of possible personality difficulties and character pathology can then be undertaken and long term treatment planning can be undertaken.

Conclusions

Although it is only three years since the promulgation of the DSM-III concept of dysthymia, epidemiologic and clinical evidence indicate that this is a disorder with wide prevalence and clinical importance and based upon clinical and research experience an approach to planning treatment is provided.

REFERENCES

Akiskal HS: Dysthymic disorder: Psychopathology of proposed chronic depressive subtypes. Am J Psychiatry 140:11-20, 1983.

Keller MB, Shapiro RW: "Double depression": superimposition of acute depressive episodes on chronic depressive disorders. Am J Psychiatry 139:438-442, 1982.

Klerman GL: Long-term treatment of affective disorders. In M.A. Lipton, A. DiMascio, and K.F. Killam (eds.) Psychopharmacology: A Generation of Progress. New York, Raven Press, 1303-1311, 1978.

Klerman GL: Other specific affective disorders. In H.I. Kaplan, A.M. Freedman, and B.J. Sadock (eds.) Comprehensive Textbook of Psychiatry, Vol 2, 3rd Edition. Baltimore, Williams & Wilkins, 1332-1338, 1980.

Kraepelin E: Manic Depressive Insanity and Paranoia. Edinburgh, E & S Livingstone, 1921.

SUBTYPES OF CHARACTEROLOGICAL DEPRESSION

Ted. L. Rosenthal and Hagop S. Akiskal

Affective Disorders Program
University of Tennessee College of Medicine
Memphis, Tennessee   38163, USA

INTRODUCTION

Current evidence indicates that chronic depression, what DSM-III has termed "dysthymic disorder,"[1] represents a heterogeneous group of disorders.[2] For example, chronic low-grade depression may be the residuum of one or recurrent, fullblown, usually late-onset unipolar episodes.[3] Likewise, demoralization secondary to incapacitating chronic medical illnesses or to nonaffective psychiatric disorders often lead to fluctuating dysphoric symptoms.[4,5] We exclude these kinds of chronic depressions, and instead will focus on dysphorias of longstanding developmental origin, typically beginning in the early teens or before.

The early-onset dysphorias, which are our central concern in this paper, are not sequelae to well-defined affective disorder, nor to serious medical conditions. Sustained or intermittent low-grade depression is a prominent feature. Clinicians often describe such patients as suffering from "characterological depression."[6] This hybrid term refers to the weaving of depression and character pathology so intimately that it is often virtually impossible, on clinical grounds alone, to decide which is the primary illness. Based on evidence from a series of 65 probands, we have separated such depressions into at least two types: Those that are truly character-based, representing a spectrum of unstable characterologic disturbances, and comprising about two thirds of our series. The remaining third, instead, appeared to suffer from a temperamental disorder linked to both unipolar and bipolar illness but at milder intensity; for this reason, they were considered a "subaffective dysthymic" group, formes frustes of primary affective disorder. These dysthymias were initially, and tentatively, distinguished from

623

character-based depressions proper--henceforth designated the "character-spectrum" group--because the dysthymics showed positive clinical response to tricyclic antidepressants and/or to lithium; the character-spectrum group did not respond to these medications. This first, rough, division was subsequently validated by other differences to be described in this paper.

METHOD

Both the subaffective dysthymic and the character-spectrum groups had insidious onset before age 21; duration of at least 5 years; and fluctuating low-grade depressive symptoms on most days of the year. Further, no diagnosable nonaffective psychiatric disorder form the Feighner list[7] was present, nor was there a major chronic medical illness to account for the dysphoria. Thus, at index evaluation, selection was limited to patients whose depression was of insidious onset, of mild intensity and chronic course. We did not exclude patients who developed a full depressive episode after vague beginnings in childhood or adolescence. As mentioned earlier, we first distinguished the subaffective dysthymic from the character-spectrum patients by response to thymoleptic drugs. We then contrasted 20 of the dysthymics--showing positive response-- with 30 of the character-spectrum group--who had failed to respond-- on selected clinical, developmental, familial and Sleep EEG variables. We also compared these two groups with a control group of 40 primary unipolar depressives who met full Feighner Criteria.[7] We made many statistical comparisons among our three cohorts.[6,8] Virtually all comparisons were statistically significant. In other words, the results we have summarized below show a dominant pattern of contrast; they are not a "significant" iceberg broken off a larger, nonsignificant glacier.

CLINICAL VARIABLES

Sex. Forty-five percent of the dysthymics were men. Significantly smaller percentages of men were found in the character-spectrum and unipolar groups.

Phenomenology. Significantly more complaints of hypersomnia occurred in dysthymics (55%). In contrast, insomnia was most prevalent (over 80%) in both character-spectrum and unipolar groups.

Course. Superimposed depressive episodes that met full criteria occurred in 55% of dysthymics and 13% of character-spectrums. The large majority of the dysthymics' episodes were of the retarded-hypersomnic type, compared with the agitated-insomniac episodes in character-spectrum patients (p<.02). Further, dysthymics perceived their dysphoria as intermittent, with short periods of normalcy or even brief extraversion intervening. The character-spectrums, instead, often claimed their dysphoria was "continuous."

Personality Traits. Treating clinicians described the dysthymics
with such "stable" personality traits as compulsive and narcissistic.
In sharp contrast, the character-spectrums were given such "unstable"
personality epithets as passive-dependent, histrionic, antisocial,
or borderline. Despite the unreliability of individual personality
subtyping, this contrast between stable and unstable descriptive
traits differentiated the dysthymic and character-spectrum groups at
the $p < .001$ level.

PHARMACOLOGIC ASPECTS

Hypomania. The character-spectrum group did not respond to tricyclic
antidepressants or lithium. Not only did the dysthymics respond
well, but about one-third developed the only episodes of brief, drug-
induced, hypomania found in any of the three groups ($p<.001$).
Further, a substantial fraction of dysthymics responded to lithium
carbonate.

Alcohol and Drug Abuse. There was much alcohol and sedative-hypnotic
drug abuse by the character-spectrums (60%). Significantly less such
abuse was found among dysthymics (10%) or the unipolar controls
(15%). Likewise, there was a marginally greater abuse of psychedelic
and stimulant drugs by the character-spectrums (33.3%) compared to
dysthymics (10%) and unipolars (10%).

SLEEP EEG

Based on subsamples tested in the Sleep Disorder Center, the character-spectrums had a mean REM latency of 98.8 minutes, which is within
the range (70-110 minutes) for nondepressed controls. In contrast,
the dysthymics (mean=57.6 minutes) and the unipolars (mean=59.0
minutes) were significantly below the character-spectrums ($p<.001$).

FAMILIAL-DEVELOPMENTAL VARIABLES

Developmental Object Loss. Loss of at least one parent during the
formative years was significantly more frequent ($p<.001$) among the
character-spectrums (60%) than for either the dysthymics (25%) or
the unipolars (17.5%). There were also qualitative differences.
Most striking was that placement in a foster home or orphanage was
largely confined to the character spectrums.

+FH ALCOHOLISM. Likewise, alcohol dependence and the upheavel it
invites was most prevalent in the families of character-spectrum
patients (53%). In contrast, familial alcoholism was of lower
frequency ($p<.001$) in the dysthymics (10%) and the unipolars (17.5%).

+FH Depressions. As expected, the pattern was reversed for familial depressions. Significantly fewer (p<.05) occurred among kin of the character spectrums (3.3%) compared to the dysthymics (30%) and the unipolars (20%). Yet there were no differences in familial suicide among dysthymics (30%), character-spectrums (27%) and unipolars (22.5%). It is conceivable that the stormy adjustments and alcohol use by kin of the character-spectrums roughly equalized their exposure to familial suicide.

Parental Assortative Mating. Another factor for stormy adjustment among kin of character-spectrums was assortative mating.
More character-spectrums (47%) had parents who both had suffered psychiatric illnesses than in either the dysthymic (10%) or the unipolar (12.5%) groups (p<.01). For the character-spectrums, parental illnesses were typically alcoholism, sociopathy, and somatization (Briquet's) disorder. For dysthymics and unipolars, affective disorder was the dominant parental illness.

+FH Bipolar Disorders. The proportion of dysthymics (35%) with bipolar family histories was significantly higher than that in character-spectrum (3.3%) and unipolar (2.4%) patients (p<.001).

COMMENT

The findings reported tend to validate the existence of affective-based and character-disorder-based subgroups within the heterogeneous universe of the characterologic depressions. In particular, strong indications of primary affective disorder in the subaffective dysthymic group include shortened REM latency, favorable response to thymoleptic drugs, familial affective disorders, superimposed episodes with hypersomnic-retarded features, and hypomanic responses to antidepressant drugs.

Ten patients had bipolar family histories, 7 of which were dysthymic. Six of these had shown brief, tricyclic drug-occasioned hypomania. Such hypomania could not be documented in the 80 patients with -FH for bipolar illness (in a total sample of 90).[8] The probability of this happening by chance—that is, of drug-induced hypomania being associated with bipolar family history—is quite unlikely (p<.001). This conjoint pattern of bipolar family history and pharmacologically-mobilized hypomania has been replicated in a sample of 40 "unipolars" (with documented bipolar family history) who switched to hypomania during tricyclic antidepressant treatment.[9]

These data suggest that subaffective dysthymia itself is heterogeneous: Some may represent subaffective forms of unipolar illness, and the others, alternative expressions of bipolar illness. In any case, subaffective dysthymics seem quite distinct from the character-spectrum patients despite their shared feature of long-standing, low-grade dysphoria. Developmental liabilities, occurring in the setting of parental alcoholism and personality disorder

appear more central than primary affective processes in the pathogenesis of the character-spectrum pattern.

References

1. American Psychiatric Association: DSM-III: Diagnostic and Statistical Manual of Mental Disorders, ed 3. Washington, DC (1980)
2. Akiskal HS: Dysthymic disorder: Psychopathology of proposed chronic depressive subtypes. Am J Psychiatry 140:11-20 (1983)
3. Akiskal HS: Factors associated with incomplete recovery in primary depressive illness. J Clin Psychiatry 43:266-271 (1982)
4. Akiskal HS, Bitar AH, Puzantian VR, Rosenthal TL, Walker PW: The nosological status of neurotic depression: A prospective three-to-four year examination in light of the primary-secondary and unipolar-bipolar dichotomies. Arch Gen Psychiatry 35:756-766 (1978)
5. Akiskal HS, King D, Rosenthal TL, Robinson D, Scott-Strauss A: Chronic depressions: Part 1. Clinical and familial characteristics in 137 probands. J Affective Disorders 3:297-315 (1981)
6. Akiskal HS, Rosenthal TL, Haykal RF, Lemmi H, Rosenthal RH, Scott-Strauss A: Characterological depressions: Clinical and sleep EEG findings separating "subaffective dysthymias" from "character-spectrum" disorders. Arch Gen Psychiatry 37:777-783 (1980)
7. Feighner JP, Robins E, Guze SB, et al: Diagnostic criteria for use in psychiatric research. Arch Gen Psychiatry 26:57-63 (1972)
8. Rosenthal TL, Akiskal HS, Scott-Strauss A, Rosenthal RH, David M: Familial and developmental factors in characterological depressions. J Affective Disorders 3:183-192 (1981)
9. Akiskal HS, Walker PW, Puzantian VR, King D, Rosenthal TL, Dranon M: Bipolar outcome in the course of depressive illness: Phenomenologic, familial and pharacologic predictors. J Affective Disorders 5:115-128 (1983)

PSYCHOSOCIAL PREDICTORS OF CHRONICITY IN DEPRESSION

Heinz Katschnig and Eva Egger-Zeidner

Psychiatric Clinic, University of Vienna
Währinger Gürtel 74-76
A-1090 Wien

INTRODUCTION

The data presented here stems from a research project carried
out on depressed psychiatric inpatients at the Psychiatric Clinic
of the University of Vienna and at the Psychiatric State Hospital
of Gugging-Klosterneuburg near Vienna. Rigorous selection criteria
were applied to ensure the homogeneity of the sample (no alcohol
and other substance abuse, no schizophrenia, and no psycho-organic
disorders). The characteristics of the population studied are
similar to those in comparable samples with a preponderance of
females (68 %), a mean age of 45 years, and a proportion of 70 %
married patients.

The main aim of this project was the validation of different
ways of sub-classifying depressed patients according to the classical
dichotomy of "psychotic/endogenous" versus "neurotic/reactive".
In the first part of this project the validation was concerned
with precipitating life stress. Data were collected by means of
the Present State Examination (PSE, Wing et al., 1974), the London
Life Events and Difficulty Schedule (LEDS, Brown, 1974), and other
methods. In applying a number of ways of sub-classifying depression,
we could not find any substantial difference between the two classical types as far as preceding life stress was concerned (Datschnig
et al., 1981; Katschnig, 1984).

In a follow-up study of the original sample of 176 depressed
inpatients, 127, i.e. 73 % of the original sample, were reinterviewed 2 to 3 years after discharge, and the further development of the disorder in terms of both psychopathological
symptoms and measures of social adjustment was elicited for the

629

follow-up period. The data presented here are concerned with a precise two-year follow-up.

SYMPTOMATOLOGY AS OUTCOME MEASURE

11 patients of the original sample, i.e. 6,3%, had died during these two years; 9 thereof were suicides (= 5,1 %). 127 patients could be re-interviewed. 35 (27,6%) of all patients included in the study had not completely recovered from the depression within one year after discharge; 24 patients (18,9%) had not regained mormal psychological functioning within two years after discharge (Table 1).

Table 1.

Original sample N = 176

Dead 2 years later	11 (6,3 %)
Suicide 2 years later	9 (5,3 %)
Re-interviewed	127 (77 %)
Not recovered 1 year later	35 (27,6%)
Not recovered 2 years later	24 (18,9%)

An "index of chronicity" (IC) was one of the many outcome criteria developed for this project. This index was defined by a percentage of less than 10% of the follow-up period for which individual reported complete freedom from psychiatric symptoms, i.e. for less than 73 days of 730.

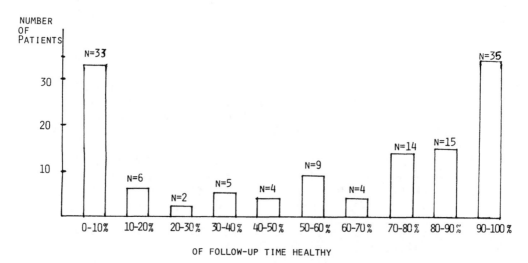

Figure 1. Number of patients according to percentage of follow-up time (2 years) for which the patient reported complete psychological health

Figure 1 shows a U-shaped distribution of the "percentage of time healthy in the follow-up period", i.e. most patients were either very healthy or very sick during the follow-up period with a relative scarcity of persons in the intermediate ranges. 33 patients of the 127 interviewed, i.e. 26,0%, belonged to the "chronic group", if the index of chronicity defined in this project was applied. At the other end of the spectrum 35 patients, i.e. 27,6% of the total sample, belonged to the "very healthy group", which comprised all patients who reported having been free of symptoms for more than 90% of the follow-up period. Here we will be mainly concerned with predicting whether a patient belongs to the chronic group but will occasionally contrast the results with those of the healthy group.

RESULTS

The following five groups of predictor variables were distinguished:

1. Diagnostic subclassification of depression
   (endogenous/psychotic versus reactive/neurotic)
2. Course criteria up to index episode
   (age of onset, bipolar, chronic course etc.)
3. Personality factors
4. Psychosocial factors characterising the living
   situation of the patient and his past experiences
5. Life stress variables
   (life events and chronic difficulties)

Diagnostic subclassification as a predictor variable

Eight different ways of subclassifying depression into 2 types were used: the RDC-definition (Spitzer et al., 1978); the CATEGO subdivision into classes N on the one hand and classes R or D on the other (Wing et al., 1974); the Viennese research criteria (Berner et al., 1983); the results of a cluster analysis (Katschnig et al., 1981); the International Classification of Diseases in its 8th revision (WHO, 1967) as provided by the doctors on the wards. Furthermore, two simple ways of subclassifying our patients into those who a) either did or did not report that they regarded their depression as being triggered by psychosocial factors ("subjective life stress"), and b) those in whom we had or had not found a triggering event in the last 4 weeks before the onset of the episode in question ("objective life stress"). Finally, a "core group" of "endogenous patients" on the one hand and "situational patients" on the other was defined, consisting of all patients who fulfilled at least five of the seven definitions of either endogenous or situational depression.

Table 2. Diagnostic Subclassification: Percentage Patients
With Chronic Course 2 Years After Discharge

DIAGNOSTIC CRITERIA	ENDOGENOUS	NON-ENDO-GENOUS	
VIENNESE CRITERIA	26,0%	26,0%	N.S.
CATEGO D/R=END.,N=NON-END.	22,9%	34,5%	N.S.
RDC ("DEFINITE")	27,3%	40,0%	N.S.
CLUSTER ANALYSIS	25,0%	27,3%	N.S.
OBJECTIVE LIFE STRESS(LEDS)	27,5%	22,2%	N.S.
SUBJECTIVE LIFE STRESS	31,4%	19,3%	N.S.
ICD-8	23,5%	30,6%	N.S.
CORE GROUP	29,7%	33,3%	N.S.

No significant differences emerged between any of the subtypes
for the development of chronicity. If at all, there is a slight
tendency for situational depression, defined on the basis of cross-
sectional symptomatological information, to lead more frequently
to chronicity than its endogenous counterpart. On the other hand,
if depression is subdivided on the basis of preceding life stress
a tendency to develop lower chronicity can be found in those patients
whose depression had been triggered by life events.

The degree of severity of the index episode measured by the
Index of Definition (Wing and Sturt, 1978) showed no correlation
with chronicity.

Course characteristics before the index episodes as predictor
variables

A number of variables were chosen for describing the course
of depression up to the index episode. As we had not only taken
first-ever episode variables, such as duration since the first
episode and the age of onset, pre-existing manic episodes and pre-
existing chronicity had to be taken into consideration. With the
exception of pre-existing chronicity none of these variables
correlated with chronicity during the follow-up period. Pre-
existing chronicity, however, had a very high predictive power
(p < .001) (Table 3).

Table 3. Course Characteristics Before Index Episode
Percent Patients With Chronic Course
2 Years After Discharge

	CHRONIC (10% HEALTHY)	HEALTHY (90% HEALTHY)	
CHRONIC OR HEALTHY IN YEAR BEFORE ONSET	50.0%	16.9%	p < 0.001
	BIPOLAR	UNIPOLAR	
BIPOLAR UP TO INDEX EPISODE	20.8%	27.2%	N.S.
AGE AT ONSET (YEARS)	-40 YRS. 25.6%	41+ YRS. 26.8%	N.S.
DURATION OF ILLNESS (YEARS)	-5 YRS. 21.9%	6+ YRS. 30.2%	N.S.

Personality variables as predictor variables

Personality variables were taken from a personality inventory developed for a German speaking standard population, the "Freiburger Persönlichkeitsinventar" (FPI, Fahrenberg et al., 1970) which was applied after the first depressive edpisode had receded. With this inventory each patient can be described on twelve dimensions using a scoring system from 1 to 9. Only a sub-population of 101 patients of the total sample of 127, i.e. 79,5%, had provided adequate information on this inventory. In addition to the FPI the clinical judgment of the interviewing psychiatrist was used to sub-divide the cohort into a group with a disturbed and a group with a healthy premorbid personality.

With regard to personality factors, a tendency emerged for the development of a chronic course in those patients who showed the following characteristics: high nervousness, high aggressivity, high depressivity, high irratibility and high emotional lability (similar to "neuroticism" in other personality inventories), but low sociability, low openness, low extraversion and low masculinity. Only two of these relationships are, however, significant (sociability: p < 0,01; neuroticism: p < 0,05). The psychiatrist's judgment about the premorbid personality of the patient did not predict chronicity (Table 4).

Whereas relatively few variables could be identified for pre-

Table 4. Personality Variables:
Percent Patients with Chronic
Course 2 Years After Discharge

FPI	LOW (SCORE < 3)	HIGH (SCORE < 7)	
FPI-1 NERVOUSNESS	12,5%	38,8%	N.S.
FPI-2 AGGRESSIVITY	13,8%	37,5%	N.S.
FPI-3 DEPRESSIVITY	0,0%	36,4%	N.S.
FPI-4 IRRITABILITY	16,7%	41,7%	N.S.
FPI-5 SOCIABILITY	40,0%	8,3%	p<0,01
FPI-6 CALMNESS	37,8%	37,5%	N.S.
FPI-7 DOMINANCE	28,6%	28,6%	N.S.
FPI-8 SELFCONSCIOUSNESS	0,0%	35,9%	N.S.
FPI-9 OPENNESS	30,3%	18,8%	N.S.
FPI-E EXTRAVERSION	40,9%	21,1%	N.S.
FPI-N NEUROTICISM	0,0%	39,5%	p<0,05
FPI-M MASCULINITY	31,6%	25,0%	N.S.
	DISTURBED	NOT DISTURBED	
PREMORBID PERSONALITY	31,4%	23,9%	N.S.

Table 5. Personality Variables
Percent Patients Healthy During
The 2 Years Following Discharge

FPI	LOW (SCORE < 3)	HIGH (SCORE < 7)	
FPI-1 NERVOUSNESS	50,0%	20,0%	N.S.
FPI-2 AGGRESSIVITY	34,5%	43,8%	N.S.
FPI-3 DEPRESSIVITY	66,7%	20,0%	p<0,05
FPI-4 IRRITABILITY	11,1%	25,0%	N.S.
FPI-5 SOCIABILITY	14,3%	54,2%	p<0,01
FPI-6 CALMNESS	11,1%	62,5%	p<0,001
FPI-7 DOMINANCE	14,3%	28,6%	N.S.
FPI-8 SELFCONSCIOUSNESS	57,1%	15,4%	p<0,05
FPI-9 OPENNESS	24,2%	56,3%	p<0,01
FPI-E EXTRAVERSION	11,4%	42,1%	p<0,01
FPI-N NEUROTICISM	50,0%	18,4%	N.S.
FPI-M MASCULINITY	15,8%	62,5%	p<0,01
	DISTURBED	NOT DISTURBED	
PREMORBID PERSONALITY	14,3%	32,6%	p<0,05

dicting a chronic course of depression, a substantially greater number of variables predicted more or less complete health during the follow-up period. Personality variables which especially proved to be associated with a very good prognosis, were: low depressivity ($p < 0.05$), high sociability ($p < 0.01$), high calmness ($p < 0.001$), low selfconsciousness ($p < 0.05$), high openness ($p < 0.01$), high extraversion ($p < 0.01$) and high masculinity ($p < 0.01$) (Table 5). A healthy premorbid personality (psychiatrist's judgment) predicted health ($p < 0.05$).

Psychosocial variables as predictors for chronicity

A wide range of psychosocial variables was tested for predictive power. None proved to have any predictive power, with the exception of a few variables reflecting personal attitudes rather than objective psychosocial facts, such as work satisfaction or regarding one's partner as a confidant (also more or less reflecting satisfaction with the relationship).

Life stress as a predictor for chronicity

The last group of predictor variables consited of life stress data, collected for the time before the onset of the index episode. Both life events elicited for different time periods before the onset and chronic psychosocial difficulties were not correlated with chronicity or lack of chronicity.

Multi-variate analyses

The best single predictors identified so far were selected for carrying out multi-variate analyses in order to identify possible combined effects. The variables chosen were pre-existing chronicity before the index episode, a number of personality variables, and satisfaction with partner relationship and work. With these variables a step-wise multiple regression analysis was carried out. The results were rather disappointing: although all the single variables chosen had significant relationships to a chronic course, only two variables (pre-existing chronicity before the index episode and low sociability) of those selected for the multiple regression equation gave a multiple regression coefficient of .44 for predicting chronicity during the follow-up period.

A cluster analysis was carried out using both measures of chronicity, that of the index episode and that of the follow-up period, and seven personality variables. From the five, four and three cluster solutions provided we have chosen the three cluster solution for illustrative purposes.

The largest cluster contained 54 patients who were neither chronic before the first episode nor during the follow-up period. Apart from a slightly raised value for "depressivity", all other personality variables were within the normal range. In a second cluster, comprising 27 patients, who on both occasions, before the index episode and during the follow-up period, were classed as chronic, personality characteristics departed to a high degree from the normal values. These patients were very high on nervousness and depressivity and very low on sociability and calmness. (Table 7)

Table 6

"HEALTHY" CLUSTER (N=54)	
Pre-Episode Chronicity	no
Post-Episode Chronicity	no
FPI-1 Nervousness	normal
FPI-3 Depressivity	high
FPI-5 Sociability	normal
FPI-6 Calmness	normal
FPI-8 Self-Consciousness	(normal)
FPI-E Extraversion	(normal)
FPI-N Emotional Lability	(normal)

Table 7

"CHRONIC" CLUSTER (N=27)	
Pre-Episode Chronicity	yes
Post-Episode Chronicity	yes
FPI-1 Nervousness	very high
FPI-3 Depressivity	very high
FPI-5 Sociability	very low
FPI-6 Calmness	very low
FPI-8 Self-Consciousness	(high)
FPI-E Extraversion	(very low)
FPI-N Emotional Lability	(very high)

The mean values for nervousness, depressivity, sociability and calmness were significantly different the first, the "healthy" cluster and the second, the "chronic" cluster. Self-consciousness, extraversion and emotional lability also showed normal values in the healthy and abnormal values in the chronic cluster. However, the differences did not reach statistical significance.

Table 8

"HIGH RISK" CLUSTER (N=20)	
Pre-Episode Chronicity	no
Post-Episode Chronicity	yes
FPI-1 Nervousness	high
FPI-3 Depressivity	high
FPI-5 Sociability	low
FPI-6 Calmness	low
FPI-8 Self-Consciousness	high
FPI-E Extraversion	low
FPI-N Emotional Lability	high

The last cluster contained 20 patients who had been healthy for most of the time before the index episode, but developed chronic depression during the follow-up period. The values for personality factors had intermediate values for this cluster (Table 8).

SOCIAL ADJUSTMENT AS OUTCOME MEASURE

22,8% of the total population were seen to suffer during the follow-up period of two years from a so-called major difficulty, i.e. a difficult living situation in the non-health area which had lasted for the whole of this period. The concept of "major difficulty" was taken form the "Life Event and Difficulty Schedule" (LEDS) of Brown (1974); it implies all chronically difficult living situations scoring from 1 to 3 on a 6-point rating scale, where 1 stands for the maximum threat and 6 for the least threat implications of the difficulty in question.

Leaving aside the complex problem of the concept of "social adjustment"(see Katschnig, 1983), and also the difficult question of whether the symptoms caused maladjustment, maladjustment caused the symptoms, or both were independent from each other, the result that nearly a quarter of the total population was constantly living in such a difficult situation is in itself significant, especially if therapeutic and management problems are the focus of interest. Concerning the prediction of social maladjustment in the follow-up period, we first looked for the predictive power of the different diagnostic subdividions. Among the 7 diagnostic subdivisions chosen for this analysis, 4 showed a significant relationship, with "neurotic" depression being more frequently associated with social maladjustment than "endogenous" depression. (ICD-8, RDC, cluster analysis, and depression regarded by the patient to be psychosocially triggered).

A chronic course of depression in the year before admission proved to be a significant factor for predicting social maladjustment: 44% of those with this history suffered from a major difficulty in the follow-up period, as opposed to only 15,4% of the 65 patients who were depressed for less than 10% of the total pre-index episode time.

It is noteworthy that none of the personality dimensions tapped by the personality inventory FPI proved to be a significant predictor for maladjustment in the follow-up period. However, of those 35 patients whom the research psychiatrist had judged to have had a premorbid personality disorder, 40% were found to be socially maladjusted in the follow-up period, as opposed to only 16,3% of the 92 patients whom the psychiatrist had judged as having had a more or less healthy premorbid personality.

None of the social demographic variables, such as age, sex,

marital status, housing situation, education, social class, low measures of quality of relationship (such as having a confidant or not) or, finally, "childhood variables", such as the death or divorce of parents during childhood, proved to be a significant predictor for social maladjustment.

On the other hand, severe life events and major difficulties before the onset of the index episode proved to be highly significant predictors of social maladjustment in the follow-up period. On an average 50% of persons who had at least one severe life event in different time periods before the onset of the index episode were maladjusted during the follow-up period.

CONCLUSION

The main result of our study consists in the finding that the prediction of chronic symptomatology on the one hand and of social maladjustment on the other hand follows different patterns (see table 9).

Table 9. Prediction of "course of symptoms" and "maladjustment"

| Predictor Variables | Predicted Variables | |
	Symptomatology	Maladjustment
Diagnostic subclassification	0	++
Preexisting chronicity	+++	+++
Personality variables	+++	0
Social factors	(+)	0
Life stress	0	+++

Diagnostic subclassification is of no value in predicting a chronic course in symptomatology, whereas neurotic depression is significantly more strongly associated with social maladjustment in the two years following discharge than endogenous depression. Preexisting chronicity, i.e. a chronic course already before the index episode, is the strongest single predictor we could identify: Both chronic symptomatology and social maladjustment are highly associated with preexisting chronicity. A number of personality variables, such as depressivity, sociability and extraversion, show a high correlation with symptomatological course criteria but no correlation with social maladjustment. Psychosocial factors, describing the actual living situation of a patient, and psychosocial history data are, by and large, neither associated with chronic symptomatology nor with social maladjustment. Finally, stress, operationalized as life events or chronic difficulties preceding the onset of the index episode, shows no association with subsequent symptomatological chronicity but a clearcut relationship with social maladjustment.

References

Berner, P., Gabriel, E., Katschnig, H., Kieffer, W., Koehler, K., Lenz, G.,and Simhandl, Ch., 1983, "Diagnostic Criteria for Schizophrenic and Affective Psychoses: Vienna Research Criteria", American Psychiatric Press, Washington.

Brown, G.W., 1974, Meaning, measurement and stress of life events, in: "Stressful Life Events: Their Nature and Effects", Dohrenwend, B.S. and Dohrenwend, B.P., eds., Wiley, New York.

Fahrenberg, J., Selg, H.,and Hampel, R., 1970, "Freiburger Persönlichkeitsinventar", Hogrefe, Göttingen.

ICD, 8th Revision, WHO Manual of the International Statistical Classification of Diseases, 1967, WHO, Geneva.

Katschnig, H., 1983, Methods for measureing social adjustment, in: "Methodology in evaluation of psychiatric treatment", Helagson, T. ed., Cambridge University Press, Cambridge.

Katschnig, H., 1984, The independence of syndrome type from life events in depression, Integrative Psychiat.2:77-79.

Katschnig, H., Brandl-Nebehay, A., Fuchs-Robetin, G., Seelig, P., Eichberger, G., Strobl, R.,and Sint, P.P., 1981, "Lebensverändernde Ereignisse, Psychosoziale Dispositionen und Depressive Verstimmungszustände", Psychiatrische Universitätsklinik, Wien.

Spitzer, R.L., Endicott, J.,and Robins, E., 1978, Research Diagnostic Criteria: Rational and reliability, Arch. Gen. Psychiat., 35:773-782.

Wing, J.K., Cooper, J.E.,and Sartorius, N., 1974, "The Measurement and Classification of Psychiatric Syndroms", Cambridge University Press, London.

Wing, J.K.,and Sturt, E., 1978, "The PSE-ID-CATEGO System", Supplementary Manual, Medical Research Council, London.

This work was supported by research grant No. P4123 of the "Fonds zur Förderung der wissenschaftlichen Forschung", Vienna.

THE DIAGNOSIS OF DEPRESSION: 20 YEARS LATER

Per Bech

Psychochemistry Institute
Rigshospitalet
Copenhagen - Denmark

In 1962, Beck and his group in Philadelphia published three studies on the reliability of psychiatric diagnoses. They found a level of agreement of 54% for specific diagnostic categories (e.g. schizophrenia and endogenous depression) which was not conceived as acceptable for research purposes. In contrast to other studies in this field the Philadelphia group made an attempt to analyse the reasons for the diagnostic disagreement. Only 5% of their disagreement was found due to inconstancy on the part of the patient. Inconstancy on the part of the interviewer was found to be more critical for the disagreement (32%). The most serious factor seemed to be differences in the diagnostic weight or loadings attributed to signs and symptoms found present, whereas differences in interviewing technique played only a minor role. However, the Philadelphia group found that around 63% of the disagreement was due to inadequacy of DSM-I. On the basis of these results the Philadelphia group suggested the following strategy to improve the reliability of psychiatric diagnoses, especially in the field of depression:
1) to revise DSM-I in respect to precise criteria for combining signs and symptoms into diagnostic categories that are mutually exclusive
2) to supplement, but not to replace, the DSM with a multidimensional assessment system which would not require that individual syndromes be mutually exclusive, but rather would assume that more than one dimension may be present in a given patient.

During the last 20 years the Hamilton Depression Scale (HDS) has been a scale most frequently used for measuring the severity of depressive states. There is, however, a basic difference in

Hamilton's and Beck's view of how to use symptom rating scales for depression. According to Hamilton symptoms are only meaningful in the context of the diagnosis. The HDS was, therefore, originally devised for use only on patients already diagnosed as suffering from depression. The Hamilton point of view is, of course, derived from the classical, medical model of disease, namely that it is the disease which biologically bears the symptoms. On the other hand Beck has a phenomenological point of view, namely that the symptoms have their own phenomenological existence for research. Thus, Beck holds that the cluster of depressive symptoms can identify depressed patients independently of the diagnosis. The Beck Depression Inventory (BDI) is, as a self-rating scale, completed by patients who have no knowledge of their own diagnosis.

During the twenty years which have passed since the development of HDS and BDI both types of scales have demonstrated that it is possible to measure symptoms in psychiatry with an accepteble degree of inter-observer agreement independently of the diagnosis. We have analysed the HDS as a one-dimensional scale for measuring depressive states of patients with different diagnoses, and found that a subscale of the HDS constituted a one-dimensional depression continuum. On the basis of this scale we have developed our Melancholia Scale.

The clinical assessment systems for depression brought together during this symposium have all been constructed after the development of the HDS and BDI. According to their correspondance between item definitions and item combination they can be ordered as the following

Item definition	Item combination
SADD	ICD-9
SADS	RDC
Not developed	DSM-III
Newcastle scales	Newcastle scales
PSE	PSE
AMDP	AMDP
Not developed	Multiclad
-------------------------------	-------------------------------
DSM-III	DSM-IV
ICD-10	ICD-10

We have made an analysis of the inter-observer reliability of the Melancholia Scale, the Newcastle Scale, Feighner criteria for definite depressive episode, RDC and DSM-III criteria for major depression and for endogenous depression. We found an acceptable agreement, more accepteble than the results published twenty years ago, but not better than there still is room for improvements.

THE NEWCASTLE RATING SCALES

M. Roth, C. Gurney*, and C.Q. Mountjoy

Department of Psychiatry University of Cambridge and *
St. Nicholas Hospital, Gosforth

INTRODUCTION

Rating scales have three main applications in clinical and
scientific work in psychiatry. They may be employed to measure
the severity of illness and thereby response to different forms of
treatment. Secondly they can be applied to predict the course of
illness or the outcome of treatment, and thirdly they can be used
to assist differential diagnosis. These three types of scale have
to be differentiated from each other. For when the multivariate
techniques from which they have been derived are examined it is
apparent that their mathematical derivation differs. Severity
rating scales are derived from the main general component, extracted by principal component analysis, when this method is applied
to investigate the clustering of features within homogenous or
closely related disorders. The weights accorded to the different
items are derived from their loadings on the main general factor
extracted. The second type of scale, that intended to provide an
instrument for the prediction of outcome is derived from a stepwise
multiple regression analysis of the items that characterise a
uniform group of patients whose progress has been systematically
recorded over a period. In the case of discriminating scales such
as the anxiety/depression scale the scores of the different items
are derived from a bipolar factor on which features characteristic
of each of the pair of overlapping disorders under investigation,
show scores of opposite sign. The first step in this case is to
attempt to secure the greatest possible degree of separation
between the pair of conditions whose continuity or independence
is under investigation. This is accomplished by the application
of discriminant function analysis or some related technique. Any
dichotomy secured by this means is of course tentative and

643

requires confirmation from fresh samples and as far as possible
validation by independent criteria such as biochemical variables,
course or treatment response. Validation is easier to achieve in
the case of scales that rate severity than for discriminating
scales. In the case of the former the correlation of the scores
with response to one or more methods of treatment with clinical
observation with self ratings and relatives ratings can be
undertaken. The possibilities of validation are more restricted
in the case of discriminating scales. To invoke clinical observations is to reason in a circle. Differences in outcome and
treatment response in parallel with the diagnostic discrimination
predicted may provide validating evidence. But different disorders may respond in a closely similar manner to the same
treatment (as in the case of corticoids and antibiotics) or pursue
similar courses. The scales developed in Newcastle in relation to
affective disorder have been of the classificatory and predictive
type.

THE NEWCASTLE SCALES FOR THE DIAGNOSIS OF DEPRESSION

The first of these published in 1965 by Carney, Roth and
Garside[1] provided a scale which differentiated depressions into
endogenous and neurotic types and a second scale which predicted
outcome following E C T. On the basis of the distributions
derived from discriminant function analysis the cut off score for
endogenous depression was set at +6 or greater and for neurotic
depression 5 or less. The bimodailty of the distribution has been
shown to be independent of severity[2] in that patients classified
as neurotic or endogenous by the diagnostic scale did not differ
in respect of severity of depression as measured by the Hamilton
Depression Rating Scale. The weightings of the items for the E C T
predictive scale are very different from those of the diagnostic
index. A score of 1 or more indicates a good outcome and a score
of 0 or less a poor outcome with E C T.

The second Newcastle depressive diagnostic scale is one of a
series of scales for the differentiation of disorders of affect
developed from the results of enquiries into the relationship of
anxiety states and the depressive illnesses[3][4][5][6] It was published by Gurney (1971) and is described in the next section which
is devoted to anxiety depression scales.

Scales for Differentiation between and within
Anxiety and Depressive States

The first scale to emerge from the Newcastle investigations
to which reference has been made was developed with the aid of
principle component and discriminant function analyses applied to
a group of patients diagnosed as depressive, anxiety or mixed -
uncertain disorder. The anxiety/depression discriminating scale

644

allocates patients to the anxiety or depressive class of affective disorders. The cut off point for diagnosis lies between a score of 2 and 3. A score of 2 or less is consistent with a diagnosis of depressive illness and a score of 3 or more with a diagnosis of anxiety state.

Patients allocated to the depressive disorders on the basis of their scores on the anxiety/depression scale or patients given a clinical diagnosis may be divided into endogenous or neurotic (reactive) depressions by means of the depression diagnostic scale. A number of the items which figure in the anxiety/depression diagnostic scale recur in the depression diagnostic scale but carry different quantitative weights. The cut off point for depression lies between -19 and -20. A score of -20 and below is indicative of endogenous depression and of -19 and above of neurotic (reactive) depression.

Similarly patients allocated to anxiety states on the basis of their scores on the anxiety/depression scale or those judged clinically to be suffering from an anxiety state can be differentiated into the group of simple anxiety, or into the class of agoraphobic states with the aid of the anxiety diagnostic scale. Here again items which may have figured previously in the other scales are to be found in the anxiety scale but with different quantitative weights. The cut off point for anxiety states is 68 or below and for agoraphobia 69 and above.

Reliability and Validity

The inter-rater reliabilities have been found to be satisfactory (The Spearman Rank correlation coefficient for the sum of weighted scores is equal to 0.91, n = 13 p = 0.0091[8]). A recent study shows the inter-rater reliability agreement to be 90% for the Carney and 91% for the Gurney scale[9]. The intraclass coefficients were high for both scales: for the Carney et al. r = 0.82 and 0.77 for the Gurney scale[9]. The Carney diagnostic scale has been validated by its ability to predict improvement following E C T although the E C T predictive scale was of greater value in this respect[1]. The results have been replicated in a separate study[10] which also yielded a bimodal distribution of scores on the diagnostic scale, a low miclassification rate compared with initial diagnosis (8%), and a correlation between diagnostic scale score and reduction of severity of depression as measured by the Hamilton depression scale following E C T. The anxiety/depression scale is validated by the differences in outcome and on performance in psychometric tests between those patients allocated by the scale to the class of anxiety states and those assigned by the scale of the depressive group[11,5].

The Relevance of Rating, Discrimination and Predictive
Scales for diagnosis and classification in psychiatry

Scales for rating severity and for diagnostic discrimination
and prediction incorporating questionnaires and comprehensive rating
scales have played an important part in the development of
psychiatric research in the past few decades. A common feature
of these methods is that they seek to evaluate clinical phenomena
according to set rules and operational definitions. They
facilitate the testing and replication of experimental findings
eliminating the subjective components that are liable to enter in
the absence of standardization.

Despite the well known limitation of discriminant function
analysis which have been stressed here some of the scales have
been found to be value in relation to a wide range of clinical
problems. The sub-division of depressive disorders that can be
made by application of the Carney scale has been shown to
correlate significantly with a number of biological measures
and with prediction of improvement with treatment. Patients
classified as endogenous by the scale have been shown to have
significantly increased excretion of urinary free cortisol[12],
have lower skin conduction levels[13] and also significantly more
abnormal dexamethasone suppression tests[14] [15]. A study of
cognitive therapy in depression showed reduction in negative
thought frequency to correlate significantly with scores on the
Carney scale, being greater for neurotic depressions[16]. The
intermediate score range (4 - 8) has been found to predict the
best response to amitriptyline[17] and an endogenous score has been
reported to be a successful predictor of favourable outcome
following E C T[1, 10, 18]. One would have expected a predictive
scale derived from the outcome of treatment with E C T to prove
of little or no value when applied to other forms of therapy.
This follows from the fragility and sensitivity of discriminant
function and related techniques. However, the E C T prediction
scale has also proved valuable in forecasting outcome with antidepressant drugs and to be a better predictor of E C T response
than the D S T[19]. In the case of the anxiety/depression scale the
separation in the initial study was replicated in experiments in
which endogenous cases were excluded[20]. It would appear that the
rule according to which no general significance can be attached
to any scales derived unless patient populations and items identical
with those in the original cohort from which the scale has been
derived is not upheld in practice.

Rating scales and reference diagnosis have already made a
valuable contribution to a narrow but important range of problems
relating to diagnosis and classification. They have introduced
stringency and objectivity into many kinds of scientific exercise
including the investigation of treatment response and the predic-

tion of outcome, facilitated communication between different scientists and made it possible to compare different methods of description and classification. But employed alone they are not the sole or ideal instrument for every kind of scientific investigation in psychiatry that seeks to characterise clinical phenomena. Both in relation to clinical practice and scientific research various types of rating and quantified scales can be used with advantage as adjuncts to clinical diagnosis (which has benefited from the objectivity and stringency of rating scales) rather than as a substitute for it.

New disorders and new classifications are unlikely to emerge from more valid and reliable forms of rating clinical phenomena. They will probably come in the future, as they have done in the past through the perceptions and insights of gifted psychiatric observers.

REFERENCES

1. M. W. P. Carney, M. Roth, and R. F. Garside, The Diagnosis of Depressive Syndromes and the Prediction of E C T Response, Brit. J. Psychiat.111, 659-674 (1965)
2. P. Bech, L. F. Gram, N. Reisby and O. J. Rafaelsen, The WHO Depression Scale, Relationship to the Newcastle Scales, Acta psychiat. scand. 62, 140-153 (1980)
3. M. Roth, C. Gurney, R. F. Garside and T. A. Kerr, Studies in the Classification of Affective Disorders, The Relationship between Anxiety States and Depressive Illnesses - 1, Brit. J. Psychiat. 121, 147-61 (1972)
4. C. Gurney, M. Roth, R.F. Garside, T. A. Kerr and K. Schapira, Studies in the Classification of Affective Disorders, The Relationship between Anxiety States and Depressive Illnesses-11, Brit. J. Psychiat. 121, 162-66 (1972)
5. T. A. Kerr, M. Roth, K. Schapira and C. Gurney, The Assessment and Prediction of Outcome in Affective Disorders, Brit. J. Psychiat. 121, 167-74 (1972)
6. K. Schapira, M. Roth, T. A. Kerr and C. Gurney, The Prognosis of Affective Disorders: The Differentiation of Anxiety States from Depressive Illnesses, Brit. J. Psychiat. 121, 175-81 (1972)
7. C. Gurney, Diagnostic scales for affective disorders. Proceedings of the Fifth World Conference of Psychiatry, Mexico City, p.330 (1971)
8. P. Kragh-Sorensen, C. E. Hansen and M. Asberg, Plasma Levels of Nortriptyline in the Treatment of Endogenous Depression, Acta psychiat. scand. 49, 444-456 (1973)
9. P. Bech, A. Gjerris, J. Andersen, S. Bojholm, P. Kramp, T.G. Bolwig, M. Kastrup, L. Clemmesen and O. J. Rafaelsen, The Melancholia Scale and the Newcastle Scales, Item-combinations and Inter-observer Reliability, Brit. J. Psychiat. 143, 58-63 (1983)

10. M. W. P. Carney and B. F. Sheffield, Depression and the New-castle Scales Their Relationship to Hamilton's Scale, Brit. J. Psychiat. 121, 35-40 (1972)

11. T. A. Kerr, K. Schapira, and M. Roth Measurement and prediction of outcome in affective disorders. Proceedings of the Royal Society of Medicine, 63, 235-8 (1970)

12. P. Milln, M. Bishop and A. Coppen, Urinary free cortisol and clinical classification of depressive illness. Psychological Medicine 11, 643-645 (1981)

13. A. M. Mirkin and A. Coppen, Electrodermal Activity in Depression: Clinical and Biochemical Correlates. Brit. J. Psychiat. 137, 93-97 (1980)

14. A. Coppen, M. Abou-Saleh, P. Milln, M. Metcalfe, J. Harwood and J. Bailey. Dexamethasone Suppression Test in Depression and other Psychiatric Illness. Brit. J. Psychiat. 142, 498-504 (1983)

15. N.L. Holden, Depression and the Newcastle Scale. Their Relationship to the Dexamethasone Suppression Test. Brit. J. Psychiat. 142, 505-507 (1983)

16. J. D. Teasdale and V. Rezin, The effects of reducing frequency of negative thoughts on the mood of depressed patients - tests of a cognitive model of depression. Br. J. soc. clin. Psychol. 17, 65-74 (1978)

17. V.A. Rama Rao and A. Coppen, Classification of depression response to amitriptyline therapy. Psychological Medicine 9, 321-325 (1979)

18. D.N. Vlissides and F. A. Jenner, The Response of Endogenously and Reactively Depressed Patients to Electroconvulsive Therapy. Brit. J. Psychiat. 141, 239-242 (1982)

19. C. L. E. Katona and C. R. Aldridge. Antidepressant effects of electroconvulsive therapy. Brit. Med. J. vol. 286. 1443 (1983)

20. C. Q. Mountjoy and M. Roth. Studies in the Relationship between Depressive Disorders and Anxiety States. Journal of Affective Disorders 4. 127-147 (1982)

STUDIES OF DEPRESSIVE DISORDERS USING THE PSE-ID-CATEGO SYSTEM

P. Bebbington, E. Sturt, and N. Kumakura

MRC Social Psychiatry Unit, Institute of Psychiatry
De Crespigny Park
London SE5 8AF

ABSTRACT

The PSE-CATEGO-ID system and its approach to the sub-classification of depression is described. The principle of sub-classification partly corresponds to the empirical relationships between symptoms of affective disorder. Comparison of CATEGO and DSM III demonstrates that major differences of classification can arise because of differences of the classificatory algorithm even though similar lists of symptoms are used. Empirical studies of the PSE-CATEGO-ID system are described and their importance in providing evidence for a rational choice between classificatory system is emphasized.

This paper describes the classification of the affective disorders and its use in empirical research. It is argued that different classifications of depression may have little overlap and that we are a long way from any general acceptance of a particular system.

The Present State Examination (PSE) is by now widely known and its 9th Edition (1). It is a semi-structured interview designed to determine the presence of commonly acknowledged psychiatric symptoms and signs. It is an attempt to standardise the method of corss-examination normally used ty psychiatrists to establish a description of the mental state.

The structure of the interview means that the phenomenal ground is covered in a standardized way. The establishment and rating of items is standardized by the provision of rating instructions and a glossary of differential definitions, and also by attendance of raters on training courses.

Since the development of the PSE itself, it has been extended by the two optional computer programs for handling the output
of the interview. The first is CATEGO. This condenses the information from the interview in a series of steps until each case is
alloted to one final symptom-based class. As this is based solely
upon the symptoms present in the month before interview, it cannot
be a diagnosis, but within this considerable limitation the class
can be expressed as the equivalent of an ICD category. There is
also provision for adding information from the clinical history
by means of the syndrome checklist and aetiology schedule.

Such a classificatory program will classify any input provided by the investigator. It works best when all the symptoms
required for a clinical diagnosis are present, as for example
with most in-patients and out-patients. However, the PSE has also
been found useful in surveys of general populations (2 - 9).
Many people in the community experience a few neurotic symptoms
which would not ordinarily be regarded as sufficient evidence for
the existence of disorders such as those seen in the clinic. For
this reason, an Index of Definition (ID) program was developed,
specifying levels below which too few symptoms are present to make
classifications comparable with those of out-patients and inpatients (10). The program allocates subjects to one of eight confidence levels. The procedure is essentially a symptom-count with
added weight being given to specific symptoms such as depression
or anxiety. Level 5 is a threshold level set deliberately low,
while levels 6 to 8 are increasingly definite. Community surveys
which have used the program have taken level 5 and above to represent cases. The CATEGO program can then be applied.

When surveys are made of psychiatric disorders in the community, most of the prevalence is accounted for by minor affective
disorders. The CATEGO program uses a partially hierarchical principle in arriving at classes of symptomatic disorder. This reflects a prevalent strategy of clinical psychiatric diagnosis
and has been strongly argued by Kendell (11) in the case of depression. Thus, once organic conditions have been discounted,
most clinicians in Europe will regard the presence of certain
symptoms as indicative of a diagnosis of schizophrenia despite
the presence of symptoms of mania, depression or anxiety. If there
are no symptoms characteristic of schizophrenia, the psychiatrist
will then consider the possibility of major affective disorder.
If there are no grounds for this, account is next taken of symptoms
of more minor depressive disorder and anxiety. Some psychiatrists
allow depressive disorder to take diagnostic precedence over
anxiety states, others regard anxiety and depression as requiring
assessment each on its own merit, forming categories which are not
mutually exclusive.

The CATEGO program permits either approach. In the production of the final class, significant symptoms of depression do take precedence over symptoms of anxiety clinical judgement into the balance. It is possible, however, to use output at an earlier stage to retain subclasses of anxiety and depression. The same is true of other symptoms. It is possible to use a profile of eight symptom sub-classes rather than one overall classification. The final class has, however, been found to match clinical diagnosis fairly well in several international studies.

This flexibility means that the PSE-CATEGO-ID system can be used for a wide variety of purposes. It ia also necessary in view of the uncertainty surrounding the status of minor affective disorders and the practicalities of their subclassification.

The CATEGO program uses four classes to cover depression and anxiety states. Class D is depression accompanied by delusions, the equivalent of disorders most psychiatrists classify within the ICD category 296. Class R contains cases which are not delusional but have symptoms of pathological guilt, retardation or agitation. Class N covers cases with depressive symptoms other than those above. Class A includes anxiety and phobic states, conditions which may also be characterised by secondary or minor depressive features. Class N and Class A cases come within ICD category 300. The position of Class R depression is equivocal as some psychiatrists would include it in category 296 while others would employ category 300. To a certain extent this depends upon the purposes of the researcher.

The first question that may be asked is whether this subdivision of the affective states corresponds to an empirical reality. Is there a hierarchical relationship between the symptoms which determine classification into different categories? If the idea of a hierarchy is taken in a logical sense, this is obviously untrue: the presence of pathological guilt does not absolutely guarantee that worrying or muscular tension will also be present. However, in a probabilistic sense, a hierarchy does exist. Sturt (12) examined the distribution of symptoms within a general population sample from South London. Rarer symptoms such as pathological guilt predicted a high score on the PSE, indicating the presence of the commoner, often non-specific, symptoms which go to make the overall picture of affective disturbance. Commoner symptoms, in contrast, did not predict high PSE scores. In this sample class D depressions did not occur, but it is clear that symptoms determining Class R depression were high in the hierarchy relative to those sufficient only for Class N depression. Somewhat surprisingly, the symptom of depressed mood was less predictive of other symptoms than generalised anxiety was. It appears that the hierarchical principle invoked in the CATEGO classification of depression does correspond to some extent to an empirical relationship between symptoms, but that there may not be great justification for applying it to the distinction between 'neurotic' depression and anxiety states.

A number of systems of subclassifying depression now exist. To what extent do the various sets of rules, whatever the underlying principles, result in a given case being classified similarly? Dr. Kumakura has studied two systems which rely upon quite similar lists of symptoms to establish their classification of depression, namely CATEGO and DSM III. The CATEGO system, however, lays particular weight on certain special symptoms whereas DSM III places greater reliance on simple symptom counts. Kumakura used symptoms taken from Maudsley case notes to make the classification, and it is possible that there might have been more convergence using more complete date derived from interviews. However, his findings give no cause for complacency as can be seen from the large areas of disagreement in these Venn diagrams. His conclusion is that the discrepancy must arise because of the difference in alogrithms rather than in the symptoms used. The problem is, of course, that the number of alogrithms which could be constructed to classify depression is very large indeed, particularly if a hierarchical approach is chosen. The appropriate course is to test the empirical validity of those we have.

One way in which this can be done is by using the classifications to test emperical hypotheses about depression. Griesinger (13), for instance, made the claim that depressive disorders with more unusual symptoms were less likely to be those which were preceded by a major psychosocial stress. In our work, we corroborated this hypothesis by comparing categories composed of R and D depressions with Class N and Class A disorders. (Table 1, see also 14). Currently we are engaged in a study of depressed patients in which the interaction of social and genetic factors is being examined in different CATEGO classes.

The subclassification of depression has far to go before the general acceptance of any particular system. Whilst different instruments may be necessary for different purposes, a sufficient number of systems of classification now exists. It is easy to be dissatisfied with these systems, and all too easy to develop new alternatives. In the authors' view, this tendency should be constrained by the discipline of using the ones we have in an adequate number of empirical studies of the kind described here.

TABLE 1

(Bebbington)
STANDARDISING COVERAGE

| Sectional Organization | Optional Probes |
| Obligatory Questions | Cut-off Points |

REFERENCES

1. Wing J.K., Cooper, J.E. and Sartorius, N. (1974). The Measurement and Classification of Psychiatric Symptoms. Cambridge University Press: Cambridge.
2. Bebbington P., Hurry J., Tennant C., Sturt E. and Wing J.K. (1981a). The epidemiology of mental disorders in Camberwell. Psychological Medicine, 11, 561-80.
3. Brown G.W. and Harris T.O. (1978). Social origins of depression. Tavistock. London.
4. Brown G.W. and Prudo R. (1981). Psychiatric disorder in a rural and an urban population: 1. Archiology of depression. Psychological Medicine, 11, 581-599.
5. Costello C.G. (1982). Social factors associated with depression: a retrospective community study. Psychological Medicine, 12, 329-39.
6. Henderson A.S., Byrne D.G. and Duncan-Jones, P. (1981). Neurosis and the Social Environment. Sydney. Academic Press.
7. Lehtinen V. and Vaisanen E. (1981). Epidemiology of psychiatric disorders in Finland. A five-year follow-up. Soc. Psychiat. 16,171-180.
8. Orley J. and Wing J.K. (1979). Psychiatric disorders in two African villages. Archives of General Psychiatry, 36, 513-520.
9. Surtees P.G., Dean C., Ingham J.G., Kreitman N.B., Miller P.McC. and Sashidharan S.P. (1983). Psychiatric disorder in women from an Edinburgh community: associations with demographic factors. British Journal of Psychiatry, 142, 238-46.
10. Wing J.K., Mann S.A., Leff J.P. and Nixon J.N. (1978). The concept of a 'case' in psychiatric population surveys. Psychological Medicine, 8, 203-217.
11. Kendall R.E. (1976). The classification of depressions: a review of contemporary confusion. British Journal of Psychiatry, 129, 15-28.
12. Sturt E. (1981). Hierarchical patterns in the incidence of psychiatric symptoms. Psychological Medicine, 11, 783-794.
13. Griesinger W. (1861). Die Pathologie und Therapie der psychischen Krankheiten. (Second edition). Braunschweig. Wreden. Translated as Mental Pathology and Therapeutics by Robertson, C.L. and Rutherford, J. (1867). London. New Sydenham Society.
14. Bebbington P.E., Tennant C. and Hurry J. (1981b). Life events and the nature of psychiatric disorder in the community. Journal of Affective Disorders, 3, 345-66.

DEPRESSIVE SYNDROMES AND SCALES IN THE AMDP-SYSTEM

A. Pietzcker and R. Gebhardt

Psychiatrische Klinik der
Freien Universität Berlin
Eschenallee 3
D - 1000 Berlin 19
F. R. G

The Association for Methodology and Documentation in Psychiatry was founded in 1965 by a group of psychiatrists from Germany, Switzerland and Austria. It developed a uniform and comprehensive system for the documentation of psychopathological, somatic, and anamnestic findings, the AMP-System. In 1979 a revised system was introduced, the AMDP-System (5).

1. SYNDROME SCALES IN THE AMDP-SYSTEM

The sheets "psychopathological symptoms" and "somatic signs" of the AMP-System contain 180 items. A data-reduction by means of factor-analyses seemed desirable for the examination of syndromes which are postulated as a result of clinical experiences; further-more, it seemed necessary not only to examine clinical syndromes but also to make suggestions as to syndrome scales.

Thus, the scales based on factor-analyses are further evaluated by means of the methods of classical test-theory. There are five different syndrome solutions in the AMP-System, calculated in five different samples of four different clinics with not identical methods (1). In spite of this, most authors have interpreted nine factors which show a good comparability across the 5 solutions. In our own factor analysis, the symptoms of 2269 patients on admission to the clinic of Berlin were factor-analysed to build syndromes of psycho-pathology. The syndromes could be cross-validated, they satisfy test-statistical criteria.

In order to obtain final AMDP scales right after the revision

of the AMP-System into the AMDP-System in 1979, the AMDP group decided to combine data from the Psychiatric Clinic of the University
in Munich with data of the Psychiatric Clinic of the Free University
in Berlin. In this way, a sufficient number of patients was available for the data analysis. Further, it was possible to define them
sufficiently sample-independent and to cross-validate them. All the
140 AMDP items of psychopathological and somatic data of all 2313
patients documented routinely in 1980 on admission to the clinics,
were included in the analysis. The diagnostic composition of the
sample was wide-spread: organic psychoses 8 %, schizophrenia 33 %,
affective psychoses 21 %, neuroses 15 %, alcohol and drug dependence
6 %, all other diagnoses 17 %.

Principal component analyses were calculated as factor extraction
methods. The subsequent rotation was made with the orthogonal Varimax method. A symptom was selected as marker item for a syndrome
only if it was possible to associate it unequivocally with a factor
in the majority of the various factor analyses carried out in the
Berlin sample and separately in the Munich sample as well as in
randomized split-halfs of these samples. Subsequently, item analyses
were computed. (For details of the samples, methods used and results
see 2, 3.)

Altogether 70 items are associated with the syndromes. A comparison of factor structure between the Munich solution and the
Berlin solution showed an extremely high similarity of the results
of the factor analyses of both samples: the similarity S between
both factor matrices reached a value of S = 0.989.

Eight syndromes could be extracted from the different factor
analyses: the paranoid-hallucinatory (PARHAL), depressive (DEPRES),
psychoorganic (PSYORG), manic (MANI), hostility (HOST), autonomic
(AUTON), apathy (APA), and the obsessive-compulsive (OBSESS) syndrome.

In order to make the syndromes constituted by different item
numbers comparable, the raw scores were transformed into T-values
($\bar{x}$ = 50, s = 10).

A comprehensive description of the psychopathology (and partly
of the somatic findings, too) of each patient or patient-group is
best made by a syndrome profile comprising all eight syndromes.
There is a high similarity of the syndromes in the AMP-System with
the syndromes in the AMDP-System (3).

2. DISCRIMINATION OF DIFFERENT DEPRESSIVE DISEASES BY AMDP SYNDROME
   PROFILES

We shall concentrate upon the most discussed problem in this area, the discrimination of depressive neurosis from endogeneous depression; these diagnoses were set at discharge by the physician in charge of the patient. The shape of the syndrome profiles of both groups are rather similar. But the endogeneous depression has higher mean-values especially in the depressive, psychoorganic and apathy syndrome, lower values in the autonomic syndrome.

We carried out a discriminant analysis. Each diagnostic group was randomized in two split-halfs, in the first half the discriminant functions were calculated, the classifications were cross-validated in the other halfs (and vice versa).

If the discriminant function is calculated in the first half, there are 84 % of the patients correctly classified, but only 67 % in the cross-validation in the second half. The results are better if the discriminant function is calculated in the second half and validated in the first half: 81 % resp. 83 % correct classifications.

As it was expected just by inspection of the syndrome profiles, the depressive, the psychoorganic, and the autonomic syndrome have the highest loadings on the discriminant function. These results demonstrate that it is possible to classify merely by means of the AMDP syndromes most patients into the both clinical-diagnostic groups, but in 12 % to 33 % of the patients this is not possible. Nevertheless, these results of classification by psychopathological syndromes are remarkably good, if one considers, that the syndromes are calculated on the basis of the data of patients with all psychiatric diagnoses for a comprehensive description of all kinds of psychiatric patients and were not constructed especially to discriminate different depressive diseases.

3. CLASSIFICATION OF DIFFERENT DEPRESSIVE PATIENT-GROUPS BY CLUSTER ANALYSIS

However, as the results of the discriminant analyses have indicated, there is a considerable overlap between the diagnostic groups, set up clinically according to ICD - or otherwise stated, the diagnostic groups are heterogeneous in respect to the psychopathology of the patients grouped together.

In order to obtain more homogeneous groups of patients, cluster analysis is a suitable method to classify patients in homogeneous groups regarding psychopathology independently of nosological concepts.

We have carried out extensive studies using cluster-analytic methods on the basis of the AMP-System (4), and shall give only some examples pertinent to the classification of depressive states.

By comparing different cluster-analytical methods, we decided to select a non-hierarchical K-centroid method using r-metrics as measure of similarity. We carried out the analyses in our above mentioned sample of 2269 patients, who were analysed simultaneously altogether on the basis of the AMP syndromes. As best solution by statistical and clinical criteria we have chosen a cluster structure with K = 46 clusters, with a mean homogeneity of 0.55 within the clusters and no overlap between the clusters. 23 clusters contain at least 20 patients, 91 % of the whole sample are grouped into these 23 clusters. Out of these 23 clusters, 7 are characterized by a depressive symptomatology.

These "depressive" clusters have characteristic and distinct syndrome profiles, cluster 2 e. g. being a moderately "depressive-apathetic" cluster, cluster 5 is similar in shape but with more depressive and less apathetic features, and cluster 13 is characterized by extremely high values in the depressive, apathy, and stuporous syndrome.

The depressive neurosis in comparison shows a syndrome profile which resembles closely cluster 5, having only slightly lower mean values in the depressive syndrome and slightly higher values in the other syndromes.

The clusters are far more homogeneous in psychopathology than the diagnostic groups according to ICD, by discriminant analyis the patients were correctly classified almost all to 100 %. If the diagnostic composition of the clusters is inspected, the overlap of diagnostic groups becomes evident. In cluster 2 neuroses and depressive psychoses are grouped together in equal proportions. In cluster 5 which resembles depressive neuroses in syndrome profile, the latter diagnostic group is over-represented, but the cluster contains also 20 % depressive psychoses. Cluster 13 with the most severe depressive symptomatology contains the greatest proportion of depressive psychoses (64 %) but also 18 % schizophrenias, mainly severely depressed paranoid schizophrenics.

By a global evaluation, this classification of psychiatric patients by cluster analysis could not be proved to be more valid than the classification by ICD-diagnoses (4). Nevertheless, using in addition other data derived from the AMDP-System, including e. g. anamnestic data, cluster analysis seems to us a promising approach for the improvement of classification in psychiatry, also in the field of depressions.

4. CONCLUSIONS

The AMDP-System is a comprehensive documentation system for psychiatric data with elaborated instruments for the assessment and classification of psychiatric patients, including depressed patients. The discrimination of depressive diseases is possible to a remarkable degree in spite of the fact, that the AMDP-System was developed for the description of all kinds of psychiatric patients and not especially for depressive states. The system avoids some shortcomings of other systems by its comprehensiveness, it has obviously its own shortcomings, e. g. in so far it is more suitable for the assessment of psychoses than of neuroses. The AMDP-System cannot solve the difficult problem of classification of depressions, but it can serve as a suitable tool for this purpose.

REFERENCES

1. U. Baumann, A. Pietzcker, B. Woggon,
   Syndromes and Scales in the AMP System,
   in: "The AMDP-System in Pharmacopsychiatry",
   D. P. Bobon, U. Baumann, J. Angst, H. Helmchen,
   H. Hippius, eds., Modern Problems of Pharmacopsychiatry
   Vol. 20, Karger, Basel (1983)
2. R. Gebhardt, A. Pietzcker, A. Strauss, M. Stöckel, C. Langer,
   K. Freudenthal,
   Skalenbildung im AMDP-System,
   Arch. Psychiatr. Nervenkr. 233: 223 (1983)
3. A. Pietzcker, R. Gebhardt, A. Strauss, M. Stöckel, C. Langer,
   K. Freudenthal,
   The Syndrome Scales in the AMDP-System,
   in: "The AMDP-System in Pharmacopsychiatry",
   D. P. Bobon, U. Baumann, J. Angst, H. Helmchen,
   H. Hippius, eds., Modern Problems of Pharmacopsychiatry
   Vol. 20, Karger, Basel (1983)
4. A. Pietzcker,
   Psychiatrische Klassifikationen. Empirische Untersuchungen zur psychiatrischen Diagnostik und Klassifikation auf der Grundlage des AMP-Systems.
   Habilitationsschrift, Berlin 1983
5. D. P. Bobon, U. Baumann, J. Angst, H. Helmchen, H. Hippius, Eds.,
   "The AMDP-System in Pharmacopsychiatry",
   Modern Problems of Pharmacopsychiatry Vol. 20,
   Karger, Basel (1983)

ICD-10 AND DEPRESSION

Norman Sartorius

Director, Division of Mental Health
World Health Organization
Geneva, Switzerland

Perhaps the most spectacular change over the last twenty years
is the increase in both incidence and recognition of depression as
a major public health problem. With an estimated 100 million people
suffering from the condition and likely to benefit from qualified
help, depression has come into the forefront of efforts of
psychiatrists and general health practitioners. The availability
of relatively effective treatments has undoubtedly made a major
contribution to the acceptance of depression as a disease of public
health importance with which all members of the health service
should be able to deal.

The increased recognition of the importance of depression is
also reflected in changes of the classification of depressive disorders between the 8th and 9th Revision of the International
Classification of Disease. As Stengel said many years ago, an
international classification must be a servant rather than a master
of international communication. In this instance, the role of
servant was played by increasing the number of categories for the
classification of depressive conditions so that the many different
diagnoses used for depression can all be accommodated. There are
eleven categories into which a depressive condition can be classified
in the ICD-9. It is difficult to know how useful these categories
have been until a full analysis of the use of ICD-9, chapter 5, at
national level is available. Such evidence could help to eliminate
some of the categories which are used extremely rarely as well as
categories which seemed to be used only in one specific geographical

or language area. In such instances, the placement of specific
diagnosis will have to be in national classifications with a translation into the international one.

The principles by which ICD-10 will be developed are similar
to those used for ICD-9. They will include conservatism unless
definite evidence is provided showing that it is necessary to
include a new category into the classification. There will be an
emphasis on retaining some measure of continuity between ICD-8,
ICD-9 and ICD-10 to facilitate longitudinal analysis and technical
arrangements for reporting at national level.

The revision will be based on points of agreement among mental
health professionals and between them and the other users of the
classification. It will not aim at replacing national classifications; rather it will attempt to ensure that its structure facilitates
translation of national or local schemes into the international
reference classification. It will include definitions for each of
the terms used, probably in an operational language. Terms which
cannot be translated into the different languages will be accepted
with reluctance.

The main preparatory activity for ICD-10 formulation will be
the collection of data on use and usefulness of categories in ICD-9
and in other systems. It is likely that it will also be necessary
to carry out special multicentric studies to clarify specific points
or to obtain complementary evidence.

The WHO international study on depressive disorders which seems
to confirm the usefulness of a small number of categories for the
classification of depressive disorders will continue to provide
data since it is planned to continue the follow-up of the cohorts of
depressive patients in five cultures to gain knowledge about
cultural influences (or lack of them) on the course and outcome of
depression. Other multicentric and multinational studies which
have been carried out by WHO coordinated networks are also likely
to yield useful hints for the new revision. These are in particular
the WHO studies in biological psychiatry (e.g. on the value of the
dexamethasone suppression test in which some 1000 patients will be
included in nine centres) and WHO studies on the effects of antidepressant treatment in different cultural groups involving patients
in seven different countries.

Two other developments are likely to be important in the process
of preparation of ICD-10. First, are the results of a WHO task
force on definition of psychiatric terms which is in the process of
providing definition for a large variety of terms used in the
description of depressive states. The second are the results of a

new WHO initiative, which will lead to an expanded programme of WHO coordinated research and in the course of which it is hoped that a number of research teams in developing countries will come into existence.

WHO's studies and efforts are at all times the result of good will and collaboration of the leading experts and institutions from all over the world. We hope that through continued collaboration with all those who can make contributions to the improvement of classification and their use it will be possible to develop proposals for the classification of depression in ICD-10 which will be valid, acceptable to all and useful for the purposes of international communication and improvement of care for the mentally ill, their families and communities.

ASSESSMENT SCALES FOR DEPRESSION: THE NEXT 20 YEARS

Per Bech

Psychochemistry Institute
Rigshospitalet
Copenhagen - Denmark

The assessment systems presented during this symposium have been selected because of their clinical importance for the diagnosis of depression. They can be ordered on a one-way axis starting with national names and descriptions for depressive disorders, going through the international names given by ICD-9 or DSM-III and ending with the various types of research criteria and rating scales. This axis is a one-way axis because it is, as also noted by Roth et al. (1983), unlikely that new disorders will emerge from rating scales. Such scales must be regarded as instruments constructed for objectivity and reliability on the basis of observations obtained by psychiatrists who had demonstrated their skills in making masked symptoms palpaple, and thereby named the identified disorder.

At the moment there exists only a few studies in which assessment scales for depression have been mutually compared. When analysing inter-scale agreements expressed in percent, it is, however, as important as when analysing inter-observer agreement, to take the chance agreement into account. Kappa statistics are recommended, and the sensitivity and specificy of each scale should, then, be calculated.

We have compared the research criteria (Feighner, RDC, DSM-III) with depression rating scales (Melancholia and Newcastle) and found that the inter-scale agreement expressed by Kappa values was very poor, although they all were of statistical significance. During the years to come, comparative studies of this kind should be carried out, however, especially with weight on external criteria of validity, e.g. prediction of outcome.

It is at the moment, of course, difficult to predict the systems which most successfully will survive the next 20 years. From a logical point of view, however, there should be less need for choosing among the various assessment systems, if cut-off scores within each system can be transformed to the three basic elements in the classification of depression for which there seems to be a growing:

(1) The hierarchical element by which organic mental disorders and schizophrenia are excluded

(2) Quantitative scales by which the depressive states are defined (e.g. major versus minor depression)

(3) Qualitative scales by which the diagnosis of depression are defined (e.g. endogenous versus reactive depression)

When evaluating states versus traits, personality scales are often needed. During the next 20 years observer scales for personality traits or disorders will, undoubtfully, be constructed.

In the attempt to increase the international communication in the field of depression it was suggested to follow some guidlines for standardizing the assessment procedure which included: Applicability, administration, comprehensiveness, item definitions, item combinations, type of interview, length of interview, length of observation period, validity, and reliability.

INTRODUCTION: HISTORY AND PROBLEMS

OF ORGANIC PSYCHOSYNDROMES

Uwe Henrik Peters

Professor and Chairmann
Dpt. of Psychiatry and Neurology
University of Cologne, W.-Germany

Not many areas of psychiatry have been criticized as much as organic psychiatry: it is said to have no real terminology and no validity. It is even difficult to present a wider concept that could be generally understood. If one looks at the programs of today's symposiums, then the criticisms would rather be justified than be disproved. Organic psychiatry speaks many languages and can be categorized under many viewpoints which contradict each other.

Historically speaking, however, we find ourselves on very old soil of medical science. The fundamental distinctions known to us today between physically based psychic disorders on the one hand and endogenous psychoses on the other hand was even known in ancient times. AURELIANUS of the 5th century A.D. made on the one hand a distinction between phrenesia - an acute exogenous psychosis - and madness on the other hand. He explicitly makes the point that a fever precedes the psychic changes in phrenesia. Fever is interpreted as a sign of brain fever whereas the psychic symptoms are interpreted as a consequence of brain fever. Furthermore AURELIANUS explicitly states that an insane person on the contrary would never show any organic disorders. If an insane person who is excited for example, gets a fever, then this would be a result of his excitement and thus not a sign of a somatic disease of the brain.

At the end of the middle ages we also find a minute analysis of what is termed nowadays as the clouding of consciousness. Even the terminology is similar to the one used today, although one has to be aware that the history of terminology always takes on a different development to the history of clinical observation regarding this terminology.

667

The overall term is sopor (clouding of consciousness). The sopor is divided into three degrees namely, somnolence, coma and carus.

There are more wider terms such as lethargus. This term signifies the mental changes that occur in organic brain diseases. The general condition consisting of fever, delusion and the resulting memory gaps is comprised in this term. Other organic-psychiatric terms whose meanings have been changing over the centuries, are catochus and stupor.

If there is really such a rich historical development of organic psychiatry, of which I can only present a few short examples here, then one should indeed pose the question, why is it that we do not have any accepted theory of organic psycho-pathology today, neither in international, nor in any of the national psychiatries.

I think that there are two important and closely connected reasons for that. My thesis is as follows:
The beginning of the segregation of the previously homogeneous structure of medicine into several individual disciplines also led to the fact that the treatment of patients with organically caused mental disorders was now undertaken by a number of different disciplines. Hence, psychiatrists are partially responsible for the care of such patients, and mainly only then, when irreparable intellectual damages and the resulting social consequences demand that the patient be transferred into an asylum.

Within psychiatry there has never been a classical organic psychiatry. I understand the term classicism as the development of a generally accepted and at least understandable language and systematics. Perhaps such an opportunity existed foremostly in Germany. But even this opportunity was lost. KRAEPELIN, who created such a classicism for the area of non-organic madness, describes organic-psychic disorders in an entirely conventional way, i.e. with all the contradictions of the pre-classical period of psychiatry.

On the contrary BONHOEFFER had been developing his own theory of organic psychopathology in Berlin since the beginning of this century. At the crux of BONHOEFFER's theory is the principle of the unspecific nature of his so called exogeneous reaction types. According to this, all exterior causes of diseases that invade the brain (infections, intoxication and others) despite their large numbers and differences produce a small number of symptoms. This thesis of BONHOEFFER which was first formulated in a short essay in 1908 was presented only one more time in a thin volume, "The symptomatic Psychoses" (1910). Unfortunately BONHOEFFER never ever condensed his thesis in a special textbook, so that up to today it can not be read in a comprised form, not to mention the fact that

BONHOEFFER for that reason has never been translated into another language. As a result he remained largely unknown outside of Germany. Added to this come the tragic circumstances that BONHOEFFER's short monography appeared in 1910 in the same year as the 2nd volume of the 8th and last edition of KRAEPELIN's "Textbook of Psychiatry" which was dedicated to organic-psychic disorders. KRAEPELIN therefore could not have considered BONHOEFFER's theory any more, even though there are doubts as to whether KRAEPELIN would have shown the right understanding for it.

Is a symposium at a world congress for psychiatry able to replace the missing classicism? Presumably not. However the organizers hope to achieve two things: They hope that the classic of organic psychopathology may still be sitting unnoticed amongst the participants. Or if this would not be the case, then they hope that international discussion would be stimulated and perhaps this would lead to a gradual forming of a mutual language.

BRAIN DAMAGE, MENTAL DISORDERS AND DSM-III

Kalle Achté and Jouko Lönnqvist

Department of Psychiatry
University of Helsinki
SF-00180 Helsinki 18, Finland

Organic mental disorders arise from temporary or permanent disorders of cerebral function. The disorder may be associated with a disease or with the administration of one or more chemical substances. Diagnosis must be based, not only upon psychiatric symptoms but also upon evidence relating to aetiology or pathogenetic factors, but the diagnosis can also be established even when the clinician is otherwise convinced of the organic character of the disorder. Here, only mental disorders caused by brain damage are considered, to some extent critically.

Classification and assessment of organic mental disorders arising from traumatic brain damage.

The significance of organic factors in the diagnosis and treatment of mental disorders has until recently clearly been underestimated (Lipowski, 1980a). The incidence of organic mental disorder in the work-load of each psychiatrist naturally varies greatly. Brain damage following head injury lies behind only a small proportion of all organic mental disorders.

Organic mental disorders are disorders of mental function and behavior caused by permanent damage to or temporary dysfunction of the brain, or both. The differences in clinical presentation reflect differences in the location, mode of onset, progression, duration, and nature of the pathological process. According to the third edition (1980) of the American Psychiatric Association's Diagnostic and Statistical Manual of Mental Disorders (DSM-III), the organic mental disorders comprise seven syndromes, which fall into three groups (Lipowski, 1980b). The classification which follows is slightly different from the DSM-III classification but

671

corresponds to Lipowski's classification. (However, it reflects the basic criteria of the DSM-III classification).

1. Global cognitive impairment
   - Delirium
   - Dementia

2. Circumscribed cognitive impairment
   - Amnestic syndrome
   - Organic hallucinosis

3. Personality or functional disorders
   - Organic affective syndrome
   - Organic delusional syndrome
   - Organic personality syndrome

Traumatic brain damage can give rise to all the syndromes mentioned. At the acute stage of head injury, delirium and the amnestic syndrome are prominent. In contrast, late effects of head injury manifest themselves primarily as an organic personality syndrome and, in the most severe cases, as dementia.

The organic affective syndrome includes lability of affect. It is very common for patients to display involuntary laughter and crying. Particular emphasis needs to be placed upon the fact that motor automatic crying or laughter is associated with an emotional component in only a small proportion of patients. In some cases, it obviously merely occurs if, for example the person finds him or herself in a situation in which he or she is exposed to stimuli, whether happy or sad.

A very interesting observation is that in cases of injury of the nondominant cerebral hemisphere, emotional colouring may disappear from speech. The individual can no longer use implict expressions. Loss the emotion may also reveal itself in expression. Some patients cannot smile but can grin normally and have normal facial movements. This disorder is related to aprosody and is analogous to it. Gestures and the ability to imitate are often also damaged.

The organic personality syndrome is frequently associated with more severe brain damage. The essential feature is a marked personality change. The syndrome is characterized by emotional lability (explosive outbursts of temper, sudden crying), impairment of control of impulses or social judgement and marked apathy and indiffenrence. The border with dementia is blurred. In some instances the diagnosis has to be changed to dementia when intellectual impairment becomes the predominant feature.

672

The symptoms of brain damage naturally have to be understood in relation to the overall situation of the individual. Differentation between organic and psychogenic symptoms is difficult and may even, in some respects, be unnecessary. The condition of the patient can be influenced in different ways, regardless of how it has arisen. Symptoms of purely organic permanent damage can also be treated, and the patient rehabilitated by psychological and social means. On the other hand, differentiation between causes is important for the achievement of optimal results. In addition, assessment of the organic origins of symptoms, however difficult it may be, is an element if good clinical examination.

The location of brain damage, especially as regards frontal and temporal injuries, in relation to the frequency and nature of mental disorders has been widely discussed in the literature. In his study concerning persons who suffered brain injury during the war, Hillbom (1960) stated that injury to the left hemisphere was significantly more common among patients with mental disorder (52 %) than in the group studied as a whole (42 %). Lishman (1968) also concluded that injuries to the left hemisphere constitute a greater psychiatric hazard than injuries to the right hemisphere. However, the opposite has also been reported. In addition, the conclusion from both studies mentioned above was that the more severe mental disorders are particularly linked to temporal and, to some extent, to frontal injuries. In Hillbom's study, personality disorders in association with frontal injury were prominent as were psychoses with temporal injury. In both studies, occipital injury was clearly under-represented among those suffering mental disorder. In general, associations between a site of injury and the nature of a psychiatric disorder are made with reservation.

In his study on civilian brain damage, Roberts (1979) found organic mental disorders in 66 % of patients (Table 2) who had recovered from head injury associated with unconsciousness or amnesia lasting at least one week. Brain damage occured with frontal lobe personality change alone in 21 patients, with dysmnesia in addition in 34 and dysmnesia and irritability in another 50, i.e. in a total of 105 out of 291 patients (36 %). On the basis of reports in the literature, Roberts (Table 2) related the following features to frontal personality change: euphoria, disinhibition, irresponsibility and childishness, a blunting of emotional responsiveness towards children or spouse, loss of former drive and initiative, apathy and anergia or a change to greater energy effectiveness. Persistent mild impairment in day-to-day memory, without evidence of personality change or impairment of other functions, was found in 35 patients.

According to Blumer and Benson (1975), lesions affecting the frontal areas tend to leave intellectual function intact while causing marked alterations in personality. The two types of personality changes involved may be designated pseudodepressed (apathy and indifference) and pseudopsychopathic (puerility and euphoria). The pseudodepressed appear to have lost all initiative and are slow, indifferent and apathetic. Pseudopsychopathic patients are characterized by lack of adult tact and restraint.

Hecaen and Albert (1975) also include affective disorders and disorders of motor activity and cognitive functions as well as certain paroxysmal disorders in the clinical frontal lobe syndrome. A conspicuous feature of the patient's behavior is an increase in affective tone occurring episodically and manifesting itself through euphoria and lack of concern for the present or the future. However, there is apathy in the background. Outbursts of irritability on the part of the patients may cause problems from the therapeutic point of view. These outbursts are sometimes violent and may compel institutionalization. The reason for the change in motor activity is inability spontaneously to initiate an intended or automatic motor task. In the background to defects of cognitive functions there are disorders of attention and recent memory as well as a tendenct to forgetfulness. Given enough time, however, these patients will recall items and events.

They may be coarse, irritable, facetious, hyperkinetic, promiscuous, paranoid or grandiose. They may commit antisocial acts in marked contrast to their previous behavior. These post-traumatic frontal lobe personality changes are most often transient but may be permanent. The pseudodepressed type of personality change relates to lesions of the cortical convexity and the pseudopsychopathic type to lesions of the orbital surface. Bilateral damage can result in frontal personality disorder. In recent years, views of relationships between sites of injury and psychiatric symptoms have changed considerably, following the discovery that deep-lying structures can cause organic symptoms previously regarded as cortical.

Brain injury only rarely gives rise to sexual promisquity, shop-lifting or lack of interest in various areas of life. Impotence, if it occurs, is more likely to be associated with a decrease in self-confidence following brain injury. Suspicious or paranoiac behavior, though it may form a background to personality changes, occurs, in my opinion, in most cases, via a psychological mechanism rather than as a result of brain damage. An abrupt change of social role is usually associated with injury, and may, in some cases, result in a severe crisis of self-confidence.

DSM-III is only a rough framework within which various organic symptoms can be placed. When considering the relationship between DSM-III and brain damage it needs to be stressed particularly that both local and global symptoms of brain injuries have to be indicated in detail in the medical statement. In DSM-III the

emphasis lies on the global changes. Is visual coordianation
lacking or does the patients suffer from aphasia or other verbal
disorders? Is visual agnosia present? Are spatial disorders
present?

Somatognostic disorders which change the feedback from the
body cause distortions of body image are also of psychiatric
significance. Anosognostia for one's own symptoms is also possible.

Is sign blindness or hemi-inattention present? Disturbances
of voluntary motor movements are quite common for example visuo-
constructive disorders. Can so-called dynamic, spatial, postural
or classic apraxia be observed? Is memory disorder axial (of the
Korsakoff-type) or cortical, i.e. partly agnosia? In all of these
groups there are several disorders, differentiation between which
is often useful for diagnosis and rehabilitation.

It should be borne in mind that particular disorders are, in
most cases, present without dementia. In DSM-III, symptoms have
been classified only in association with dementia. The investigator
has personally met several people with capacity and intelligence
of a high level suffering from limited particular disorders.
There was no dementia in such cases.

Difficulties arising from particular disorders in relation to
internal control, effects on self-image etc. may explain some of
the reactive symptoms.

The accurate analysis of symptoms of brain injuries is
difficult and time-consuming although neuropsychological
clarifications based on psychological tests are available and, in
many cases, vital.

REFERENCES

American Psychiatric Association, 1980, DSM-III, Diagnostic and
    Statistical Manual of Mental Disorders, 3rd ed., Washington,
    D.C.
Blumer, D. and Benson, D.F., 1975, Personality changes with frontal
    and temporal lobe lesions, in: Psychiatric Aspects of
    Neurological Disease, F.D. Benson and D. Blumer, eds., Grune
    & Stratton, New York.
Hecaen, H. and Albert, M.L., 1975, Disorders of mental functioning
    related to frontal lobe pathology, in: Psychiatric Aspects of
    Neurological Disease, F.D. Benson and D. Blumer, eds., Grune
    & Stratton, New York.
Hillbom, E., 1960, After-effects of brain-injuries. Acta Psychiat.
    Neurol. Scand., Suppl. 142.
Lipowski, Z.J., 1980a, A new look at organic brain syndromes.
    Amer. J. Psychiatry 137:674-678.

Lipowski, Z.J., 1980b, Organic mental disorders: introduction and review of syndromes, in: Comprehensive textbook of Psychiatry /III, H.I. Kaplan, A.M. Freedman and B.J. Sadock, eds., Williams & Wilkins, Baltimore-London.

Lishman, W.A., 1968, Brain damage in relation to psychiatric disability after head injury. Brit. J. Psychiatry 114:373-410.

Roberts, A.H., 1979, Severe Accidental Head Injury. An Assessment of Long-term Prognosis. Macmillan Press, London.

ADAPTATION TO HEAD INJURY

Jouko Lönnqvist

Department of Psychiatry
Helsinki University Central Hospital
Tukholmankatu 8 C, 00290 Helsinki 29, Finland

INTRODUCTION

In most cases, head injury occurs without warning, and the
abruptness of the event alone leads easily to a crisis of adaptation.
In addition, head injury as a traumatic event is usually severe
enough to be outside what is regarded as the normal range of human
experience. Symptoms occur during the first few days and weeks
following injury, but may also continue as an indication of a chronic
crisis of adaptation. If the symptoms continue for more than six
months, the question is one of chronic posttraumatic stress disorder.

A patient experiencing posttraumatic stress disorder is always
affected by unwelcome reliving of the traumatic event in a variety
of ways. Some individuals have recurrent painful recollections of the
event, dreams, or dissociative-like states during which the traumatic
event is vividly relived. A patient may complain of feelings of
detachment or estrangement from other people, of loss of ability to
become interested in activities previosly enjoyed or of inability
to feel emotions of any kind. This diminished or restricted
responsiveness has been described as psychic numbing or emotional
anesthesia. Nearly all patients with posttraumatic stress disorder
develop symptoms of excessive autonomic arousal, such as hyper-
alertness, an exaggerated startle response, or difficulty in falling asleep. Among other symptoms, disturbances of sleep, memory,
and capacity to concentrate, as well as various degrees of
depression, anxiety, irritablity, impulsiveness, and feelings of
guilt may occur in addition.

Head injury occupies a special position in relation to many
other injuries because the possibility of disturbance to cerebral

677

function is a very emotive question for the patient and relatives. Brain injury usually results in concentration on feelings of helplessness, worthlessness, and general dependence. Many patients strive to maintain the balance of their self-esteem by means that are maladaptive in nature and lead to ever increasing difficulties. Such maladaptive means of adaptation include excessive use of drugs or alcohol, other self-destructive behavior, a tendency towards isolation and deliberate control and manipulation of relationships within the family. Such development leads, before long, to premature decline. In its most severe form, maladaptive development leads to psychotic desorganization or to suicide.

Optimal adaptation requires accurate appreciation of the injury and realistic orientation of life on this basis, The chance of successful adaptation is linked to several factors, including the brain injury and how it is treated, together with rehabilitation, but also to factors such as current life situation, social environment, and pretraumic personality. Brain injury is not only a severe adaptational challenge but also implies a deterioration in the capacity to adapt.

Return of function after brain injury takes place over the first few years. According to most studies, limitation of psychosocial functioning is the greatest obstacle to rehabilitation, not so much the neurological symptoms which are surprisingly little in evidence, even after severe injury. Reduction in function correlates most obviously with both age and degree of injury.

ADAPTATION AFTER BRAIN DAMAGE - TWENTY-FIVE YEAR FOLLOW-UP

In order to elucidate adaptation to brain damage in more detail over a lengthy period, twenty-three brain-damaged war veterans who formed a random representative sample of brain-damaged men living in the Helsinki area, were studied more thoroughly twenty-five years after injury (Table 1). Assessment was based on the original case histories and documentary data throughout the follow-up period as well as on an intensive, semistructured interview lasting several hours.

The adaptation of patients proved to be better in this unselected group than among brain-damaged individuals who had sought treatment. Eleven had a profession before they were injured, and fourteen sought work after injury similar to that in which they had been engaged. After injury, six individuals had engaged in strenuous physical work, nine in light physical work, and eight in intellectual work. All patients surviving twenty-five years after injury had resumed work and only one retired during the first twenty years. Fourteen were still working at the time of the study.

Definite psychiatric invalidism had been involved following

Table 1. Brain Damage in 23 War Veterans

	Per cent
Open injury	52
Duration of unconsciousness:	
no information	4
not unconscious	13
less than one hour	43
more than one hour	39
Post-traumatic epilepsy	43
Degree of disability	
mild (10-25 %)	13
moderate (30-65 %)	39
severe (70-100 %)	48
Hospitalization after primary care of injury:	
less than 3 months	39
3 to 5 months	35
more than 6 months	26

injury at some stage in nineteen of patients out of a total of twenty-three. In the majority, mental difficulties manifested themselves even in the first few years after injury. The principal mental symptoms included insomnia (76 %), anxiety (76 %), aggressiveness (52 %), and depression (48 %). Paranoid traits occurred in one quarter (26 %) of the patients and clearly psychotic symptoms in four (17 %). Some of the disabled still took psychoactive drugs, and a few were also compelled to take analgesics in large quantities. In addition, there were cases (17 %) with definite alcohol problems. All had required hospital care after primary treatment but, on the whole, their needs had been surprisingly modest. One third felt there was a lack of understanding within their evironment as regards their disability.

All those injured were married, over a third prior to disablement. Patients' marriages proved more stable then expected, although definite conflicts continued to occur in some, both with wife and children. About one fifth (22 %) of patients were hostile or overtly violent within their marriage. During the interview study, a fairly reliable image of the sex life of the disabled could be formed. Two had lost interest in sex immediately after injury and four suffered immediate problems with potency. In other subjects reduction of both libido and potency only began to show itself with age. Nine individuals classed their libido and potency as remaining normal and unchanged, One quarter had no further sex life and another quarter had intercourse one to three times a week.

It is important to support the spouse and children, not only for the sake of their own mental health, but also because interrelationsships within the family are of extreme great significance in the adaptive process of the brain-demaged individual. The patient's difficulties impose great demands on other members of the family and, during the acute stage, can make them readily prone to mental crisis and later to depression. External support reduces the incident of these complications and also indirectly supports the patient himself.

STUDY ON TREATMENT OF BRAIN-DAMAGED PATIENTS

In order to clarify the problems of brain-damaged patients 197 consecutive patients were studied,who visited a rehabilitation center for brain-damaged war veterans for treatment and rehabilitation, i.e. twenty-five years posttraumatically, on average. The patients' conditions were assessed before treatment, during treatment, six months after treatment and ten years later. The majority (68 %) sought treatment on their own initiative, the rest were referred by a physician.

The subjective symptoms in patients immediately before seeking treatment are shown in Table 2. We were struck by the frequency of mental symptoms. Of the patients, 27 % considered the mental invalidism caused by their injuries to be greater than the physical invalidism, while in 61 per cent of cases, the reverse was true. Twelve per cent regarded mental and physical invalidism as equal.

From the point of view of treatment and rehabilitation, the patients with severe mental symptoms formed a separate group. Half suffered from relatively deep depression. These were significantly more lonely and withdrawn than the others and also exhibited more difficulties within the family. Deep depression also correlated significantly with unemployment and financial difficulties. In addition, these patients, more than others, tended to use drugs excessively. It is also noteworthy that they felt significantly more often than the others that the attitudes of the others towards their injuries were not understanding, while even the experts had, in their view, rated the degree of invalidism resulting from the injury too lightly.

Rehabilitation took place under comfortable conditions in a small institute in the country. On the basis of physical examination, interview and documentary records at the stage when the patient reported for treatment, an individual four-week rehabilitation program was drafted, the central elements of which were physiotherapy and various occupations designed to maintain activity, which progressed gradually into agreeable spending of leisure time. The patients also had an opportunity for supportive psychotherapy. Table 3 shows the patients' sujective assessment six months later of how useful they had found the

680

Table 2. Symptoms in 197 Male Brain-Damaged Patients

Symptom:	Per cent
Headache	93
Tiredness	93
Dizziness	88
Pains of different kinds	86
Nervousness	85
Depression	85
Insomnia	76
Very depressed and dissatisfied with the life	50
Very lonely	33
Problems with wife	25
Problems with children	19
Excessive use of drugs	12
Excessive use of alcohol	2

particular form of therapy concerned. Forms of treatment requiring more activity physical effort, concentration and attentiveness were less popular and resulted most often disappointments. Almost everyone found physiotherapy useful.

Virtually all patients (98 %), however, considered this type of treatment had, on the whole, been of benefit. The effect of therapy on capacity for work was, however, significant only among those who had retained their capacity for work and, in the majority, the effect lasted less than four months. It is interesting that the benefits of rehabilitation were concentrated particularly on mental problems and symptoms in 38 per cent of patients and on purely somatic complaints in 41 per cent while 21 per cent considered both mental and somatic benefits as significant.

In the light of the present study, it would seem that this kind of therapy supplements the capasity for adaptation of brain-damaged individuals when it is acutely impaired. Most patients benefit from therapy, but its value is restricted with regard to time. Consequently, most feel an annual rehabilitation period of few weeks might be arranged.

About half (54 %) of those who sought treatment had already totally retired from work and the rest worked either occasionally (22 %) or regularly (24 %). Those at work were, naturally,

Table 3. Subjective Assessment of Treatment

Form of Therapy	Participated %	Dissatisfied %	Beneficial %
Mixing with others	96	6	86
Physiotherapy	96	2	97
Sauna	93	9	76
Outdoor exercise	87	10	85
Swimming	80	12	77
Light gymnastics	77	6	87
Ball games	55	30	55
Crafts	53	25	57
More strenuous gymnastics	46	34	49
Massage	40	14	75

significantly younger, but a higher occupational status also distinguished them from those in retirement. The beginning of incapacity for work correlated both with the subjective degree of severity of disablement and the objective degree of invalidism. Those incapable of work never considered that rehabilitation might restore their capacity for work, but nevertheless regarded rehabilitation as important for their own function, and were more desirous of rehabilitation services than those capable of work.

The finding that the patient's own estimates of their future capacity for work proved wholly correct over the ten-year follow-up period is interesting. Similarly, their subjective concept of the degree of severity of their injury correlated significantly with risk of death, although brain damage was not an important immediate cause of death during the ten-year follow-up period. The patients who regarded their work as suiting them, those whose work was intellectuas in nature and the disabled individuals who felt the greatest degree of invalidism resulting from the injury to be mental retained their capacity for work significantly longer.

PERCEPTION OF COGNITIVE IMPAIRMENT AMONG ALCOHOLICS

David Davis

Department of Psychiatry, School of Medicine
University of Missouri-Columbia
Columbia, Missouri, U.S.A

INTRODUCTION

The traditional view is that chronic alcoholics tend to show
impaired performance on a variety of psychological measures
indicating neuropsychological deficit as in the work of Fitzhugh,
Fitzhugh and Reitan (1) and the review of the subject by Tarter (2):
furthermore, the association between depression and alcoholism
continues to be examined eg. by Schuckit (3) and on the other hand,
there appears to be some evidence that some cases of sociopathy
may arise from "abnormal" or "altered" brain function - Guze (4).
In an effort to clarify the possible associations among these
various conditions, I would like to describe two studies.

FIRST STUDY

First, an intensive investigation of eight subjects conducted
by the author at the National Center for Prevention and Control of
Alcoholism of the National Institute of Mental Health which tended
to suggest an association between depression and cognitive defect
in alcoholics. In this study the subjects consisted of eight
volunteer chronic alcoholics of mean age 35.7 years and a mean
average spree-drinking history of 16 years. They were recruited
from a rehabilitation center for alcoholics. All had a history
of withdrawal symptoms and had no evidence of current major
physical illness, psychosis, nor use of medications. No subject
had ingested alcohol for at least two weeks prior to the study.
The subjects participated in a free-choice drinking program on the
inpatient alcoholism research ward and alcohol study unit for 20
days which time was divided into (A) a baseline period of five

days during which physical and mental status examinations, laboratory studies, breathalyzer tests, self-reported assessments of
mood and cognitive functioning using a Q-sort derived from the
Lorr-McNair mood adjective checklist were carried out; (B) a
drinking period of five days during which chips were given to each
subject to be inserted into a dispenser to obtain 50% grain alcohol
and (C) a withdrawal period of five days. 60 cards in sets were
sorted, and consisted of nine which contained depression items,
nine with feeling carefree items and five with cognitive functioning
items. The depression factor consisted of items "sad", "down-
hearted", "worthless", "unhappy", "useless", "depressed", "blue",
"troubled", and "lonely". The carefree factor consisted of items
"happy", "full of pep", "carefree", "at ease", "active", "cheerful",
"satisfied", "lively", and "efficient". The cognitive factor items
included items "confused", "able to think clearly", "forgetful",
"able to concentrate", and "alert". Four extra cards were
duplicates and four more contained instructions to ascertain that
each subject was, in fact, reading and understanding what was
printed on the cards. Three total sets of cards with different
duplicates and instructional cards were used according to a predetermined schedule. The cards were sorted into a box divided
into four compartments labelled "not at all", "a little", "quite
a bit", and "extremely". The results of this sorting process
during four times daily is shown on the following figures.

Figures I-VIII

If one looks at the shape of the histogram and its relation
to the blood alcohol level it is interesting to note the reciprocal
relationship between the "carefree" factor and the "depression"
factor which tends to add to the reliability and validity of the
scales. A statistical comparison of non-drinking and drinking
periods shows a decrease in scores on the "carefree" factor
(P= $<$.05) and the "cognitive" factor (P= $<$.01) for all eight
subjects. In six of the subjects figures I—VI the decrease in
the "carefree" factor and the increase in the "depression" factor
is paralleled by a similar decrease in the "cognitive" factor but
in the last two subjects figures VII and VIII where the effect on
the depression scale is minimal, the effect on the cognitive scale
is also minimal.

Since this study in 1971 a number of investigators have
continued to examine cognitive defects in alcoholics - Kleinecht
and Goldstein (6), Freund (7), Parker et al (8), Brandt et al (9),
Marlatt and Rohsenow (10), and in a recent study of dysphoric
psychopaths by Weiss, Davis, Hedlund and Cho (11) in which the
author was a co-investigator. This is the second study on which I
would like to comment.

684

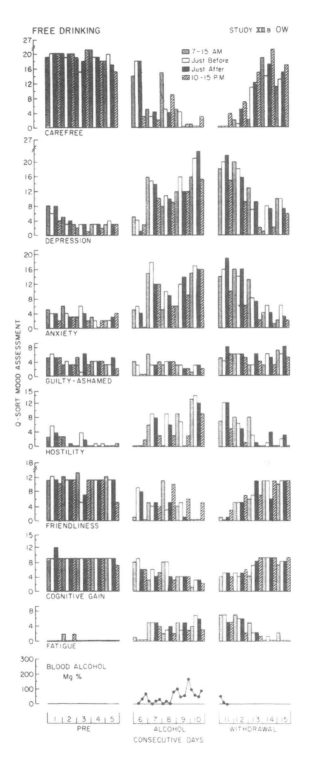

Figure I

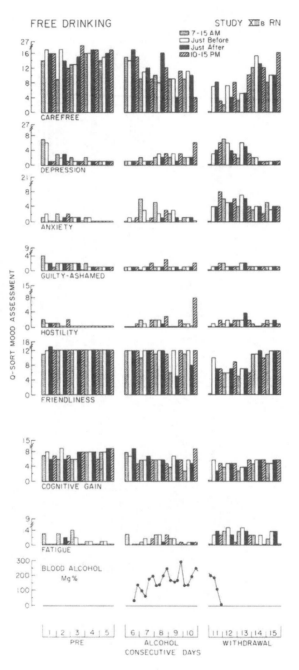

Figure II

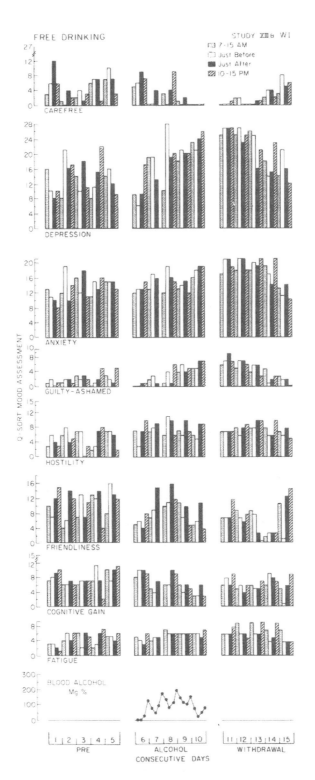

Figure III

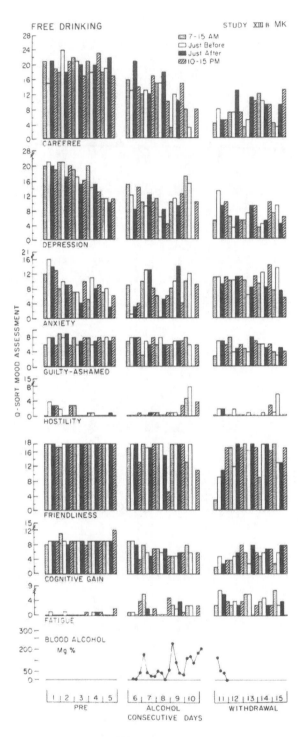

Figure IV

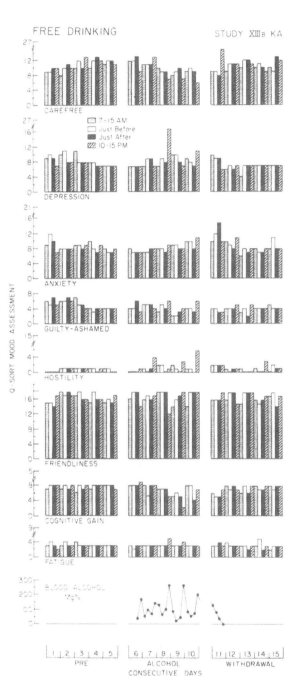

Figure V

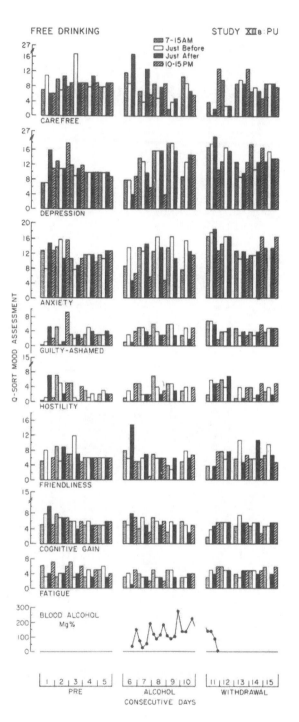

Figure VI

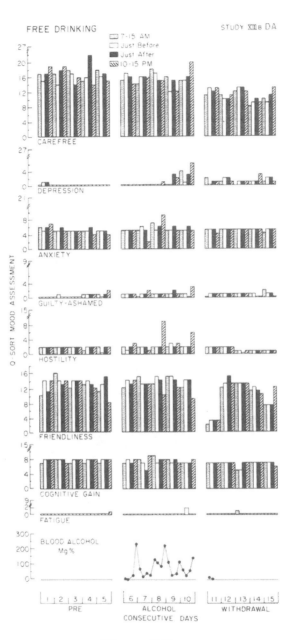

Figure VII

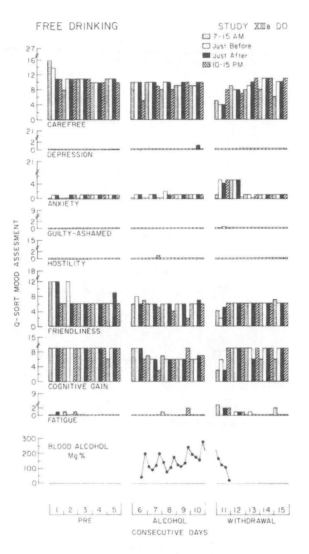

Figure VIII

SECOND STUDY

We selected from the Missouri Department of Mental Health Automated Patient Data Base all first admission inpatients and outpatients (from 1972 to 1980) who had an automated mental status examination and a positive psychiatric diagnosis of antisocial personality. A matched control group of psychiatric patients without antisocial personality disorder was drawn from the data base using the first preceding cases that matched each experimental subject. From the 1,032 patients with a diagnosis of antisocial personality and the 24,289 patients with other psychiatric diagnoses, 524 pairs of experimental and control subjects were matched. Of the 120 mental status items, 37 were found to be significantly different for psychopaths versus controls. A sub-group of dysphoric psychopaths was delineated which would appear to constitute as many as a quarter of all patients with antisocial personality disorder seen in public psychiatric hospitals and outpatient clinics. Such dysphoric patients seem to be depressed, anxious, agitated, and irritable with suicidal thoughts and difficulties in intellectual functioning. Mental status items having to do with "depressive ideation" (ie. suicidal thoughts and plans, ideas of hopelessness and worthlessness, and ideas of guilt), exclusive of depressive mood per se, were significantly more frequent among the psychopaths than the controls. Of the 524 patients with a diagnosis of antisocial personality disorder 131 evidenced depression by mental status criteria --393 did not-- and of the 524 matched controls 159 similarly evidenced depression.

Figure IX

Another factor identified in the psychopaths and controls was called "difficulties in intellectual functioning". This variety of items was scattered among different factors but the cluster which appeared most consistently to characterize the dysphoric psychopath included irritability, poor memory, inability to concentrate, feelings of unreality and apathy. These items were significantly more common among the depressed psychopaths figure X than either non-depressed psychopaths or non-psychopathic depressed controls.

Figure X

It was found that by comparing diagnoses made at index admission with latest diagnosis that approximately one-quarter of both the antisocial group and the matched controls had received an additional diagnosis of alcoholism.

Figure IX

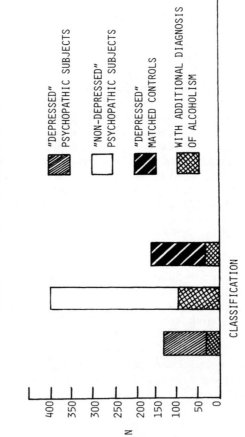

NUMBERS OF "DEPRESSED" AND "NON-DEPRESSED"
PSYCHOPATHS VS. "DEPRESSED" MATCHED CONTROLS.

"DEPRESSED"
PSYCHOPATHIC SUBJECTS

"NON-DEPRESSED"
PSYCHOPATHIC SUBJECTS

"DEPRESSED"
MATCHED CONTROLS

WITH ADDITIONAL DIAGNOSIS
OF ALCOHOLISM

CLASSIFICATION

N

Figure IX

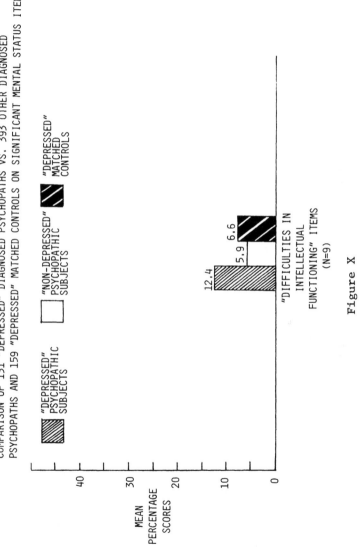

COMPARISON OF 131 "DEPRESSED" DIAGNOSED PSYCHOPATHS VS. 393 OTHER DIAGNOSED
PSYCHOPATHS AND 159 "DEPRESSED" MATCHED CONTROLS ON SIGNIFICANT MENTAL STATUS ITEMS

"DEPRESSED"
PSYCHOPATHIC
SUBJECTS

"NON-DEPRESSED"
PSYCHOPATHIC
SUBJECTS

"DEPRESSED"
MATCHED
CONTROLS

MEAN
PERCENTAGE
SCORES

40

30

20

10

0

12.4

5.9

6.6

"DIFFICULTIES IN
INTELLECTUAL
FUNCTIONING" ITEMS
(N=9)

Figure X

695

If the figures for the various "depressed" and "non-depressed" psychopaths and control group are held constant for alcoholism at approximately 25% in each group, the proportions relating to cognitive deficit still remain unchanged.

CONCLUSIONS

Thus, cognitive impairment as perceived on mental status examination or measured by a self-rating Q-sort does not appear to be associated in a necessary relationship to either alcoholism, depression or antisocial disorder alone (except perhaps in the extreme or chronic cases of the first two conditions). Rather, cognitive impairment is likely to be manifested when some moderate to severe degree of clinical depression is found in association with either alcoholism or antisocial personality disorder, or both.

This pecular set of relationships suggests some alteration in brain function (rather than on an experiental basis). The newer evidence by Schulzinger (12) indicating a clear genetic diathesis for psychopathy (as modified by experience) and the work of Winokur and his colleagues (13, 14) in depression and alcoholism suggesting that neurobiological systems may be altered in all three of these conditions indicates some disturbance of balance. Recent work with the drug, Zimelidine, suggests a further relationship between alcohol, depression and cognitive function. It may well be that it is not just the drinking effects alone that cause the cognitive decrease but the concomitant presence of depression, especially in persons who have a history of repetitive antisocial or violent behavior which may be an additional pre-disposing or exacerbating factor in the cognitive impairment.

REFERENCES

1. Fitzhugh EC, Fitzhugh KB, and Reitan RM. Adaptive Abilities and Intellectual Functioning of Hospitalized Alcoholics: Further Considerations. Quart. J. Alc. 26:402-411, 1965.
2. Tarter RE. Psychological Deficit in Chronic Alcoholics: A Review. Internat. J. of Addictions 10:327-368, 1975.
3. Schuckit M. Alcoholic patients with secondary depression. Am. J. Psychiatry 140:711-714, 1983.
4. Guze SB. Criminality and Psychiatric Disorders. Oxford University Press Inc., New York, 1976.
5. Davis D. Mood changes in alcoholic subjects with programmed and free-choice experimental drinking. In Mello N and Mendelson J (Editors) Recent Advances in Studies of Alcoholism: An Interdisciplinary Symposium. Rockville, MD., NIMH, NIAAA 1971.

6. Kleinecht RA and Goldstein SG. Neuropsychological deficits associated with alcoholism. Quart. J. Stud. Alc. 33:999-1019 1972.
7. Freund G. Chronic central nervous system toxicity of alcohol. Ann. Rev. Pharmacol. 13:217-227 1973.
8. Parker ES, Alkana RL, Birnbaum IM et al. Alcohol and the disruption of cognitive processes. Arch. Gen. Psychiat. 31:824-828 1974.
9. Brandt J, Butters N, Ryan C, Bayog R. Cognitive loss and recovery in long-term alcohol abusers. Arch. Gen. Psychiat. 40:434-442 1983.
10. Marlatt GA and Rohsenow DJ. Cognitive processes in alcohol use: expectancy and the balanced placebo design. In Mello N (Ed.) Advances in Substance Abuse, JAI press Inc., Greenwich, Conn. 1:159-199 1980.
11. Weiss JMA, Davis D, Hedlund JL, Cho DW. The dysphoric psycho-path: a comparison of 542 cases of antisocial personality disorder with matched controls. Comprehensive Psychiatry 24:355-369.1983.
12. Schulsinger F. Psychopathy: heredity and environment. In Biosocial Bases of Criminal Behavior. Mednick S and Christiansen KO (Eds). Gardner Press Inc. New York 1977 pp. 109-125.
13. Winokur G, Reich T, Rimmer J and Pitts FN. Alcoholism III, diagnosis and familial psychia-ric illness in 259 alcoholic probands. Arch. Gen. Psychiat. 23:104-111 1970.
14. Winokur G. et al. Relationship of genetic factor to course and drug response in schizophrenia, mania and depression. Genet. Psychopharmacol. Med. Probl. Pharmacopsychol. 10:1-11 1975.

SCHNEIDERIAN FIRST RANK SYMPTOMS IN ORGANIC PSYCHOSES

Andreas Marneros

Universitäts-Nervenklinik
5000 Köln 41
W.Germany

The desire of psychiatric research workers for diagnostic criteria which are as uniform and as reliable as possible has led to renewed interest in Kurt Schneider's first rank symptoms (FRS) since the early 1970's. Their nontheoretical, pragmatic character and their high reliability make them indispensible for empirical clinical research. According to Kurt Schneider's concept, FRS occur both in schizophrenic and in organic psychoses. He writes: "Where such types of experience are definitely present and no bodily basic disease can be found, we speak clinically - in all humility - of schizophrenia. It is important to know that they can all occur in psychotic states based on bodily disease: in the alcoholic psychoses, in the epileptic twilight state, in anaemic and other symptomatic psychoses, and in widely differing cerebral diseases" (1).

Kurt Schneider found only a low incidence of FRS in organic psychoses: in the clinical department of the Psychiatric Research Institute in Munich, of which he was Director, his co-worker Leibig found in 1006 organic psychoses only 16 cases with FRS, i.e. approximately 1.6 % (2). Jörn Weitz, another of his co-workers, later found an even lower incidence, with FRS in only 9 patients out of 1930 cases of organic psychoses, i.e. approx. 0.5 % (3). These sparse findings were the reason for Kurt Schneider's statement that he had earlier overestimated the importance of "symptomatic schizophrenia". It occurred to us, however, that in many aetiologically defined groups, the numbers of cases occurring in the material of the Psychiatric Research Institute in the period studied was very low. Thus in Schneider's material, which was very similar to Leibig's one, for instance there were only 11 cases of delirium tremens and alcoholic hallucinosis, 8 cases of Korsakoff's psychosis, and only 102 cases of all internal diseases and infections together. Weitz, too, admitted that for many diagnoses, in which first rank schizophrenic symptoms are known to occur not infrequently, the number of cases in his material was low, for instance only 19 cases of acute psychosis of chronic alcoholics.

MATERIAL AND METHODS

We asked ourselves how the incidence rate of FRS would have appeared if the material had contained larger numbers of aetiologically defined cases. In other words: does the incidence of Kurt Schneider's FRS depend on the aetiological classification of the particular organic psychosis? Is it possible to speak of the frequency of FRS in organic psychoses in general, or do we need to differentiate separately between the frequency in alcoholic psychoses, for example, or in intoxication psychoses or in epileptic psychoses and so on? In our follow-up investigations of patients with suspected schizophrenia, we have particularly studied this question. With the object of testing the value and reliability of the FRS as a diagnostic tool, we have investigated the incidence and structure of FRS in all forms of psychoses, including the organic psychoses. For various reasons the patients of the Cologne University Psychiatric Hospital form a very suitable collective for answering the above questions. For thirty years the hospital was directed by a pupil of Kurt Schneider, Prof. Dr. Werner Scheid, who regards himself as an orthodox Schneiderian. In the 30 years from 1950 to 1979, the Schneiderian concept was the sole diagnostic concept used in the hospital. The diagnoses and their documentation were controlled by the director of the hospital, either personally or through his senior assistants, who themselves all strictly apply Kurt Schneider's diagnostic criteria and of whom two underwent part of their training under Kurt Schneider himself. The findings were usually very extensively documented, so that there is no difficulty in using 190 items per patient.

The material used for this study is the case records of 1208 patients hospitalized for schizophrenia for the first time ever and 1181 case records with the discharge diagnosis organic psychosis. The comparison and combination of 190 items per patient was carried out with the aid of a computer system.

With the aim of avoiding descriptive inaccuracies - a danger which is always present in retrospective studies based on case records - we classified the first rank symptoms into six groups as follows:

1. delusional perceptions
2. "first rank auditory phenomena", i.e. hearing voices talking to one another, hearing voices commenting on the patient's own actions or omissions, or the patient hearing his own thoughts spoken aloud (Gedankenlautwerden)
3. thought insertion
4. thought withdrawal

5. thought broadcasting
6. other feelings of being influenced by outside forces

RESULTS

The group "organic psychoses" includes all usable case histories of psychoses in the following aetiologically defined groups: 1. disorders of internal secretion, 2. arteriosclerosis, 3. intoxications, 4. infections, 5. post-operative psychoses, 6. Wernicke-Korsakoff psychoses, 7. acute nondelirious alcoholic psychoses, 8. 154 acute delirious alcoholic psychoses, randomly selected, 9. psychoses after contusio cerebri, and 10. all epileptic psychoses occurring in a total collective of 9002 epileptic patients.

Productive psychotic symptoms, i.e. delusions and/or hallucinations and/or disturbances of experience of the self, were presented by 745 of the organic psychosis patients, i.e. 63 %. Of the schizophrenic patients, productive symptoms were presented by 81 %.

Figure 1 shows that around 37 % of the organic psychosis patients showed no productive symptoms, around 54 % showed second rank productive symptoms, and around 9 % showed FRS. The difference between productive and nonproductive forms in the organic psychoses is highly statistically significant in favour of the productive forms, as is likewise the difference between first and second rank symptoms in favour of the second rank symptoms. In comparison with this, as figure 1 shows, in schizophrenia FRS occur significantly more frequently than second rank symptoms and nonproductive phenomena.

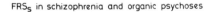
FRSs in schizophrenia and organic psychoses

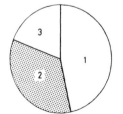 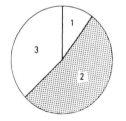

FRSs in Schizophrenia   n=1208   FRSs in organic psychoses   n=1181

1) FRSs   (n=567 – 47 %)   1) FRSs   (n=109 – 9 %)
2) other productive symptoms   (n=411 – 34 %)   2) other productive symptoms   (n=636 – 54 %)
3) non-productive symptoms   (n=230 – 19 %)   3) non-productive symptoms   (n=436 – 37 %)

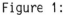
Figure 1:

Table 1:

First rank symptoms in organic psychoses n=1181			Schizophrenia n=1208	
Delusional perception	11	0,9 %	229	19 %
First rank auditory phenomena	81	6,9 %	263	22 %
Thought broadcasting	8	0,7 %	76	6 %
Thought withdrawal	5	0,4 %	44	4 %
Thought insertion	4	0,3 %	70	6 %
Other feelings of being influenced	31	2,6 %	186	15 %

Forms of FRS in organic psychoses (Table 1)

In the organic psychoses, delusional perceptions were recorded for 11 patients (almost 1 %); first rank auditory hallucinations for 81 patients (almost 7 %); thought broadcasting, thought withdrawal and thought insertion each less than 1 %; other feelings of being influenced from the outside - usually bodily influence - for 31 patients (almost 3 %). The findings in schizophrenia, by comparison, were: delusional perceptions 19 %; first rank auditory hallucinations 22 %; thought broadcasting 6 %; thought withdrawal 4 %; thought insertion 6 %; other feelings of being influenced by outside forces 15 %. This comparison shows that the trend of the incidence of FRS is almost the same in organic and in schizophrenic psychoses, except for the delusional perceptions.

Table 2 shows the frequencies of the FRS in the different aetiological forms of organic psychosis. This shows a very wide variation in incidence between the different aetiological groups. Thus FRS are found in less than 1 % of patients with contusio psychosis, but in 40 % of the epileptic psychoses and in 45 % of the acute nondelirious alcoholic psychoses, but no FRS in delirious acute alcoholic psychoses.

Frequency of first rank symptoms in correlation with the patient's state of consciousness

If we exclude the epileptic psychoses, in which there were some intrinsic uncertainties regarding the state of consciousness, then, of the remaining 1131 patients, 610 (54 %) showed disturbances of consciousness in the sense of clouded consciousness, while the remaining 521 showed no changed state of consciousness. Of the patients with disturbed consciousness, only less than 3 % showed FRS, as against over 14 % of patients with unimpaired consciousness. Of the patients with FRS and disturbed consciousness, 11 of 17 cases showed FRS during their nondisturbed periods. The other 6 patients

Table 2:

FRS_S in organic psychoses

Kinds of psychoses		FRS_S	
Disorder of int. secretion	(n= 31)	3	10 %
Arteriosclerosis	(n= 120)	8	7 %
Contusio cerebri	(n= 139)	1	1 %
Intoxication	(n= 362)	38	11 %
Non-delirious acute alcoholpsychoses	(n= 64)	29	45 %
Delirious acute alcoholpsychoses	(n= 154)	0	0
Wernicke-Korsakow-Syndrom	(n= 104)	3	3 %
Infection	(n= 104)	4	4 %
After operation	(n= 53)	3	6 %
Epileptic psychoses	(n= 50)	20	40 %

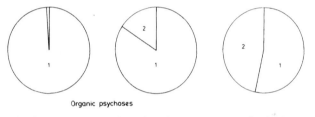

Organic psychoses

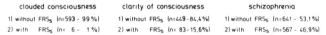

clouded consciousness	clarity of consciousness	schizophrenia
1) without FRS_S (n=593 - 99 %)	1) without FRS_S (n=449 - 84,4%)	1) without FRS_S (n=641 - 53,1%)
2) with FRS_S (n= 6 - 1 %)	2) with FRS_S (n= 83 - 15,6%)	2) with FRS_S (n=567 - 46,9%)

Figure 2:

(i.e. less than 1 %) showed slight-degree alterations in state of consciousness (disorientation, reduced comprehension, or reduced attention). If we reclassify these 11 patients into the group with unimpaired consciousness, then almost 16 % of the unimpaired consciousness patients showed FRS as against 1 % of the patients with disturbed consciousness (Figure 2).

CONCLUSIONS

It can be seen from the above findings that the frequency of FRS in the organic psychoses depends on the aetiological classification of the psychoses and on the clarity of consciousness. This means that we cannot speak of "the frequency of FRS in organic psychoses" in general, but we must distinguish according to the particular aetiology and form of the organic psychosis in question.

This fact seems to us to be of major theoretical importance. Interpretations can be linked either to the ideas of Huber (4) and his co-workers on the "substrate-related basic symptoms", or to those of Janzarik (5) on the "dynamic reaction type". Huber et al. regard the FRS as "highly complex schizophrenic end-phenomena" which "are produced, through psychoreactive mediation, working-over and re-forming processes, from initially noncharacteristic, basic symptoms". According to Huber, such basic symptoms can sometimes occur in phenomenologically identical form in cases of organic brain disease. The "dynamic unsteadiness" which characterises the schizophrenic psychosis can, according to Janzarik, also sometimes be activated by toxins or other organic causes, presenting similar to endogenous psychoses.

It seems likely that acute organic psychoses with unimpaired consciousness fulfill the conditions necessary for "substrate-related basic symptoms" to develop into "highly complex end-phenomena" in Huber's sense. Our findings show differences in the relative frequency of the various forms of FRS between schizophrenic and organic psychoses. We were also able to confirm the findings of U.H. Peters (6) that it is not only possible but indeed imperative to distinguish psychopathologically between the two forms of psychosis from their constellations of symptoms. This is however to be expected if we consider, that the disturbance of the "representative part of the personality", in Janzarik's terms (5), determines the psychopathological clinical picture in organic psychoses, so that exogenous and endogenous syndromes show a different colouring.

We think that the relatively high incidence of FRS in certain groups of organic psychoses under certain conditions compels us to assume that FRS are "psychotic reaction patterns" whose substrate-related basis runs right across the spectrum of endogenous and exogenous psychoses.

References
1. K. Schneider, "Klinische Psychopathologie", 10. Auflage, Thieme, Stuttgart, 1973
2. K. Schneider, Fünf Jahre klinische Erfahrung an der Forschungsanstalt für Psychiatrie, DMW 25 (1937) 957-973
3. J. Weitz, Zur Statistik der Symptomatischen Schizophrenie, DMW 72 (1947) 38-39
4. G. Huber, Das Konzept substratnaher Baisissymptome und seine Bedeutung für Theorie und Therapie Schizophrener Erkrankungen Nervenarzt 54 (1983) 23-32
5. W. Janzarik, "Dynamische Grundkonstellationen in endogenen Psychosen, Springer, Berlin-Göttingen-Heidelberg, 1959
6. U. H. Peters, "Das exogene paranoid-halluzinatorische Syndrom" Karger, Basel-New York, 1967

PSYCHOPATHOLOGICAL TYPES AND NEURORADIOLOGICAL

CORRELATIONS OF ORGANIC PSYCHOSYNDROMES

Gisela Gross and
Gerd Huber

Psychiatric Clinic of the University of Bonn
D-5300 Bonn 1

Computed tomography (CT) has many advantages against earlier neuroradiological methods (1,3,4). It is less susceptible to artefacts than f.i. pneumoencephalography (PEG); in spite of it, false interpretations are quite often in the diagnostic of cerebro-atrophic syndromes. In the opinion of most authors it is possible to demonstrate and interpret the cortex, especially localization and expansion of cortical atrophies, much better than by PEG. In spite of it, the danger of <u>misinterpretations</u> is high, especially at the cortex in the sense of false-positive findings of a cortical atrophy. Cortical atrophies were diagnosed too often as we published earlier (1,2). Considering the possibilities and limits of the cranial CT with regard to neuropsychiatric diseases, the most important question with reference to the theme of this symposion is whether there is any <u>correlation to the presence or absence</u> of clinical-psychopathologically demonstrable irreversible organic psychosyndromes and their degree or not. Up to now, there are no investigations that had tried to correlate systematically psychopathological and CT findings in all psychiatric diseases.

Previous clinical PEG studies have shown significant positive correlations between irreversible psychosyndromes of known brain diseases and brain atrophy. Furthermore, certain types of atrophic brain syndromes could be correlated to certain types of irreversible psychosyndromes. More <u>generalized and cortically accentuated atrophy</u> seems to correspond with organic dementia processes, whereas <u>internal cerebral atrophy</u> in the area of the ventricular system is correlated to more isolated (not associated with severe organic dementia) organic personality disorders ("organische Wesensänderung") and irreversible pseudoneurasthenic syndromes. On the basis of PEG and echoencephalographic investigations we concluded that in neuroradiological-clinical studies no correlations could be expected between certain groups of diseases, e.g. epilepsy, multiple sclerosis or schizophrenia as a whole, and findings by PEG or CT (4). But correlations exist in definable organic psychoses as well as in endogenous schizophrenic and affective psychoses if irreversible psychosyndromes of an organic character are present.

Up to now, the problem of normal data in CT has not yet been solved. Especially regarding the cortex, the risk of faulty judgement, i.e. false-positive findings, is considerable. In probands who were not older than 50 years and without neurological or psychiatric diseases we found an average third ventricle diameter of 4.2 mm without age-correlated increase in size. In this group of variations in psychic reactions and personality in the sense of K. SCHNEIDER (psychic-reactive disturbances and psychopathic personality disorders), there were no significant differences with regard to average diameter of the third ventricle in patients younger than 50 years of age. According to GÖTZE et al. (s. in 1), the normal width of the third ventricle show deviations between 2.0 and 5.5 mm. In our material of 34 cases with variations of psychic being, these sizes varied between 2.0 and 6.0 mm. Therefore, up to the 50th year of age we considered a transverse diameter of the third ventricle of 7 mm and more as pathological. On the lateral ventricles more markedly changes of the shape in frontal segments, cella media, and at the cortex, a 3 mm width of the sulci or more were considered pathological. For judging the brain cortex, more basically situated sulci in various slices have to be taken into consideration, whereas the sulci of the three highest slices near the vertex (just as the cysterns, the interhemispheric fissura, and pacchionian granulations) were not considered.

Cortical and/or subcortical cerebral atrophy are non-specific and not characteristic for certain diseases. Nearly all brain diseases can cause a cerebral atrophy and a cerebro-atrophic syndrome, demonstrable by CT, which is always nonspecific. In an earlier study in Heidelberg patients we had confirmed by correlations between neuro-radiological and psychopathological findings that a cortical atrophy usually (in 80 %), but not without exception, corresponds with an irreversible organic psychosyndrome.

706

So-called compensated brain atrophies, i.e. atrophies without irreversible psychosyndromes, were seen chiefly on the basis of posttraumatic or postdystrophic brain damages respectively defect states. On the other hand, irreversible organic psychosyndromes occur without any brain atrophy (23 %; s. in 3).

The results obtained earlier in Heidelberg by PEG were examined by CT in Bonn patients. Our investigation is based on 451 inpatients (276 males, 175 females) of the Neuropsychiatric University Clinic of Bonn who were admitted during 1978-1980 with various psychiatric diagnoses. Of the whole sample of 451 patients, 40 patients were diagnosed as psychopathic personality disorders, 151 patients as endogenous psychoses, and 260 patients (167 males and 92 females) as characterized brain damages and brain diseases. All anamnestical and clinical data, especially the psychopathological syndrome at the time of CT investigations, were documented with the intention to answer the question of correlations between CT and psychopathological findings. The actual organic psychosyndrome was subdivided according type and degree of severity of the psychopathological syndrome in conformity with our earlier distribution (1,2,3) as described in the following:

Degree 0: No psychopathological syndrome at all. – Degree 1: Chronical pseudoneurasthenic syndromes. They were observed most frequently in posttraumatic, postencephalitic and postdystrophic brain damages and in vascular brain diseases. They can be considered as slightest form of an organic personality disorder and correspond with the so-called "weak cerebral function". The psychopathological picture is determined by slight, noncharacteristic and etiological ambiguous psychosyndromes of "neurasthenia", characterized by disturbances of affective reactivity, i.e. increased emotional lability and excitement and a reduction of mental energy level with complaints about weakness of concentration and derangement of the capacity to register, increased exhaustibility and fatigability in connection with vegetative-vasomotoric disorders. All complaints remain in the subjectivity and fluctuate extremely. A differential diagnosis against psychopathic and neurotic neurasthenias and asthenic pure residues after remission of endogenous psychoses is difficult and often only possible considering clinical data, somatic findings and the long-term course. – Degree 2: Organic personality disorders. This psychosyndrome is characterized chiefly by alterations of the dynamic part of the personality, e.g. disorders of the mental ability to react, increased excitability, affective lability or incontinence, diminution of initiative, psychomotor delaying, decrease of impulsion, derangement of task set, perseveration and adhesitivity. - <u>Degree 3: Dementia</u>. This organic psychosyndrome is less frequent than the degrees 1 and 2. It is determined f.i. by intellectual and mnestic deficits, a reduction of comprehension, deficient judgement, lack of discrimination, pronounced disorders of logical thinking, memory and ability to combinate. Often can be observed a disturbance of the memory for recent events, disorientation and irreversible Korsakoff's syndrome (5).

In our patients with brain diseases (260 cases) 29 % (75 cases) show no psychopathological alterations, 26 % (68 cases) an irreversible pseudoneurasthenic psychosyndrome, 37 % (95 cases) an organic personality disorder and only 5 % (13 cases) a dementia. Among 1.474 patients of a former study in Bonn with irreversible organic psychosyndromes pseudoneurasthenic and slight organic personality alterations have been more frequent (62 %) than pronounced organic psychosyndromes (33 %) and dementia (5 %; s. in 5).

Practically it is very important that pseudoneurasthenic syndromes and slight organic personality alterations, causing a lot of differential diagnostic difficulties, are the <u>most frequent irreversible organic psychosyndromes</u>. Considering groups of diagnoses it is important that dementia processes are most frequent in primary cerebro-atrophic processes, whereas pseudoneurasthenic syndromes and organic personality alterations predominate in diseases of the brain vessels and in posttraumatic brain damages.

The rate of pathological cerebro-atrophic findings in the whole sample of <u>definable brain diseases</u> and <u>brain damages</u> reaches 81 % in patients with irreversible organic psychosyndromes, whereas patients <u>without psychopathological alterations</u> show only in 13 % pathological changes in CT. The differences between these both subgroups is highly significant. Thus there is a statistically significant positive correlation between brain atrophy, proofed by CT, and irreversible organic psychosyndromes. - Patients with vascular brain diseases predominantly show irreversible organic psychosyndromes (87 %). The rate of pathological CT findings is 37 % in patients without irreversible psychosyndromes, but 88 % in those <u>with irreversible</u> organic psychosyndromes. In this subgroup the rate of pathological CT findings in cortex and ventricles increases from 76 % in patients with pseudoneurasthenic syndromes to 93 % in patients with organic personality

708

disorders and finally to 100 % in patients with dementia.

The pathological CT findings show a different distribution in the three groups with irreversible psychopathological psychosyndromes: In pseudoneurasthenic syndromes pathological findings concern most frequently the third ventricle which is usually enlarged isolated. Organic personality disorders reveal beside pathological findings at the third ventricle additional pathological changes of lateral ventricles. In the group with dementias prevail generalized brain atrophies accentuated at the cortex.

Our findings emphasize also the problem of the concept of multiinfarct-dementia. In our patients with vascular brain diseases the so-called apoplectic forms with neurological losses were missed. Circumscript neurological deficits and infarctions in CT show only 1/5 of our subgroup with vascular brain diseases and irreversible psychopathological syndromes; predominantly these patients show only psychopathological changes without neurological deficits and without criteria of encephalomalacia in anamnesis or in CT. In patients without neurological deficits and without infarctions (65 cases) demonstrable in CT, irreversible organic psychosyndromes were observed in 86 %, but in the small subgroup (13 patients) with neurological deficits or infarctions in 92 %. Our investigation emphasizes that irreversible organic psychosyndromes in vascular brain diseases are not obligatory connected with neurological findings or encephalomalacias detectible in CT.

Summarizing, we emphasize that the neuroradiological findings of a brain atrophy, however, is always nonspecific concerning a certain brain disease or a certain brain damage. All kinds of etiological heterogenous diseases and damages of the brain can lead to an atrophy of the internal or external spaces of the brain, demonstrable in CT. But the brain atrophy is not correlated regularly with irreversible psychopathological syndromes. Principally there is a difference between the statement of a cerebral atrophy by neuroradiological criteria and its clinical-psychopathological relevance. The pure finding of cerebral atrophy demonstrated by CT does not mean anything reliable; only in connection with other results, especially with psychopathological findings and results of psychological tests, the diagnosis of a brain disease with an irreversible organic psychosyndrome, often important in regard to clinical, social and forensic aspects, can be verified. On the other hand, a normal CT without atrophic findings does not exclude persistent psychopathological

alterations in the sense of organic personality disorders
or even of a dementia. - In spite of the considerable differences between neuroradiological and psychopathological
findings in some cases, the correlations, however, concerning the majority of patients are easily to be seen (3,4).
Also by CT a correlation of high significance can be
proved concerning irreversible psychosyndromes and brain
atrophy. Certain types of irreversible brain atrophies are
associated with certain types of irreversible psychosyndromes: Well defined dementias are related to generalized
cerebral atrophy, often accentuated in the cortex. Isolated personality disorders without severe intellectual deterioration and pseudoneurasthenic syndromes are corresponding with an atrophy close to the ventricular system.
There exist also a positive correlation between the degree
of severity of irreversible psychosyndromes and the degree
of the brain atrophy. Statistical correlations exist between the degree of reduction of brain substance but they
are not obligatory for the individual case. That is why
treatment is always indicated, even the therapy of chronic conditions of cerebral atrophy is not hopelessly because they often include some amount of reversibility. -
Finally, we want to emphasize that the pseudoneurasthenic
syndromes and not the dementia are of high importance for
the early diagnosis of neuropsychiatric diseases; these
relatively less marked and often noncharacteristic psychosyndromes are the essentials of our diagnostic and false
diagnostic.

References

1. Gross, G., Huber, G., and Schüttler, R., 1982, Computerized tomography studies on schizophrenic diseases. Arch.Psychiat.Nervenkr. 231: 519-526
2. Gross, G., Huber, G., and Schüttler, R., 1982, Psychopathologische und computertomographische Befunde
   bei neuropsychiatrischen Alterserkrankungen,
   Fortschr.Neurol.Psychiat. 50: 241-246
3. Huber, G., 1964, Neuroradiologie und Psychiatrie, in:
   "Psychiatrie der Gegenwart," vol.I/1, H.W.Gruhle,
   R.Jung, W.Mayer-Gross, M.Müller, eds., Springer,
   Berlin Göttingen Heidelberg
4. Huber, G., 1972, Klinik und Psychopathologie der organischen Psychosen, in: "Psychiatrie der Gegenwart,"
   vol.II/2, 2.ed., K.P.Kisker, J.E.Meyer, C.Müller,
   E.Strömgren, eds., Springer, Berlin Heidelberg
   New York
5. Huber, G., 1981, "Psychiatrie. Systematischer Lehrtext
   für Studenten und Ärzte," 3.ed., Schattauer,
   Stuttgart New York

PSYCHOPATHOLOGY AND PSYCHODIAGNOSTIC FINDINGS IN

PATIENTS WITH FRONTAL LOBE TUMOURS

G. Ransmayr, F. Gerstenbrand and S. Plörer

University Clinic for Neurology
A-6020 Innsbruck, Austria

INTRODUCTION

The symptomatology of frontal lobe lesions of different
origin was already discribed in the last century. In
1934 KLEIST differentiated the semiology of lesions of
the frontal lobe convexity and the frontobasal region.
In 1949 KRETSCHMER published the changes of personality,
character and vegetative functions after fractures of
the base of the skull and comprised these symptoms as
orbital brain syndrome and diencephalic syndrome.
SCHMIEDER (1968) described the symptoms of the post-
traumatic frontoconvex syndrome. GERSTENBRAND (1970)
differentiated the posttraumatic frontoconvex and the
posttraumatic frontobasal syndrome. ANGELERGUES et al.
(1955) and LURIA et al. (1964) published detailed clinical findings as well as experimental psychodiagnostic
results of patients with frontal lobe tumours. Their
conclusions are of great importance for the understanding
of the frontal lobe psychopathology.

Materials and Methods

Since 1979 the University Clinic for Neurology of
Innsbruck analyzed 10 male and 16 female patients
with primary tumours of the frontal lobes in
order to correlate the clinical symptomatology
and the psychodiagnostic findings with the morphological lesions by the use of the CAT. The ages
of the male patients ranged from 26 to 62, with

711

a mean age of 49,2 yrs., and of the female patients from 18 to 75, with a mean age of 46,3 yrs.. In 22 of the 26 patients a histological diagnosis was achieved by operation. Eight patients suffered from a glioblastoma (in 3 of them the tumour originated in the corpus callosum), 3 of an astrocytoma I-II and 3 of grade III — IV. Two of them had an oligodendroglioma, 1, an oligoastrocytoma II (classification of KERNOHAN and SAYRE), 1, a monstrocellular sarcoma (classif. ZÜLCH) and 4 pts. a meningioma. In 4 pts. an operation was impossible because of contraindication. According to the CAT-findings it was assumed that 1 of the non-operated pts. had a meningioma, 1, a glioblastoma of the corpus callosum, and 2, an oligodendroglioma. In 7 pts. the tumour was situated merely in the left frontal lobe and in 4 pts. in the right. In 9 pts. the tumour originated in the left frontal lobe and extended to the right, in 4 pts. vice versa. In 2 pts. the tumour was localized in the midline. The tumour was predomi-nately localized in the frontobasal region of 7 pts., in the frontoconvex of 8,and in the frontopolar of 4. In 7 pts. the tumour comprised the whole frontal lobe of one hemisphere from the basis to the convexity. The largest diameter of the tumour was more than 5 cm in 14 pts.. In 18 pts. there occured either a lateral displacement of the frontal midline of more than 5 mm, or a perifocal brain edema or a compression of the anterior part of one side-ventricle. Epileptic seizures had appeared in 17 pts.. Premorbid brain damage was not known in any of the patients. Twenty-three pts. were right-handed.

The investigations consisted of an elaborate history taking from the patient and outside persons, a clinical neu-rological and a psychiatric examination, EEG, CAT, transfe-moral cerebral angiography and neuropsychodiagnostic ex-amination, consisting of the Reduced WECHSLER ADULT INTEL-LIGENCE SCALE, flicker-fusion-frequency-analysis, BENTON VISUAL RETENTION TEST and the RORSCHACH TEST.

Results

According to 22 outside sources psychiatric symptoms had been observed in 16 pts. (table 1). They had appear-ed for the first time three weeks to four yrs., mean 42 weeks, before the admittance. Ten pts. realized mental changes themselves. Neurological symptoms, reported by the patient or outside persons had appeared in 24 pts. 3 weeks to 8 yrs., mean 60 weeks before the first clini-cal examination (table 2).

Table 1: History of psychiatric symptoms: N = 26

Outside sources: N = 22   16 pts. pos.
                            6 pts. neg.

apathy	9	loss of concentration	4
psychomotor slowing	8	loss of appetite	4
loss of initiative	8	nervousness	3
forgetfulness	7	facetiousness	2
disorientation	6	euphoria	2
depression	4	dysphoria	1

Table 2: History of neurological symptoms: N = 26

Outside + patients' information: N = 26

24 pts. pos., 2 neg.

epileptic seizures	17	anosmia	4
tiredness	9	nausea	4
headache	6	blurred vision	3
dizziness	6	dysphasia	2
paresis	6	dyspraxia	2

According to outside sources the psychiatric symptoms dominated the neurological in 11 cases.

At the admittance of the clinic all patients were alert. The most frequent neurological symptoms were frontal signs, mild pyramidal signs, mild hemiparesis and anosmia. The mental state revealed a mild frontal lobe syndrome in 9 pts., a medium in 7 and a severe in 10 pts.. (range of symptoms listed according to frequency talbe 3). The symptoms of the frontal lobe syndrome could be categorized as disturbance of incentive, highest mental function, memory and orientation, mood and behaviour (table 4).

The severity of the frontal lobe syndrome did not correlate to histology, side and localization in the

Table 3: <u>Mental state in frontal lobe tumour:</u> N = 26

psychomotor slowing	14	perplexity	7
disturb. of initiative	12	depression	6
apathy	10	confusion	5
loss of insight	10	facetiousness	2
distractability	10	dysphoria	2
disturb. of memory	9	loss of criticism	2
red. assoc. thinking	8	impulsiveness	2
disorientation	7	euphoria	1

Table 4: <u>The frontal lobe tumour syndrome</u>

Disturbance of:

<u>Incentive</u>:	apathy, disturbance of initiative, psychomotor slowing
<u>Highest mental functions</u>:	loss of insight and criticism, facetiousness, perplexity, impaired associative thinking
<u>Memory and orientation</u>:	forgetfulness, disorientation, confusion
<u>Mood</u>:	depression, euphoria, dysphoria
<u>Behaviour</u>:	impulsiveness, tactlessness

frontal lobe, but to the size of the tumour and the age of the patients (p < 0,01). In 4 pts. the symptomatology resembled the frontobasal and 14 the frontoconvex syndrome. Eight pts. demonstrated a mixture of both. There is no unequivocal correlation between the frontobasal and the frontoconvex syndrome and the exact localization of the tumour.

In 13 pts. neuropsychodiagnostic examinations were performed. Five pts. had a predominantly frontoconvex, 5, a frontobasal and 3, a frontopolar localization of the tumour. The Reduced WAIS and its sub-tests as well as the FFFA did not reveal differences between the sub groups. The values of the Red. WAIS were borderline to low ones. The Benton Visual Ret. was gen. reduced, showed significantly lower values in the frontoconvex group compared to the frontobasal one (p < 0,05). In the Rorschach Test the number of responses was significantly higher in the frontobasal compared to the frontoconvex group (p < 0,05). Whole blot percentage was significantly higher in the frontopolar group compared to the frontobasal group (p < 0,05). The percentage of forms of good quality was significantly higher in the frontoconvex group compared to the frontobasal one (p < 0,05). (For the statistic evaluation of U-Test of MANN and WHITNEY was used). Generally the Rorschach Test revealed an organic pattern.

Summary

In frontal lobe tumours the frontal lobe syndrome nearly obligatorily appears. Its severity depends on the size of the tumour and the patients' age. In most cases the frontal lobe tumour syndrome resembles the frontoconvex syndrome and in fewer cases the frontobasal syndrome. A strict correlation between the symptomatology and the localization of the tumour does not exist. (see also HECAEN 1978, POECK 1982).

Conclusion

Apathy, psychomotor slowing and disturbance of immediate and recent memory, depression, euphoria or dysphoria, facetiousness and loss of criticism without gross neurological symptoms are suspect of a frontal lobe process and demand special attention.

REFERENCE

Kleist, K., 1934: Zusammenfassung der Ergebnisse über Störungen der Ichleistungen und ihre Lokalisation im Orbitalhirn, Cingulum und Zwischenhirn. Gehirnpathologie. Barth, Leipzig.
Kretschmer, E., 1949: Die Orbitalhirn- und Zwischenhirnsyndrome nach Schädelbasisfrakturen. Arch.Psychiat. Ztschr.Neurol. 182, 452-477
Schmieder, F., 1968: Psychiatrische Rehabilitation traumatischer Hirnschäden. Wien.Med.Wschr. 38, 779-782.
Gerstenbrand, F., Grünberger, J., 1970: Klinische Erfahrungen mit Mesoridazin in der Therapie und Rehabilitation von traumatischen Frontalhirnschäden. Wien.Med.Wschr. 42/43, 732-737

Angelergues, R., H. Hecaen, J. De Ajuriaguerra, 1955:
    Les troubles mentaux au cours de tumeurs du lobe frontal.
    Ann.med.-psychol. 2, 577-642
Luria, A.R., K.H. Pribram, E.D. Homskaya, 1964: An
    experimental analysis of the behavioural disturbances
    produced by left frontal meningioma. Neuropsychologia
    2, 257-280
Hécaen H., M.L. Albert, 1978: Human Neuropsychology.
    John Wiley and Sons, New York.
Poeck K., 1982: Klinische Neuropsychologie. Thieme
    Verlag Stuttgart - New York.

EVALUATION OF PSYCHO-ORGANICITY IN HEALTH DISASTERS-

THE TOXIC OIL SYNDROME EXPERIENCE

Juan J. López-Ibor Jr, José M. López-Ibor, Adela
Alonso, Angela Hoz, P. Fuentes and Berta Rios

Centro Ramón y Cajal and C.S. Primero de Octubre
Carretera de Colmenar, Km. 9, Madrid (34), Spain

From early May 1981, an outbreak of a previously unknown
disease occurred in central Spain. The epidemic reached a peak by
mid June, when more than 600 daily hospital admissions due to the
disease were recorded. Illegally sold denatured rapeseed oil has
been accepted as the most probable cause. Therefore the illness has
been called Toxic Oil Syndrome (TOS). By December 1982, a total of
336 deaths had occurred, the total number of cases recorded had
reached 20,178.

The TOS has been considered a natural catastrophe, that is to
say an inevitable **disaster.** However, catastrophe is also synonymous
with an unfortunate **denouement** , that is, there is always a
previous history in which the disaster has been slowly forging
ahead, ignored by its protagonists up to the moment of the
unraveling. Therefore every catastrophe provokes the feeling that
it in itself or its consequences were not inevitable.

The TOS consists of an acute (toxic) and a chronic (toxic and
probably inmunological) phases. During the acute phase there is
fever, eosinophilia, skin rash, pruritus, malaise, myalgia,
arthralgia, dispnoea, non-cardiogenic pulmonary oedema, and
nonspecific gastrointestinal symptoms. The chronic phase,
developing insidiously over a period of months, is characterized
mainly by peripheral neuropathy with muscle atrophy, skin tautness
of schleroderma type, xerostomia and xerophthalmia (sicca syndrome)
and pulmonary hypertension. The observed progression of some of the
lesions suggests that the total perspective of chronic effects has
yet to develop. Fewer than 2% of patients with TOS have died. The
clinical course of the majority of cases so far has been that of a

slow, spontaneous resolution. In a small proportion of patients the severe chronic changes described above have developed, and in a few patients these have not resolved. In a significant proportion of patients an almost stable reduction of diffusion capacity of the lungs and/or increase of liver enzyme levels remain.

The TOS received from the beginning extraordinary public attention. The mass media were during months concerned with it in a preferential manner and the TOS was an important topic in the political battles between the political parties in and out of Parliament. Not everything was to the benefit of the patients, since the mass media often became an anxiety provoking factor (for example, the newscast on television began, during practically the whole second half of 1981, with the number of deaths the day before and one of the most circulated newspapers in Spain, announced in October, 1981 when the number of affected was over 15.000, that all of them were hopelessly condemned to death). Political deliberations weren't always appropriate either, since measures were taken which favoured the proliferation of a rent neurosis, although initially it was thought to avoid these by means of generous subsidies and preferential care, based on the slogan "the only limit is the demand". One of the lessons derived from the TOS catastrophe is that the psychological repercussions are not lessened by generous or special measures, not is the differentiation between psychiatric stress reactions and malingering made easier by them, on the contrary, some can be harmful to the doctor-patient relathionship.

Just to give an idea, up to now the TOS has cost around 21 billion pesetas, that is, around 150 million US dollars. For instance, every family has received between 1 and 1.5 million pesetas (10,000 US dollars) per deceased member, subsidies up to three times the minimum salary, and other subsidies for domestic help or for compensation of family enterprises or farming.

PSYCHOLOGICAL AND PSYCHIATRIC ASPECTS

From the beginning of the epidemic, psychological alterations were present whose importance grew, as much in patients as in particular wards where the drama of the illness, the pressure from the mass media and the anxiety itself of the patients caused a growing stress upon the staff. The psychopathology detected in the acute phase was represented by acute psychological reactions (depressive, anxious or phobic) to the situation of their illness, by the drama of the setting in which they received the care (initially in isolated wards) and also by the fear of immediate death. The illness affected usually several members of the same family, or people of the same neighbourhood. Together with these symptoms acute brain syndromes secondary to ventilatory insufficiency or deteriorated physical condition appeared.

During the chronic phase other complaints appeared: insomnia, severe and chronic pain in the limbs, difficulties in doctor-patient relationships and chronic psychological reactions.

The cases referred to the psychiatrists were studied by a specially appointed team of 25 psychiatrist and 25 psychologists in 15 hospitals and 3 out-patient units, and their findings documented with the aid of the Unified Clinical Record (HCU), a computerized Clinical Record that we describe elsewere in this Congress. Over 4,000 patients (20% approx.) have been referred to psychiatrists and the findings of 1,338 have already been analyzed. TOS patients tend to show a predominence of women, of low socio-economic levels and little education. These trends were more accentuated in the cases referred to the psychiatrists, where for instance, 14% of illiterate people were found.

The reactive disaster psychic syndrome is a neurotiform reaction to stress, consisting of the following symptoms: almost 1 patient in 2 shows sadness, depression, anxiety, insomnia and irritability, and in 1 out of 4-5 loss of concentration, loss of short term memory, feelings of personal inadequacy and incapacity and despair or fear. Some family members of those affected by the TOS referred to the psychiatrists present more or less the same symptoms with almost the same frequency, with the exception of a lower incidence of sadness, depression, loss of short term memory and a higher one of vegetative symptoms.

THE PROBLEM OF ORGANIC BRAIN DAMAGE:

During the acute phase, coinciding with the pulmonary syndrome, psychiatrists detected in 10% of the patients, alterations of the level of conciousness and deterioration of the intellectual and instrumental functions. Later on such alterations did not become present and were attributed to a brain syndrome secondary to respiratory insufficiency, malnutrition, associated infections, medications or vascular disturbances, and toxic oedematous encephalopaty.

During the chronic phase the presence of the neurological symptoms mentioned and the appearance throughout 1982 of mioclonias muscular cramps, contractions and rigidity, trembling and crisis which could be atributed as well to motor unit hyperactivity as to central disfuntions brought out the fear of a possible brain damage. This coincided with the presence of complaints such as insomnia, lability of emotions and above all a lack of concentration and memory disturbances. To study this aspect several teams of psychologists were formed. The research into this aspect is getting to be very complex due to: the interference of psychological factors and the mimicry of the symptomatology of patients who are treated in special units and coincide very often in the hospitals, the interference of the the reactive disaster psychic syndrome mentioned, the low socio-cultural and educational level, the not always positive attitude towards the examinations of patients who have been examined countless times without brilliant results on his clinical state. Another important reason is that we are dealing with a new illness whose natural history has an uncertain future. The appearance of a single case where it could be demonstrated without a doubt a direct affectation of the Central Nervous System in the TOS would be sufficient to recognize this affectation and forsee the appearance of new cases.

We have followed two independent paths to try to solve this problem: the study of the clinical symptomatology of the patients and to perform neuropsychological examinations.

Study of the clinical symptomatology: Taking advantage of the data of the H.C.U., we have made a filtration in several stages:

a) **Patients with a possible organic brain affectation.** We have considered such those that presented some of the following characteristics or data: convulsive crisis, abnormal behavior and attitudes during the inteview, speaking disturbances in general, disturbances in the rythm and modulation of speech, aphasias, alterations of conciousness, disorientation, disturbances of attention and memory, hypersomnia, that they had a point count of less than 28 in the mini-mental state examination or that they had been diagnosed as having organic transitory psychosis (ICD9-293), other chronic organic psychosis (ICD9-294) or specific mental non-psychotic disturbances following organic encephalic lesions (ICD9-310). In total 555 patients, (41%) fulfilled this condition.

b) **Doubtful organic cases:** From the above list we eliminated those cases with a psychiatric pathology previous to the TOS: alcoholics with organic deterioration, hyperkinetic syndromes in childhood, epilepsy, subnormality, very intensive depressive and anxiety syndromes, psychogenic confusion and all those in which the symptoms mentioned were not taken into account in the final diagnoses of the patient. A group of 30 (2.2% of the total) patients remained which were re-examined and in 14 cases it was found that an acute confusional state was psychogenic. The detailed study of the Clinical record showed up the existence of a previous brain pathology (craneal trauma, presenile dementia and cerebral vascular accidents) in 3 cases. In 5 cases the cognitive deficits were attributed to depressive states. What was left then was 8 cases in which the patient had been diagnosed of an organic brain syndrome, psychotic or non-psychotic, present or doubtful in its relation to the Toxic Oil. In none of these 8 cases was it clear if the affectation, present or doubtful, was or was not a direct or indirect consequence of the intoxication. Two presented important respiratory insufficiency, another had a great loss of weight with

720

doubtful findings in the neurological examination, CT Scanner and visoperceptive tests; another was illiterate and one other showed normal results of a neuropsychological examination.

Neuropsychological examination: A pilot study carried out on 13 patients referred to the psychiatrist with a modified neuropsychological battery because of the motor disturbances of the patients. A psychodiagnostic study of Rorschach was included. The results obtained were the following: in 12 cases alterations of attention-concentration were present in a mild or moderate degree, not attributed by its character to an organic brain affectation, rather to interference by factors of anxiety and depression; in another patient in addition disturbances of speech and apraxias because of peripheric disfunction were present. Another female patient had had previously a brain infarct and she therefore showed signs of cerebral organicity. These 13 patients have been or will be re-examined for a control of evolution of their states.

In July of 1982, a more detailed investigation was designed in which the following tests were applied:

-Specific questions in a standard interview.
-Benton right left discrimination and finger localization test.
-Drawing of the human figure.
-Laterality
-Bender's gestalt test.
-Weschler's Intelligence Scale for Adults: WAIS.
-Rorschach's Psychodiagnostic Test.
-Luria-Christensen's Protocol of Neuropsychology, adapted.

Up to now 34 patients have been examined, selected among the most suspected of presenting symptoms of motor hyperactivity (mioclonias, etc.) or were receiving psychiatric attention because of complaints predominantly of loss of memory. A study is being carried out of 2 control groups of TOS patients with peripheric neurological symptoms and and no psychiatric complaints and another group of TOS patients without clinical neurological affectation.

The average time of the application of the tests varies between five and a half hours and seven and a half hours. Including the corrections the average time employed in the study of each patient is 13 hours. During the application of the tests we observed difficulties in the examination. While 23 patients were acceptably helpful, 5 presented an open agressive attitude and 6 demonstrated an indirect agressivity. And on the other hand and in general, the low cultural level, the characteristics of a very primitive personality, an attitude of demand for recognition and compensation and definitely, the special status of the affected patients, are facts which make it extraordinarily difficult to analyze and evaluate these patients.

The results obtained up to now are partial. In only 4 patients were we able to detect alterations that could correspond to a possible psychoorganic syndrome, of which a 50 year old patient is a chronic alcoholic with a psychiatric history. Another, a 46 years old woman is a neurotic personality, a low cultural level and is illiterate, which makes his evaluation very difficult achieve, the third, 42 years old woman, suffered a previous brain infarct and there appeared signs of cerebral organicity. And the last one, 52 years old woman, had presented before the TOS a psychotic episode and subsequent psychic and behavioral disturbances which makes us suspect that the deficit detected dates to before the TOS.

In three patients we were able to detect a doubtful psycho-organic syndrome. In a 59 year old male and a 46 year old female we detect deficits difficult to affiliate, since in her there exists a hypochondriac and pathomimic attitude, and in him a severe depressive picture. A follow-up study was normal in both. In the third patient we detect a component of anxiety reactive to his illness and economic uncertainty which could interfere with his performance during the tests. These 7 patients are pending a follow-up study after a period of several months.

In the rest of the patients studied, there didn't appear at present from the tests applied, signs of organic brain affectation. On the other hand, the data obtained in relation to an elevated percentage of traits of anxiety and depression stands out.

CONCLUSIONS

We only have provisional conclusions which are: as shown, the subjective complaints of the patients are analogous to those of the family members not affected by the intoxication, but in which is present a psychic syndrome secondary to the intoxication. The neuropsychological examination of these patients is extremely complicated because of the interference of peripheric motor affectations, psychological factors (anxiety, demand, malingering or factitious disorders) and social factors. The subjective complaints of patients suffering from the reactive disaster psychic syndrome mimic the complaints and symptoms of psycho-organic syndromes making this differentiation very difficult, but at the same time very important. Anyhow, up to now there hasn't appeared any case in which it can be accepted with certainty that the toxic substance had affected directly the higher nervous functions. But if one is found it would be enough to prove that the TOS can also affect the higher centers of the Central Nervous System.

COMPARING FRENCH AND INTERNATIONAL CLASSIFICATION SCHEMES :

V. DSM III AND THE FRENCH POSITION ON ORGANIC BRAIN SYNDROMES

Charles B. Pull and Pierre Pichot

Centre Hospitalier, 1210 Luxembourg and
Clinique des Maladies Mentales et de l'Encéphale
75014 Paris

I INTRODUCTION

The rational underlying DSM III is widely known by now.[1]
The implications of the DSM III approach to classification are
particularly apparent in the chapter on organic mental disorders.[2] Major traditional dichotomies, such as psychotic/non-
psychotic and acute/chronic have been eliminated. The whole
class of conditions caused by or associated with cerebral
disease or dysfunction is designated "organic mental disorders".
The disorders are defined on the basis of (1) the presence of
one or several extensively described organic brain syndromes
and (2) the reference to a known or presumed organic etiology
or pathophysiological process.

The French classification [3] is based on traditional
French nosology. Established in 1968 by the Institut National
de la Santé et de la Recherche Médicale (INSERM), the INSERM
classification constitutes an attempt to systematize diagnostic
practices that are commonly accepted by French clinicians. It
is a simple nomenclature, which is not accompanied by a
glossary and which does not provide any additional information.
It contains 20 categories which are subdivided into up to 10
sub-categories. There are 6 categories pertaining partly or
exclusively to organic mental disorders. The classification
criterion in this field is etiological. Owing to the fact that
the classification is uni-axial, it has to rely to a large
extent on so-called "combination categories" for coding combined mental and physical disorders. The situation is particularly apparent in those categories termed "symptomatic mental
disorders" (2 categories) or "mental disorders of epilepsy".

French textbooks, on the other hand, clearly individualize specific organic brain syndromes and the possible etiological factors are listed separately. As a consequence, the following account will be based on textbook descriptions [4,5,6,7,8,9].

II SYNDROMES IN DSM III AND IN FRENCH TEXTBOOKS

DSM III identifies 7 purely descriptive clusters of psychological or behavioral signs and symptoms, without reference to a specific etiology, referred to as "organic brain syndromes" : Delirium, Dementia, Amnestic syndrome, Organic hallucinosis, Organic delusional syndrome, Organic affective syndrome and Organic personality syndrome. To make a diagnosis of a given syndrome, DSM III requires : (1) the presence or absence of clearly defined inclusion and exclusion criteria and (2) evidence of a specific organic factor judged to be etiologically related to the disturbance. Each organic brain syndrome may be due or associated with a variety of physical disorders. Delirium, dementia and amnestic syndrome make up the bulk of the organic mental disorders. The diagnostic criteria defining the various DSM III syndromes are not reproduced in the following.

French textbooks identify most of the syndromes listed in DSM III. With one exception, concerning "mental confusion", the terminology is basically the same.

A. MENTAL CONFUSION

The concept of "mental confusion" was introduced in 1851 by DELASIAUVE [4] who described a psychopathological state characterized by clouding of consciousness, spatio-temporal disorientation, impaired memory and perception. In 1895, CHASLIN [4] developed the concept of "primitive mental confusion" which he separated from symptomatic and secondary mental confusion, and which was to become a nosological entity with different etiologies, both organic and functional. In 1915 , the same author changed his position in two important directions : (1) mental confusion was now considered a syndrome and (2) the etiology of which was predominantly organic. Finally, REGIS [4] related mental confusion to oneiric delusional states and insisted on its almost systematic association with intoxication or infection.

1. Current Views on Mental Confusion.
In all current textbooks, mental confusion is clearly described as an acute syndrome, with the term "syndrome" appearing in every single description.

a) Diagnostic criteria. Current diagnostic criteria are identical with those suggested by REGIS and as such insist upon clouding of consciousness, disorientation, impaired memory and perception, oneiric delusions and hallucinations and evidence of organic dysfunction.

b) Causative Factors. The most important factors judged to be etiologically related to the disturbance are intoxication, infection, neurological, endocrine and metabolic disorders. In exceptional cases, the disturbance may be due to externe psychological stress such as natural disasters or military combat. Mental confusion associated with an organic factor is termed non reactive mental confusion in the INSERM classification, and reactive mental confusion in association with psychological stress.

c) Course. Onset is acute or subacute. Duration and complications are a function of the underlying causal process. In most cases, prognosis is favorable, but complications such as chronic delusional state or chronic and demential confusion are possible.

d) Subtypes. Besides symptomatic subtypes (depending on the predominance of one of the symptoms of the syndrome), French clinicians describe a rare malign confusional state, termed "delire aigu" characterized by (1) profound confusion or intense oneiric delusions and (2) severe somatic disturbance with hyperthermia, dehydration and hyperuremia and (3) generally fatal course.

2) Comparison with DSM III
The current French acceptance of mental confusion corresponds closely to the DSM III concept of delirium. One major difference is that DSM III precludes the possibility of extreme psychological stress as a sufficient causative factor, but this possibility is considered extremely rare by French clinicians as well. A second difference concerns "délire aigu" which is not considered in DSM III.

B. DEMENTIAL STATES

In traditional French psychiatry, the term dementia implied a chronic, i.e. progressive and irreversible course. This definition is, however, no longer accepted in recent French textbooks.

1. Current Views on Dementia.
   Most current French textbooks prefer the term "demential
   states" to the term "dementia", the former term permitting to insist upon the existence of a broad spectrum
   of clinical states produced by acquired impairment of.
   intellect, as well as upon the heterogeneity of the underlying pathology. The term "demential states" presents
   no connotation as to prognosis.

   a) Diagnostic criteria. Current diagnostic criteria
      insist on memory impairment, difficulties to sustain
      attention and to understand, temporal and spatial
      disorientation, impairment of abstract thinking and
      judgment as well as other disturbances of higher cor-
      tical function such as aphasia, apraxia or agnosia.

   b) Causative Factors. Etiological factors are subdivided
      in degenerative (Alzheimer's disease, Pick's disease,
      Creutzfeld-Jacob's disease, artériopatic disease)
      and secondary (infectious, vascular, toxic, traumatic,
      endocrine, tumoral).

   c) Course depends upon the underlying pathology and the
      availability of effective treatment.

2) Comparison with DSM III.
   The current French acceptance of demential states is
   identical with the DSM III concept of dementia.

C. KORSAKOFF'S SYNDROME

1. Current views on Korsakoff's syndrome.
   Most French textbooks differentiate between Korsakoff's
   disease (used as a synonym for polyneurotic psychosis)
   and Korsakoff's syndrome, the latter being viewed as the
   amnestic component of the former. This is most apparent
   in the concept "Korsakoff's amnestic syndrome" used by
   one of the authors [7].

   a) Diagnostic criteria. Insistence is on anterograde
      amnesia, no or only mild retrograde amnesia, no im-
      pairment in immediate memory or in intellectual abi-
      lities, no clouding of consciousness. Confabulation,
      false recognitions and disorientation may be asso-
      ciated.

   b) Causative Factors. Alcoholism and other causes of
      thiamine deficiency, hypoxia and other intoxications,
      head trauma, brain tumor or any other cause interrup-
      ting Papez's circuit.

2. Comparison with DSM III.
The current French acceptance of Korsakoff's amnestic
syndrome is identical with the DSM III concept of amnestic disorder.

D. HALLUCINOSIS

1. Current Views on Hallucinosis.
According to EY [4] and POROT [6], the term hallucinosis
has three different meanings in the French literature.
(1) Hallucinosis without further specification refers
to hallucinations of any kind and which are immediatly
recognized as abnormal phenomena by the individual who
criticizes the disturbance and who is aware that it does
not correspond to reality. The phenomenon is considered
to be a neurological symptom permitting to localize pathological processes in the brain or sensory organs.
(2) Used in connection with "alcohol hallucinosis", the
concept pertains to auditory and, to a lesser degree,
visual hallucinations, associated with delusional conviction of their reality, but without further elaboration
of the delusional material. Duration is usually brief
with complete recovery. In exceptional cases, the disturbance becomes chronic and develops into chronic alcoholic
hallucinatory psychosis. (3) Finally, "pedoncular
hallucinosis" defines a rare syndrome, associated with
damage of the meso-diencephalon, in which the individual
assists passively to the appearance of particular visual
hallucinations.

2. Comparison with DSM III.
The DSM III criteria for organic hallucinosis encompass
all three meanings of the French acceptance of hallucinosis. The French concept is more restrictive in what
concerns the etiology of the disturbance. With the
exception of "alcohol hallucinosis", the French concept
is directly related with a neurological disturbance. In
particular, the term would not be associated with
hallucinogenes or with sensory deprivation, blindness
and deafness.

E. OTHER SYNDROMES

Organic Delusional, Affective and Personality disturbances
which may be related to a specific organic factor are described
in the various French textbooks in connection with a number of
disorders. There is, however, in comparison with DSM III, no
reference in this context to the existence of specific syndromes underlying a variety of organic mental disorders.

SUMMARY AND CONCLUSION

The common organic brain syndromes described in DSM III
are almost identical with syndromes described in recent French
textbooks. Delirium has its correspondant in mental confusion,
dementia in demential state and amnestic syndrome in
Korsakoff's syndrome. Organic hallucinosis encompasses different French acceptances of hallucinosis but is less specific
in what concerns etiology. Organic delusional affective and
personality syndrome are not described as specific syndromes
in France.

REFERENCES

1. American Psychiatric Association, ed, Diagnostic and
   Statistical Manual of Mental Disorders (3rd edn,
   DSM III), APA, Washington D.C. (1980)
2. Z. J. Lipowski, Organic Mental Diseases, in : Comprehensive Textbook of Psychiatry/III, H. I.
   Kaplan, A. M. Freedman, B. J. Sadock, ed, Williams
   and Wilkins, Baltimore/London (1980)
3. Institut National de la Santé et de la Recherche Médicale, ed, Classification française des troubles
   mentaux, Bull de l'INSERM, 24, Suppl. to N° 2
   (1969)
4. H. Ey, P. Bernard, Ch. Brisset, Manuel de Psychiatrie,
   5e édit. revue et corrigée, Masson, Paris (1978)
5. Encyclopédie Médico-Chirurgicale, Psychiatrie Clinique et Thérapeutique, Editions Techniques, Paris
   (published periodically)
6. A. Porot, Manuel alphabétique de Psychiatrie, 4e ed.
   remaniée et mise à jour, P.U.F., Paris (1969)
7. J. D. Guelfi, Eléments de Psychiatrie, 2e éd. revue
   et augmentée, Ed. Méd. et Univ., Paris (1979)
8. T. Lemperière, A. Féline, Psychiatrie de l'Adulte,
   Masson, Paris (1977)
9. C. Koupernik, H. Loo, E. Zarifian, Précis de Psychiatrie, Flammarion, Paris (1982)

MEMORY FUNCTION IN ORGANIC BRAIN DISEASE

V.A. Kral

Clinical Professor
The University of Western Ontario
London, Ontario   Canada

It has become clear, over a century of memory research, that one of the best ways to understand memory function in the human is to study the clinic and pathology of the various forms of memory dysfunction in organic brain disease.

The most frequently encountered type of memory dysfunction in chronic brain disease is the amnestic syndrome as described by Korsakoff in chronic alcoholics. At the present time the amnestic syndrome is most frequently found in senile dementia of the Alzheimer type and Alzheimer's presenile dementia.

Symptomatologically, it is characterized by shortened retention span, loss of recent memory, retroactive loss of remote memory, disorientation first in time, later also as to place and person. In some cases the syndrome is accompanied by confabulation. In Alzheimer's disease the onset and progress is usually gradual. Clinical research of recent years, however, has shown that it may have, in some cases, a sudden onset. It may develop out of stress induced confusional states. Although most of these stress induced confusional states of the aged clear up completely, in some of them only the level of awareness reverts to normal while memory function remains impaired (1) particularly in patients who had already suffered confusional states, once or twice before, from which they had recovered. This course bears a remarkable similarity to alcoholic Korsakoff's psychosis which also frequently develops in patients who had gone through one or more

729

episodes of delirium tremens from which they had recovered.

Gamper (2) had shown that the main anatomical lesions in alcoholic Korsakoff are to be found in the brain stem mainly in the corpora mammillaria which are connected by the fornix with the hippocampus. He concluded that these structures must in some way be related to the character-istic memory dysfunction of the amnestic syndrome. The first definite proof of the association of the amnestic syndrome with hippocampal lesions was the observation by Glees and Griffith (3) who reported on a woman who clinic-ally presented an amnestic syndrome and whose brain con-tained hemmorhagic cysts in both hippocampal areas. Since then a number of cases of amnestic syndrome associated with bilateral lesions involving the hippocampus-fornix-mammillare system have been reported. Kral (4) showed that the system involved in the amnestic syndrome is identical with the circle described by Papez (5) as the site of "the harmonious mechanism of the emotions".

In Alzheimer's dementia we also find the character-istic lesions, the tangles, plaques, granulovacuolar degeneration, Hirano bodies and the neruonal loss mainly in the posterior part of the hippocampus on both sides. (6) However, the same histological lesions can also be found, although in much smaller numbers, in other areas of the brain cortex and this explains the signs of neocortical deficit which we find in many Alzheimer patients.

Remembering is also involved in many activities of our daily life without our realizing it. This is the case in recognition in all sensoric areas and in all automatized functions of daily living, like speaking, writing, washing, using spoon, knife and fork and many others. Although the capacity to remember was needed in acquiring these gnosopractic functions their constant repitition leads to ultimate automatization and one for-gets the difficult memorial processes involved in learn-ing them. It is only when one or more of these skills are lost that the memory loss involved is being recognized. The memories underlying the gnosopractic functions are being called "partial memories" in contrast to the "personal memories" lost in the amnestic syndrome.

Clinico-pathological research has documented that the loss of these partial memories is independent of the loss of personal memories. A patient with alcoholic Korsakoff's psychosis may present an amnestic syndrome of considerable severity, but is able to talk, to under-stand spoken language, to write, read and to perform most

of the normal activities of daily living. On the other
hand, a patient after a stroke or in the early stages of
a brain tumor may not show any loss of personal memories
but be severely impaired in one or more partial functions.
He may suffer from expressive aphasia, agnosia and so on.
There is also a great number of cases where personal, as
well as partial memory functions, are lost as in many
cases of Alzheimer's dementia and in some cases of multi-
infarct dementia.

Special investigation showed that loss of partial
memories could be found only in cases with focal cortical
lesions or with diffuse cortical involvement as in Alzheimer's dementia (7). Partial memories were found preserved in cases with amnestic syndromes without any indication of neocortical involvement.

The lesions, leading to loss of partial memories,
may be of different kind as, f.i. an embolic or throm-
botic infarction or a hemorrhage or a traumatic brain
damage, a neoplasm or even a diffuse process as in Alzheimer's dementia.

Another type of memory dysfunction is "benign senescent forgetfulness". This is characterized by the inability of the subject to recall, on occasions, a detail
of an experience such as a name or a date while the event
itself of which the "forgotten" detail was a part can be
recalled. The missed detail, however, can be recalled
on other occasions, mostly when not immediately needed.

This occasional failure of retrieval may occur at
any age and is usually explained by psychodynamic factors
which interfere with recall because of an unconscious
negative emotional loading. Why it occurs more frequently
in the aged is not quite clear. It may be that with
increasing age the process of retrieval is more susceptible to interference by dynamic factors perhaps due to
the general slowing of the mental processes in old age.

Long-term observation showed that old people with
the benign type of forgetfulness,as a group, did not
show a significantly shortened survival time and an increased death rate as was found in a matched control
group of patients with the "malignant type of senescent
frogetfulness". This was the reason for calling this
type of forgetfulness benign in contrast to the malignant
type, the amnestic syndrome, as found in senile dementia
of the Alzheimer type. (8)

The question was raised whether the memory loss of of the amnestic syndrome is due to an inability to register or an inability to recall. In modern terms, is it a difficulty of encoding or of retrieval? The shortened retention span of the amnestic syndrome seems to indicate that the essential impairment is an inability to consolidate short-term engrams into permanent ones. In the benign form, on the other hand, permanent memory traces are present but not available at certain times. This seems to be a failure of retrieval.

These clinical findings, taken together, allow for some inferences regarding the memory process itself. It would seem that the various sensoric elements of an experience are, at first, registered in the relevant cortical areas; visual, acoustic, tactile, kinesthetic, etc. Engrams are formed and may even be consolidated in loco due to enforcement by repitition and thus lead to permanent partial memories. But the total personal experience is multisensorial and does not repeat itself in its totality. Therefore, consolidation of the total situation by repitition alone does not take place. For the consolidation of memories of a total situation another mechanism seems necessary. The amnestic syndrome seems to indicate an answer to this problem. It seems that the hippocampo-fornix-mammillare system, which is part of Papez's "harmonious mechanism of emotions", has to be involved in order to consolidate short-term to long-term memories of personal experiences. Only these experiences which carry an emotional charge can be consolidated into a permanent engram of a total situation. It is the emotional charge which makes the event to a personal memorable experience. (9)

The emotional charge may also be a factor in forgetting. It may interfere,although only temporarily, with recall as in the benign type of forgetfulness while in an amnestic syndrome retrieval of recent experience is impossible because they were not consolidated and the remote experiences that had already been encoded and consolidated cannot be retrieved because they have lost their connection with the most recent ones. (10)

Our considerations are restricted to what the clinician, interested in memory research, can actually observe at the sick bed and to the inferences he is allowed to draw from these observations. The interesting findings of biochemical research particularly in the field of neurotransmitter function are not dealt with here. It is hoped that this research will offer us clinicians some

tools to help our patients and even to prevent conditions
like those described above.

REFERENCES

1. V.A. Kral,"Confusional States in Modern Perspectives
    in the Psychiatry of Old Age", J.A. Howell, ed.,
    New Yor, Brunner/Mazel (1975)
2. E. Gamper, "Zur Frageder Polioencephalitis haemorr-
    hagica der chronischen Alkoholiker", Dtsch Ztsechf
    f. Nervenhk, 102, 122-124 (1928)
3. P. Glees and H.B. Griffith, "Bilateral Destruction
    of Hippocampus (Cornu Ammonis) in a case of Dementia",
    Monschft, f. Psychiatr. & Neurol., 123, 193-204
    (1952)
4. V.A. Kral, "The Amnestic Syndrome", Montschft,
    Psychiat. and Neurol., 132, 65-80 (1956)
5. J.W. Papez, "A Proposed Mechanism of Emotion, Arch.
    Neurol. Psychiat., 38, 725-743 (1937)
6. M. Ball, "Alzheimer's Disease", Arch. Pathol. Lab.
    Med., 106, 157-162 (1982)
7. V.A. Kral and H.B. Durost, "A Comparative Study of
    The Amnestic Syndrome in Various Organic Conditions",
    Am. J. Psychiat., 110, 41-47 (1953)
8. V.A. Kral, "Benign Senescent Forgetfulness in
    Alzheimer's Disease, Senile Dementia and Related
    Disorders", R. Katzman, R.D. Terry and K.P. Bick,
    eds., New York Raven Press (1978)
9. V.A. Kral, "Memories and Engrams", Can. J. Psych.,
    24, 423-430 (1979)
10. T. Lidz, "The Amnestic Syndrome", Arch. Neur. and
    Psychiat., 47, 588-605 (1942)

NEUROTIC SYMPTOM FORMATION : A PSYCHOANALYTIC APPROACH

D. Widlöcher

Professor of Psychiatry

Salpêtrière Hospital - PARIS

The concept of neurosis as it is known to-day, first appeared at the end of the last century. Clinical expressions somatic or mental of psychic suffering were then specified on the basis of Cullen's very unclear description. This discovery, initiated by Charcot and Breuer, was the work of Janet and Freud. In spite of noticeable differences, their approaches had in common the hypothesis of an unconscious (or subconscious) mental activity, similar in nature to conscious thinking. This hypothesis was validated by therapeutic change which, after Breuer and Freud's preliminary communication (1893), may be formulated in the following manner : the symptom is suppressed when the subject becomes conscious of the unconscious formation. Such was the criterion on which the nosological frame of neuroses was built, putting together the clinical entities of hysteria, phobias and obsessions that up until then were considered unrelated. Free-floating anxiety completed the picture, constituting so to speak a pure form in which anxiety appeared as the direct expression of internal conflict.

We are now faced with a radical questioning of this model. The general framework of neuroses has been pulled apart by D.S.M. III classification. On the one hand, the concept of hysteria is divided into somatically expressed syndroms included in Somatoform Disorders and thought disorders included among other dissociative disorders. The concept of phobia and obsession are included in the general group of Anxiety Disorders.

One can wonder why the framework of neuroses, which receives so much support from psychoanalytic theory and practice, did not resist this questioning. Essentially, the psychoanalytic model is

based on two criteria closely related to the therapeutic practice
of psychoanalysis. The first criterion relies on the idea that neurotic symptom formation derives from defense mechanisms against an
internal conflict between two incompatible thought formations
(defense neuro-psychosis). The other criterion rests on the idea
that, in the course of the treatment, internal conflict is displaced
into one of attachment to the therapist (transference neurosis).
It is important to recall the close initial complementarity between
the theory of neuroses and that of psychoanalytic treatment. One
could caricature this by describing it as a tautological reasoning :
defense or transference neuro-psychosis defines a mental state that
can be modified through psychoanalysis which in turn constitues
the specific treatment of psycho-neuroses.

We emphasize these classical data because there is a relationship between the rejection of the concept of neurosis and the extension of the applications of psychoanalysis. Psychoanalysis is now
seldom used in typical neurotic states, but more often in character
disorders, severe narcissistic personality disorders, etc. This
change in treatment practices has had consequences on psychoanalytic
theory. But it did not alter the fundamental paradigms of psychoanalytic therapy. They have therefore lost their specificity for
neuroses. The concepts of defense and transference neurosis can no
longer be considered as criteria for the psychoanalytic model of
neurosis.

To the consequences of these extended applications of psychoanalysis, must be added those of the relative decrease in the
recourse to psychoanalytic therapy of neuroses. This decrease is
related to the use of chemiotherapy, symptom-focused behavioural
therapies, systemic therapies centered on family interactions.
These approaches shed light on other aspects of neurotic pathology :
the role of anxiety, depression, secondary gains turned into primary
mechanisms, etc.

I would like to stress here the fact that D.S.M. III neurosis
classification is neither "neutral" nor merely descriptive. While
it reflects the rejection of all references to psychoanalytic
pathology, it also marks the influence of new pathogenic views. By
linking all phobias and obsessive manifestations to anxiety disorders, D.S.M. III emphasizes the role of the latter trait in symptom
formation. Chemiotherapy and behavioural therapy also focus on
anxiety. Moreover, somatic symptoms in histeria are no longer lipked
to thought disorders (Dissociative Disorders) but are isolated
within Somatoform Disorders on the basis of their relation to a
significant external event and the existence of secondary gains.
The latter criteria are more consistent with the goals of systemic
therapy than with those of psychoanalysis.

736

My purpose is neither to criticize the D.S.M. III classification nor to defend that of the psychoanalytic approach. I only wish to suggest that any nosology is the reflection of a pathogenic theory which in turn is related to a therapeutic practice. Our practice aim at bringing about a change in the patient's behaviour. The theories which underlie them should define the processes of change and resistance to change that these practices allow us to observe. Our descriptions, classifications, explanations theories of mental disorders are closely dependant on theses theories.

Now we may well ask ourselves if the psychoanalytic conception of neuroses deserves to be discarded. From a practical point of view, we have no ground to do so. But we must also wonder what really specific neurotic features, not found in other pathologies, can be observed through psychoanalysis. I believe such a specificity resides in the mechanism of symptom formation and, more precisely, in the substitutive function (Ersatz Bildung) it plays with regard to the unconscious fantasy. My hypothesis is that in symptomatic neuroses specifically the unconscious pathogenic fantasy constitutes an intense source of pleasure, derivating a significant part of sexual excitement and that the production of the symptom indicates that this pleasure has been reached. The difficulty of the psychoanalytic treatment of neuroses lies not only in the existence of an internal conflict but also in the unconscious pleasure of which the subject will be deprived by the treatment.

In other words, the origin of the symptom must be distinguished from its function. The origin of neurotic symptoms is completely heterogeneous. Neurotic attitudes have a normal finality but their nature can be very diverse : a way of reasoning, avoidance behavior and, in hysteria, a state of transe or of possession. The first two may be observed in everyday life but the third is seldom seen in western culture, in normal social life.

These attitudes can combine with other traits and enter a pathological system. Their function or finality is from then dependant on motivations belonging to that system. Obsessive symptomatologies may have a specific finality in psychotic illness or after cranial trauma. Phobic or hysteric symptoms may have different functions, finalities in "border-line" pathology or after a severe psychic trauma.

In this context, psychoanalytic theory can be conceived as a description of the relationship which established itself between an attitude turned into a symptom and the unconscious fantasy. From that point of view, attitudes which had nothing in common at first sight take on a meaning which brings them closer to one another. The body, space or thought become the place where the scenario of internal conflict, the unconscious scene, is being played. More specifically, the unconscious act expresses itself either in the form of a mental act, as in obsessive thinking, or with a physical gesture, as in hysterical conversion. Phobia essentially represents an intermediate state in which an avoidance behaviour develops when a situation of danger is faced, the danger residing either in a thought (obsessive impulse) or in a potential action (fear of fainting).

To conclude, the psychoanalytic theory of neuroses confers a unity to diverse clinical states in so far as, and only in that, these states play the role of substitutes for an unconscious pleasure. If other functions are considered, a completely different nosological classification may be adopted.

THE ROLE OF DIAGNOSIS IN BEHAVIOR THERAPY

Frederick H. Kanfer

University of Illinois
Department of Psychology
Champaign, IL 61820, U.S.A

Traditional psychiatric diagnosis is based on the assumption that the various psychiatric disorders are due to distinctly different pathological processes and that all members in the category show similarities in etiological factors, in the course of the disorder and in prognostic outlook. This model of psychological disturbances defines the task of the clinician and of the researcher. Their work centers on discrimination of significant symptom patterns on one hand, and discovery of causal factors and the nature of the disease process on the other. The clinician perceives a syndrome, derives a prognosis and selects an appropriate treatment. The researcher's task is to refine the conceptualization of the mechanisms by which the disorder originated, study the nature of its course as it affects normal procedures that stop or reverse the pathological process. Unfortunately, this view of direct (single or multiple) causes, universal disease processes, and similarities in reactions to treatment among patients who manifest similar syndromes has been supported only for a small fraction of disturbances, those that are linked to pathophysiologic or organic processes. In recognition of the inadequacies of this underlying model, DSM-III has provided additional diagnostic axes. Axis 3, 4 and 5 include some individual characteristics that influence prognosis and treatment.

In contrast to the taxonomic and normative orientation of traditional psychiatric diagnosis, the behavioral analysis for dysfunctions focusses on analysis of the patient's idiosyncratic behavior patterns, the variables that control their occurrence and how these patterns interfere with effective functioning of the patient in the daily life-setting. This orientation, to which we subscribe, raises the question of "diagnosis for what purpose."

739

That is, our analysis always includes a comparison of a current
unsatisfactory state (A) with a future goal-state (B)-that would
restore effective psychological functions and reduce distress.
When the purpose is individual treatment, the analysis includes
assessment of available resources to implement the change from
state A to state B. For administrative or social planning purposes
it includes a full statement about the problematic state A since
these are most relevant to the administrator's or planner's task.
From this point of view, the diagnostic process for use in therapy
is seen as one that is future-oriented. Diagnosis is conceptualized
as a recursive problem-solving and decision-making sequence. As
we have pointed out in detail in several papers (Kanfer and Saslow,
1965; Kanfer and Grimm, 1977, 1980; Kanfer and Busemeyer, 1982),
the clinician is faced with the problem of answering the question:
"What needs to be changed to move state A toward state B?" The
changes can be biological, psychological or social. Diagnosis
provides the basis for a therapeutic plan. Since assessment and
treatment are closely interrelated and since each treatment intervention alters the client's life situation, often in unforeseeable
ways, the diagnostic process must be viewed as a dynamic, recursive
and iterative enterprise, extending over the entire span of treatment. That is, at various times, and often only as a result of
initial interventions, different features of states A and B take on
diagnostic and prognostic significance. Taxonomy-based Diagnosis
is a static characterization of an individual in relation to a
normative population. Behavioral analysis tends to characterize
the current functioning of a person in a specified milieu (socio-
cultural as well as biological) in relation to some specified
desirable future scenario.

The implied theory of human behavior presumes that actions,
thoughts and emotions are the result of three sets of continuously
interacting influences, namely, biological, environmental and cognitive. We propose that a general-systems or field model can best
describe these complex interactions, rather than a model that
limits itself to processes within the person. The data on the
close interrelationships between cognitive and biological processes
on the one hand and their relationship to socio-cultural factors
on the other strongly support such a model.

Thus we consider personality disorders and neuroses as conditions that gradually evolve from a long-standing dynamic and reciprocal interaction of biological predispositions and the patient's
social and physical environment. But in addition their impact on
subjective experiences and behavior is strongly moderated by self-
regulatory processes that guide the individual response to the
biological and environmental inputs.

A therapist is most concerned whether intervention at the
somatic or behavioral or sociocultural level will be most effective.

Practicality dictates intervention at the level that contains the processes responsible for the most serious consequences to the person (or to society). But a future-oriented, closed-loop feedback model suggests in addition that treatment be selected not only for immediate effectiveness but also to bring the patient closer toward the specified goal state (B) in the long run. It should also consider both beneficial and detrimental effects on the person as well as on other persons in his social system. For example, psychopharmacological intervention in depression affects not only the patient but also the reaction of others in his social environment, leading in turn to different demands and expectations and requiring further adjustments by the patient as a result. Behavior therapy for agoraphobia not only reduces the patient's fear; it also enables him to engage in a wider range of activities and thereby may present new problems due to skill deficits or inability to cope with previously avoided situations. Clearly, such a view also considers the potential impact of therapy on a patient's partner, work setting and other family members. From this viewpoint treatment is not limited to alleviating the presenting complaint. It aims toward establishing a more effective and satisfying harmonious balance in the patient's cognitive, emotional and behavioral functions in relation to himself and to his environment. Regardless of the diagnosis or treatment mode, therapy aims at remedial actions that are appropriate for the particular patient and his present and future life circumstances. The main differences between taxonomic diagnosis and a problem-solving assessment are summarized in Table 1.

In addition to the focus on the patient, behavioral researchers are also giving increasing attention to the study of the clinician. In the process of diagnosis a clinician's judgments are influenced by personal history and training. But as a human being, the selection and processing of information, the making of inferences, predictions and decisions is also influenced by universal characteristics. Experiments by decision theorists and cognitive psychologists indicate, for example, that predictive judgments are biased by the context, the difficulty of the task, the judge's theory and the similarity of a case to a category model. Since clinicians are required to operate under time pressure and with incomplete information, normative formal models of decision-making are not appropriate. Instead, in medical and psychiatric diagnosis, decision aids and heuristics need to be developed for counteracting known biases and allowing flexibility and revision. Current taxonomic schema of diagnosis do not fit this requirement. Their static quality tends to bias the clinicians to search for confirming evidence once a diagnosis is made. The underlying logic of diagnosis should be based on utility criteria, not on criteria of accurate category assignment. The focus of such research therefore is on understanding and improving clinical judgments and decisions, not only on developing a better classification system. Our view

TABLE 1

COMPARISON OF TRADITIONAL DIAGNOSIS AND BEHAVIORAL ANALYSIS

TAXONOMIC DIAGNOSIS	PROBLEM-SOLVING ANALYSIS
1. ASSIGN PATIENT TO CATEGORY	1. ASSESS CURRENT STATE (A) IN RELATION TO GOAL-STATE (B)
2. DIAGNOSIS RELATIVELY CONSTANT OVER TIME-STATIC	2. PROBLEM-DEFINITION CHANGES OVER TIME-DYNAMIC
3. DIAGNOSIS INDEPENDENT OF SETTING AND CLINICIAN'S PURPOSE	3. ANALYSIS IN CONTEXT OF CURRENT SETTING AND PURPOSE
4. SYNDROME IMPLIES ETIOLOGY AND PROGNOSIS-GENERIC (COMMON CAUSES)	4. SYNDROME IN CONTEXT OF INDIVIDUAL LIFE EXPERIENCES AND SUBCULTURAL NORMS -IDIOSYNCRATIC (INDIVIDUAL CAUSES)
5. INTERVENTION FOCUSSES ON PATIENT AS TARGET	5. INTERVENTION TARGETS ANY COMPONENT OF SYSTEM (SOCIAL, BEHAVIORAL, BIOLOGICAL)
6. THERAPY AIMS TO REMOVE CAUSES OF SYNDROME-RESTORATIVE, REMEDIAL	6. THERAPY AIMS TO IMPROVE PATIENT'S HEALTH AND EFFECTIVENESS-PROACTIVE FUTURE-ORIENTED
7. OUTCOME VIEWED AS PRODUCT OF DIAGNOSIS PLUS TREATMENT CRITERIA UNIVERSAL	7. OUTCOME CRITERIA VARY FOR EACH PATIENT-THEIR SELECTION INFLUENCE TREATMENT GOALS AND METHODS

suggests that young psychiatrists must be trained to make decisions on the basis of incomplete data. Therefore huam weaknesses in processing such data need to be studied and remedied by use of decision aids.

To summarize, I have suggested (1) that diagnosis in psychiatry is best approached as a problem-solving task in which each step toward resolution requires reassessment of strategies and goals; (2) that a systems approach best fits the analysis of human behavior; and (3) that cognitive science research can assist in developing improved heuristics for training and making diagnostic statements that have maximal treatment utility.

References

Kanfer, F. H., and Saslow, G., 1965, Behavioral analysis: An alter-
    native to diagnostic classification. Archives of General
    Psychiatry, 16:593-602.

Kanfer, F. H., and Grimm, L. G., 1977, Behavioral analysis:
    Selecting target behaviors in the interview. Behavior
    Modification, 1:7-28.

Kanfer, F. H., and Grimm, L. G., 1980, Managing clinical change:
    A process model of therapy. Behavioral Modification,
    4:419-444.

Kanfer, F. H., and Busemeyer, J. R., 1982, The use of problem-
    solving and decision-making in behavior therapy. Clinical
    Psychology Review, 2:239-266.

THE PERSONALITY FROM THE MEDICAL-PSYCHIATRIC POINT OF VIEW

Francisco Llavero

Antonio Maura 12
Madrid (14) Spain

If we want to understand, accept or rectify a concept or model of the personality from the medical-psychiatric anthropological point of view which permits overcoming the lamentable, schismatic and chaotic confusion that prevails in the psychiatric disciplines on a world scale, I consider it indispensable to begin to remember some basic questions.

Medical psychiatry bears the original singularity most accentuated and demanding of all branches of knowledge and learning, delving into that existential enigma: man such as he is, healthy and ill, with his individual experiential capacity and mutations of conscience throughout history. Those biosomatic, pathogenic processes which cause bodily sufferings, are subject to management, laws and causal and lineal principles inherent in the positive-explanatory sciences with a primary reality: this medical-organicist pathology has many parts in common with veterinary pathology.

A very different question is that concerning medical-anthropological psychiatry because this bears also and at the same time, another dimension inseperable from the first:the psychic dimension, which is the most specifically human.

In the face of this original singularity, that is, faced with the reality of a continuity of the constitutive unit of man, with his freedom of decision, the scholar, the researcher, the philosopher, the physician, but above all the medical-psychiatrist as such, always come up against, compellingly, -in theory and in practice- the "secret of the sphinx" living, thinking and feeling.

This great secret compels them to ask time and time again, attracted by the magnetism of the unknown: what "bond", what kind of "correlations" and "parallelisms"? what type of "relationship" exists or should exist between dimensions of such a different nature as are the somatic and the psychic? How do they "articulate" between themselves? Does there exist some "functional frontier" or "seam" -as Spinoza would say- between the biosomatic and the dimensions of the qualities? Whoever doesn't ask questions doesn't investigate fully.

In any event, I think there doesn't exist a question, a query with more antiquity and that has promulgated more rivers of ink. However, the reality of living and feeling man is there, impenetrable and defiant, be what may the advances in neurology and biogenetics.

In this situation of impotence and desideratum conceptual in the foundation of psychiatry, the advances in the positive sciences in the field of medicine, biochemistry, biogenetics, in psychopharmacology, biological rythms, neurophysiology, cybernetics, and so on, emerge. The scholars find themselves with an "accumulation of valuable data" and they made a "recount" -as Jaspers says- but without a structural and integrated sense in a superior reality.

At the same time as this anarchy originated by the constant advances of the positive sciences and also because of the lack of that "superior integrated reality" to place each one of these advances in the corresponding position, another complication of enormous importance is produced. It is the central idea of the scientific-natural causality, to which man owes nothing more nor nothing less than the power over the thing -as Lorenz would say- a causality based on occidental thinking since the time of Linneo, as is for example, **Natura non facit saltum, causa aequate effectum.** It is an idea which today cannot be maintained in an exclusive way. It is necessary to have, therefore, a new doctrine of causality in psychiatry, as I explain in another place(1).

In this alternating and chaotic struggle between the advances of positivist knowledge and the so-called sciences of the spirit -today looking back- we should listen to the authorized warning of a pioneer in psychiatry, K. Schneider, when he says: "It is possible to develop neuropathology without metaphysics, it is possible to develop psychopathology without metaphysics, but psychiatry, which seeks to fuse both, permanently runs into metaphysical problems."

In the last decades, three have been the more outstanding attempts, totally or partialy unsuccessful, to overcome this situation. First, accepting the "medical model" by the influence of positivism, and with it the so-called "biological psychiatry" is brought up to date with independent pretensions; at the same time psychology is "biologized" as before that somatic medicine "freudially psychologized", giving rise to that "hybrid" product also called "psychosomatic medicine", today in a slump.

A second attempt would, paradoxically, lie in a renunciation: to abide by a syndromic or symptomatic psychiatry, empiric and pragmatic "in the American style" with an "anencephalic" behavioristic socio-psychiatry and psychiatric care "in the Italian style" on the basis of "angelical community utopias" and furthermore subject to "politization" with the chaotic consequences that we are seeing; the rest would be "speculations", philosophies which would have nothing to do with psychiatric illness. Faced with the repeated failure of all these attempts, the most alerted scholars thought, and with reason, that we should have available, at least a "navigation chart" or "mental scheme" in this jungle of problems. With a rare unanimity the researches directed their efforts towards a conclusion or concept of personality.

To the engagement came outstanding representatives of psychoanalysis, of psychology, beginning with Freud, Jung and the constitutionalists with Kretschmer at the head, behaviorists, sociologists among many more. However, at the end of innumerable publications, one has to return to ask oneself: What is personality? Are the "models" valid, the conceptions that appear in world literature in relation to the exigencies -theoretical-practical- inherent in psychiatric bidimensional illness according to the actual state of our knowledge? And in relation to the modwern treatments based on psychotropic drugs and their undeniable problems of causality?

Summing up, how can a psychiatrist, researcher and therapist manage beyond a blind empiricism, without conception or scheme of the personality, be what it may, but whose dynamics responds to a minimum of the exigencies noted in acordance with actual knowledge? I should acknowledge that in literature we cannot find founded answers to these questions in topics so crucial -now and always, theoretical and practical- to the psychiatric disciplines.

Since my conception on the personality from the medical-psychiatric, anthropological point of view and its internal dynamics, cannot be explained here -I put at the disposal of the interested party my publications- I will limit myself to defining it as "the individual human totality more all inclusive with regards to a substantial unit, constitutively bidimensionsl -psychic and biosomatic- in permanent evolution in the healthy individual and in regression in the patient, above all with regards to the individual and social experiential capacity."

This definition bears some exigencies that I will summarize in these eight:

1. In the conception, scheme and structure of the personality, all the components of its total and constitutively bidimensional unit, should remain integrated or prone to integration.

2. It should keep its operational individuality, in theory and in practice, without having to resort to the schemes of the present or future psycholigical classifications.

3. To permit the establishment of "functional frontiers" -with possible modifications- between the specific and the unspecific in the medical-psychiatric events, with didactic, clinical, therapeutic, operational ends in practice and in research.

4. To permit establishing correlations between the dimensions of the qualities and the biosomatic ones, conserving the constitutive unity and surpassing the Cartesian dualisms, without taking refuge, prematurelym, in totalized "monisms" such as "asylum ignorantiae".

5. Permitting to delimit -at least virtually- the biocerebral participation as an instrumental cause of the qualities and biogenetic potentialities in relation to the psychic dimension, healthy or ill, without letting it be pulled by the confortable but false epiphenomenic conceptions or basis of the lineal and direct causality.

6. To permit to delimit the fields of action of the so-called somatic disturbances and of the pharmacological and psychotherapeutic treatments in psychiatric illness not originated by lesions or organic brain processes, that is, by an "alteration".

7. To facilitate the understanding of the influences of the changing historic and cultural process on the evolution of the healthy or ill personality and on the point of experiential individual seriousness along the different epochs in the biographical evolution. Let us remember those realities formulated by Kant with an accurate phrase: "Man is always himself, but never the same."

8. Finally, that the scheme of the personality which we manage permit us to integrate the new findings -scientific, clinical, therapeutical, anthropological- which procede from the different branches of medical-psychiatric knowledge and borderline fields, without violoting the constitutive but bidimensional unit of man; the "Cartesian dualism" necessary and operating in practice, and the aristotelic "substantial unity" or "totality" structured or

gestaltic, should not be incompatible with our dynamic conceptions or open scheme of the personality.

REFERENCES

Llavero, F. Symptom und Kausalität. Grundfragen der Neurologie und Psychiatrie. Georg Thieme, Stuttgart, (1953).

Llavero, F. El encuentro de la Medicina y de la Psiquiatria. Folia Neuropsiquiátrica., No. 3,(1966).

Llavero, F. Psiquiatría y proceso histórico-cultural. Folia Humanística, 9, No. 98, (1971).

Llavero, F. and V. Conde,Tratamientos medicopsiquiátricos. Criterios, fundamentos y aplicación. Liade, Madrid, (1970).

López-Ibor Jr., J.J., C. Ruiz Ogara, and D. Barcia, Psiquiatría, Vol. I, Toray, Barcelona, 1982.

THE REHABILITATION OF PATIENTS

WITH PERSONALITY DISORDERS

Walter Goudsmit

Psychiatric University Clinic
State University Groningen - Holland
P.B. 30001, 9700 RB   Groningen, The Netherlands

It was with great relief that I heard this morning on the
wireless that a large majority of the British House of Commons
voted against the reinstatement of the death-penalty. I mention
this here, because the work about which I am to report, partly
concerns exactly those patients who, in many countries, are either
put to death or imprisoned for life.

In the following, I should like to remark upon the concept of
personality disorder, upon symptomatology, upon aethiology, and
upon diagnosis.

Then I should like, in this context, to show you the three
levels of rehabilitation of patients with personality disorders,
as I see them and as they are generally regarded in the
Netherlands; then I should like to make some remarks about
rehabilitation in various social systems and cultural patterns,
and finally a short but unusual final remark.

1. The concept of personality disorders: remarks about symptomatology, aethiology, and diagnosis

The beginning of every medical treatment is the examination,
the basis of every diagnosis. I make a distinction here between
primary and secondary diagnosis, in which the latter is the further
diagnosis during a prolonged observation or treatment. Often, the
true diagnosis can only be made in the secondary diagnostic phase,
especially when the patient has a strong defense-mechanism, when
there is a clear case of a "mask of sanity", or when the patient
leads the examiner astray by attractive pseudo-adaptation.
Especially with this group of patients such things frequently

751

occur. Many wrong diagnosis are made when the examiner is too much preoccupied with the phenotypical behaviour of the patient, when he interprets the social anamnesis one sidedly, or when he has prejudices, for instance, that personality disorders only occur in the lower classes of society and in social marginal groups.

The descriptions, which are listed in the DSM-III under "personality disorders", show a rich and very diverse variety of symptoms. One symptom occurs with most patients, namely the failure to adapt to society as a result of the personality disorder; the deranged contacts with society and the ensuing conflicts, which often lead to a great vicious circle.

As regards the aethiology of these disorders, opinions are still divided. However, it is certain that a great part of the serious personality disorders is the result of very early development-disorder, often going far back into the first year of the patient's life. Added to this are organic disorders and a great number of social factors which influence the already disordered development further in a negative way. As concerns the micro- and macro-environment, it is mostly the chronicness of the trauma's that most seriously affects the development and leads to the worst symptoms. Often described, but not adequately ascertained, are the genetic connections.

Before entering into the matter of the three levels of rehabilitation, please allow me some introductory remarks.

The variety of clinical pictures considered as "personality disorders" makes clear that the treatment and rehabilitation of these patients cannot be carried out uniformly either. With the rehabilitation of the group of patients we discuss today, one is faced with the fact that, apart from the factors already mentioned, these patients are often discriminated against and serve as scapegoat, and moreover, that these patients call up aggression to which society reacts, which leads to the already mentioned vicious circle. A further factor is that many psychiatrists do not yet know the possibilities of a treatment; even in very recent manuals of psychiatry hardly anything if found about this.

The first level of rehabilitation understandably starts in that part of society where the conflict of these patients takes place. Without a minimum of understanding within society for the fact that certain "social disturbers" are patients with severe adaptation-disorders, the rehabilitation of these patients is impossible. One can not treat and discriminate at the same time.

About the question whether a socially maladapted person is a patient or not, opinions are divided. At the same time, we see how dependent psychiatric science is from the prevailing opinions

and principles in various societies. Also, adaptation to the social
system can never be a criterion of psychiatric disease, but in most
cases a symptom at the very most. There are, in fact, cases where
the adaptation itself to the prevailing social system is pathological. In general however, a clinical picture can only be
determined when it is carefully examined. As the symptoms are poly-
morphous and the origins multicausal, the examination of these
patients must be done by an interdisciplinary team whenever possible.
The first level of rehabilitation begins with finding understanding
from the health-authorities and the Departments for the fact that
these diagnosed patients need treatment rather than punishment.
One also has to be prepared for and to be capable of bringing
together the necessary means for a rehabilitation; that one has
the necessary well-trained and experienced co-operators at on's
disposal. What has been said so far, demonstrates that the first
level of rehabilitation of these patients is the most difficult.

The second level of rehabilitation is that of social treatment in its widest sense. It is impossible to even attempt to go
into the many aspects of social treatment.

I should like to only mention a few strictly necessary stipulations without which social treatment is not possible.
1. The requirements, as named in the first level of rehabilitation,
   must have been met.
2. A dependable multidisciplinary and multidimensional diagnosis
   must have been made as a basis for further rehabilitation or
   treatment.
3. A therapeutic milieu must be warranted.
4. Well-trained and experienced co-operators (psychiatrists,
   psychotherapists, clinical psychologists, social workers) must
   be available.
5. For the various co-operators in the team, experienced atten-
   dants and supervisors should be available for the intramural
   conduct or treatment. It is our experience that the attendance
   of the various co-operators in the disciplines is more important
   than methodical psychotherapy, because the therapy as such can
   come to nothing when the other co-operators do not support the
   therapeutic milieu, or often even damage it.
6. In case of intramural treatment, there must be enough time for
   the members of the team to communicate.
7. It is necessary to be open towards the patient under attendance
   or treatment: only openness from the therapist in social work
   leads to openness from the patient.
8. One's attitude towards the patients must be flexible, and must
   be oriented on the possibilities they have during the
   rehabilitation-period. In practice, this means that, at first,
   one should make few demands upon him, and one should not
   confront him too much with himself or his situation within
   society, because in general the confrontation-tolerance of

these patients is very low. Only in the course of further
attendance or treatment should one adapt the confrontation, as
well as other demands from the patient, to his growing
possibilities.
9. One of the difficulties of prolonged intramural treatment is
    the appearance of hospitalization-symptoms. Whenever it is
    not possible to treat the patient ambulatorily, because of
    danger to the patient, it is much to be desired that within the
    institution where he is treated, he keeps as many contacts as
    possible with persons from society.
10. The integration into society must be very flexible, and requires
    much patience and thought. One of the greatest difficulties is
    the assessment of the patient's social risks. For this, we
    unfortunately do not yet have psychological tests, and we must
    needs rely upon prolonged very intensive observation of the
    patients.
11. Still too little is done for patients with personality disorders
    that are not "social disturbers" and that do not represent great
    social risks, although it is precisely for this group that very
    positive possibilities of treatment exist.

The third level of rehabilitation represents the actual methodical psychotherapy. Unfortunately, so far there are but few
therapists who are well up in the necessary knowledge and in the
necessary modifications of therapeutic techniques, and who have the
necessary experience. To experiment with enthusiastic but untrained
and inexperienced co-operators usually leads to failure. New methods
should be tried very carefully, because, especially with this
group of patients, failure of treatment also means negative repercussions on the method of treatment.

It is not always necessary that the three levels of rehabilitation follow one another. There are patients with less conspicuous
symptoms, who qualify for a treatment without many socio-therapeutic
measures.

The methodical use of treatment-techniques has to be modified
in the cases of many patients. Thus, in most cases it is pointless,
and often even harmful, to point from the start to an analytical
psychotherapy or, in less cases, an analysis. More than with other
therapies, it is important to establish a therapeutic relationship
first. At first, all else is subordinate. Also, the contact-therapy
I mentioned or pre-therapeutic treatment serve at first solely to
build a diadic relationship, without which no therapy is possible.

About rehabilitation in different social systems

The rehabilitation and treatment of patients that we discuss
today, and the way in which this is done in the Netherlands, is

expensive. It is not difficult to realise, however, that not to
treat them could be more expensive. Yet, such a treatment-model
can not simply be exported. In other countries, there are different
norms, different opinions about health-politics, and also different
laws. It is clear that the intensive treatment of such patients as
it is done in the Netherlands is up till now impossible in most
European countries. It is therefore necessary for each country to
find their own forms of rehabilitation with due observance of
their present ideas, habits, and laws. At any rate, experiments
in the Netherlands have shown that it is very rewarding to treat
such patients.

An unusual final remark

Over two-thousand years ago, one of the wise men of this world,
the Chinese poet Tsjung-Tse, wrote a short poem that I should like
to quote:
A person stealing a tie is called a thief,
A person stealing a country is called a hero.
Without further explanation, it will be clear to all of you that
these short lines are just as true today as they were when they
were written. It is not exaggerated to claim that our generation is
witness to what may be the greatest crime against humanity of all
history: such incomprehensibly large amounts of money are spent
yearly on the destruction of life on earth, that we are therefore
not capable of fighting hunger and disease; that we can therefore
not afford the comparatively modest costs for a further humanising
of society. The question is: are we really all that helpless?

GROWING POINTS IN THE STUDIES OF AGORAPHOBIA, PANIC DISORDERS AND
ANXIETY STATES

Sir Martin Roth
Department of Psychiatry
University of Cambridge

Classification and Aetiology

New classifications relating to a group of disorders in
psychiatry often embody new hypotheses or theories about their
character and aetiological basis. It is perhaps worth taking a
look at the section of DSM lll relevant to the subject matter of
this Symposium to ascertain whether it is informed by a novel
concept. A glance at the classification of anxiety disorders shows
our expectations to be upheld. They are divided into three main
groups of which two are relevant for this symposium. The phobic
disorders and anxiety states comprise six main groups: Agoraphobia
(with and without panic attack), Social phobia, Simple phobia, Panic
disorder, Gereralised anxiety disorder and Obsessive-compulsive
disorder. This grouping reflects the role of central importance
allocated by Klein and his colleagues to the panic attack as the
precursor and primary syndrome from which the more severely disabling
agoraphobic disorder evolves as a secondary development.

Agoraphobia is a specific form of anxiety neurosis and one
general feature of this form of affective disturbance is manifest
in its anticipatory quality in extreme form. Darwin first pointed
out that anxiety was concerned with the future, with coming ordeals
demanding a special effort. In agoraphobics this is found as an
anguished anticipation that the danger the patient rationally
recognises as remote is nonetheless certain to materialise. The
danger is that of collapsing, losing control, being seen prostrate
and helpless. The controversial issues that have recently emerged
regarding the classification and treatment of agoraphobia stem in
part from three distinct types of aetiological theory regarding the
nature and origin of agoraphobic disorder. According to one theory,

757

this syndrome or panic disorder and its sequel in agoraphobia constitutes a genetically determined medical condition expressed as a biochemical abnormality in the central nervous system. Panic disorder is regarded as the central core of the disorder (Sheehan 1982). Phobic avoidance behaviour develops as a result of conditioning, cognitive reappraisal or stimulus generalisation determined by the circumstances surrounding the early panic attacks. The successes achieved by pharmacological treatment are cited as validating evidence for this hypothesis. Leaving aside treatment effects which are discussed at a later stage this theory appears to oversimplify the evidence regarding the genetics of anxiety and phobic disorder. It overlooks the many features which have been found to differentiate agoraphobic patients from other neurotic and control subjects: family circumstances, developmental history and personality traits. It also ignores the limitations of pharmacological treatment. The second theory is the more sophisticated successor of earlier views which explained agoraphobic states in terms of classical conditioning or learning theory and the reinforcement of phobic behaviour. Modern theorists using purely psychological paradigms recognise that the whole range of disabilities of agoraphobics and the manner in which change occurs during behavioural treatment cannot be explained in terms of theories of learning. But in their use of behavioural treatment, they implicitly regard the phobic symptoms as being the whole disease. All other observations regarding the agoraphobic patient are irrelevant for therapy. These theories tend to overestimate the extent of the success achieved by behavioural methods in the total population of agoraphobic patients and overlook the constrained disabled and limited lives even of those patients who have derived some symptomatic relief from behavioural therapy. Thirdly, there are theories that stem from psychoanalytical and psychodynamic viewpoints. These regard the symptoms as the manifestation of a defective character structure which has originated from conflicts engendered in early childhood. This is manifest in all aspects of life adaptation - sexual, marital, interpersonal, social, all of them integral parts of the disorder. They precede the phobic symptoms and are not merely the consequence of them. A historical perspective is in the view of this writer indispensable for the understanding and management of agoraphobia. But psychoanalysis can neither provide explanation for the abrupt interruption of the discontinuity of emotional and personal life that begins with the onset of agoraphobia nor can they explain why this change is so very difficult to reverse. Psychodynamic therapies used as the sole method are certainly ineffective to this end.

Taken in isolation none of these three theories is free from objection. Yet each is consistent with a certain amount of evidence and tells us something about one aspect of causation. They may therefore contain some of the elements from which scientifically valid aetiological theories may be developed in future.

The Phenomena requiring explanation

One step towards the formulation of a valid hypothesis that can be taken is to describe the main phenomena that need to be explained.

The first experience of panic or the first episode of phobic anxiety may be followed rapidly and often in step wise fashion by a complicated network of avoidance behaviours. There may have been a sudden attack of terror in a crowded store or a syncopal attack or near-faint in the WC of a friend's house. Within a short time the patient may be confined to her home and unable to walk by herself for a distance more than 50 yards from it. It is reasonable to seek for some underlying physiological process that generates and sustains such a sudden dramatic change in behaviour and adaptation. But no plausible explanation for this stage in the development of agoraphobic disorder has come to light. It cannot follow in an ineluctable manner from a succession of severe panics for these occur also in other disorders with high levels of anxiety.

The second aspect is that neither panics or phobias emerge out of an entirely clear sky. The great majority of patients have a high level of trait anxiety and a substantial proportion have an actual anxiety state before the emergence of disabling phobias. There is evidence in favour of a hereditary predisposition to anxiety and panic disorder but a major Mendelian gene is unlikely to be responsible. A whole range of adverse circumstances differentiates agoraphobic patients from other affective disorders and control subjects. They include an unstable family background, a poorer relationship with parents, a higher prevalence of early neurotic traits and a less effective social adjustment together with more pre-morbid personality traits of anxiety, immaturity, dependence and instability than non-phobic, anxious, and depressed patients. As a group agoraphobics have proved to be significantly more introverted and to score higher in neuroticism than controls and other emotional disorders. The evidence in relation to pre-morbid traits of emotional dependence of agoraphobic patients is not unambiguous. But some of the evidence points to it. It is difficult to explain the almost total relief from phobic anxiety and panic afforded by the presence of some supportive figure such as spouse or mother unless one postulates exaggeration during illness of a pre-morbid tendency to feel insecure, fearful and alone in the world when supportive figures are beyond reach. This may underlie what some workers have called the agoraphobic's "external locus of control."

The sequence of historical events in agoraphobia contain some clues regarding the nature and aetiology of the disorder. Three main stages may be defined (1) Neurotic traits are found in excess in these patients in childhood. But a number of systematic studies show clearly defined phobias to be uncommon. School phobia before the age of nine or ten is rare and conversely its long term prognosis is known to be good. When it begins later in the teens school phobia

759

pursues a more chronic course and may continue into adult life to
form a small minority of agoraphobic and social phobic disorders of
great severity. One or other parent (usually the mother) is anxious
or phobic but the phobia is well camouflaged. Yet adoption studies
will be needed before we can interpret the facts as testifying wholly
in favour of genetical factors. For as work of neurophysiologists
Hubel and Wiesel (1977) Kandel (1981) as also of ethologists Hinde
and McGinnis (1977) have shown learning, habituation and deprivation
at this stage give rise to long lasting change in behaviour which
probably derive from biochemical or structural changes at synapses.
These may powerfully influence personality development but they are
not necessarily irreversible. (2) In the early teens anxiety of a
more or less circumscribed nature makes its appearance. Anticipatory
anxiety prior to examinations and other ordeals is commonly pronounced but is usually concealed and compensated at this stange. Most
agoraphobic disorders begin after patients have established themselves
in an independent home with a husband or consort and the term
"housebound housewife" has been translated into many languages.
Early in marriage anxiety about competence in a maternal note is
common and in about 12% of a recent series of female patients,
phobias had made their appearance during the first year after child-
birth. At some phase in the middle or late twenties anticipatory
anxiety escalates, increased tension is manifest in anxious
preoccupation with everyday difficulties. Transient phobic symptoms
readily surmounted with an effort make their appearance. (3) At
this stage the patient has become sensitised to any steep escalation
of anxiety. This will be experienced as an attack of panic. The
first attack develops almost invariably when the individual is at
some distance from home and alone or with strangers. After one or
more panics in which attempts to surmount the desire to take flight
are made, avoidance behaviour develops. Leaving home, entering
shops, crowds, queues, public transport, going to the hairdresser,
keeping a fixed appointment become impossible without some supporting
presence. Avoidance and dependant behaviour are reinforced by flight
and by the presence of external support. Only in a small minority
of severely incapacitated cases do panics occur with any frequency
when the patient is alone in her own home.

Both behavioural methods of treatment such as exposure in vivo
and pharmacological therapy may owe their effects to the influence
they exert upon step like change in mental functioning and behaviour
ushered in by the first panics and phobias. They enable patients
to acquire new strategies for handling severe anxiety or making
better use of old ones. Conversely, it is perhaps their failure to
make any impression on the psychological infrastructure in which the
condition is rooted that accounts for the residual disabilities and
relapses. Dynamic forms of psychotherapy on the other hand may
exert little influence because they have no concepts for handling
the abrupt step like leaps in behaviour and adaptation manifest in
the history of agoraphobic disorder. They view the condition as a
progressive unfolding of the behaviour patterns in a personality
flawed by conflicts unresolved in childhood. But agoraphobia does

760

not evolve as a continuous, linear unbroken sequence in psychological development from childhood to adult life. But this should not be taken to mean that phobias constitute the entire disorder or that psychodynamic factors are irrelevant.

Advances in Treatment

The behavioural treatments of agoraphobia constitute a significant advance in the management of this group of conditions. It is rapid exposure in vivo over an adequate period of time to the situations feared by the phobic patient that has proved the most effective method of treatment. It has also become clear that practice in exposure between therapeutic sessions goes far to decide the quality of the results achieved. A number of self-help manuals which provide detailed instruction regarding the steps to be adopted in practice have provided a valuable adjunct to treatment. A number of follow up studies have established that improvements achieved in the course of behavioural treatment can endure for as long as two to seven years. These are significant achievements. But the number of patients studied remains relatively small. It is also difficult in some studies to judge how much selection or self selection has been entailed in recruitment to trials and controlled investigations have been few in number. Many severely agoraphobic patients remain disabled, others relapse after treatment and there is a group whose phobias show marked fluctuations in severity. There are few large psychiatric clinics without their burden of such cases. And there is good reason for questioning whether improvements registered on existing scales in respect of specific treatments provide an accurate picture of the extent to which the lives of patients remain limited and constrained.

As far as Pharmacological treatment is concerned some evidence from controlled investigations favours the efficacy of both tricyclic compounds and monoamine oxidase inhibitors in the treatment of panic disorders. The important investigation by Klein and his colleagues (Zitrine et al) comparing the results of Imipramine with behaviour therapy, imipramine with supportive psychotherapy and placebo with behaviour therapy over a twenty six week period is well known. Each method that incorporated a tricyclic compound proved significantly superior to methods without an active pharmacological agent. The results were attributed to the beneficial effects of imipramine on spontaneous panic, causing anticipatory anxiety and avoidance behaviour to recede. However, as the effects of tricyclics are judged to be confined to panic anxiety and without direct effect on avoidance behaviour, the failure to demonstrate any advantage of behaviour therapy over supportive psychotherapy is surprising: that exposure is effective in some measure in the treatment of avoidance behaviour is well established. In one enquiry, phenelzine has proved superior to imipramine (Sheenan et al 1980). But in another investigation, imipramine has been found to be ineffective in the treatment of agoraphobia (Marks et al 1982) and there is independent evidence that its beneficial effect is proportionate to its influence

761

upon concomitant depression. The robe of depressive disorder in causation and symptom response in agoraphobia need to be studied. Certain other problems are in particular need of further investigations. Dropouts in the main enquiry (Zitrine et al 1981) ranged from 20 - 26% in the agoraphobic cases and 22% of the patients were in relapse at the end of the year. Follow ups over longer periods have been few and on the whole suggest that the effects of treatment with tricyclic compounds are not well sustained (Cloninger et al 1981). There is also a need for more information about the disabilities that continue after pharmacological treatment at the end of clinical trials, ratings in the published accounts tend to show agoraphobic patients to be substantially above the bottom of the ordinates that represent their scores.

Conclusion

Agoraphobia may be regarded as a paradigm of neurotic disorder. The final stage, that is the emergence of the disabling neurotic illness, often evolves rapidly. In the case of agoraphobia the symptoms may be influenced up to a point and sometimes substantially, by behavioural therapies on the one hand or pharmacological treatments on the other. These are significant advances which have opened up fresh seams of scientific enquiry and also relieved the sufferings of many patients. From the successes there have issued psychological theories in terms of learning and cognition on the one hand and in terms of a conventional genetical bio-chemical disease model on the other. These theories have focussed on the disabling symptoms that have recently evolved and viewed them as an illness. Their successes call into question the traditional psychoanalytic theories of agoraphobia for a number of reasons. These theories regard phobias as surface manifestations of a deeper malady. Treatment directed at such symptoms would be doomed to failure because the old disabilities are bound in due course to be superceded by new ones. But the recorded results of behavioural and pharmacological treatments have shown any successes achieved are not marred by a fresh crop of symptoms. Although psychoanalytic theories view agoraphobia as evolving in continuous linear fashion from the early years to adulthood, the development of the disorder tends to be rapid and often explosive rather than continuous. The results of both behavioural and drug treatment can account for the known facts up to a certain extent, but both have obvious defects when presented as complete theories. And we do not understand except in a shadowy manner the links between the two different types of explanation. Moreover, we must in a realistic spirit acknowledge the limitations and failures of each of the two forms of treatment from which these theories derive, if scientific knowledge about agoraphobia is to be advanced. And for all the limitations of the psychoanalytical viewpoints there are developmental and psycho-dynamic aspects which cannot be left out of account in the management of patients and, ultimately, of scientific theories.

It is to be hoped that the theories of the future will be able to draw upon fresh concepts and new languages to bring these three dimensions, the neuro-biological the psychological and the developmental into a single integrated explanation that will bring to light their inter-relationships and promote greater success in treatment.

DIAGNOSIS AND MORPHOLOGY OF PANIC AND OTHER ANXIETY DISORDERS

Isaac Marks

Professor of Experimental Psychopathology

Institute of Psychiatry, London, SE5 8AF

The Greek God Proteus eluded capture by constantly changing his
shape. Panic disorder is the latest in a long line of labels for a
group of problems whose protean manifestations have been well
described for more than a century. Each label has reflected a
particular focus. One of the earliest, agoraphobia, denotes a fear
of public places, and is still one of the commonest terms for these
problems. It was coined by Westphal (1871) to describe 3 men whose
(SLIDE)

> "..agony was much increased at those hours when the
> particular streets dreaded were deserted and the shops
> closed. The subjects experienced great comfort from the
> companionship of men or even an inanimate object, such as
> a vehicle or a cane. The use of beer or wine also allowed
> the patient to pass through the feared locality with
> comparative comfort. One man even sought, without immoral
> motives, the companionship of a prostitute as far as his
> own door... some localities are more difficult of access
> than others; the patient walking far in order not to
> traverse them.. in one instance, the open country was less
> feared than sparsely housed streets in town. One case
> also had a dislike for crossing a certain bridge. He
> feared he would fall into the water. In this case, there
> also was apprehension of impending insanity. "

Later labels have included (SLIDE) anxiety hysteria,
illustrating the dramatic form the anxiety can take and the hidden
fears they were thought to have, neurasthenia, phobic-anxious state
and phobic-anxiety-depersonalization syndrome, which focussed on the
exhaustion, free-floating anxiety and depersonization which plague

765

sufferers, neurocirculatory asthenia, cardiac neurosis and soldier's heart, which concentrated on the palpitations, tachycardia and fear of fainting, dying or having a heart attack, platzschwindel - denoting the frequent dizziness and fear of falling, street fear, barber shop fear or locomotor anxiety, which described loci or precipitants of anxiety, and prostitution fear, which seized on an occasional fantasy expressed by sufferers.

Recent focus on panic disorder is yet another attempt to solve a puzzle from which most pieces are still missing. However, we have reached the stage where a concerted program of research could answer important questions to reduce our ignorance and lead to more rational classification. Ideally a classification should 'carve nature at the joints'. Most clinicians are interested in identifying the joints of etiology, course and treatment of the disorder in question.

For panic and other anxiety disorders we know next to nothing about etiology and a bit about course and treatment though there is still no consensus. Locating the joints is especially difficult because we are not yet sure which body of data we are trying to dissect, there are no standard measures of relevant data, and important sampling differences between localities can occur even when the same diagnostic label is used (Marks 1983). Not only do clinic populations differ across centers, but there may be substantial variation among inpatient, outpatient, primary care and community samples in the same locality. Last but by no means least, disorders can not be properly understood solely from cross-sectional analysis at one point in time but need to be followed up for years to see what coheres with what.

Without a longitudinal perspective the link between primary, secondary and tertiary syphilis might never have been discovered. The difficulty is a bit like that involved in tracing bundles of wool strands twisted together along the length of a skein. Raters may agree well about identifying anxious patients from apparently distinct categories of pathology at any one time (e.g. DiNardo et al 1983), yet years later those very patients who were so reliably distinguished from one another may come to look identical or fit into fresh slots merely because of the natural history and they might earn the label panic disorder at one point, agoraphobia with panic attacks at another, then agoraphobia, and, still later, depressive disorder.

Some continuities over time have been found. Followup over 4-5 years has shown that neither phobic nor obsessive-compulsive disorders change into some other problem (Marks 1971; Munbey & Johnston 1980; Emmelkamp 1981), though episodes of depressed-anxious mood punctuate the course of many patients of this kind.

A long-term view of a community sample affords the clearest picture of a disorder, though such data is expensive to collect. The most systematic work on these lines so far is the excellent study of Angst's (1983) team which is still in progress but has already produced some important findings which need replication elsewhere and in older subjects. It deals with anxiety, panics and phobias in normal 19-20 year olds from the 1.1 million people living in the canton of Zurich (SLIDE). About 50% of the men aged 19 and women aged 20 were screened with the SCL-90. From the 6000+ replies (response rate was 100% of males, 75% of females), 300 men and 300 women were studied over the next 3 years. Of these, one-third were selected from subjects scoring in the 15% lowest percentiles of the SCL-90 and two thirds were selected who scored in the highest 15% percentiles. A year after screening they were interviewed for $1\frac{1}{2}$-2 hours each. Two years after screening they had questionnaires again, and three years after screening they were reinterviewed.

The various anxiety symptoms were summarised into 6 overlapping 'syndromes' which overlapped by 24% . These were (SLIDE)-1. generalized anxiety, 2.anxiety and panic attacks 3.panic, 4.phobia, (simple or social + panic attacks) 5.agoraphobia without panic attacks, 6.agoraphobia with panic attacks.

These syndromes had some specific patterns of scores on the SCL-90 slide. Agoraphobics with or without panic attacks scored highest on most of the SCL-90 subscales, especially on interpersonal sensitivity, phobia and depression. The frequency of interpersonal sensitivity in agoraphobia agrees with other findings of frequent social anxiety in such populations (Marks, 1969). On the SCL-90 depression scale high scores were also obtained by subjects who had anxiety or panic. Panic attacks (total n = 99) usually occurred with generalized anxiety (n=40) or agoraphobia (28) and less often on their own or with other phobias.

At initial interview all syndromes showed considerable overlap between anxiety and depression, 24% of subjects having depressive episodes of at least 2 weeks duration and/or severe social consequences. Even excluding these, most subjects who had agoraphobia with panic attacks also had depressive symptoms such as anhedonia, sadness, sickness of living, loss of interest and performance, feelings of inferiority and difficulty in falling asleep (SLIDE). In each of the 3 years of study all syndromes taken together were significantly associated with depression (Cramer's V = .24, .29, .27), and slightly less so with headache, intestinal symptoms, hypochondriasis and exhaustion. It was impossible to find two distinct classes of depression and anxiety states which would exclude each other. This same intimate association between anxiety and depression at the levels of both symptom and syndrome has been found in numerous other studies in the US and UK (Marks 1983b), and variations in this association may account for much of the disagreement about the role of antidepressants in different anxiety syndromes (reviewed by Leibowitz 1983; Marks 1983).

The point prevalence of anxiety disorders in this community sample of young adults was high for both men and women, but especially so for women. Combining men and women with social impairment from the problem, the 4-week prevalence was 5.8%. The one-year prevalence was no less than 8.4% of the population. The 4 week prevalence (with social impairment) of anxiety disorders was 1.5%, of panic attacks 1.1%, and of the combination, 0.6%. With the criterion of avoidance behavior being present, the 4 week prevalence of agoraphobia was 1.1% with and 0.4% without panic attacks, and of other phobias 1.1%; the one-year prevalence was very similar.

Much lower than the one-year prevalence was the one-year treatment prevalence - 1.7% for men and 1.1% for women (1.4% for both together). There was thus a large pool of untreated sufferers in the community. We do not yet know much about what distinguishes those who ask for help in the clinic from the rest, but clearly the characteristics of a clinic population cannot be extrapolated in unqualified fashion to the entire pool of sufferers. One survey of 1000 agoraphobics found that untreated subjects were less able to confide in others than were treated patients (Marks & Herst 1971).

A final finding from the study of Angst and coworkers is the frequency of phobias and complex phobias without panic attacks (SLIDE). Fully two-thirds of the agoraphobics had no non-phobic panic. This highlights a point made by Mathews et al (1982, p.10) about the emphasis of Klein and others (Mendel & Klein 1969, Zitrin et al 1980, Sheehan et al 1980) on spontaneous panic attacks as the central focus in agoraphobia for treatment by antidepressant drugs (SLIDE): "Klein and his colleagues have never formulated a definition of panic attacks that allows them to be distinguished clearly from acute anxiety experienced in response to phobic stimuli".

Avoidance of feared situations is crucial from the standpoints of handicap and of treatment. Social impairment largely stems from avoidance of situations that evoke phobias and compulsive rituals. An agoraphobic becomes housebound not because of spontaneous panics but because she avoids public situations that trigger fear. A compulsive washer becomes restricted once he avoids the discomfort engendered by supposed 'dirt', reducing that discomfort by hours of washing. Behavioural treatment by exposure effectively reduces phobias and compulsive rituals up to 4-7 years followup (Marks 1971; Emmelkamp 1981; Munby & Johnston 1980; McPherson et al 1980). In agoraphobics exposure treatment not only reduces phobic avoidance but also spontaneous panics (Marks et al 1983). As yet behavioural treatment is only consistently useful in anxiety disorders complicated by avoidance. In assessing a patient it is thus vital

768

to delineate his avoidance profile. What situations is he consistently avoiding because they produce discomfort? Mapping the avoidance profile immediately allows the clinician to help the patient successfully carry out exposure therapy. If there is no avoidance, exposure therapy is not indicated. When avoidance is present exposure treatment is lastingly effective in phobics even if self-administered with the help of a brief manual or appropriate computer program (Ghosh et al 1984). Overcoming avoidance is the single most important step in reducing handicap. Patients can be taught to live unimpaired in the presence of other problems like spontaneous panic, though these also commonly improve after exposure therapy.

Antidepressant drugs help many sufferers from anxiety disorders, though there is lively debate about whether such drugs are useful in the absence of depressed-anxious mood (an issue separate from the diagnosis of depressive disorder). Four controlled studies in agoraphobics found that antidepressants did not reduce phobic avoidance (Solyom et al 1981; Marks et al 1983; McNair & Kahn 1981; Telch 1983). In the first 2 studies patients began with normal mood. Telch's patients had depressed-anxious mood that improved with imipramine, but imipramine did not reduce phobias in the absence of exposure therapy. McNair & Kahn also found that imipramine improved depressed mood but not agoraphobia, though it did reduce panics (SLIDE). In addition, a substantial proportion of phobics and obsessive-compulsives have normal mood, and in them a drug effect is questionable. Even where antidepressants are helpful in these conditions, many studies report that relapse is common on stopping even prolonged medication. Moreover, the drugs are not without side effects.

It is important to settle the role of antidepressant drugs in these conditions by controlled research with relevant measures and with followup for at least a year after stopping the drug. Our understanding of panic and other anxiety disorders and their link with minor affective disorders would greatly increase if future studies carefully measured 5 dimensions repeatedly over several years with and without treatment (SLIDE). Each of these 5 dimensions reflects a name given to one or other syndrome. They are 1) spontaneous phasic panics independent of being in or thinking about a phobic situation, 2) non-phasic tonic anxiety independent of being in or thinking about a phobic situation, 3) depressed mood, 4) phobic avoidance, 5) obsessive ruminations and compulsive rituals. Given this data recent methods of longitudinal multivariate analysis could help us better identify the coherent patterns of pathology.

Even after such a research program many conundrums will remain e.g. why depressed-anxious mood is so much more frequent among agoraphobics and compulsive ritualizers than among specific phobics, why spontaneous panic is common in agoraphobics but not in ritualizers, why the subjective component of the pathology is usually anxiety with phobics but discomfort with obsessive-compulsives, why some people with spontaneous panic and/or depressed-anxious mood never become phobic or obsessive-compulsive, why there is such a female preponderance in most of these conditions except for social phobias. Despite the many intriguing questions remaining about these disorders, however, we are fortunately able at last to help many sufferers.

MINIMUM MEASURES NEEDED FOR FUTURE RESEARCH
<u>Measures to be repeated over years</u> (and at least a year after stopping drugs)

1. Spontaneous phasic panics   when <u>not</u> in phobic situation
                                              or thinking of it
2. Non-phasic (free floating) anxiety   "   "   "   "   "

3. Depressed mood (Hamilton, Beck)

4. Phobic avoidance (Marks & Mathews) of situations

5. " discomfort if anticipating (thinking of entering) phobic
                                              situations
6. Obsessive ruminations and compulsive rituals

Table 1

DEFINITION

SYNDROME	SCL-90	SPIKE - Interview
Generalized anxiety	23. Suddenly scared for no reason	Dread of being alone Fear of the coming day
Panic	72. Spells of terror or panic	Anxiety attacks Panic Cardiac panic/anxiety Heart beating Shortness of breath with anxiety
Agoraphobia	13. Feeling afraid in open spaces or on the streets 25. Feeling afraid to go out of your house alone 47. Feeling afraid to travel on buses, subways, or trains 70. Feeling uneasy in crowds, such as shopping or at a movie.	
Social phobia	73. Feeling uncomfortable about eating or drinking in public 82. Feeling afraid you will faint in public	
Simple phobia		Situational phobia Animal phobia

Table 2

SYNDROMAL CONFIGURATION OF ANXIETY DISORDERS

Anxiety disorder	Syndromes					Subjects
	GENANX	SOCPHO	SIMPHO	AGOPHO	PANIC	
1 ANX	+					54
2 ANXPAN	+				+	40
3 PAN					+	22
4 PHO			+			23 ⎫
		+	+			5
		+	+		+	2
	+		+			6 ⎬ 48
	+		+		+	5
	+	+	+			5
	+	+	+		+	2 ⎭
5 AGO				+		1 ⎫
			+	+		13
		+	+	+		16 ⎬ 41
	+		+	+		1
	+	+	+	+		10 ⎭
6 AGOPAN			+	+	+	1 ⎫
		+	+	+	+	1 ⎬ 28
	+		+	+	+	8
	+	+	+	+	+	18 ⎭
Total						233

Table 3

ANXIETY DISORDERS, SOCIAL IMPAIRMENT, AVOIDANCE
BEHAVIOR, AND EXCLUSION OF DEPRESSION

Anxiety disorder	Subjects	Socially impaired	Avoidance behavior	without Depression
1 ANX generalized anxiety disorder	54	36	-	30
2 ANXPAN generalized anxiety and panic attacks	40	27	-	19 } 69
3 PAN panic attacks (no other syndromes)	22	13	-	10
4 PHO simple phobia a/o social phobia	48	26	17	11
5 AGO agoraphobia (no panic attacks)	41 } 29 / 62	24	19	14
6 AGOPAN agoraphobia and panic attacks	28	21	18 54	14
Total	233	147	130	98

773

REFERENCES

ANGST J & DOBLER-MIKOLA A. Anxiety states, panic and phobia in a
    young general population: results of the Zurich study.
    Awaiting publication.
COHEN S D, MONTEIRO W, MARKS I M. (1983). Two year followup of
    agoraphobics after exposure and imipramine.
    Arch.Gen.Psychiatry. (In press).
DINARDO et al. (1983). Arch Gen Psychiatry. (In press).
EMMELKAMP P. Behavioural treatment of obsessive-compulsive patients
    Paper to Learning Theory Symposium, Crete, April 1980.
KAHN R J et al. (1981). Effects of psychotropic agents in high
    anxiety subjects. Psychopharmacology Bulletin, 17, 97-100.
LEIBOWITZ M. (1983). Review of antidepressants in anxiety
    disorders. Awaiting publication.
MARKS I.M.(1969) Fears and Phobias. Academic Press.
MARKS I.M. Are there anticompulsive or antiphobic drugs? Review of
    the evidence. Br.J.Psychiatry. 1983. (In press).
MARKS I.M. Phobic disorders 4 years after treatment. Br.J.of
    Psychiatry, 1971, 118, 683-688.
MARKS I M. (1983). Stress and other risk factors in anxiety
    disorders: in Goldston S & Goldman H. NIMH Publication.
MATHEWS A M, GELDER M G & Johnston D. (1982). Agoraphobia: Its
    nature and treament. Guildford Press, NY.
MCNAIR D M & KAHN R J. (1981). Imipramine compared with a
    benzodiazepine for agoraphobia. In Anxiety: New Research and
    Changing Concepts (eds.DF Klein & J Rabkin), 69-80, New York,
    Raven Press.
McPHERSON F M, Brougham L. & McLaren. (1980). Maintenance of
    improvement in agoraphobic patients treated by behavioral
    methods. 4 year followup. Beh.Res. & Ther. 18, 150-152.
MENDEL, JGC & KLEIN DF. (1969). Anxiety attacks with subsequent
    agoraphobia. Comprehensive Psychiatry, 10, 190-5.
MUNBY, M & JOHNSTON, D W. Agoraphobia: Long term follow-up of
    behavioural treatment. Br.J.Psychiatry, 1980, 137, 418-427.
SHEEHAN D, BALLENGER, J, JACOBSEN G. (1980). Treatment of
    endogenous anxiety and phobic, hysterical and hypochondriacal
    symptoms. Arch.Gen.Psychiatry, 37, 51-9.
TELCH M. (1983). Ph.D. Dissertation. Stanford University,
    California.
WESTPHAL C. (1878): Zwangvorstellungen. Archiv.Psychiat.Nervenkr.,
    8, 734-750.
WESTPHAL C. (1871-2): Die agoraphobie: eine neuropathische
    erscheinung. Arch.fur Psychiatrie und Nervenkrankheiten, 3
    pp.138-171, pp.219-221.
ZITRIN C M et al. (1980). Treatment of agoraphobia, with group
    exposure in vivo and imipramine. Arch.Gen.Psychiatry., 37,
    63-72.

PANIC AND OTHER ANXIETY DISORDERS: DIAGNOSIS AND TREATMENT

David V. Sheehan

Massachusetts General Hospital
Harvard Medical School
Boston, MA. 02114, U.S.A

Anxiety, phobic and hysterical disorders have long been areas of distressing diagnostic confusion. In an attempt to clarify some of the confusion in this area the DSM III [1] classification attempted to operationalise definitions for anxiety and related disorders with precisely defined criteria in a way that reflected then current views about these disorders. The result was a significant proliferation in the number of anxiety related disorders that were felt to be distinct. What was anxiety neurosis in previous classifications was broken up into two groups 1) generalised anxiety disorder and 2) panic disorder. What was previously phobic neurosis was broken down into 1) simple phobia 2) social phobia 3) agoraphobia with panic attacks 4) agoraphobia without panic attacks. And there were many others. The rationale behind breaking up anxiety neurosis into two groups appeared to be that the severe anxiety disorder associated with spontaneous panic attacks responded well to antidepressant medication[2,3] and poorly to benzodiazepines, while the milder anxiety disorder associated with chronic tension and autonomic hyperactivity appeared to respond to benzodiazepines and antidepressants were not needed. The evidence behind this distinction was merely suggestive but on close examination does not inspire much confidence. In the absence of any definitive evidence one way or another it was decided to create 2 disorders where one existed before and to study the apparent differences over the following years.

Similarly the prevailing view in the 1970's was that phobic disorders with or without spontaneous panic attacks and including the agoraphobic syndrome responded well to behavior therapies particularly exposure treatments.[4-6] Closer examination supports the view that these behavioral methods do facilitate the extinction of phobic avoidance behavior. But the evidence that such treatments were effective against other symptoms in the cluster of agoraphobia eg the spontaneous anxiety attacks is weak (it is only recently that instruments measuring the panic attacks have been used). Yet because they appeared on the surface to respond to different treatments, this reinforced the diagnostic distinction.

A number of developments are now blurring these neat categorisations. Indeed they are casting the entire organisation of the anxiety classification into question. First the majority of patients with agoraphobia and social phobias and some simple phobias like claustrophobia have spontaneous attacks in addition to their situational panic attacks. Treating these patients with behavior therapy alone yields incomplete and unstable recovery. Treating them with antidepressants delivers more substantial recovery and controls the core spontaneous anxiety attacks. Indeed in a head to head comparison of these treatments the results favoured antidepressant drug treatment.[7] Clinicians who treat these disorders with frequency have noted that many cases of "generalised anxiety disorder" who only get incomplete results with benzodiazepines often respond in a satisfactory manner to antidepressants. However more systematic studies are needed to establish this with more certainty. More recently a new triazobenzodiazepine, alprazolam is being found effective against agoraphobia with panic attacks and panic disorder.[8-10] This further clouds meaningful distinctions between generalised anxiety disorderand panic disorder and between panic disorder and agoraphobia. Another recent study on patients with severe panic attacks and extensive phobic avoidance eg agoraphobia found that those patients satisfied symptom criteria for the diagnosis of several DSM III anxiety related diagnoses simultaneously. This suggests that there may be major category overlap among these disorders as defined and that they are not inherently mutually exclusive.[11,12] . In another study (elsewhere in this volume[13]) 119 patients with panic attacks and agoraphobia were asked to review the natural history of their disorder from its first onset and 'to rank order stages they may have passed through during its course. The majority passed through the stages in a particular sequence and these stages each corresponded to a different diagnostic category as defined in DSM III. This suggests that several of these DSM III disorders as defined may only be stages in the natural history of one pathological anxiety disorder.[14,12] As outlined elsewhere the currently established diagnostic delineation of these disorders may not be the more efficient economical one, nor the best predictor of treatment response.[11,12,13,14] Is there an alternative diagnostic classification that will serve as a better predictor of treatment response.

An Alternative Diagnostic Classification
The decision tree for an alternative diagnostic approach is outlined in Fig. I below.

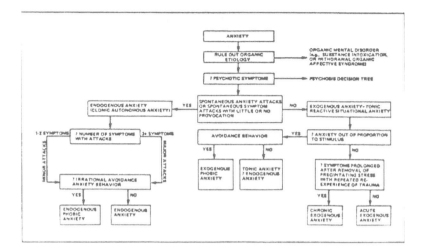

Figure 1. Diagnostic Decision Free for Anxiety and Phobic Disorders.

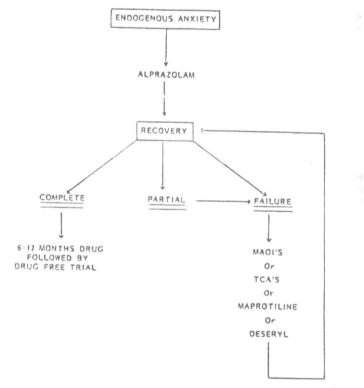

Figure 2. Management Strategy for Endogenous Anxiety.

Fig 1

The diagram illustrates that the first step is to rule out any
organic medical illness and then any psychotic disorder. The
central pivotal diagnostic distinction (but by no means the only one
eg see diagnostic criteria for endogenous anxiety in Ref. 14) is
whether the patient has or has ever had spontaneous anxiety or
spontaneous symptom attacks during the natural history of their
disorder. If they have then it is likely they have endogenous anxiety
(anxiety spectrum disorder). Only if they fail to satisfy criteria
for endogenous anxiety (anxiety spectrum disorder) are they assigned
to the residual category of exogenous anxiety.This may be either
acute or chronic. If the anxiety is associated with one phobia
only then it is called exogenous phobic (a phobia occuring in the
absence of spontaneous attacks). Endogenous anxiety can be subdivided for treatment purposes into two major subtypes: 1) The
early milder form of the disorder before it is complicated by phobias
when it is called endogenous anxiety or 2) the later more chronic
severe form of the disorder when it is called endogenous phobic
anxiety. The reason for this distinction clinically is that in
both the spontaneous attacks respond to antipanic medication, but
the endogenous phobic anxiety requires additional behavior therapy,
particularly exposure treatments after the drug is effective to
extinguish any residual phobias. Endogenous anxiety (anxiety
spectrum disorder) can be staged along a continuum of severity and
chronicity from its mild early symptoms to its late severe, chronic
and disabling manifestations (as outlined elsewhere in this volume[13]).
This staging embraces into one pathological anxiety disorder a
spectrum of anxiety related disorders previously regarded as distinct
entities. The older classifications adopted a cross sectional view
at different points in the natural history of the disorder. What is
recommended here is the adoption of a longitudinal perspective of
this one disorder. Viewed in this way the treatment strategies that
work best become logical extensions of this diagnostic approach.

Treatment Strategies

Endogenous anxiety

Fig 2

Patients with endogenous anxiety alone may be started on any one of
several antipanic drugs. At this time alprazolam appers to be the most
rapidly effective. Its merits in relation to the tricyclic antidepressants and MAO inhibitors for this disorder is currently under study
in double blind controlled studies. If after 3 to 4 weeks on a
satisfactory dose (a mean final dose of 6·5mgs/day was needed in
our studies for good antipanic effect) the therapeutic response is
not satisfactory or only partial then the patient is switched over
to an MAO inhibitor, a tricyclic antidepressant, a tetracyclic, or
zimelidine or trazadone. Trials of each of these for at least 6 to
8 weeks at optimal therapeutic doses are indicated before abandoning
that drug for the next in the sequence for a further trial of 6 to

8 weeks. If recovery is complete continue the regimen for 6 to 12 months and very slowly taper the dose. The relapse rate is high.

Endogenous phobic anxiety

Fig 3

The treatment strategy is very similar to that for pure endogenous anxiety in Figure 2. However because in its severe chronic form the spontaneous panic attacks have precipitated extensive phobic avoidance behavior, a further ingredient-behavior therapy- is added to the treatment package. The drug therapy usually controls the core spontaneous panic attacks and anxiety symptoms. However some phobic avoidance behavior may remain, until the patient is encouraged to reenter the situation and successfully cope with it without being overwhelmed by anxiety. This repeated invivo exposure appears to be the "active ingredient" in all behavior therapies directed at overcoming phobias.[4-6] As in Fig 2, the arrows are followed until a satisfactory therapeutic result is achieved.

Exogenous Anxiety

Fig 4

Patients with an exogenous phobia require a different treatment approach to those with acute or chronic exogenous anxiety. The treatment of choice for an exogenous phobia is behavior therapy, especially invivo exposure (usually graduated) and prevention of the usual flight response.[5] Medication is rarely necessary. However if after a reasonable trial of effective behavior therapy, satisfactory improvement is not achieved, a trial of one of the effective antipanic drugs listed for endogenous anxiety may be indicated. When this has been regulated, the invivo exposure is repeated. What appeared at first as an uncomplicated exogenous anxiety, may later turn out to have been a low grade endogenous anxiety complicated by one or two phobias only.

In patients with acute or chronic exogenous anxiety the treatment is to identify the stresses that precipitated or continue to aggravate the symptoms. Usually psychotherapy is effective in working through these difficulties. Medications eg benzodiazepines are often prescribed but not always necessary. If reasonable psychotherapeutic intervention fails to resolve the patients problems within three to six months and unless there are extenuating circumstances, treatment with one of the effective antipanic drugs should be considered in addition to the psychotherapy.

Because of renewed interest in pathological anxiety, it is likely that significant advances in our basic understanding of the underlying mechanisms will soon occur. This will inevitably lead to further refinements in our diagnostic precision and treatment strategies.

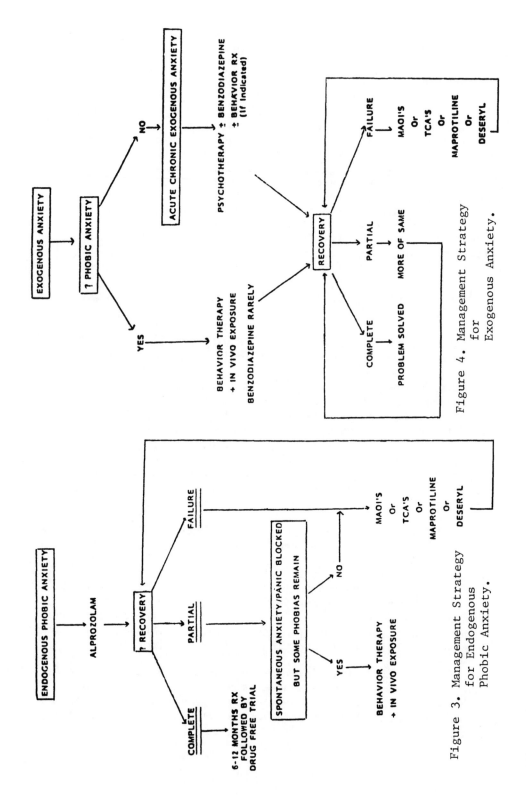

Figure 4. Management Strategy for Exogenous Anxiety.

Figure 3. Management Strategy for Endogenous Phobic Anxiety.

REFERENCES

1. Diagnostic and Statistical Manual of Mental Disorders DSM
    III. 3rd ed. American Psychiatric Association. 1980.
2. Klein,D.F. Importance of psychiatric diagnosis in prediction
    of clinical drug effects. Arch. Gen. Psychiatry,16:118-126.
    1967.
3. Sheehan,D.V., Ballenger,J., Jacobson,G. The treatment of
    endogenous anxiety with phobic, hysterical and hypochondriacal
    symptoms. Arch. Gen. Psychiatry,1980:37:51-59.
4. Sherman,A.R. Real life exposure as a primary therapeutic
    factor in the desensitisation treatment of fear. J. Abnorm.
    Psychol.1972: 79:19-28.
5. Marks,I.M. The current status of behavioral psychotherapy:
    Theory and practice. Am. J. Psychiatry. 1976:133:253-261.
6. Marks,I.M. The cure and care of neuroses. Wiley. New York.
    1981.
7. Zitrin,C.M., Klein D.F., Woerner,M.G. Behavior Therapy,
    supportive psychotherapy, imipramine, and phobias. Arch.
    Gen. Psychiatry.1978: 35:307-316.
8. Sheehan, D.V., Coleman,J.H., Greenblatt, D.J., et al. Some
    biochemical correlates of agoraphobia with panic attacks
    and their response to a new treatment.J. Clin.Psychopharmacol.
    in press.
9. Shader,R.I., Goodman,M., Gever,J. Panic Disorders: current
    prespectives. J. Clin. Psychopharmacol. 1982:2:Suppl.2S-10S.
10. Sheehan,D.V., Uzogara,E., Coleman,J.H. Treatment of panic
    states. paper presented at American Psychiatric Association
    annual meeting. Toronto, Canada. May 1982.
11. Sheehan,D.V., Sheehan, K.E. The classification of anxiety and
    hysterical states. Part I. Historical review and empirical
    delineation. J. Clin. Psychopharmacol.1982:2(14):235-244.
12. Sheehan,D.V., Sheehan, K.E. The classification of phobic
    disorders. Int.J. Psychiatr. Med.1982-83:12(4):243-264.
13. Sheehan,D.V., Sheehan,K.E. Classification of anxiety disorders
    proceeding of VII World Congress of Psychiatry. Plenum.
    London,1983.
14. Sheehan,D.V.,Sheehan,K.E. The classification of anxiety and
    hysterical disorders,Part II. Towards a heurestic class-
    ification. J.Clin.Psychopharmacol. 1982:2(6).386-393.

ANXIETY DISORDERS:
CONSIDERATIONS FROM THE PERSPECTIVES OF
PRIMARY MENTAL HEALTH CARE

Carlos A. León

Department of Psychiatry
Universidad del Valle
Cali, Colombia

I. INTRODUCTION - SIZE OF THE PROBLEM

Even though there is a paucity of epidemiological studies dealing with prevalence of mental disorders in Latin America, a few
well designed surveys conducted in different places point to the
presence of rates of mental disorder quite similar to those found
in developed industrial countries. What follows is a brief review
of some studies which include data dealing with anxiety disorders
and other related problems as observed in populations covered by
primary health care services.

In a survey conducted in Bogotá[1] using an adaptation of the
Langner 22 items[2], in a sample of 1502 persons between 15 and 50
years of age it was found that 34.4% complained of "restlessness;"
15.3% of "nervousness and irritability;" 3.6% of "palpitations"
and 30.8% of "hot flashes." In a similar survey conducted in Cali[3],
aimed at identifying the level and distribution of symptoms of
mental disorders in a sample of 681 community residents, using also
the Langner 22 items, it was found that the average score for males
was 6.0% and for females 8.8%. These figures are much higher than
those found in the U.S.A., but otherwise consistent with several
studies that suggest higher prevalence for Latin American as opposed
to North American populations[4]. The proportion of respondents in
Cali answering affirmatively to questions related to anxiety was
quite high: "restlessness" 38.2%; "nervousness," 23.2%; "palpitations,"
8.4%; "hot flashes," 28.3%. Women reported a larger number of symptoms than men and higher proportion of scores for several types of
symptoms.

In a study involving 17 municipal health centers   (public facilities providing primary health care) serving a population of approximately 700,000 inhabitants in Cali[5], it was found that during a 10 month period a total of 84,203 persons aged 15 years and above had received primary health attention. Among them were 1,130 cases who were given a <u>main</u> diagnosis of mental disorder by the attending physician and were recorded as suffering from mental disorder <u>only</u> (a proportion of 1.34%). Anxiety was the most frequent generic diagnosis in this group, with a total of 436 cases, which represents 38.6% of all the psychiatric cases recorded.

In a recent W.H.O. study[6], a sample of 1,624 persons was collected sequentially among people attending primary health facilities in 4 developing countries (Colombia, India, Philippines and Sudan). Among them, a total of 222 (13.9%) were identified by primary health workers as suffering from mental disorders, through the use of instruments capable of detecting the presence of psychiatric morbidity. The screening process for cases was carried out independently of the usual consultation-treatment process. The health workers, following their habitual procedures, were able to correctly detect only about one third of the psychiatric cases diagnosed as such by a psychiatrist. In the same sample, a diagnosis of anxiety neuroses was made in 30.9% of the cases identified as psychiatric cases. Another important finding in this study was that the majority of patients with mental disorders complained primarily of physical symptoms, some of which are those usually regarded as potentially "psychosomatic."

A health promoter working in a rural area of 1,068 inhabitants in Colombia was able to detect, in the course of one year, a total of 55 persons suffering with diverse types of mental disorders[7]. Among these cases, 26 (47%) complained of "nervousness," "restlesness," "fears" or "excessive worrying" as one of the presenting problems. On subsequent examination by a psychiatrist who reviewed all cases, 42 (76%) were found to present anxiety among their current symptoms. However, because other symptoms were more prominent, anxiety as such was used as a generic diagnosis by the health promoter only in 9 cases (16.3%), all of which were confirmed by the psychiatrist. In general, the level of agreement or correspondence of generic diagnoses made by the health promoter and the specific diagnosis made by the psychiatrist was very satisfactory.

In a prevalence study conducted in a rural area in Colombia by a group of student health promoters[8], a total of 31 cases of mental disorder was detected in a sample of 128 persons aged 15 years and above (a total prevalence rate of 24.2%). Among these 31 cases, 21 (68%) complained of subjective feelings of anxiety; 22 (71%) complained of being easily frightened or over-reacting to stimulii; 21 (68%) described cardio-respiratory autonomic symptoms and 19 (61%) other types of autonomic symptoms. A diagnosis of anxiety neurosis was made in 6 cases. (Estimated prevalence rate for the population: 4.6%).

II. CLINICAL ILLUSTRATIONS

The following cases have been deliberately selected to exemplify not only typical conditions of frequent occurrence in our communities, but also variants of the anxiety disorder as they appear at diverse stages of the process of symptom formation in the pathological picture.

Case # 1. Clara, a 26 year old married woman and mother of 2 children (5 and 2), is unable to leave her house because she fears that she may collapse and die in the street. Her heart pounds, she trembles and becomes dizzy whenever she hears a knock at her door and she locks herself in a room if any person outside the family is to come to the house. The case was detected by a public health auxiliary nurse, in the course of her work in a maternal and child health program. It was found that the trouble had started about one year and a half ago, when the patient lived in a different neighbourhood. At that time the house next door was being repaired by 2 workers who impressed her as mischievous and insolent. One of them, especially, seemed to constantly stare at her and smile in a seductive way. They knocked at the door and tried to get into the house, using any excuse. She did not mention anything to her husband for fear of his jealous reaction. One day, on leaving her house, Clara saw that the worker moved in her direction and seemed to whisper some words. She immediately felt dizzy and fainty, her legs became weak, her heart stopped for a moment, then it started beating very fast and she choked gasping for air... With a supreme effort of her will, she was able to return home and collapsed in bed. Since then, she developed an intense fear of leaving the house and has not improved at all despite having moved to another place and tried different treatments suggested by friends and relatives. She suspects that the man put a jinx on her, to retaliate for her lack of response to his advances. There is no history of any previous emotional of mental problem.

Case # 2. Bernardo, a 19 year old student, comes to the out-patient clinic referred from a health center with the complaint that for the last 2 months he is unable to feel anything, as if he "were not a person" or "did not exist at all." He can look at his hands or parts of his body, or look at his face in a mirror, but somehow he can not capture the feeling that he is himself; it is as if he was looking a stranger. He can use expressions such as "I feel" but they lack meaning altogether, and even the word "I" sounds empty and useless. Asked to recount how the problem started, he informs that one night as the family gathered to eat supper, all of a sudden he felt a great fear and had the impression that the walls in the room were coming together; he tried to run away but his movements became "uncoordinated" and purposeless and at the same

time he felt as if something inside his head was going to "snap."
His heart was throbbing and he panted for air. He thought that he
was about to have a heart attack or an epileptic fit or that he was
"losing" his mind... His astonished relatives thought the same and
took him immediately to the emergency room of the hospital. He was
given sedation and sent home. On the following day he continued to
feel restless, uneasy and tense; however, he managed to attend
classes yet he could not concentrate. In the middle of a lecture
he had the feeling that he was about to have another attack and
that all of his classmates seemed to be aware of what he was
experiencing. He describes the situation as "the beginning of an
attack of fear, plus the terror and shame of having it in front of
all those people..." Using all his self-control he tried to keep
quiet but he noticed that he was breathing very fast and that his
vision became blurred. He then felt a tingling sensation starting
in his hands and going up the arms. An instant later, he felt his
body becoming lighter and lighter, until he seemed to be floating
in midair, while experiencing at the same time a curious feeling of
detachment "as if nothing mattered any longer." He felt numb and
distant and continued, from then on, to experience a sense of
estrangement which he can only describe as "being unable to feel
himself." However, the attack of fear was aborted and has never
occurred again. On careful questioning about the circumstances
preceding the initial attack, he informs that on that day he had
attempted to have intercourse with a prostitute, but failed to have
an erection. The prostitute became angry and accused him of being
a masturbator. He felt intense shame and anger and on leaving her
place he had the feeling that people around seemed to know what had
happened. Later, at home, he tried his best to forget the incident
and engaged in several chores to keep himself busy, until dinner
time, when he experienced the attack.

Case # 3. Eduardo is a 23 year old single man brought to the
health center by the police, friends and relatives who informed that
while attending a charity fair he had an "ataque de rabia" (rage
attack). During the episode, he "acted crazy;" screamed, yelled,
fought and struggled violently, hitting out and kicking indiscrim-
inately at everybody around. When he was finally subdued, after
great efforts, he was "shaking all over," "breathing heavily" and
"foaming at the mouth." At the center, he showed "generalized
tremors" and "hyperventilation," and seemed to be in a state of
exhaustion, and cloudiness; but he was able to answer questions
and complained of an intolerable "desesperación" (desperateness).
After given parenteral sedation, he became relaxed and was able to
give an account of what had happened. From the information collected from relatives and from the patient himself, it was found that
for the last 2 or 3 weeks, Eduardo had been feeling nervous and
jumpy, unable to sleep and worrying excessively about everything,
but must of all about his girl friend; he became obsessed by
jealous thoughts and had the need to check her whereabouts

786

constantly. On the day of the fair he felt increasingly nervous and had to keep moving from one place to another; then, all of a sudden, he felt overwhelmed by intense fear as if "struck by lightning;" he felt as being in terrible danger, "like going to die, or about to be killed." His vision became blurred, he could not breath and he was about to collapse. Then, in a sudden flash, he thought that he may have been poisoned in a drink he had taken and that this could be the result of a conspiracy plotted by a rival. At that very moment, he looked around and seemed to detect expressions of mocking contempt in several people's faces; he went into a blind rage, decided that he "should die fighting" and from that moment on he only has a faint recollection of what happened. This case exemplifies a type of disorder which is found rather frequently in Latin American populations under such names as "ataque," "ataque de rabia," "mal de pelea" (fighting illness) and the misnomer of "Puerto Rican Syndrome." Because of its paroxysmal features, it is often regarded as an epileptic or epileptiform disorder, but the dramatic and gaudy nature of its presentation is also suggestive of hysteria. What must be emphasized about this case (and probably other similar) is that the rage reaction is <u>immediately preceded by a panic state</u>, which because of the dramatism of the attack of rage, goes initially undetected and is not systematically explored.

III. COMMENTS

Anxiety represents not only a very common complaint among people with mental disorders, but also a frequent finding in general populations, as well as in a sizeable proportion of persons seeking primary health care. But, before we can accept the results of prevalence studies and surveys, with a degree of confidence, it would be desirable that the characteristics of a case had been defined and ascertained in a reliable way, which unfortunately seldom happens. The comparison between studies is particularly hazardous because of the conceptual differences and divergent clinical orientation of the researchers, not to mention the methodological heterogeneity of the study designs and the socio-cultural differences of the populations investigated. One of the intriguing findings in transcultural comparison is the consistently higher scores obtained by Latin American respondents to screening questionnaires, as mentioned above. Yet, it is not clear whether this corresponds to a truly greater degree of pathology or to a disposition to admit more readily or openly the presence of symptoms. There seems to be a definite need for the use of valid and reliable instruments administered in a standard way to different types of populations, preferably through collaborative studies conducted in various socio-cultural settings, in different parts of the world.

It may also be appropriate to emphasize the need for familiarity with the socio-cultural background of the patient such as mores, attitudes, beliefs, traditions and expectations, each of which may play an important role, not only in giving shape to a disorder, but also on its course and outcome. The successful handling of a case may demand certain complementarity between the notions and needs of the patient and the disposition, or ability, of the therapist to function within a pertinent and meaningful frame imposed by the prevailing cultural conditions, so that a true therapeutic alliance may emerge.

REFERENCES

1. M. Gonzalez, et al. "Epidemiología de los trastornos mentales en Bogotá". Ediciones Tercer Mundo, (1978).
2. T.S. Langner. A twenty-two item screening score of psychiatric impairment. J. Health Soc. Behav. 3:269 (1962).
3. M. Micklin and C.A. León. Life change and psychiatric disturbance in a South American city: The effects of geographic and social mobility. J. Health Soc. Behav. 19:92 (1978).
4. P. Haberman. Ethnic differences in psychiatric symptoms reported in community surveys. Public Health Reports 85:495 (1970).
5. C.A. León. Resultados de un cursillo de actualización psiquiátrica al personal médico de centros de salud en Cali. Presented to the Second Ecuadorean Congress of Psychiatry. Quito March 11-14 (1976).
6. T.W. Harding et al. Mental disorders in primary health care: A study of their frequency and diagnosis in four developing countries. Psychol. Med. 10:231 (1980).
7. C.A. León. Classification of mental disorders in a primary health care setting. Presented to the World Psychiatric Association Regional Meeting. New York October 30-November 3. (1981).
8. C.A. León. Barefoot researchers: The potential role of rural students as mental health promoters performing prevalence surveys. Bull.Pan.Am. Health Org. 15:361 (1981).

THE OVERLAP OF THE SPECTRUM OF ANTIANXIETY AND ANTIDEPRESSANT DRUGS: A MULTIVARIATE APPROACH*

Giovanni B. Cassano**, Luciano Conti,
Gian FRanco Placidi and Liliana Dell'Osso
Institute of Clinical Psychiatry
University of Pisa
Via Roma, 67 - 56100 Pisa, Italy

INTRODUCTION

The relationship between anxiety and depression, the delimitation of the two phenomena and the area of overlap between them is not only of theoretical, but also of clinical and therapeutic significance.

Although an attempt was made in DSM-III[1] to differentiate affective from anxiety disorders it seems to have ignored a wide area of overlap where the two types of clinical phenomena coexist[2] . A satisfactory definition of specific antianxiety and antidepressant compounds presupposes a precise psychopathological delimitation of these two areas. However in every day practice, these compounds are often used interchangeably to treat depressed patients showing symptoms of anxiety or anxious patients showing symptoms of depression. Any decision as to which of the two psychopathological phenomena is primary or secondary is not easily made on clinical grounds. Thus, for both psychopharmacologists and clinicians alike, patients suffering from a mixture of depression and anxiety present a difficult challenge. It

---

* This study was supported by NIMH Grant no. 1UO1 MH33922-03.
** 2nd Chair of Clinical Psychiatry - Institute of Clinical Psychiatry of Pisa University.

would therefore appear difficult to arrange for a clinical psychopharmacological study to treat pure anxiety
disorders or pure depressive ones given the significant
overlap between anxiety and depression. Although the
most recently devised rating scales for anxiety disorders
are mainly focused on typical symptoms of anxiety, the
most widely used rating scales for depression assess
symptoms of both depression and anxiety. This situation
further confounds the description as to which drugs are
specifically anxiolytic or specifically antidepressant.
As a result, anxiolytic and antidepressant properties are
often ascribed to both categories of drugs. Thus, no
adequate separation between the spectra of activity of
the two classes of compounds has so far been achieved.

In the treatment of depression, benzodiazepines
are often combined with tricyclic antidepressants. The
most commonly stated justification for the use of the
anxiolytic compounds is that they may possess a particularly rapid therapeutic activity on a wide range of
symptoms of anxiety and agitation during the first few
days of treatment; by contrast, two or more weeks should
elapse before tricyclic antidepressants make a major
impact on depression. If this is so, the properties of
tricyclic antidepressants and benzodiazepines should be
most marked during the first week of treatment. It was
therefore thought worth carrying out a comparative
analysis on data recorded during the early phase of
treatment with benzodiazepines and tricyclic antidepressants in two populations of depressed patients.

MATERIAL AND METHOD

Data organized who underwent treatment with
benzodiazepine anxiolytics or tricyclic antidepressants
in a double-blind controlled clinical trial were
selected and retrieved from the data banl of Biometric
Laboratory Information Processing System/Data Bank for
Psychopharmacology (BLIPS/BDP) operating at the Institute
of Clinical Psychiatry of the University of Pisa. The
benzodiazepines used included nitrazepam, oxazepam,
temazepam, diazepam, chlordiazepoxide, medazepam,
pinazepam and camazepam. The triciclic drugs was either
imipramine or amitriptyline. The subjects utilized were

consecutive inpatients who had all experienced a major
depressive episode by DSM-III criteria and all had an
initial HAM-D total score at at least 18.

The data were processed at the Center for Clinical
Psychopharmacology Data Documentation (CCPDD) of the
Institute of Clinical Psychiatry utilizing the statistical
routine of BMDP (Biomedical Computer Programs P-Series
1979) available at the CNUCE Institute of CNR of Pisa.

RESULTS

178 patients treated with benzodiazepines (BNZ) and
209 patients treated with a tricyclic antidepressant
(TCA) were selected (Table 1). However, it was clinically
necessary to give PRN hypnotics during the first week
of treatment to one-fifth of those under the tricyclic
regimen.

The mean age of the BNZ group (49.64) was modestly
lower than that of the TCA group (54.33), and in both
groups there were fewer males than females. The initial
clinical judgement of severity did not differ in the two
groups, ranging from "moderate" to "severe" (a mean of
6.5 refers to a degree of clinical intensity intermediate
between "moderate" and "severe").

Table 1. Characteristics of the two samples.

Variables	Treatment	
	BNZs	TCAs
No. of subjects	178	209
Age (mean + SD)	49.64 (+13.27)	54.33 (+11.24)a
Sex (males %)	12.9%	20.8%
Initial severity of illness (mean + SD)	6.50 (+1.18)	6.57 (+1.23)
Initial HAM-D total score (mean + SD)	25.10 (+14.89)	26.68 (+16.13)a
Hypnotics at night (%)	–	22.18

a) Student t-test: p < .05, two-tailed.

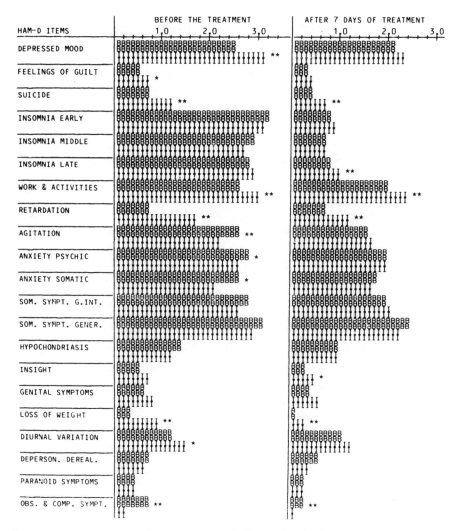

Figure 1 - HAM-D items: profile of the two treatment groups (Benzodiazepines (BB) and Imipramine or Amitriptyline (II) at the beginning and after 7 days of treatment. * = p < .05; ** = p < .01 (Student t-test).

The initial mean total score of the HAM-D was 25.10 for the BNZ group and 26.68 for the TCA group; this difference was statistically significant, given the large simple size, but it is obvious that from a clinical standpoint both groups had nearly equal severity of illness.

The pre-treatment profiles of the two groups are

Table 2. Covariance analysis on HAM-D item scores at the beginning and after 7 days of treatment with Benzodiazepines and with Imipramine or Amitriptyline (Significant differences).

HAM-D	Before	7 day	Diff.	Before	7 day	Diff.	Covar. anal. F-value	P
Depr. Mood	2.51	2.05	-0.46	3.04	2.25	-0.79	3.94	.05
Agitation	1.29	0.78	-0.51	1.07	0.84	-0.23	6.05	.05

shown in figure 1. The TCA-treated group has significantly higher scores in depression items such as "Depressed Mood", "Guilt", "Suicide", "Work and Activities", "Retardation", and "Loss of Weight". By contrast, the BNZ-treated group exhibited significantly higher scores in such anxiety items as "Agitation", "Psychic Anxiety", "Somatic Anxiety", and "Obsessive Symptoms". After 7 days the BNZ group showed a mean improvement of 7.63 and the TCA group of 7.29 on the HAM-D total score; these values were not significantly different. Nor did the end score differ significantly between the two groups (17.47 vs 19.39, respectively) after one week of treatment.

The HAM-D profiles changed markedly after 7 days of treatment in both groups (Fig. 1). The item scores for "Suicide", "Work and Activities", "Retardation", and "Loss of Weight" were still significantly higher in the TCA, and that for "Obsessive Symptoms" in the BNZ groups respectively.The items "Late Insomnia" and Insight", which were not different between treatment groups and baseline, were significantly lowered in the BNZ-group afte 7 days of treatment.

When covariance analysis was performed on the item scores before and after 7 days of treatment, significantly higher improvements appeared in the "Depressed Mood" item for the TCA group and in the "Agitation" item for the BNZ group (Table 2).

As displayed in figure 2, discriminant analysis on the differences between the initial and 7 day HAM-D item

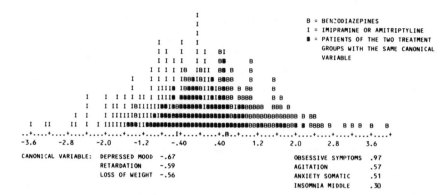

Figure 2 - Discriminant analysis on differences between initial and 7 day HAM-D item scores of patients treated with Benzodiazepines and with Imipramine or Amitriptyline. Distribution of subjects according to the canonical function.

scores isolated the items "Depressed Mood", "Retardation", and "Loss of Weight" in the canonical variable characterizing the therapeutic activity of BNZs. The overlap area is shown by the distribution of the patients along the canonical variable derived from discriminant analysis on the improvement obtained in the first 7 days of treatment. On the basis of the canonical variable, 36.0% of the BNZ-treated patients could be re-classified as assimilable to the group treated with tricyclic antidepressants, and 30.7% of the TCA-treated patients could be re-classified as assimilable to the BNZ group.

DISCUSSION

According to SCHATZBERG and COLE[4] in clinical practice as well as in a controlled therapeutic setting, BNZs are known to improve not only anxiety, but also sleep, agitation, and depressive mood, even if the benefits are limited. However, the findings which suggest that they may have positive effects in treating anxious depression are not sufficiently compelling to justify a change in their labelling.

On the other hand, several clinical studies[5,6,7,8,10,11,12] have been carried out to establish whether TCAs can adequately treat symptoms of anxiety. Besides the widely recognized efficacy of antidepressants in panic attacks, these studies have suggested that TCAs may be more effective than BNZ in other types of anxiety states[13].

While a number of studies have compared BNZs with TCAs in anxiety disorders, research comparing old and new BNZs with TCAs in depressive patients is still needed. In future research, the anxiolytic effects of antidepressants as well as the antidepressant effects of anxiolytics should be carefully evaluated.

The present study aimed to compare the therapeutic spectrum of activity of anxiolytics and TCAs has been carried out on clinical data recorded from population of subjects and made available by the Data Bank in the Clinical Psychopharmacology Data Documentation Center of Pisa.

The initial differences in psychopathological profiles, which showed a greater degree of anxiety in the BNZ group and a greater degree of inhibition in the TCA group, were accepted as a feature of this study favoring a better characterization of each treatment by reducing the overlap area between the two spectra of activity.

In our sample, changes in symptoms were quantified by means of the HAM-D. After 7 days of treatment the BNZ group showed a mean improvement of 7.63 and TCA group a mean improvement of 7.29; the difference between these figures was not significant.

When such improvement in the two groups was analysed comparatively by means of covariance analysis on the HAM-D item scores, only the item "Depressed Mood" displayed a significantly greater improvement in the TCA group, and only the item "Agitation" showed a significantly greater improvement in the BNZ group. This demonstrated that there is a wide overlap area in the initial therapeutic effects of the two treatments.

Thus, even when the items on the HAM-D most specific to depression were singled out for analysis, this did not allow the two drugs to be distinguished on the basis of their initial effects on the most typical symptoms of depression.

These findings seem to confirm the common view that the use of BNZs in depressives is justified because they take effect more rapidly than TCAs on a wide range of anxiety symptoms that are often found clinically in cases of depression.

The significant improvement rapidly produced by both treatments on the total score and on various items of depression and anxiety confirms that there is a vast area of overlap in therapeutic effect ranging from "Diurnal Variation", "Suicide", "Work and Activities" and "Retardation" to psychic and somatic anxiety. A visual image of this overlap is given by the distribution of the patients along the canonical variable, which reveals a considerable group of patients (about 30% of the subjects in each group) for whom the spectrum of activity of the two treatments was indistinguishable.

The psychotherapeutic profile of a drug is related not only to its chemical structures and to its pharmacodynamic properties, but also to the phenomenological characteristics of the patients treated.

If a compound produces an improvement both in depressed patients and in anxious ones, it may be called 'antidepressant' when given to melancholic patients and 'anxiolytic' when given to anxious ones[14]. When such a drug is tested on a strictly selected and uniform sample (purely anxious or purely depressive) which has been assessed with a very specifically targeted rating scale, its possible effects on the other psychopathological phenomenon are likely to be overlooked, in which case the definition of its spectrum of activity would appear in an incomplete form.

Comparative analysis of the improvement produced by the two different types of treatment - with TCAs or BNZs - on patients with an anxiety-depression complex, makes it possible to give a more comprehensive definition of these compounds' initial spectrum of activity.

In conclusion, these data again confirm previous findings[15] showing that anxiolytic drugs such as BNZs

possess a more powerful initial effect and a wider
spectrum of activity than TCAs on symptoms of anxiety
and agitation, and that there is a large overlap area
between the initial effects of the two classes of drug
on both depressive and anxious symptoms. It is an open
question whether the improvement in anxiety induced by
TCAs is secondary to their primarily antidepressant
effect, and, similarly, whether the improvement in
depression induced by BNZs is secondary to their
primarily anxiolytic effect.

REFERENCES

1. American Psychiatric Association: Diagnostic and
    Statistical Manual of Mental Disorders (Third
    Edition). Washington, D.C., APA (1980).
2. M. Roth and C.Q. Mountjoy, The Distinction between
    Anxiety States and Depressive Disorders, in:
    "Handbook of Affective Disorders", E.S. Paykel
    ed., pp. 70-92, Churchill Livingstone, Edinburgh,
    London, Melbourne, New York (1982).
3. H.M. Rhoades and J.E. Overall, The Hamilton
    Depression Scale: Factor Scoring and Profile
    Classification, Psychopharmacol. Bull. 1:91
    (1983).
4. A.F. Schatzberg and J.O. Cole, Benzodiazepines in
    Depressive Disorders, Arch. Gen. Psychiat. 35:
    559 (1969).
5. M. Roth and D.H. Myers, Anxiety Neurosis and Phobic
    States: Diagnosis and Management, Br. Med. J.
    1:559 (1969).
6. C.M. Zitrin, D.F. Klein and M.G. Woerner, Behavior
    Therapy, Supportive Psychotherapy, Imipramine
    and Phobias, Arch. Gen. Psychiat. 35:307 (1978).
7. D.S. Haskell, J.D. Gambill, G. Gardos, D.M. Mc Nair
    and S. Fisher, Doxepin or Diazepam for Anxious
    and Anxious-depressed Outpatients, J. Clin.
    Psychiat. 2:135 (1978)
8. D.V. Sheehan, J. Ballanger and G. Jacobsen, Treatment
    of Endogenous Anxiety with Phobic, Hysterical
    and Hypocondriacal Symptoms, Arch. Gen. Psychiat.
    37:51 (1980).

9. D.M. Mc Nair and R.J. Kahn, Imipramine compared with Benzodiazepine for Agoraphobia, in: "Anxiety: New Research and Changing Concepts", D.F. Klein and J. Rabkin ed., Raven Press, New York (1981).

10. D.V. Sheehan, J. Ballanger and G. Jacobson, Relative Efficacy of Monoamine Oxidase Inhibitors and Tricyclic Antidepressants in the Treatment of Endogenous Anxiety, in: "Anxiety: New Research and Changing Concepts", D.F. Klein and J. Rabkin ed., Raven Press, New York (1981).

11. A. Bjertnaes, J.M. Block, P.E. Hafstad, M. Holte, I. Ottemo, T. Larsen, R.M. Pinder, K. Steffensen and S.M. Stulemeijer, A Mulricenter Placebo-controlled Trial Comparing the Efficacy of Mianserin and Chlordiazepoxide in General Practice Patients with Primary Anxiety, Acta Psychiat. Scand. 66:199 (1982).

12. H.G. Nurnber and E.F. Coccaro, Response of Panic Disorder and Resistance of Depression to Imipramine, Am. J. Psychiat. 8:1060 (1982).

13. M.R. Liebovitz, Tricyclic Therapy of the DSM-III Anxiety Disorders: A Review with Implication for Further Research, Unpublished data.

14. W.W. Zung, The Role of Rating Scales in The Use of Antidepressants, Dis. Nerv. Syst. 37:22 (1976).

15. G.B. Cassano and L. Conti, Some Considerations of the Role of Benzodiazepines in the Treatment of Depression, Br. J. Pharmac. 11:235 (1981).

COMPARING FRENCH AND INTERNATIONAL CLASSIFICATION SCHEMES : IV. COMPARISON OF ANXIETY DISORDERS IN FRANCE AND THE UNITED STATES

C. B. Pull, M. C. Pull, and P. Pichot

Centre Hospitalier, 1210 Luxembourg and
Clinique des Maladies Mentales et de l'Encéphale
75014 Paris

INTRODUCTION

In a number of reports concerning comparisons of French and international classification schemes, the present authors have relied on a variety of different methods : evaluation of video-taped interviews[1], comparison of diagnostic stereotypes[2], computer programs[3], phenomenological classification[4], national enquiries[5] or investigations[6], and analysis of textbook descriptions[7]. Recent French studies in this field are based on Lists of Integrated Criteria for the Evaluation of Taxonomy (L.I.C.E.T.)[8,9].

Up to now, however, there are no empirical data on the field covered by the DSM III[10] category of Anxiety disorders and it would be hasardous, in this changing area, to base an account on what is described in psychiatry textbooks. It is for those reasons that the authors of the present report decided, "faute de mieux", to adopt an original, but hardly scientific method to compare DSM III and the French classification of Anxiety disorders.

METHOD

All three authors have been extensively involved with DSM III since 1978, first by participating in one of the field trials, and then in the French translation. It rapidly became apparent that the new American classification had taken a significant step towards traditional French nosology on several major positions, which consequently were perfectly understandable to French clinicians. Other positions were bewildering,

and among those the chapter on Anxiety disorders was probably
the most intriguing. For eighteen months, the translation group
met regularly and adopted four successive positions on Anxiety
disorders. Initially, the new DSM III category seemed to depart
radically from other classification schemes, and in particular
from the French one. After some time, the category was considered new in style but hardly in substance. A third examination
was necessary to identify the fundamental changes introduced
in this field by DSM III, which in turn led to a questionning
about the reasons that produced them.

In the following, the four successive phases experienced
by the French translation team will serve as a guideline to
the comparison of anxiety states in France and in the United
States.

PHASE I : Bewildered

For French clinicians, a first approach to the DSM III
chapter on Anxiety disorders can only lead to complete bewilderment. In French nosology, anxiety is considered to be part
of a number of disorders, but not to be a disorder in itself,
even if it dominates the clinical picture. As a consequence,
the mere existence of this chapter comes as a surprise. The
second shock is provided by the terminology adopted to classify the different anxiety disorders. DSM III introduces a number
of new concepts, not to be found in any French psychiatry
textbook. Moreover, some of these new terms simply can not be
translated into correct French. The French translators decided,
after many discussions, to adopt a litteral translation and
thus to sacrifice good French. Prominent translation problems
and possible solutions retained in the French translation of
DSM III are given in table 1.

Table 1. French translation problems for anxiety
disorders

Anxiety disorders = Troubles anxieux
Panic disorder = Trouble : Panique
Panic attacks = attaques de panique
Generalized anxiety disorder = Trouble : Anxiété généralisée
Post-traumatic stress disorder = Trouble : Etat de stress
post-traumatique

The fact that the term neurosis has either been discarded
to qualify the disorders listed in this chapter or relegated
between brackets for some of them will probably be a matter of
great concern to many French clinicians, but this would seem
to apply to many American clinicians as well. The reasons for
this major change in terminology are, however, extensively

discussed in the introduction to DSM III. They may not necessarily be accepted by French clinicians, but they could hardly be misunderstood.

PHASE II : Reassured

One of the great advantages of DSM III concerns the fact that every category is described by clearly defined operational criteria. Moreover, DSM III provides a very thorough preliminary description for every category, with in particular clear indications concerning its differential diagnoses. On the basis of these descriptions and diagnostic criteria, it rapidly became apparent to the translation team that cases of anxiety disorders as described in DSM III could easily be classified in one or the other subcategory listed in category 10 "Neuroses and neurotic states" to the French classification of Mental Disorders [11] (table 2).

Table 2. Initial equation of DSM III and
French categories

Agoraphobia, with or without panic attacks, social phobia and simple phobia would be classified in the single category "Phobic Neurosis" (INSERM 102).

Panic disorder and Generalized anxiety disorder would be classified in the simple category "Neurotic anxiety states. Anxiety neurosis" (INSERM 100).

Obsessive-compulsive disorder obviously corresponds to "Obsessional neurosis" (INSERM 103).

Finally, post-traumatic stress disorder, acute and chronic or delayed would be classified under "Acute or chronic reactive state with neurotic symptomatology" (INSERM 106 and 107).

There are, however, no diagnostic criteria nor any other definitions included in the French classification of mental diseases. The French classification, established by the Institut National de la Santé et de la Recherche Médicale (INSERM) is a simple nomenclature without glossary, and as such may lead to erroneous conclusions when compared directly with more explicite classification schemes.

On the other hand, the use of a glossary might not be sufficient to recognize immediately what is basically new in the DSM III classification of anxiety disorders. ICD-9 [12] categories pertaining to this field would probably be equated to DSM III concepts in a way similar to the one presented above.

PHASE III : Intrigued

In course of time, it became apparent to the members of the translation team that the four equations presented above could not be maintained.

French clinicians adhere to the psychoanalytic concept of phobic neurosis as a specific structured neurosis in which anxiety is deplaced to an object or situation symbolizing unconscious conflict. In this acceptance, agoraphobia, social phobia and simple phobia are basically equivalent symptoms characterizing a single disorder. DSM III, on the contrary, subdivides phobias into three separate categories. The reasons provided in DSM III concern "differing clinical pictures, ages at onset, and differential treatment response". This is a new position, which departs radically from the French acceptance of the phobias.

The same applies to the separation of Panic disorder and Generalized anxiety disorder. According to DSM III, there is compelling evidence that Panic disorder, as a distinct entity, has differential treatment response as compared with other disorders in which anxiety is prominent. The French concept of anxiety neurosis combines the two preceding categories and anxiety attacks are viewed as acute, diffuse physical and mental manifestations of anxiety occuring on a chronic state of persistent anxiety. The approach taken in DSM III may thus not be equated with traditional French nosology.

The description provided in DSM III for Obsessive-compulsive disorder corresponds closely to the French acceptance of "Obsessional neurosis". There is, however, in the latter a reference to psychoanalytic theory and defense mechanisms that has been discarded in the DSM III description.

In the end, the equation concerning Post-traumatic stress disorder was the only one of our four initial equations that could be maintained without restraint.

PHASE IV : In search of a rationale

The inadequacy of the three first equations established in phase II and the identification of what is fundamentally new in the DSM III classification of Anxiety disorders led of necessity to a search for the rationale underlying the changes introduced in the new American classification.

Part of the rationale is clearly exposed in DSM III itself. The general approach taken in DSM III is atheoretical with regard to etiology or pathophysiological process. Although

the terms "neurosis" and "neurotic" possibly might be defined
in a purely descriptive way, they are obviously used as well
by most clinicians to indicate the etiological process defined
by psychoanalytic theory. In addition, a number of other
theories have been developed in this field, during the last
decades, such as social learning, cognitive, behavioral, and
biological, for which the neutral term "disorder" might be more
appropriate.

On the other hand, the subdivision of phobic disorders in
agoraphobia, social phobia and simple phobia is a classic subdivision in learning theory, and the DSM III statement about
differential treatment response would make little sense outside
of behaviour therapy. It would thus appear that DSM III is not
completely devoid of any theoretical orientations and that
learning and behaviour theories in particular had an impact on
its development. The composition of the advisory committee
(Marks, Gelder, Saslow) on anxiety and dissociative disorders
is revealing in this context.

The fact that DSM III might not be as atheoretical as
stated in the introduction also emerges in the position adopted
on Panic disorder, its separation from Generalized anxiety disorder, and its implication on the development of Agoraphobia.
Although there is no reference to either tricyclic treatment
or to lactate metabolism and its possible relation to anxiety
in DSM III itself, the classification approach adopted in this
field is probably best suited for biological theories on
anxiety. In this context, the presence of D. F. Klein on the
committee could hardly be a coincidence.

CONCLUSIONS

The disorders assembled under "Anxiety disorders" in
DSM III represent a radical departure from traditional classification schemes in what concerns their grouping as such, their
terminology, and their sub-divisions. Without intending to
take position on the theoretical and practical implications of
the DSM III approach in this field, the authors of the present
report would advise not to equate the new American categories
to traditional concepts of other classifications, but to assess
their validity and reliability through both empirical and comparative studies.

REFERENCES

1. R. E. Kendell, P. Pichot, M. von Cranach, Diagnostic
   criteria of English, French and German psychiatrists. Psychol. Med., 4, 187 (1974)
2. P. Pichot, R. Bailly, J. E. Overall, Les stéréotypes

diagnostiques des psychoses chez les psychiatres
français. Comparaison avec les stéréotypes américains, in : Proceedings of the 5th C.I.N.P.,
H. C. Cole et al., eds., Excerpta Medica, New
York (1967)

3. C. B. Pull, P. Pichot, J. E. Overall, Comparison of
French and American Diagnostic Practices for
Schizophrenia and Depressive Disorders, Psycho-
pharmacol. Bull., 16, 43 (1980)

4. C. B. Pull, P. Pichot, J. E. Overall, Une classification syndromique des maladies mentales. III :
Comparaison des stéréotypes français avec les
stéréotypes américains, Ann. Méd-Psychol., 1,
109 (1977)

5. P. Pichot, Definitions of the limits of the schizo-
phrenia in France, in : World Issues in the
Problems of Schizophrenic Psychoses, T. Fukuda,
H. Mitsuda, eds, Igaku-Shoin, Tokyo (1979)

6. C. B. Pull, M. C. Pull, P. Pichot : Etude Nationale
sur les Critères de Diagnostic des Psychiatres
Français dans les Psychoses Non-Affectives : Pre-
miers Résultats, Comptes rendus du Congrès des
Psychiatres et Neurologues de langue Française,
P. Sizaret, ed, Masson, Paris (1981)

7. C. B. Pull, P. Pichot, Comparing French and International Classifications Schemes. V : DSM III
and the French position on organic brain syndromes, Proceedings of the VII World Congress of
Psychiatry, P. Berner, ed, Plenum Press, London
(1982)

8. C. B. Pull, M. C. Pull, P. Pichot, LICET-S : Une
Liste Intégrée de Critères d'Evaluation Taxinomi-
ques pour les Psychoses Non-Affectives, J. Psych.
Biol. Thérapeut., 1, 33 (1981)

9. C. B. Pull, M. C. Pull, P. Pichot, LICET-D : Une
Liste Intégrée de Critères d'Evaluation Taxinomiques pour les dépressions, Psychol. Méd. (in press)

10. American Psychiatric Association, Diagnostic and
Statistical Manual of Mental Disorders (3rd edn.,
DSM III), A.P.A., Washington D.C. (1980)

11. Institut National de la Santé et de la Recherche Médicale, ed, Classification française des troubles
mentaux, Bull. de l'INSERM, 24, Suppl. to N° 2
(1969)

12. World Health Organization, Mental Disorders, Glossary
and Guide to Their Classification in Accordance
with the Ninth Revision of the International
Classification of Diseases, W. H. O., Geneva
(1978)

THE DELUSIONAL MISIDENTIFICATION SYNDROMES: CONCEPTUAL

FRAMEWORK AND AREAS OF RESEARCH

George N. Christodoulou

Department of Psychiatry
Athens University, Medical School
Eginition Hospital, 74,Vassilissis Sofias Avenue,Athens

INTRODUCTION

The ancient Greek myth of Alcmene's "innocent" infidelity has apparently provided the original denomination of the syndrome of Capgras, the most frequently encountered delusional misidentification sub-type.Capgras and Reboul-Lachaux (1923)termed this syndrome Illusion des "Sosies" and it was 6 years later that the syndrome acquired the denomination "syndrome de Capgras", after the distinguished French psychiatrist Joseph Capgras.

Σωσίας (sosie, double) was the servant of Amphitryon, husband of Alcmene and King of Tiryns. Zeus, who was notorious for his infidelity, once decided to have a love affair with Alcmene, famous for her beauty but also, by an unfortunate coincidence, for her virtue. In order to succeed in his erotic operation Zeus asked Hermes to assume the appearance of Sosias (and thus Hermes became the double of Sosias) and Zeus himself, disguised as Amphitryon succeeded, according to one version in having a sexual relationship with Alcmene which resulted in the birth of Hercules. The ancient Greeks projected their own image in their Gods and this explains the human "weaknesses" of Zeus.

The syndrome des "Sosies" should perhaps more appropriately be called the syndrome of Hermes, because Hermes was the one who underwent changes in order to look like Sosias and not Sosias. Thus, Hermes was the double of Sosias and not vice versa.

Four syndrome sub-types are included in the framework of the delusional misidentification syndromes :

1. The syndrome of Capgras (described by Capgras and Reboul-Lachaux in 1923), the best known variety. This syndrome is a delusional negation of identity of a familiar person (or persons). The patient believes that a person well-known to him, or more often to her, has been replaced by a replica double.

2. The syndrome of Frégoli (described by Courbon and Fail in 1927). This variant is characterized by false identification or a familiar person (usually the patient's persecutor) in various strangers.

3. The syndrome of Intermetamorphosis (described by Courbon and Tusques in 1932) is similar to the Frégoli syndrome. It differs from it in that the patient claims that the persecutor and the misidentified strangers have not only psychological similarities (as in the Frégoli syndrom) but also physical similarities.

4. The syndrome of subjective doubles (Christodoulou, 1978). This sub-type is characterized by the patient's delusional conviction of other people's physical transformation into his own self.

Very often various combinations of these syndrome sub-types occur in the symptomatology of the same patient.

The setting in which the delusional misidentifications develop is always that of a psychosis (either functional or organic).

Vié (1930) distinguished the syndrome of Capgras from the syndrome of Frégoli, characterizing the former as illusion of negative doubles and the latter as illusion of positive doubles. Similarly, the present author (Christodoulou, 1976, 1977)· regards the syndrome of Capgras as a hypoidentification and the syndrome of Frégoli, the syndrome of Intermetamorphosis and the syndrome of subjective doubles as hyper-identifications.

The delusional misidentification syndromes have been studied extensively from the clinical and the psychodynamic points of view and, in recent years, from the point of view of organic participation in their pathogenesis.

The pathogenetic rôles of depersonalization-derealization phenomena, false memories of familarity, of the déjà vu and déjà vecu type and autoscopic experiences (with reference to the syndrome of subjective doubles) have been pointed out in the literature. Psychological mechanisms, such as projection, ambilalence, splitting of the object and concretization of mental representation have been proposed by psychodynamically oriented authors, the rôle of archaic modes of thought has been stressed, organic factor such as cerebral dysrhythmia, cerebral ischaemia, head trauma, hypothyroidism, pseudohypoparathyroidism, ECT prosopagnosia, reduplicative paramnesia, have been proposed as aetiological or contributory factors and reduced MAO activity has been suggested as a possible biochemical marker.

Some of the above aspects will be presented and discussed in the presentations that follow this introduction.

The delutional misidentification syndromes are important not only on account of their spectacular and colourful clinical presentation but also because through them, the mechanisms involved in the genesis of delusions can be more fully understood. Additionally, although the existing evidence does not justify their consideration as markers of organicity, yet, their frequent occurence in association with organic states helps to orientate the physician towards a careful search for (and management of) organic pathogenetic contributors.

REFERENCES

Capgras, J., Reboul-Lachaux, J., 1923, Illusion des "Sosies" dans un délire systematisé chronique, Bull. Soc. Clin. Med. Ment., 11:6.

Christodoulou, G.N., 1976,Delusional hyper-identification of the Frégoli type. Organic pathogenetic contributors, Acta Psychiat. Scand., 54:305.

Christodoulou, G.N., 1977, The Syndrome of Capgras, Br.J.Psychiatry, 130:556.

Christodoulou, G.N., 1978, Syndrome of subjective doubles, Am.J. Psychiatry, 135:249

Christodoulou, G.N., 1978, Course end prognosis of the syndrome of Doubles, J. nerv. ment. Dis. 166:68.

Courbon, P., Fail, G., 1927, Syndrome d' illusion de Frégoli et shizophrénie. Bull. Soc. clin. Med.Ment., 15:121.

Courbon, P., Tusques, J., 1932, Illusion d' intermétamorphose et de charme. Ann. Med. Psychol. 90:401.

Enoch, M.D., Trethowan, W.H., 1979,"Uncommon psychiatric syndromes", Wright, Bristol.

Vié , J., 1930, Un truble de l' identification des personnes. L' illusion des sosies. Ann. Méd. Psychol., 88:214.

Bogousslavsky, J., Salvador, A., 1981, Le syndrome de Capgras, Ann. Méd. Psychol., 139:949.

Merrin, E.I., Silberfarb, P.M., 1976, The Capgras phenomenon, Arch. Gen. Psychiat., 33:965.

CAPGRAS IN HIS DAY,

AN INTRODUCTION TO AN EPISTEMOLOGY OF THE SYNDROME

Luauté J.P., Bidault E., and Forray J.P.

Centre Hospitalier Service de Psychiatrie Générale
Boulevard Rémy Roure
26100 Romans France

When Joseph Capgras and his assistant Reboul Lachaux reported in 1923 about "l'illusion des sosies dans un délire systématisé chronique" they had probably no idea of the interest that the syndrome identified by the name of Capgras would awaken in the subsequent generations of searchers and this symposium is, sixty years afterwards, a form of tribute to him.

Joseph Capgras' three reports [3,4,5] about this matter gave the impulse to the description of other delusional misidentification syndromes and to a number of studies referring to the psychodynamical significance of these disorders.

In fact, and from the very beginning, the syndrome will have offered a preferred field of application for this type of interpretation, so much the patient's affectivity is committed in this particular process of non recognition of his closiest relations and so much delirium assumes by this reason a clearness, even a significance whose evidence is likely to convince of the correctness of the interpretation.

In our opinion this impulse was originated in Capgras' postulate to the effect that there was no perceptive nor mnesic disorders, as the syndrome was to be understood from purely psychogenic data.

Most of those who will study the syndrome then will adopt this postulate and with the exception of a few isolated writers only in recent years was the initial concept reconsidered to some extent after the frequency of organic brain lesions had been evidenced, thereby giving rise to new possibilities of interpretation.

The examples of such a change in evaluation are very few, with the possible exception of Kanner's autism, it shows the high interest that some organicist psychiatrists give the syndrome that continues in arousing a passionate attraction in those who believe in psychodynamical psychiatry for easily understood reasons.

We have thought it might be of interest to seek in Capgras' works how he was led to this specific concept and the extent to which it was accounted for by the then prevailing ideas.

We do not think that we shall prejudice Capgras'credit by observing that the fact that the word "sosie" in its usual meaning exists in the French language was probably a favourable factor permitting the expression of this type of disorder by patients and its identification by psychiatrists as a delirium thema.

This word of the French language literally designates a person who is an accurate copy of another person.

In the practice such a likeness which would correspond to the idea of "double" cannot exist (with the exception of identical twins), and in the usual language, sosie means a person whose likeness with another person is very great.

In our opinion, when patients use the word sosie they give it the meaning we have just explained and this relative likeness is an explanation to the fact that the original person and the sosie – an impostor – TODD[10] are distinct persons and hence this search for differentiating features which is one of the unique characteristics of this syndrome.

Joseph CAPGRAS was born in 1873. He had a very successfuel school career in Toulouse and was a resident medical student there. Next, he came to Paris to be a resident student at Asiles d'Aliénés de la Seine (he was number one at the competitive examination of 1898). Let us not forget that he was Paul Sérieux' student and preferred assistant and by this reason he was a further link in a line of famous mental specialists, since Sérieux has been an assistant and follower of the great Magnan.

In France, Joseph Capgras is not known so much by his syndrome but above all as the co-author (with Paul Sérieux) of a masterly work issued in 1909 "Les Folies Raisonnantes" (Reasoning Madness)[9] with the subtitle "Le Délire d'Interpretation" (the Delusion of Interpretation).

This monograph was the result of research work initiated by
Sérieux as early as 1890 at Magnan's suggestion. It is an essential
factor if the syndrome defined later is to be understood. The
authors report about a chronic systematized psychosis, that is
characterized by its mechanism a "delirious interpretation". The
work is well in line with the French psychiatric tradition and is
one of its masterpieces ; the clinical description is the major
part of the work and it is noteworthy to notice that the section
"origin and causes" is reduced to a few pages only.

When describing the mechanism of a delirious interpretation,
the authors make an analogy with the physiological (sic) interpretations which are typical of passionate states.

The conventional comparison : passion — madness is discussed
with reference to many writers and more particularly to Théodule
Ribot and large abstracts of his work "La logique des sentiments"
are quoted. Their object is to explain the evolution of mental
illness by an "emotional reasoning, a logic of feelings". The
origin is an emotion that fixes an idea, withdraws it from any
logical evaluation resulting in an "idéa-emotional complexus",
developed on an anomaly, an aberration of the personality, of
paranoia kind. Like Kraeplin, the authors stress the fact that
intellectual functions are not altered ; it cannot be otherwise.

With this psychogenic theory of paranoia, Sérieux and Capgras
take a pattern and formulas first introduced by RIBOT and link up
with the preceding views of the initial dynamic psychiatry,
ELLENBERGER[6] but they acknowledge BLEULER's concept of idea-emotional
complexus — Bleuler had just published in 1906 a work on affectivity
and paranoia — and in this way they already refer to Jung ans the
newborn psychoanalysis.

Now, if we examine 1923 editio principe[3], we find the basic
definition of the syndrome as agnosia of identification. The
original individual vanishes and is substituted by a sosie from
whom he differs — as mentioned above — by particulars.

Capgras and Reboul Lachaux give for this the following pathogenic
interpretation : first, they give a short summary of the normal
mechanism of recognition, using the concept of image that was at
the basis of the associationist idea in the views of Taine, Binet,
Ribot and Bergson as mentioned later.

They complete the previcus pattern with the idea of a conflict
between the emotional elements that accompany sensorial and
mnemonic images.

This conflict leads to recognition with more or less ease, depending on the prevalence of feelings of familiarity (when near relations are concerned) over the feeling of strangeness. In the case under study, as the latter feeling is very strong, both images, although they are identical cannot coincide by reason of a different emotional factor, they are not identified despite their likeness ; this interpretation involves both a recognition (thereby eliminating any perceptive and mnesic deficience) and a non-recognition that can be caused by an emotional factor only.

Intellectual integrity is absolutely necessary, the wrong emotional judgment is the key of the case.

The mechanism of recognition is most probably taken from BERGSON ; we were able to check that Capgras'library included the famous work "Matière et Mémoire" [2], published in 1896 In this work, the eminent philosopher discussed the idea of a double recognition :

- automatic and instantaneous recognition, in consequence of the feeling of familiarity

- attentive recognition which requires the use of memory images.

But the basic model of the work published in 1923 is "Les Folies Raisonnantes", by the way, the reference is stated clearly, and "l'illusion des sosies" is in fact acknowledged as a delirious interpretation based "first on emotional condition, then a turn of mind". The latter idea - used in "Les Folies Raisonnantes" corresponds to the paranoiac frame of mind "strong inclination to be suspicious, careful search of the slightest details".

This interpretation by means of paranoia and affectivity is confirmed yet with slight alterations in the paper published one year later in cooperation with Lucchini and Schiff [5]. This work is quite noteworthy by the importance given to organicity, most congruous and paradoxical since the "illusion des sosies", regarded as "the conclusion of a mental effort based on the analysis of correctly observed particulars", is found with a female patient suffering from a nevrotic syphilis that caused a mental, basically mnesic, deterioration.

In the same manner, the paper published by CARRETTE [4] in the same year "illusion des sosies et complexe d'Oedipe" scotomizes the part played by organicity even though the female patient is a probably deteriorated mentally deficient person with a primitive basedow. In this case, the illusion des sosies is invented in order to hide incestuous thoughts towards the father. The aim was to evidence the correctness of the Freud theory (by the way, Dr. de Saussure, a Freud follower had been requested to give his opinion). In the discussion of the paper, Hesnard – a psychoanalyst pioneer in France – has the satisfaction to comment that, owing to cases of the kind, there is a beginning of control of the psychoanalytic theory which permits to find the signification of delusion as opposed to "the disorder and incoherency that psychiatric tradition had assumed until then".

We saw in this connection that "Folies Raisonnantes" revealed an effort in order to understand the evolution of delirium, its pathogenesis, not its signification. Well, between a psychogenic concept of paranoia, accepted by most authors of the time and an illustration of the signification of a delirous syndrome by Oedipus complex, there was a gulf. Did Capgras allow himself to be led away by his assistants who co-operated to his works ? We have to admit that prevailing ideas at that time could not but push him towards this direction.

As a matter of fact, 1923 was the year of the official introduction of psychoanalysis in France since the yearly report of the Association des Médecins Aliénistes et Neurologistes was devoted to psychoanalysis and prepared by HESNARD. In 1924, HESNARD[8] writes "nowadays there is no psychiatric publication that does not include some hint to Freud ideas and no meeting of mental specialists where psychoanalysis is not discussed".

In his paper about "l'illusion des sosies et complexe d'Oedipe" Capgras provides data about the nosological position of the future syndrome by including it in the pattern of systematical non-recognition. By doing so, he established points of similarity with other events of same kind he had been interested in : pseudo-amnesia, repudiation of memories, more or less voluntary forgetfulness, feelings of "jamais vu". Later this concept was adopted immediately by another clinician full of genius : Gaëtan Gatian de CLERAMBAULT.

During this historical meeting, he joined in the discussion to claim that systematical non-recognition should be isolated and studied and furthermore to suggest an interpretation of the case under study based on the idea of love chagrin. It was a clear hint to another "basically French syndrome" FERDIERE[7] this syndrome will be designated by de CLERAMBAULT name and outlive him : erotomania or the delirious illusion that one is loved.

In the years 1920-1923, de CLERAMBAULT had read his famous papers on erotomania to the Society. CAPGRAS who was interested in the matter used to comment occasionally, which could give rise to lengthy controversial discussions. It is noteworthy to observe that there is nowadays a strong tendency to stress the frequency of an erotic or erotomaniac component in patients with Capgras'syndrome, and it is not unfrequent that both syndromes are associated.

At the end of this short survey, we believe it is quite a significant fact that Capgras and his followers were able, in the period 1923-1924 to produce a masterly description of the new syndrome on the one hand and prepared the way for the psychodynamic interpretation to come, on the other hand, that will be prevailing for years. In fact, the period concerned was at the end of the great classical period characterized by the search for entities and syndromes, by the genius of description, by a triumphant clinical approach - CAPGRAS was a heir to this tradition - it was also the beginning of the modern period tending to a generous search for significations, associated with the resort to doctrinal systems, BERCHERIE[1].

As a conclusion, we will quote an excerpt by the famous French-Catalan psychiatrist, TOSQUELLES "despite the fact that delusion of sosie is exceptional, its careful and polydimensional study makes a genuine princeps case in any approach to the psychopathological event and its complexity "He added : "not by reason of interest in folklore events have most conscientious and efficiency-minded psychiatrists analyzed these privileged cases".

References
1 - Bercherie P. - les Fondements de la Clinique - Ornicar ?Paris 1980
2 - Bergson H. - Matière et Mémoire - P.U.F., Paris 1970
3 - Capgras J., Reboul-Lachaux J. : l'illusion des Sosies dans un Délire Systématisé Chronique. Bull.Soc.Clin.Méd.Ment.1923,11,6-16
4 - Capgras J., Carrette P. : Illusion des Sosies et Complexe d'Oedipe - Ann.Med.Psychol.1924,82,48 - 68
5 - Capgras J., Lucchini P., Schiff P. : Du Sentiment d'Etrangeté à l'Illusion des Sosies. Bull.Soc.Clin.Méd.Ment.1924,121,210 - 217
6 - Ellenberger H.F. The discovery of the unconscicus Basic Books INC pub NY 1970
7 - Ferdière G : l'Erotomanie - Douin - Paris 1937
8 - Hesnard quoted by Bourguignon : Evol. Psychiat.1976 - 187 - 194
9 - Sérieux P., Capgras J. : Les Folies Raisonnantes, Laffite Reprints, Marseille 1982
10 - Todd. J. - the History of the syndrome of Capgras in "Historical Aspects of the Neurosciences" ; Raven Press N.Y.1982
11 - Tosquelles F. in Bieder J. : Délire des Sosies - Ann.méd. Psychol. 1973 659 - 673.

THE PSYCHOPATHOLOGY OF THE CAPGRAS SYNDROME

M. David Enoch

The Royal Liverpool Hospital
Prescot Street
Liverpool 7

In psychopathological terms the Capgras Syndrome is an intra-psychic affective conflict, resolved in an exclusive way by the splitting of the opposing feelings of love and hate and projecting the former on to an ideal object, albeit peripheral and absent, and the latter on to a double present in the patient's contemporary scene.

The delusion of doubles is the essential feature of the Capgras Syndrome. It is, in spite of often being termed the illusion of doubles, not an illusion; there is no distortion of the external object perceived. Indeed the patients themselves emphasise how identical the object is, especially initially, to the real person in all aspects.

My very first Capgras patient, which Dr. Rolf Strom-Olsen pointed out to me over a quarter of a century ago, swore that while the woman who visited him in hospital was not his wife but 'a double', she nevertheless resembled his wife in every respect. He said: "She looks like my wife, has my wife's eyes, my wife's face, she walks like my wife, but she is not my wife."

Thus the distortion occurs in the interpretation of the perceived object. The 'lesion' is within the patient.

And within the patient there is a fundamental <u>conflict of affect</u>. A love-hate clash. This state of affairs is the culmination of a deteriorating relationship between the patient and the object, usually a close relative, for example a spouse, and always a key figure in his or her emotional life.

Sometimes it is clear that there has been a deterioration in the interpersonal relationships. It may start within either, but certainly the patient becomes aware of it, and in most cases attempts to stem the tide of this deterioration by exhibiting greater zeal for it and with protestations of great love as if seeking reassurance and seeking to reassure.

This behaviour finds an echo in the alcoholic who is becoming impotent and jealous. He often shows a great increase in affection and sexual zeal and in both cases this increased zeal is counter-productive. The object tends to be repulsed and hence greater rejection ensues and greater deterioration occurs in the relationship.

There is a reality change within the patient. Feelings of rejection, anger and hatred ensue. This is in contradistinction to the previous held feeling of love, acceptance and warmth.

Here, therefore, we have the phenomenon of the fallen idol and now hate resides where love once reigned supreme. Both love and hate exist at the same time in the same person towards the one object. We have the problem of ambivalence.

The Capgras Syndrome is one exclusive, colourful way of solving the love-hate ambivalence problem. The love is projected on to an absent peripheral vague figure who is still imbued with all the good qualities which the original object, the ideal, possessed. The new hate is projected on to the person in the present situation who exists in the daily life of the patient but he becomes to be regarded as a double who has taken the place of the original object. Splitting, therefore, of the perplexing ambivalent, love-hate feeling occurs, and as Cargnello and Della Beffa have shown, the delusional experience of the patient now embraces three persons, namely the patient, the alter, the other, the person who is well known to the patient and the alias (the double or imposter).

The patient believes that it is the object that has changed where in reality it is he whose feelings have changed and who projects these on to the outside object.

Lord Brain in accepting the sense-datum theory states in his 'Mind, Perception and Science': "If objects in my perceptual world are in fact my own creation they can possess not only sensory characteristics but emotional ones too. The objects are imbued with these characteristics by a process of projection ....." He adds that, ".....much of what we perceive is our own contribution to the perceived object, and that an attitude to people may be influenced by emotional characteristics which we imagine them to possess....."

The English vocabulary emphasises this fact, for not only has it the word perception, but apperception, which is perception + emotion.

Hence, in the Capgras Syndrome, the 'bad' feelings are projected on to the object, present in the real, actual world of the patient and is regarded as the bad imposter. Indeed, often the patient himself will use the very words "double" or "imposter".

The word "imposter" implies not only a double but a great hated double. This reminds me of the beautiful Welsh poem 'The Flower-Bed' by Crwys, one of the great poets of our time, in which he describes how mother created the flower border and tended it with loving care. Then one day he noticed a change in it - in that there were weeds present in the flower-bed and he cries out: "How did these arrogant imposters know that mother was becoming old?" "Sut Wyddai'r hen droseddwr hyf, fod Mam yn mynd yn hen."

In all recorded cases, whatever the primary diagnosis, the paranoid component is present. And there is here "the kernel of disguised truth" that axiomatically forms the core of all paranoid delusions.

Often the cases show clearly the stages in the development of the classical Capgras delusion as described by Todd. At first the patient merely has an intangible or intuitive feeling that the visitor was not her daughter but a double. Later she was perfectly satisfied that this was so and advanced reasons in support of her belief, namely, that the imposter was darker and shorter than her daughter. Lastly her rationalization reached a stage when she "recognised the pretender as one of her daughter's friends". i.e. from 'a mere feeling' to partial delusion to complete delusion.

Capgras himself emphasised the initial change in feeling that occurs and is quoted by Coleman as saying "that the illusion had been determined by the occurrence of feeling of strangeness or foreignness, which was in contradistinction to that of recognition."

Coleman, one of my predecessors at Runwell Hospital, himself (quoting Courbon) describes how a change in feeling towards an object is first recognised as internal, with further deterioration the patient rationalizes the feeling to non-recognition of the object.

"In the 'Capgras delusion' as a result of the affective disorder, the subjective experience has been projected into the outer world. The psychotic now believes that it is the object which has changed and which no longer produces the same effect on him." There is affective, distorted perception. This may, and is termed by some, 'psychotic cognition'. This reminds us that usually psychotic cognition means a more generalised confusion with disorientation for time, place and person, defect in memory, lack of grasp and deficient concentration and attention; in other words the organic reaction type of syndrome with organic confusion, delirium or dementia.

However, in the Capgras delusion we may have psychotic cognition, but it is significantly narrow and selective. And this is one feature which has always intrigued me about this syndrome.

Equally important is the fact, as Stern and McNaughton have pointed out, that "the fundamental value of perception such as colour, perspective etc. are unchanged", though they add that "there is a primary change of the experience which cannot be defined further."

Brochado (63) compared these changes of experience with certain altered states of consciousness in epilepsy, for example depersonalization and déjà vu. These altered states, however, may occur in other conditions such as depression and hysterical states (Ganser Syndrome). But certainly depersonalization often occurs in the initial stage of development of the Capgras delusion.

There is a fundamental change in the reality world of the patient due directly to his disordered affect. Disordered affect leads to distorted changed reality.

As indicated above, the selective exclusiveness of the Capgras delusion is intriguing. It is suggested by Mikkelsen and Gutheil that the answer may be found in the personal familial history of the patient. They emphasise that the delusion occurs "when profound disappointments in family expectations of an object have occurred and imperfect identification of objects has been made or witnessed." They add that this proves the importance of exploring the family history and personal history of the patient in great detail.

They go on to make a striking claim that describing Capgras Syndrome as a clinical entity may detract the clinician from exploring family history and personal history in sufficient detail and depth. Their claim is based on the fact that they have noted that a great majority of reported cases and literature have been preoccupied with a diagnosis and labelling of the syndrome to the exclusion of investigating the full family and personal history and the therapeutic implications.

I accept their emphasis, that a full and detailed history is required to understand the patient's background and that it may well have therapeutic implications. I also accept the fact that they note that the Capgras Syndrome is a mode of communication. No doubt the Capgras delusion is conveying something about the patient's life, his feelings towards others and about deteriorating relationships between him and a key figure or key figures in his life.

As one who has been interested and researched into this syndrome and other rare syndromes for most of his professional life, I would also emphasise that, whereas we should not spend too much time and energy arguing about the diagnostic nosological, the position of the Capgras Syndrome whether it is a clinical entity or not, we certainly can accept it as a colourful syndrome with an exclusive psychopathology. And further, in studying it in depth and understanding it, albeit a narrow, limited, exclusive syndrome, we can find that it is a narrow gate into greater understanding of the broader spectrum of the paranoid states. In other words, in concentrating effort and research on a narrow front, we may break through and then find clues to the aetiology, psychopathology and treatment of paranoid conditions in general. And when we know the aetiology and the stages of development of these disorders, we will be more successful in our psychotherapeutic intervention for diagnosis, and the understanding of aetiology and psychopathology are merely the first steps in the successful treatment of any conditions.

OBJECT RELATIONS THEORY AND THE CAPGRAS SYNDROME

B. Frank Vogel

Director of Clinical Services
Mental Health Institute
Cherokee, Iowa   51012, U.S.A

Before I enter into the topic itself, let me give a brief
description of the syndrome and some relevant material drawn from
the object relations theory. I shall then attempt to apply this
to the Capgras Syndrome in an effort to elucidate this special
phenomenon of delusional misidentification.

The syndrome has been found particularly in schizophrenia, but
also in affective psychoses and in a number of cases of cerebral
dysfunctioning. My own clinical experience however, has been with
female schizophrenic patients. It is a relatively rare syndrome
and Wilcox and Waziri (1983) have stated that fewer than 500 cases
have been reported in the 50 years since the syndrome was first
described. The patient believes that a person, usually closely
related to him, has been replaced by an exact double. The term
"impersonator" or "impostor" rather than "double" is most often
used. The delusion assumes and maintains a nuclear dominating role
in the symptomatology even in the presence of other psychotic
features. It is a highly specific condition with a characteris-
tically constant clinical pattern (Vogel, 1974).

There has been growing interest in object relations for the
past 30 years on the part of developmental psychologists and
psychoanalysts. The contributions of Hartmann (1964), Jacobson
(1954) and Mahler (1955, 1975) have been most fruitful. Kernberg's
integrative studies (1975, 1980) also have included important contributions. Object relations theory has added considerably to the
understanding of patients with severe regressive states. This
theory can be defined as a special approach within psychoanalysis,
which examines clinical issues and metapsychological ones, in terms
of the vicissitudes of internalized object relations.

The earliest structures of the psychic apparatus evolve from successive stages of internalized object relations. These are: infantile autism, symbiosis, separation-individuation, and finally, object constancy. Object constancy is the capacity to unite the libidinal and the aggressive drives on the one hand, and to maintain the wholeness of the object on the other. When object constancy is poorly established and unstable, the individual, to protect valued parts of the self from attack by unwanted or bad parts, splits the warring elements apart and keeps them fenced off. Unconscious intrapsychic conflict always involve self and object representations. In psychosis, such dissociative mechanisms do have a stabilizing effect on the dynamic structures within an ego-id matrix, and permit contradictory aspects of these conflicts to present themselves simultaneously. Among these mechanisms the foremost are splitting and projective identification, and others include primitive idealization, denial, omnipotence, and devaluation. These defenses attempt to mitigate or to fragment intrapsychic conflicts so that the patient's painful ambivalence with significant persons is lessened.

There is most often a lack of differentiation between self and object representations in the earlier stages of ego development or, if regression takes place, there can be a fusion of those early self and object representations due to traumatic factors. This lack of differentiation of self and object representations will interfere with the maturation process and the necessary differentiation between self and object, and result in vague delimitation of ego boundaries as well as imperfect object constancy.

Frequently found in the early history is erratic mothering, with unpredictable alternation in the emotional distance between the child and the caregiver. Acceptance equally has been erratic, sometimes with a full emotional meeting and at other times with marked rejection, disparagement, disapproval and devaluation. Just as frequently, the emotional ambience is deficient and there is a long-lasting lack of adequate models for identification. In such infants, developing part-object relations progress poorly. As adults they appear to be the most devoted, long-suffering and catering of spouses, because reaction formations can be extremely powerful formations when the feared alternatives are abandonment and annihilation. They completely hold all aggression in check, and hostility seems absent even in the face of extreme provocation and hurt. Such individuals in their pre-psychotic period, have poor long-term relations with significant others. They see them as distorted and partially unreal, and they are unable to deal with them as whole people. I have also noted the appearance of overtly expressed sexual invitations to the spouse, when hate is turned into apparent syntonic lust. This seems to be a penultimate effort to change the spouse's denigrating and rejecting attitudes. When this endeavor fails, splitting and projective identification begin to

822

operate with maximum force. There is a projection of split-off parts of the self into the hated-loved person. An aim of this process is to forcefully enter into the object and control the object by parts of the self. Because of the aggression with which the object is cathected, further attempts to bring the opposed loving and hating images together, precipitate a great amount of anxiety.

Now the full Capgras Syndrome emerges, and should be seen as the resultant of many psychological vectors. To protect the fragile ego, torn endlessly between love and hate for the same object, there is a cessation of effort to fuse the contradictory aspects into one whole objdct. Splitting then becomes an active defensive operation and creates an all-good and an all-bad entity (Kernberg 1980). The all-good entity is maintained to be the true, all-loving, all-accepting spouse who has been killed or removed to a distance and who has been replaced by an impostor who is all-bad, unloving, and rejecting. It will be convenient to use Cargnello and Della Beffa's (1955) terms of "alter", for the all-good entity (the real person according to the patient) and the "alius", for the all-bad entity, (the impostor according to the patient).

This is the most stable psychopathological finding -- the un-shakeable conviction, delusional in nature, that an emotionally significant and hitherto intimate person has been replaced by a double. When this appears, a most unusual calm is exhibited by the patient. It is as if she had penetrated to the eye of the hurricane, and left the shrieking, buffeting gales without. Or, to change the analogy, as if by some act of self-exorcism, she had extruded into the alius and the alter the tearing and distressing burden she had for so long carried within her breast. Another striking observation at this phase is that the alius and alter are without life or sig-nificance for the patient, who seems to see them as removed papier-mâché figures. True, there are complaints about the alius -- the impostor -- but in almost a dispassionate way, as one might complain about poor weather interfering with an outing.

To conclude: in instances conducive to the development of Capgras symptomatology, there is, early in life, a pathological fusion or re-fusion of self and object representations, and conse-quently poor ego boundary structures and poor differentiation of self from non-self. The lack of synthesis of contradictory self and object representations into a well-functioning whole self-representation or whole object-representation interferes with estab-lishing object constancy. For the future, the train will be laid and a sufficient spark can set off the powder and a psychotic regres-sion will occur.

The Capgras Syndrome will then emerge as an ultimate, desperate holding action of immeasurable protective value. It defends against the feared fragmentation of the self. This is the ultimate fear.

It is the psychobiologic substrate of all anxiety, and is the traumatic state of psychotic helplessness feared beyond all other anxieties. (Rangell, 1983) The lesser of two evils is chosen and compartmentalization at the all-good, all bad level is a preferable and far less painful, alternative to chaotic fragmentation of good and bad concepts.

REFERENCES

Cargnello, D. and Della Beffa, A. (1955) L'Illusione del Sosia, Archivo Di Psicologia, Neurologia e Psichiatria 16:173

Hartmann, H. (1964) Essays on Ego Psychology, Int. Univ. Press, New York

Jacobson, E. (1954) The Self and the Object World: Psychoanal. Study of the Child 9:75

Kernberg, O. (1975) Borderline Conditions and Pathological Narcissism, Jason Aronson, New York.

Kernberg, O. (1980) Internal World and External Reality, Jason Aronson, New York.

Mahler, M.S. and Gosliner, B.J. (1955) On Symbiotic Child Psychosis: genetic, dynamic and restitutive aspects, Psychoanal. Study of the Child 10:195

Mahler, M.S., Pine, F., and Bergman, A. (1975) The Psychological Birth of the Human Infant, Basic Books, New York.

Rangell, L. (1982) The Self in Psychoanalytic Theory, J. Amer. Psychoan. Assn. 30:863

Vogel, B.F. (1974) The Capgras Syndrome and Its Psychopathology, Am. J. Psych. 131:922

Wilcox, J. and Waziri, R. (1983) The Capgras Symptoms and Nondominant Cerebral Dysfunction, J. Clin. Psychiat. 44:70

FREGOLI SYNDROME IN A MANIC SETTING

G.M. Triccas, A.P. Karkanias and G.N. Christodoulou

Athens University Medical School, Department of Psychiatry, Eginition Hospital, Athens, Greece

INTRODUCTION

Following its original description, by Courbon and Fail (1927), very few reports of the syndrome of Frégoli have appeared in the literature (Christodoulou, 1975; 1976).

Association of this syndrome with de Clérambault (1942) syndrome is of particular interest, in view of speculations that this association probably represents a common pathology.

A third reason that justifies presentation of this case is the appearance of the syndrome in a manic setting. To our knowledge association of the Frégoli syndrome with mania has not appeared in the literature previously. Additionally the differential response of the syndrome and the basic illness to ECT, administered to the dominant hemisphere, was thought to be of particular interest.

CASE REPORT

The patient is a good-looking, physically healthy, 18-year-old, shy and sensitive girl, with no personal history for physical illnesses and no family history for mental illness. She lived in a small village and was a high-school senior with excellent scholastic achievement.

In autumn 1981, she developed depressive symptomatology, clearly of the endogenous type, which lasted for six months. She received no treatment and being unable to cope she had to stop school. She recovered gradually and remained normothymic until the summer

825

of 1982, when she became cheerful, energetic, developed pressure of talk, psychomotor restlessness, uninhibited behaviour and erotic preoccupations. She started writing love letters and poems to a teacher of hers, claiming that he had fallen in love with her and that she was prepared to accept his marriage proposal. Her conduct inevitably led to her stopping school and, as her behaviour could not be controlled, she was admitted into hospital in a state of typical manic excitement, consistent with DSM III criteria. It was then that she first developed the Frégoli syndrome. She insisted that her therapist was in fact her hypothetical lover and, although she agreed that there was no physical similarity between the doctor and the lover, she nevertheless believed that these two persons were psychologically identical.

"Stop behaving like a stranger", she would plead her therapist. "I know you are John, only he is tall and blond and you are short and have a beard. Come on, grow up, take off your mask and take me in your arms".

At other times the patient would identify her hypothetical lover in members of the hospital staff, visitors, medical students and even persons of female sex. The patient's delusional hyperidentification occupied a central position in her symptomatology. She also misidentified various relatives of hers in nurses and occupational therapists, attributing the lack of physical similarity to the use of masks and wigs. Additionally she claimed that her own self was various different persons wearing the same face.

Routine laboratory investigation (hematological and serological tests, urinalysis) and chest and skull x-rays were normal. EEG, CAT scanning and prosopagnosia test were also normal. Thyroid scanning revealed a multi-nodular goiter but thyroid function tests (T3-T4) were normal. Rey's copy of a complex figure test and Benton's visual retention test provided some evidence of organicity but the over all picture was not conclusive. Wechsler's test revealed a difference of 35 points, between verbal and performance I.Q., in favour of the former (verbal 99 - performance 64).

The Figure shows the course of the patient's illness and the treatment she received. She failed to respond to haloperidol and carbamazepine. A course of 14 left-sided ECT sessions resulted in remission of her mania but had no effect on the Frégoli syndrome. Following ten days' normothymia, her manic symptomatology recurred, failed again to respond to carbamazepine and chlorpromazine but both her mania and the Frégoli syndrome responded to a course of eight bilateral ECT sessions. The patient was subsequently put on Lithium carbonate and remains normothymic and free from the Frégoli symptomatology.

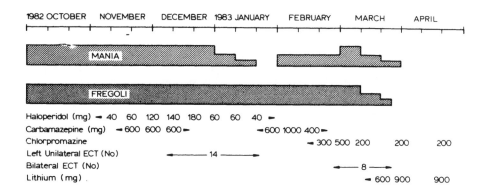

Fig. 1. Illness and treatment course of patient during hospitali-
    zation

DISCUSSION

Co-existence of the Capgras syndrome and erotomania has been
reported by a number of authors (Sims and White, 1973; Sims and
Reddie, 1976) and Pande (1981) has published a case in which there
is co-existence of incubus and the Capgras syndrome. Christodoulou
and Malliaras (1979) have drawn attention to the co-existence of
pronounced erotic admixtures in the symptomatology of patients with
the Capgras, Intermetamorphosis and Frégoli syndromes.

According to Barton (1978), this association may not be entirely a chance association. It probably indicates a common pathology, pertaining to the non-dominant hemisphere. Barton (1978) has
drawn attention to Flor-Henry's findings, which suggest that both
disordered recognition and hypersexuality are associated with right
cerebral hemisphere dysfunction.

The response of our patient to ECT merits commenting on. Since the delusional misidentification syndromes have been associated
with right hemisphere dysfunction (Wilcox and Waziri, 1983), it was

827

hypothesized that administration of ECT to the dominant hemisphere
would positively influence the patient's mental condition, but would
leave the Frégoli syndrome unchanged. This indeed proved to be the
case. On the contrary administration of bilateral ECT was equally
effective in the basic illness and the syndrome alike.

The response of the basic illness to unilateral ECT provides
some indirect evidence of left hemisphere dysfunction in mania.

The differential response of the syndrome to ECT provides e-
vidence supporting the notion of right hemisphere dysfunction in
the Frégoli syndrome. However, lack of EEG or convincing psychometric evidence, in this particular case, is not in favour of such a
hypothesis.

The lack of response of the syndrome, in contradistinction to
response of the basic illness to the initial (unilateral) course
of ECT, might alternatively be regarded as consistent with observations, which indicate that often the syndrome acquires a degree
of independence from the basic illness and that in general it tends
to respond with some latency to treatment.

REFERENCES

Barton, J.L., 1978, Neurological basis for syndromes and symptoms
        of disordered recognition? Am. J. Psychiatry 135: 1438.
Benton, A.C., 1965, Manuel de rétention visuelle. Editions du Cen-
        tre de Psychologie Appliquée, Paris.
Christodoulou, G.N., 1975, The syndrome of doubles; Associate pro-
        fessorship thesis, University of Athens.
Christodoulou, G.N., 1976, Delusional hyper-identifications of the
        Frégoli type. Organic pathogenetic contributors. Acta Psy-
        chiat. Scand., 54: 305.
Christodoulou, G.N. and Malliaras, D.E., 1979, Misidentification
        syndromes: erotic and psychomotor components, Am. J. Psychia-
        try 136: 994.
Courbon, P. and Fail, G., 1927, Syndrome "d'illusion de Frégoli"
        et schizophrenie Bull. Soc. Clin. Med. Ment., 15: 121.
de Clérambault, G.G., 1942, Les psychoses passionelles, Presses Uni-
        versitaire, Paris.
Flor-Henry, P., 1976, Epidepsy and psychopathology in: Recent Ad-
        vances in Clinical Psychiatry, Granville-Grossman K. ed.,
        New York, Churchill Livingstone.
Pande, A.C., 1981, Co-existence of incubus and Capgras syndromes,
        Br. J. Psychiatry 139: 469.
Rey, A., 1959, Test de copie d'une figure complexe. Editions de
        Centre de Psychologie Appliquée, Paris.
Sims, A. and White, A., 1973, Co-existence of the Capgras and de

Clérambault syndromes: a case history, Br. J. Psychiatry 123: 635.

Sims, A. and Reddie, M. , 1976, The de Clérambault and Capgras syndromes: a case history, Br. J. Psychiatry 129: 95.

Wechsler, D., 1958, The measurement and appraisal of adult intelligence. Williams and Wilkins, Baltimore.

Wilcox, J. and Waziri, R., 1983, The Capgras symptom and non-dominant cerebral dysfunction, J. Clin. Psychiatry, 44: 70.

AN EXPANDED CAPGRAS SYNDROME

W.A.G. MacCAllum

Purdysburn Hospital
Belfast, N. Ireland

SUMMARY

The advantages of having a wider concept of the syndrome are discussed with illustrations from cases and comparison with allied syndromes. It is the author's view that there is an organic component present in all cases. The organic component may be the dominant factor in some cases. In others it is the factor which determines the particular symptomatology of the syndrome, changing the emphasis from other aspects of schizophrenia or affective disorder towards having this substitute effect. There is a possible disadvantage in getting over-concerned about the semantics of whether to call it illusion or delusion or minimal delusion misidentification. There is an element of all of these factors present but the syndrome is amenable to the treatment of the physical condition if possible. The syndrome is beautifully placed to illustrate the necessity for psychiatrists to exhibit their general medical doctoring as well as their purely psychiatric skills.

INTRODUCTION

Capgras is to blame. He started it all and his name will stick, I hope, when others have vanished. The names of the early describers give a colourful aspect to the range of many diverse phenomenological groupings of symptoms making up the large variety of syndromes in Psychiatry.

But it should be pointed out that it has been Capgras[1] second case, published in 1924, which is sometimes taken as the caricature in a narrow portrayal of the syndrome. This schizophrenic patient, who felt that her parents had been replaced by doubles, is one of the earliest case histories published, which displays also the effect of expressed meotion, brilliantly demonstrated in the paper by Leff[2] et al. The first case published by Capgras[3] in 1923 was on a paranoid psychotic who had seen a "thousand doubles of her daughter" - rather different from those who would narrow the concept. These latter whilst writing about the syndrome using the pleural "doubles" nevertheless go on to describe "a double" - the singular e.g. Enoch, Trethowan and Barker[4] "the patient believes that a person, usually closely related to him, has been replaced by an exact double".

It has been my fortune to have come across nine cases of what to me have appeared to be within the Capgras phenomenon category. Like most others I had accepted the narrow confines of description available of the syndrome and the psychodynamic explanations. I began to have doubts about the wisdom of this. This resulted in my researches leading to the publication of the paper "Capgras Symptoms with an Organic Basis" by me in the British Journal of Psychiatry in 1973 (MacCallum[5]).

In that paper I described five cases. These have been added to by a further four whose case summaries are appended to the full paper, but the features comparatively will become obvious as I present the tables concerning all nine cases.

The first table shows that they have come from a variety of backgrounds as regards occupation, have variable marital status and are from both sexes. There is a wide range in age from a 28 year old young clerk to a 75 year old spinster. In this paper I have arranged them in chronological order by year of presentation to me. This has meant changing case number 4 of my former paper to the top of the list here.

I have shown two columns on doubling. With seven of the nine cases there were two distinct (in time) phases of doubling. So much for the frequent statements in papers that usually only one person is implicated and misidentified. It seems to me that the people or objects involved are those more closely related to the patient in the "here and now" situation rather than fanciful viewpoints trying to force upon us interpretations borrowing either from a psychoanalytical or an existential background. It would be very difficult for me to apply the theory expounded by Cargnello and Della Beffa[6] to fit my cases.

In my second table, the first few columns are to help you form the connection to the first table. I have in this table presented the main complaint or obvious feature at presentation. As is common in psychiatry, the patient himself had not been the instigator of the medical help, but instead a family or social contact. I hesitated to having orientation columns, but decided for them in view of my argument, later developed, that organic considerations now have a

TABLE 1   "DOUBLING" DATA

NO.	JOB	MAR. STA.	SEX	AGE	YR.	FIRST DOUBLING	LATER
1	Var.	S.	F	44	66	Med/nur.	Hospital
2	Fitter	Sep.	M	71	70	"Wife"	Brother
3	Clerk	S.	F	28	71	Nurses	Mother
4	Erector	M.	M	45	72	Wife	Children
5	Spinner	S.	F	75	73	Home-Help	—
6	T.U. Off.	M.	M	56	77	Wife	—
7	Baker	S.	M	21	82	Own Dr.	Psycht.
8	Tob. Work.	M.	M	36	82	Children	Wife
9	"Student"	W.	M	40	83	Parents	Sister

TABLE 2   OTHER MAIN FEATURES

NO.	JOB	SEX	AGE	OBVIOUS FEATURES	ORIENTATION		
					Tim	Pla	Per
1	Var.	F	44	Depress/Paranoid	Yes	-	+ / -
2	Fitter	M	71	Guilt/Embarrass.	Yes	Yes	+ / -
3	Clerk	F	28	Self-Awareness/ Stroke	Yes	Yes	+ / -
4	Erector	M	45	Par. Del. State	Yes	Yes	+ / -
5	Spinner	F	75	Anx./Par. Reaction	Yes	Yes	+ / -
6	T.U. Off.	M	56	Anx. - Wife's Reject.	Yes	Yes	+ / -
7	Baker	M	21	Withdrawal	Yes	Yes	+ / -
8	Tob. Work.	M	36	Exhaustion	Yes	Yes	+ / -
9	Student	M	40	Cult/Prof. Non-Adjust.	Yes	Yes	+ / -

TABLE 3   FURTHER PHENOMENOLOGY

NO.	JOB	SEX	AGE	CLOUDING	"Delusion"	Halluc.	Clin. Org.
1	Var.	F	44	Yes	Masquaraders	—	Persev. Abscess
2	Fitter	M	71	Uncertain	Imposter - Plot	—	Pneumonia Air Disease
3	Clerk	F	28	Yes	To be Poisoned?	—	Tem. R. H'plegia
4	Erector	M	45	Yes	Imperson- ators	Voices 2nd & 3rd pers.	Alc./ Chr. Path
5	Spinner	F	75	Uncertain	Food Poisoned		Malnut- rition
6	T.U. Off.	M	56	Yes	Fake Wife		Ch. Alc. G.M. Path Fits
7	Baker	M	21	—	Being Poisoned	Voices	Gr. Wt. loss

| 8 | Tob. Work. | M | 36 | Uncertain | Children Changed | Aud. Hall. | Tremor/ Sweats + + |
| 9 | Student | M | 40 | Uncertain | Masquar- aders | Pois. | Blur. Vis. Per. Neur. |

TABLE 4   ORGANIC ASPECTS AND TREATMENT

NO.	JOB	SEX	AGE	CLIN.ORG.	POS. SPEC. ORG.	TREATMENT
1	Var.	F	44	Persev.	Diabet. Glu. Tol. E.S.R. 49	Pen. Diabetic
2	Fitter	M	71	Pneumonia	Sput. B. Coli/ Sta. Aur. X-rays	Antibiot.
3	Clerk	F	28	Tem. R. Hemiplegia	EEG irreg. L R	Anaem. Treat.
4	Erector	M	45	Ac./Chr. Alc. Path.	LFT's up	Vits. Diazepam
5	Spinner	F	75	Malnutrit.	——	Shelter/ Vits.
6	T.U. Off.	M	56	Chr. Alc. Path. G.M. Fits	LFT's up, EEG R. Temp Foc.	Vits. Anti- Convuls.
7	Baker	M	21	Gr. Wt. Loss	——	Maj. Tranq.
8	Tob. Work.	M	36	Tremor/ Sweats	LFT's up	Maj. Tranq.
9	Student	M	40	Blur. Vis. Per. Neur.	——	Vits. Tranq.

TABLE 5   MAIN AETIOLOGY AND DURATION

NO.	JOB	SEX	AGE	CLIN.ORG.	MAIN FACTORS	SECONDARY FACTORS	DURATION
1	Var.	F	44	Persev, Abscess	Diabetes Mellitus	Recurr. Depress.	5 wks.
2	Fitter	M	71	Pneumonia	Toxicity	Privacy Exp.	2 wks.
3	Clerk	F	28	R. Hemi- plegia	Bas. Art. Migraine	Poss Mood Swings	10 days
4	Erector	M	45	Ac/Chr. Alc. Path.	Chr. Alc.		2 weeks
5	Spinner	F	75	Malnut.	Vit. Def.	Rehousing	10 days
6	T.U. Off.	M	56	Chr. Alc. Path. Fits	Ch. Alc. G.M. Fits	Reject. by wife	1 week
7	Baker	M	21	Gr. Wt. Ls.	Heb. Schiz.	I.Q. 71	4 wks.
8	Tob. Work.	M	36	Tremor/ Sweats +	Sleep Deprived	unusual excess Alc.	4 days
9	Student	M	40	Blur. Vis. Per. Neur.	Ac. Schiz. React.	diet. jetlag	4 weeks

definite place in the syndrome. It will be noted however that only in my first patient do I feel that the arguments for and against orientation in place are equally balanced. The others of course are in person.

Table three portrays further phenomenology. I have continued the process of keeping your orientation correct by including the same first four columns. In the column dealing with minimal clouding, I and my colleagues accepted clouding of consciousness as definitely present in four of the nine cases and probably present in four others.

I have included a column showing the main delusion expressed. Now it is I think very interesting that although there was use of the terms "wax models", "imposters" etc etc, the fact of being deluded about poisoning in four of the nine cases is significant. In British psychiatry poisoning delusions are comparatively rare in functional paranoid psychoses of different types, but instead make one suspect temporal lobe epilepsy.

I felt it necessary to include a column for hallucinations, but only three were so afflicted. Perhaps in a negative way this column is interesting in that one might have expected it to have advanced the cause of either side of the debate, but not so. My last column on this table shows the clinical organic state. It is readily seen that all the cases had organic conditions of variable severity. Some were obvious and severe but perhaps there are some psychiatrists whose clinical medicine skills have been neglected in the years of concentrating in certain extremely specialised aspects of psychiatry.

In the fourth table I have repeated some of the data to help you follow my arguments. I have inserted here the main findings of special testings carried out on patients. Only included are organic findings which are indisputably abnormal. Those showing abnormal liver function tests were very sick from that point of view indeed. I am quite sure that if proper testing had been carried out, especially in cases 5 and 9 early on before onset of multivitamin therapy etc, abnormalities in these fields would have been biochemically demonstrable. Case 7 had lost 25 kilograms in a schizophrenic apathetic withdrawn state over possibly three months and was appropriately treated as shown in the last column. The other cases were treated appropriately for their organic conditions as well as symptomatically for their anxiety symptoms etc which occur in many organic states.

In my fifth table I have linked the clinical organic state with the main and secondary factors in my Capgras syndrome cases. By this method you will notice that in the case of my first six patients, toxicity or biochemical/vitamin deficiencies or circulatory factors were the predominant features. Moreover in two of the remaining three cases the organic factors were as important almost and necessary for the syndrome development. Only in case number 7 do I feel that the weight loss was a secondary feature, but even it may have been determinant in the exact symptom-clustering of Capgras type because neither weight loss nor Capgras symptomatology has recurred in the past year.

Often authors have not commented on the duration of the syndrome - except that is in the early cases where modern treatments were unavailable. In all of my cases the doubling was of short duration. Note that in case 1 it recurred during two toxic episodes occurring until the proper diagnosis was established. Also in the last case jet lag and food inadequacies in three trips to the former home in Pakistan were involved. In all of these cases the response to the correction of the organic component was the significant factor in an early disappearance of doubling.

DISCUSSION

It would have been possible to have accepted an easy diagnosis of either affective disorder or psychotic state of schizophrenia or functional paranoid aetiology in most of these cases. I wonder has that happened to a number of cases from the past in the literature. Indeed as we tease out better understanding of the biochemical and other factors in the functional illnesses, will doubling become understandable as a transient state which in some people is called forth as a symptom grouping i.e. where the organic state or biochemistry is appropriate perhaps in some anxiety provoking situation which may indeed be produced by the organic state originally.

Christodoulou and Malliara - Loulakaki[7] (1981) surveyed 21 patients with delusional misidentification syndromes from the organic angle including 11 in a fairly tight Capgras syndrome symptomatology. Their study gave support to the organic factors, mainly from E.E.G. recordings including those cases in an apparently schizophrenic setting. In their paper they ally the Capgras syndrome with other closely related syndromes and recall as I did in my earlier paper the analogy with psychotic states in epilepsy described by Pond[8] (1957) and Slater and Beard[9] (1963).

Arieti and Meth[10] (1959) also considered this grouping of allied syndromes as did Enoch and Trethowan[11] (1979) in their updated 'Uncommon Psychiatric Syndromes' where they started acknowledging the organic contribution.

In their paper entitled 'Delusional Misidentification Syndromes and Cerebral Dysrhythmia', Christodoulou and Malliara - Loulakaki[7] grouped four rare different syndromes (as they perceived them) closely related to each other - Capgras[1,3] (1923,1924) (substitution

by doubles), Frégoli by Corbon and Fail[12] (1927) (false identification as persecutors), intermetamorphosis by Corbon and Tusgues[13]
(1932) (a Fregoli variant to include physical similarities) and subjective doubles by Christodoulou[14] (1978) (other peoples' transformation into himself). In this paper they showed the high
incidence of organic medical conditions aetiological in these
groupings. I have awaiting publication (MacCallum 1983[5]) another
related group, a syndrome where role changes by an important person
to the patient, is misconstrued by the latter. In this 'Syndrome of
Misinterpreting Role change as changes of Person' I describe my
cases of the caring daughter carrying out different duties in connection with being their husbands wives, their own professional jobs
and with being daughters etc, duties which were seen by their mothers,
who all suffered from cerebrovascular degenerative disease, as being
two or three different people.

The teasing out of these symptom-cluster formations is important, now five, but the relationship to temporal lobe epilepsy
must be very close in some. As I pointed out earlier four of my nine
cases had delusions of being poisoned which nowadays would lead me
towards a more vigorous E.E.G. investigation procedure in Belfast.
I would suspect uncal or temporal lobe irritation to be shown, where
with us delusions of poisoning are not part of a common schizophrenic
symptomatology.

I think it unnecessary for me to refer in detail to all this
recent comparative flood of papers collected by Enoch and Trethowan[11]
(1979) and Christodoulou and Malliara-Loulakaki[7] (1981), which stress
the part of organic factors in the precipitation of the syndromes of
Capgras type; and that is why now I seek an expanded concept. In
this syndrome we have a beautiful series of illustrations of the
intermixing of physiological and psychological reactions most frequently of an anxiety type. In this, the organism is trying to make
sense of a disturbed world as he sees it and is perhaps trying to
reduce his fears by partly inventing a possible escape route for his
sanity, as he sees it - a safety-first policy rather than acting out
aggressively. But factors go hand in hand, the seeing it in a be-
fuddled way and the attempt to decrease the anxiety (akin to the
being lost state of a child) by escaping into what might appear to
be a temporary delusion. Nowadays I would not be satisfied with
purely psychodynamic interpretations of Capgras syndrome. The
physical medicine side of psychiatry is at least as important and
for this condition in my opinion more so because it can then be
corrected quite quickly.

REFERENCES

1. J. Capgras and J. Carette, (1924) 'Illusion des sosies et
   complexe d'Oedipe'. Ann. Med. Psychol. Paris 82, 48.
2. J. Leff, et al. (1982) 'A controlled trial of social

intervention in the families of schisophrenic patients'.
Brit. Journal of Psych. <u>141</u>, 121-34.

3. J. Capgras and J. Reboul-Lachaux, (1923) 'Illusion des
    sosies dans un delire systematise chronique'. Bull. Soc.
    clin. Med. ment. <u>2</u> 6.

4. M.D. Enoch, W.A. Trethowan and J.C. Barker, (1967) 'Some
    Uncommon Psychiatric Syndromes'. Wright, Bristol 1 - 12.

5. W.A.G. MacCallum (1973) 'Capgras symptoms with an organic
    basis'. Brit. Journal of Psych. <u>123</u> 639-42.

6. D. Cargnello and A.A. Della Beffa, (1955) 'L'illusione del
    sosia'. Arch. psicol. neurol. e psichiat., <u>2</u> 173.

7. G.N. Christodoulou and S. Malliara-Loulakaki, (1981)
    'Delusional misidentification syndromes and cerebral
    dysrhythmia'. Psychiatria Clin. <u>14</u> 245 -51.

8. D.A. Pond (1957) 'Psychiatric aspects of epilepsy' J. Ind
    Med. Prof. <u>3</u> 1447-51.

9. E. Slater and A.W. Beard, (1963) 'The schizophrenic-like
    psychoses of epilepsy'. Brit. Journal of Psych. <u>109</u> 95-150.

10. S. Arieti and J.M. Meth, (1959) 'American Handbook of
    Psychiatry'. Vol. 1 New York, Basic Books, 548-50.

11. M.D. Enoch and W.H. Trethowan (1979) 'Uncommon Psychiatric
    Syndromes' Second ed. Wright, Bristol 1-14.

12. P. Corbon and G. Fail, (1927) 'Syndrome d'illusione de
    Fregoli et schizophrenie'. Bull. soc. clin. med. ment.
    <u>15</u> 121-24.

13. P. Corbon and Tusgues (1932) 'Illusion d'intermethamorphose
    et de charme'. Ann. Med. Psychol. (Paris) <u>90</u> 401-5.

14. G.N. Christodoulou, (1978a) 'Syndrome of subjective doubles'.
    Amer. Journal Psychiat. <u>135</u> 249-51.

15. W.A.G. MacCallum, (1983) 'Syndrome of Misinterpreting Role
    changes as changes of Person'. Awaiting Publication.

838

APPENDIX

(Cases 1 - 5 Described in Brit. Journal Psychiat. (1973) 123, 639-42)

Case 6. A 56 years old trade union official, a former patient with alcohol problems, had been admitted with a couple of grand mal fits to a general hospital. He recognised me immediately but the previous night had told his wife (and still remained convinced) that she was a fake. She had lost her temper then but to please this lady he agreed she was his wife - to her satisfaction - but he didn't believe it next day. Later when asked about it had said "My wife would not have lost her temper like she did. It was a very good fake". E.E.G. revealed a Right Sided Temporal focus and C.A.T. scan showed cortical atrophy with large ventricles. His wife just prior to his alcoholic relapse had a death of a sister and had rejected him. She accepted him again and helped him through the further relapses until he eventually entered a period of ongoing abstinence.

Case 7. A 21 year old baker was referred by a colleague who knew of my interest in the syndrome. He had claimed that the family doctor, called by the family, was a fake. When my friend Dr. Curran called he claimed that similarly for him, that he wasn't dressed like a doctor. He felt that his family was trying to poison him and kept picking out bits of bread saying that his former associates at the bakery were putting poison in the bread. He had complained of abdominal pain for six months and had withdrawn from company and had lost nearly four stones in weight. His I.Q. was 71. He heard "voices" discussing him in third person and said a voice said that both the family doctor and the psychiatrist were fakes. Eventually he gained insight on Chlorpromazine 400 mgms. daily shifting gradually to Cholpenthixole I.M. 40 mgms. fortnightly regaining improved socialisation and drive through the help of industrial therapy.

Case 8. A 36 years old tobacco factory employee had just returned from a weeks intensive part-time army training. The course had been exhaustive in preparation for dealing with terrorist activities but the camaraderie he had hoped to improve with nightly unaccustomed drinking of approximately two thirds of a bottle of Vodka (and not more than two hours sleep any night). "The children were asking questions too advanced for their ages . . .knew I was being tested by the army and police." He said he suddenly "knew" that the army had replaced his children with fakes. Later he felt that his wife had been replaced for a time. He said that they were in a radio car outside and would speak to him through the radio (which was turned off). He was in a very tense, sweaty, agitated stage. He had been knocked out in a football match four years previously and had rarely drunk alcohol. Liver function tests were grossly abnormal but we had already got him back to a regained insight settled state on Chlorpromazine before the results were obtained, and he has remained symptom free since a year ago.

Case 9. A 40 years old student of accountancy, an immigrant from Pakistan, was brought to my attention by Dr. Clenaghan, a psychiatrist colleague. He had first consulted neurologists because of blurred vision, but his sister had sought further help because he felt that someone had poisoned his sister and this masquarader of her was now attempting to poison him. He had a paranoid attitude towards food and a limited diet had produced peripheral neuritic signs. His history as he improved indicated two earlier episodes in 1975 and 1978 on journeys home to Pakistan to visit his parents. There had initially been three days confinement at the airport, querying his identity by the passport officials. He had felt that his real parents had died and been replaced by others who "adopted" him as if they were his parents. He had evidently got over the first two episodes with proper food, rest and support. On this occasion Chlopenthixol probably produced a speedier improvement.

PSYCHOMETRIC INVESTIGATION OF PATIENTS WITH DELUSIONAL

MISIDENTIFICATION SYNDROMES

Anna Kokkevi and George N. Christodoulou

Department of Psychiatry
Athens University, Medical School
Eginition Hospital, 74,Vassilissis Sofias Ave. Athens

INTRODUCTION

The term "syndrome of doubles" usually refers to the delusional negation of identity of familiar persons originally described
by Capgras and Reboul - Lachaux (1923). This rare phenomenon has
been explained on the basis of various pathogenetic frameworks summarized by Enoch et al (1967). Since the syndrome is characterized
by a separation of the normally intergrated functions of perception
and recognition, organic factors might be responsible for or might
contribute to the pathogenesis of the syndrome. This possibility has
been backed mainly by clinical observations (Gluckman, 1968; Weston
and Whitlock, 1971; Nilsson and Perris, 1971; Mac Callum, 1973; Hay
et al.1974; Hayman and Abrams, 1977) as well as by a study concerning 11 patients studied clinically and by EEG, echo-encephalogra-
phic, air-encephalographic and psychological methods (Christodoulou, 1977).

Following description of Capgras' syndrome three even more rare
clinical entities related to this syndrome have been reported, namely the syndrome of Frégoli (Courbon and Fail, 1927), the syndrome
of intermetamorphosis (Courbon and Tusques, 1932) and the syndrome
of subjective doubles or syndrome of doubles of the self (Christodoulou, 1975). Although these psychopathological conditions have
received less attention than the syndrome of Capgras there is clinical and laboratory evidence supporting the possibility of organic
participation to both the syndrome of Frégoli (Christodoulou, 1975,
1976) and the syndrome of subjective doubles.

Table 1. Characteristics of Patients with Delusional Misidentification Syndromes

Patient No	Age	Sex	Basic Illness	Syndrome	Years of schooling
1	47	F	Paranoid Schizophrenia	Capgras	12
2	52	F	Involutional Depression	Capgras	4
3	43	F	Paranoid Schizophrenia	Capgras	4
4	35	F	Hebephreno-Paranoid Schizophrenia	Capgras	0
5	40	M	Paranoid Schizophrenia	Capgras	6
6	64	F	Involutional Depression	Capgras	6
7	50	F	Paranoid Schizophrenia	Capgras	6
8	60	F	Involutional Depression	Capgras	6
9	43	F	Paranoid Schizophrenia	Capgras	2
10	18	F	Hebephreno-Paranoid Schizophrenia	Syndrome of subjective Doubles	10
11	26	F	Paranoid Schizophrenia	Frégoli	14
12	28	F	Organic Psychosis	Capgras	12
13	33	M	Paranoid Schizophrenia	Frégoli	8
14	20	M	Hebephrenic Schizophrenia	Frégoli	12
15	17	M	Hebephrenic Schizophrenia	Frégoli	9

The purpose of the present work is to investigate 15 patients presenting symptomatology compatible with three of the above syndromes with psychological tests considered useful in revealing signs of cerebral dysfunction. Since in most patients with delusions of doubles the misidentifications are primarily visual and in view of the key role of memory for the process of recognition and identification, in addition to the WAIS test, tests of visuo-spatial ability and visual memory were also used.

Brief reference to some of the psychometric findings of the Capgras and the Frégoli patients of the present material has been made elsewhere (Christodoulou, 1976, 1977). A detailed account of all the psychological test results of the entire group of patients will be presented here and the Wechsler test results of the patients will be compared to those of a control group for the purpose of rendering the results more reliable.

The present material consists of patients with three syndromes involving doubles but since all of them are in fact variations of a common psychopathological phenomenon they were grouped under a common denomination.

MATERIAL AND METHODS

Fifteen patients with delusional misidentification syndromes (10 with the Capgras variation, 4 with the Frégoli sub-type and one with the "syndrome of subjective doubles") were investigated (Table I).

The following psychological tests were used:
a) WAIS (Wechsler, 1958)
b) Benton's revised visual retention test (Benton, 1963) and
c) Rey's complex figure drawing test (Rey, 1965).

Since WAIS has not been standardized on the Greek population, this test was also administered to 15 Greek patients, used as controls. The two groups were matched for the following parameters:
a) basic illness, b) sex, c) age, d) educational level, e) urban vs. rural residence and f) I.Q.

A translated and adapted to the greek population form of the WAIS test was used. No controls were thought to be necessary for Benton's and Rey's tests because both tests can be considered as culture-free. Benton's test was administered in the following way: two forms of the test were used for each patient according to the A mode of administration (Benton, 1963). The mean number of correct points of the two forms was compared to the score expected from the I.Q. and the age of the patients. A score of two points below the expected score was considered as raising the question of impairment of the intellectual functions (±). A score of three points below the expected score was considered suggestive of impairment (+) and

843

a score of four or more points below the expected score was considered as strongly indicating such an impairment (++).

Rey's "complex figure" test was administered as follows: The
patient was first asked to copy the figure while his performance was
timed. The scoring consisted of the "type of reproduction" (level
of visuo-spatial organization) the time (copy duration) and the
points (concerning the precision of the drawing). After a period of
3 minutes during which the patient did not have access to the figure
he was asked to draw the figure from memory. The "type of reproduction" and the number of points constituted the scoring criteria.

RESULTS

a) WAIS test

Table 2 shows the mean values of the two groups as well as the
statistical comparisons between them. The mean difference between
Verbal and Performance I.Q.s was greater in the group of patients
with delusional misidentification syndromes compared to that of the
control group to a statistically significant degree (p=.02). A statistically significant difference was also noted with respect to
two subtests. The patients with delusional misidentification syndromes did worse in the picture completion subtest (t=3.14) and in
the picture arrangement subtest (t=2.22). A marked difference was
also observed with respect to the block design subtest but this difference did not reach statistical significance (t=1.91).

b) Benton's Visual Retention test

The Benton test results are presented in table 3. The performances of the patients were evaluated by comparing the score obtained
from each subject to the score expected from a) his full scale I.Q.
and b) his verbal I.Q.

Two patients (Nos 4 and 9) were unable to accomplish the test
because of their very low intelligence and one patient (No 2) accomplished only the verbal scale of the test because of defective
visual ability. Comparison of the score of each patient to the
score expected from his full scale I.Q. revealed that for four patients there was a "strong indication" of memory impairment (obtained score 4 or more points below the expected score), for three
patients there was suggestion of impairment (obtained score 3 and
3,5 points below the expected score), the scores of three patients

844

Table 2. Results on the WAIS Test of Patients with
Delusional Misidentification Syndromes
Compared to Controls

Subtests	Patients with Delusional Misidentification Syndromes		Controls			
	Mean	S.D.	Mean	S.D.	t	p
Information	9,14	2,93	7,26	3,57	2,01	.10
Comprehension	8,30	3,14	7,13	3,54	0,59	N.S.
Arithmetic	8,38	2,98	7,20	2,85	1,63	N.S.
Similarities	7,23	4,53	6,93	3,49	0,02	N.S.
Digit Span	7,07	3,06	6,13	1,12	0,56	N.S.
Vocabulary	10,00	2,94	8,80	3,46	0,61	N.S.
Digit Symbol	5,66	2,30	6,00	3,10	-1,12	N.S.
Picture Completion	4,84	2,93	6,69	3,37	-3,14	.01
Block Design	6,15	1,95	7,77	3,44	-1,91	.10
Picture Arrangement	4,30	2,65	6,08	2,90	-2,22	.05
Object Assembly	5,91	2,50	5,15	2,37	0,87	N.S.
Verbal I.Q.	89,38	17,35	83,40	17,37	0,94	N.S.
Performance I.Q.	71,15	12,72	76,92	15,83	-2,69	.02
Full Scale I.Q.	80,46	15,59	79,71	17,49	0,46	N.S.

raised the question of impairment (2 and 2,5 points below the expected score) and in two cases no evidence of memory impairment was detected. Stronger evidence of impairment was noted in some patients (Nos 13, 14, 15) when their obtained scores were compared to the scores expected from their Verbal I.Q.s.

c) Rey's "complex figure" test

Table 4 shows the results of Rey's test. With regard to the copying of the figure, all patients (with one exception, No 13) performed a poor "type of reproduction", characteristic of the 10th percentile of the general population. For seven patients, both the copy' time and the obtained score were below the level expected from the IQs of the patients.

The score of "points" for four patients was equal or even higher than the score expected from their IQs.

Table 3. Results on Benton's Test

	Points below the expected score			
Patient No	With reference to the full scale IQ		With reference to the Verbal IQ	
1	4	++	4	++
2			5	++
3	3	+	3	+
5	2,5	±	2,5	±
6	4	++	5	++
7	4	++	5	++
8	4	++	5	++
10	1	-	1	-
11	1	-	1	-
12	3	+	3	+
13	2	±	3	+
14	3,5	+	4,5	++
15	2,5	±	3,5	+

- no impairment, ± raising the question of impairment, + suggesting impairment, ++strongly indicating impairment.

The low intelligence of three of the patients (Nos 2, 4, 9) did not allow performance of the test, whilst the evaluation of the performance of one patient was not possible due to his low IQ.

Taking into account the results of all three types of scoring ("type of reproduction", "time of execution" and "points") it can be concluded that seven patients had a spatial organization defect. No evidence of impairment was found in three cases and in one case the results were inconclusive.

With regard to the reproduction of the figure from memory, for five patients an impairment was detected when the evaluation of their score was based on the expected score from their full scale IQ and for eight patients when the evaluation of their score was based on their Verbal IQ. For two patients the results were inconclusive because of their low IQs (no standards are available for IQs below 80, that is below the 10th percentile of the general population).

Table 4. Results on Rey's Test*

Patient	Copy of figure				Reproduction from Memory		
No	Type	Time	Points	General Evaluation	Type	Points	General Evaluation
1	IV	5'	34	+	IV	19	+
3	IV	3'45"	28	−	IV	7	±
5	IV	4'	34	−	I	12	±
6	IV	8'30"	9	+	VI	3	+
7	IV	6'28"	21	+	V	6½	+
8	V	4'30"	11	±	V	2	+
10	IV	2'48"	27	+	V	8	+
11	IV	2'	34	−	I	27	−
12	IV	9'	33	+	V	2	+
13	I	4'30"	35	−	I	27	−
14	IV	3'30"	32	+	V	2	+
15	IV	6'	31	+	IV	16½	+

− no impairment, + Impairment, ± results inconclusive
* The evaluation of the results is based on the score expected from
  the Verbal I.Q. of the patients.

DISCUSSION

Comparison of the WAIS test results of the group of patients
to those of the group of controls revealed a statistically greater
verbal vs performance score difference in the former group, a finding consistent with organicity (Wechsler D., 1958) and hence in
keeping with the notion that organic brain dysfunction plays a pathogenetic role in the syndrome of doubles.

In addition to the low results in the performance scale scores
the group of patients with delusional misidentification syndromes
showed particulary low scores in two of the performance scale's
subtests (the picture arrangement and picture completion subtests)
as well as a trend towards a statistically lower performance in the
block design subtest. The low performance in these three subtests
is indicative of some disturbance of visual perception and organization and since both block design and picture arrangement subtests
are considered indicators of brain damage (Wechsler D., 1958) the
possibility of organic factors interfering with the syndrome's pathogenesis is reinforced by these findings. This possibility is
further reinforced by the high frequency of disturbances concerning

the function of visual memory (Benton's test, Rey's test) and spatial organization (Rey's test) which may be interpreted as indicative of some organic dysfunction of the right posterior area of the brain.

On the other hand our patients did badly in a WAIS subtest known not to be affected by cerebral dysfunction, namely the picture completion subtest. Zimmerman and Woo-Sam (1973) have noted that "a focus on minutia without ability to differentiate can lower scores" in this subtest. In other words subjects who are concerned with details to such an extend that they end up with missing the essentials do badly in this subtest. This disturbance may in some way, be associated with the triggering mechanism of the unfamiliarity experienced by patients with the syndrome of doubles which subsequently leads to misidentifications.

In recent years a number of authors have suggested that organic brain dysfunction may be important in the pathogenesis of the delusional misidentification syndromes (Gluckman, 1968, Weston and Whitlock, 1971, Nilsson and Perris, 1971, Mac Callum, 1973, Hay et al. 1974, Hayman and Abrams, 1977) and a review of the Capgras cases which appeared in the English language literature from 1933 to 1976 revealed that 7 of the 46 reported cases were organic while at least 5 of the 28 schizophrenic cases had organic factors operating (Merrin and Silberfarb, 1976).

Our findings are in keeping with the notion that organic factors participate in the pathogenesis of the delusional misidentification syndromes and suggest that in all such cases careful search for organic pathogenetic contributors is strongly indicated.

REFERENCES

Benton, A. L., 1963, "The revised visual retention test:Clinical and experimental applications", The Psychological Corporation, New York.

Capgras,J.,Reboul-Lachaux,J.,1923,Illusion des sosies dans un délire systematisé chronique, Bull. Soc. Clin. Med. Ment., 11:6.

Christodoulou, G. N., 1975, "The syndrome of doubles", Associate Professorship Thesis, University of Athens, Athens.

Christodoulou, G. N., 1977, The syndrome of Capgras, Br. J. Psychiatry, 130:556.

Christodoulou, G. N., 1976, Delusional hyper-identifications of the Frégoli type. Organic pathogenetic contributors, Acta Psychiat. Scand., 54:305.

Courbon,P.,Tusques,J.,1932,Illusion d'intermetamorphose et de charme, Ann. Med. Psychol., 90:401.

Courbon,P.,Fail,G.,1927,Illusion de Frégoli,Bull.Soc.Clin. Med. Ment. 15:121.

Enoch, M. D., Trethowan, W., Barker, J., 1967, "Some uncommon psychiatric syndromes", Wright, Bristol.

Gluckman, J. K., 1968, A case of Capgras syndrome, Aust. NZ. J. Psychiatry, 2:39.

Hay, G. G., Jolley, D. J., Jones, R. G., 1974, A case of Capgras syndrome in association with pseudo-hypoparathyroidism, Acta Psychiat. Scand., 50:73.

Hayman, M. A., Abrams, R., 1977, Capgras' syndrome and cerebral dysfunction, Br. J. Psychiatry, 130:68.

Mac Callum,W. A. G., 1973, Capgras symptoms with an organic basis, Br. J. Psychiatry, 123:639.

Merrin, E.L., Silberfarb, P.M., 1976, The Capgras phenomenon, Arch. Gen. Psychiatry, 33:965.

Nilsson, R., Perris, C., 1971, The Capgras syndrome. A case report, Acta Psychiat. Scand., Suppl., 222:53.

Rey, A., 1965, "Test de la figure complexe", Editions du Centre de Psychologie Appliquée, Paris.

Wechsler, D., 1958, "The measurement and appraisal of adult intelligence", Williams and Wilkins, Baltimore.

Weston, M. J., Whitlock, F. A., 1971, The Capgras syndrome following head injury, Br. J. Psychiatry, 119:25.

Zimmerman, I. L., Woo-Sam, J. M., 1973,"Clinical interpretation of the Wechsler adult intelligence scale", Grune and Stratton, New York and London.

MAO ACTIVITY IN PATIENTS WITH DELUSIONAL

MISIDENTIFICATIONS

Basil Alevizos and George Christodoulou

Department of Psychiatry, Athens University
Eginition Hospital
74, Vass. Sophias Str., Athens

INTRODUCTION

Early reports suggested that Capgras syndrome is associated with functional psychoses, paranoid schizophrenia or manic-depressive illness and psychodynamic formulations for this phenomenon were reported (Capgras and Reboul-Lachaux, 1923; Courbon and Tusques, 1932). However, recent reports suggest that CNS organic dysfunction may play an important role in the pathogenesis of the delusional misidentification syndromes (Christodoulou, 1976; Prescorn and Reveley, 1978; Wilcox and Waziri, 1983).

In an attempt to further elucidate the nosological place of Capgras syndrome, Sullivan et al. (1978) reported that platelet monoaminoxidase (MAO) activity was significantly reduced in two cases of Capgras syndrome in comparison to that of psychiatric and non-psychiatric controls. The authors suggested that the low platelet MAO activity might be proposed as a potential biochemical marker of the syndrome. In addition to these two cases, a non-schizophrenic patient with delusional misidentifications, who had a primary diagnosis of organic brain syndrome, reported by Barton et al. (1980), had reduced platelet MAO activity in comparison to normal controls.

On the basis of the above reports and in order to further investigate the role of MAO activity in patients with delusional misidentifications we determined MAO activity in patients with this syndrome and compared it to that of schizophrenic and non-schizophrenic controls.

851

METHODS

The clinical material consisted of seven patients with delutional misidentifications. Six were female and only one was male.
All were diagnosed as paranoid schizophrenics. Five of the patients
were drug-free at the time of the study. Six patients manifested
delusional misidentifications of the Capgras type and one patient
showed delusional misidentifications of the Frégoli type. Sixteen
schizophrenic patients and eight normal subjects matched for sex
and age range were used as controls.

Platelet MAO activity was determined on the basis of the
method of Collins and Sandler (1971) using as substrate ^{14}-C-β-
phenethylamine in concentration 3 x 10^{-6} M. In four of the above
patients and in four normal controls plasma amine oxidase activity
was also measured according to the method of Robinson et al.(1968)
using ^{14}-C-benzylamine as substrate.

RESULTS

The results show that platelet MAO activity in the seven
patients with delusional misidentifications did not differ significantly from that of schizophrenic and non-psychiatric controls
(Table 1).

Table 1. Comparative values of platelet MAO activity in
patients with D.M. and controls (Mean ± S.D.)

	MAO activity (dpm/mg/hr x 10^{-3})
D.M. Patients (N=7)	15.05 ± 15.33
Schizophrenics (N=18)	14.90 ± 12.06
Controls (N=8)	18.02 ± 4.38

Statistical significance: NS

However, plasma amine oxidase activity was found to be significantly lower in four patients with delusional misidentifications
as compared with four healthy controls (Table 2).

Table 2. Plasma amine oxidase activity in patients with
delusional misidentifications and controls

	MAO activity (dpm/ml/hr x 10^{-3})
D.M. Patients (N=4)	16.19 ± 2.71
Controls (N=4)	30.31 ± 5.96

Stat. significance: t 4.3 ; p⟨0.01

DISCUSSION

Our findings did not confirm the previous reports on reduced
platelet MAO activity in patients with delusional misidentifications. The low activity in the two first cases reported by Sullivan
et al. (1978) might be associated with paranoid symptomatology of
patients and chronicity of their illness. These patients were
diagnosed as paranoid schizophrenics with a duration of illness
of eight and ten years respectively. Low platelet MAO activity
in chronic and paranoid schizophrenics has been confirmed by
a number of studies (Carpenter et al., 1975; Berretini et al.,1977;
Kobes et al., 1979; Schildkraut et al., 1980). The case reported
by Barton et al. (1980), although non schizophrenic, had a primary
diagnosis of organic brain syndrome for many years which could
indirectly affect platelet MAO activity. Neuroleptics and other
drugs given to these patients could also account for the low
platelet MAO activity (Takahashi et al. 1975).

MAO activity is affected by a variety of factors i.e. sex, age,
drugs and hormones, heterogeneity of platelets, substrate concentration and other methodological factors (Jackman and Meltzer, 1980).
Furthermore, a large interindividual variation with a 8-10fold
range in normals has been found and many people who do not have
a psychiatric diagnosis have low platelet MAO activity (Friedhoff
and Miller, 1980

The significantly lower plasma amine oxidase activity in four
patients with delusional misidentifications is difficult to be
explained. It could be associated with the schizophrenic symptomatology itself since a low activity is found in schizophrenics,
especially in acute, in comparison to controls (Meltzer et al.(1980).

To summarize the above, it seems unlikely that low platelet
MAO activity may represent a biochemical marker of delusional
misidentifications syndrome. Reduced MAO activity is expected to

occur in a variety of psychiatric and non-psychiatric conditions.
A great number of cases is still needed to clarify the role of MAO
in delusional misidentification syndrome.

REFERENCES

Barton, J. L., S. Chaparala, E. S. Barton, I. V. Jackson and L. G.
    Davis, 1980, Delusional misidentification and platelet momo-
    amine oxidase, Biol. Psychiat., 15/2:275.

Berretini, W. H., W. H. Vogel and R. Clouse, 1977, Monoamine oxi-
    dase in chronic schizophrenia, Am. J. Psychiat., 134:805.

Capgras, J. and Reboul-Lachaux, J., 1923, L' illusion des "Sosies"
    dans un délire systématisé chronique, Bull. Soc. Clin. Med.
    Ment., 11:16.

Carpenter, W. T., D. L. Murphy and R. J. Wyatt, 1975, Platelet
    monoamine oxidase activity in acute schizophrenia, Am. J.
    Psychiat., 132:438.

Christodoulou, G. N., 1976, Delusional hyperidentifications of the
    Frégoli type: organic pathogenetic contributors, Acta Psychiat.
    Scand., 54: 305.

Collins, G. G. S. and M. Sandler, 1971, Human blood platelet
    monoamine oxidase, Biochem. Pharmac., 20:289.

Courbon, P. and J. Tusques, 1932, Illusions d' intermétamorphose
    et de charme, Ann. Méd-Psychol., 90:401.

Friedhoff, A. J. and J. C. Miller, 1980, Platelet monoamine oxidase
    as a function of nongenetic factors, Schiz. Bull., 6:314.

Jackman, H. L. and H. Y. Meltzer, 1980, Factors affecting determi-
    nation of platelet monoamine oxidase activity, Schiz. Bull.,
    6:258.

Kobes, R. D., S. G. Potkin, C. D. Wise, T. P. Bridge, L. M. Neckers
    and R. J. Wyatt, 1979, Some kinetic parameters of platelet
    monoamine oxidase in chronic schizophrenia, Psychiatry Res.,
    1:179.

Meltzer, H. Y., R. C. Arora, H. Jackman, G. Pscheidt and M. D.
    Smith, 1980, Platelet monoamine oxidase and plasma amine
    oxidase in psychiatric patients, Schiz. Bull.,6:213.

Preskorn, S. H. and A. Reveley, 1978, Pseudohypoparathyroidism
    and Capgras syndrome, Brit. J. Psychiat., 133:34.

Robinson, D. S., W. Lovenberg, H. Keiser and A. Sjoerdsma, 1968,
    Effects of drugs on human blood platelet and plasma amine
    oxidase activity in vitro and in vivo, Biochem. Pharmac.
    17:109.

Schildkraut, J. J., P. J. Orsulak, A. F. Schatzberg and J. M. Herzog, 1980, Platelet monoamine oxidase activity in subgroups of schizophrenic disorders, Schiz. Bull., 6:220.

Sullivan, J. L., J. O. Cavenar, A. A. Maltbie and E. Silverstein, 1978, Capgras syndrome-a biochemical marker?, J, Nerv. Ment. Dis., 166:275.

Takahashi, S., H. Yamane and N. Tani, 1975, Reduction of blood platelet monoamine oxidase activity in schizophrenic patients on phenothiazines, Fol. Psychiat. Neurol. Jap., 29:207.

Wilcox, J. and R. Waziri, 1983, The Cagras symptom and nondominant cerebral dysfunction, J. Clin. Psychiatry, 44:70.

centre if suicide prevention centres did not exist and might get similar help. In this connection it is also important to emphasize that many centres, including the one in Helsinki, have an extensive training and research function.

Many suicide prevention centres are crisis intervention centres, and only some of their clients are experiencing suicidal crises.

New programmes for special target populations continue the pattern of established and developing ones in that they reflect the increasing concern for specific social problems. Thus we find programmes individualized for victims of rape, crime, sexual abuse or battery. Special settings identified with particular problems are addressed by offering crisis services to schools, jails, hospital wards and pop and folk music festivals. Specific needs are recognized in projects to assist young mothers lacking parental skills, parents who commit child abuse, and single-parent families, as well as programmes created for the needs of deaf persons and the mentally retarded. Persons with crisis-stage veneral disease have been offered a special programme, and one project has been designed specifically for those in crisis who decline referral to a crisis agency (Motto 1979).

SUICIDES AMONG THE YOUNG

What is the reason for the rapid increase in the suicide rate among the young? Is it related to unemployment? Is it associated with identification with idols who have committed suicide? Have the life habits and customs of the young changed and are they somehow involved? Further studies are needed.

A World Health Organization conference held in 1974 asserted that suicide among young people had reached epidemic proportions. In the United Stated - where the suicide rate for the entire population encreased only 8 % between 1965 and 1973 - the increase for young people who killed themselves was 71 %. During the same period in Finland, suicides among young people increased 128 %, whereas the suicide rate for the population as a whole rose only 19 % (Ross 1980).

The suicide rate in the 15-19 age group has increased explosively during the past 15 years in the Western World; in Finland it has tripled.

PSYCHOLOGY

In an important exegenesis of Freud's thoughts on suicide, Robert E. Litman traces the development of Freud's views on the subject, taking into account Freud's clinical experience and his changing theoretical positions from 1881 to 1939. It is evident from Litman's analysis that there is more to the psychodynamics of suicide than hostility. Other factors involved include the general features of human condition in Western civilization, specifically suicide-prone mechanisms involving rage, quilt, anxiety, dependency, and a great number of specifically predisposing conditions. The feelings on helplessness, hopelessness and abandonment are very important.

Suicide prevention is not a question of having command of a certain therapeutic technique, it means having the ability to deal with the problems of a person contemplating suicide critically, constructively and without fear (Böhme 1980).

More effective psychotherapy is needed in suicide prevention today. Group psychotherapy is being employed more than before. In the case of psychotherapy we need flexibility and the best possible sources of help for those in despair.

RESEARCH

The effectiveness of suicide prevention can be neither proved nor disproved on the basis of studies published in the literature on the evaluation of suicide-prevention institutions and programmes. The importance of individual factors within the complex pattern of conditions governing suicide prevention must be analysed within the framework of further studies, especially experimental ones such as appealing for help, the level and quality of the care offered, as well as amenability to influences, in order to discover ways of improving suicide-prevention care programmes (Kurz and Möller 1982).

We need more training in the methodology of suicide research, more international cooperation and greater interest in the matter.

SCOPE OF PSYCHIATRIC TREATMENT ORGANIZATIONS IN SUICIDE PREVENTION

Since suicides can be prevented merely by recourse to therapeutic measures, the first thing would be to refer anyone at risk of committing suicide for appropriate treatment. The second thing would be to correctly evaluate the risk of suicide of each patient, and thirdly to help all those needing help. We all know from everyday praxis that only parts of these three areas are covered.

The most usual feature common to all those at risk of committing suicide is depression of various degrees. It has thus been amphasized, with good reason, that every doctor should be able to identify depression in its very different forms and to treat it effectively.

860

The "causes" of suicide are usually described as social, somatic and psychological. In practice the various factors interact and form an entity in which it is difficult to differentiate the causes and consequences, and the role of a single factor as the "cause" of suicide. In terms of seeking help, however, classification of these different factors is important. If a person has somatic symptoms he contacts a doctor treating somatic diseases. In such a case it is likely that the psychological crisis in the background will not be found and will therefore remain untreated. Experience has shown that the problems of the elderly, for example those living in Helsinki, are often manifested as somatic symptoms, and their causes are often given too little attention. Aggravation of such a crisis may eventually result in suicide. The role of social factors is often not indicated sufficiently clearly during psychiatric treatment. Often it is not even possible to influence the situation. The global question is how well society's different aid organizations are able to understand the individual's life situation and help him.

Isolated examples show that by improving mental health services in general it is possible to indirectly reduce the rate of suicide to some extent. An increase in the number of services alone is probably not enough; more attention should be given to the quality of the services. How well the psychiatric treatment organization reaches different population groups and different problem groups should be investigated. The same organization should also be able to offer more specific services. These would include management of various forms of crisis, including suicidal crises, and the special treatment of those with chronic suicide tendencies.

REFERENCES

Bron, B., 1980, Neuere Aspekte des Suizidproblems. Fortschr. Neurol. Psychiat. ihrer Grenzgeb. 48:556-568.

Böhme, K., 1980, Zur praktischen Versorgung von Suicidenten. Nervenarzt 51:152-158.

Kurz, A. and Möller, H.J., 1982, Ergebnisse der epidemiologischen Evaluation von Suizidprophylaktischen Versorgungsprogrammen. Psychiat. Prax. 9:12-19.

Litman, R.E., 1971, Suicide prevention: Evaluationg effectiveness. Life-Threat. Behav. 1:155-162.

Motto, J.A., 1971, Evaluation of a suicide prevention center by sampling the population at risk. Life-Threat. Behav. 1:18-22.

Motto, J.A., 1979, New approaches to crisis intervention. Suicide Life-Threat. Behav. 9:173-184.

Ross, C.P., 1980, Mobilizing schools for suicide prevention. Suicide Life-Threat. Behav. 10:239-243.

A PRACTICAL SCALE FOR ESTIMATING SUICIDE RISK

Jerome A. Motto, David C. Heilbron, and
Richard P. Juster

University of California
San Francisco, California USA

This report details an effort to devise a scale applicable to
adults who are hospitalized due to a depressive or suicidal state.

Sample: Subjects were defined as those persons aged 18-70
admitted as inpatients to any of nine mental health facilities in
San Francisco during 1969-74, and whose admission was primarily due
to a depressive or suicidal state. The initial sample totalled
2,753. Each subject was thoroughly evaluated by means of a
clinical interview, during which information was obtained about 104
psychosocial characteristics. A subsequent annual search of the
State of California Death Registry for 1969-77 identified those
subjects who had died of suicide within two years of evaluation.
136 (4.9%) suicides were found.

Method: The sample was randomly divided into five 20% subgroups, balanced with regard to age, sex and chronicity of suicidal
ideation. By withholding each 20% subgroup in order, five 80%-20%
partitions were formed. The 80% segment served as an index set for
purposes of scale construction in each partition, with the 20%
segment serving as a validation set. Each index set totalled
approximately 2,200 subjects (108 suicides; 2,092 non-suicides) and
each validation set totalled approximately 548 subjects (27 suicides;
521 non-suicides).

Using each 80% index set, the 104 psychosocial variables rated
in the initial interview were examined for their individual associations with the outcome variable, suicide within two years. The
fifty variables showing the most significant relationship were
identified and entered into a linear logistic regression employing
a backward stepwise elimination technique, in order to produce a

863

scale of variables having a p value of .05 or less. The estimated
coefficients resulting from this procedure were applied to the 20%
validation set for each partition, to determine how well the derived
prediction equation differentiated the suicides from the non-
suicides in the independent samples. The variables derived from
all five partitions were then combined and subjected to another
linear logistic regression to produce a final set of 15 predictors
significant at the .0285 level or better when applied to the entire
sample.

Results: One criterion for "high risk," for our purpose, is
a probability of suicide in excess of 4.94%, which is the rate of
suicide in the overall sample. The validity of the estimation of
risk was demonstrated by the "high risk" subjects having an actual
suicide rate greater than 4.94%, and the "not high risk" subjects
less than 4.94%. All 5 partitions show this separation in the
independent samples, with the "high risk" group ranging from 6.8%
to 9.6% and the "not high risk" from 3.0% to 3.8%. (Table 1)

Table 1. Performance of Risk Estimators on Validation Sets*

Validation Set	Estimated Risk	Observed No Suicides	Observed Suicides	Total	Percent Suicides
1	Not High	380	15	395	3.8%
(N = 553)	High	146	12	158	7.6%
2	Not High	370	12	382	3.1%
(N = 548)	High	150	16	166	9.6%
3	Not High	355	11	366	3.0%
(N = 548)	High	166	16	182	8.8%
4	Not High	377	15	392	3.8%
(N = 553)	High	150	11	161	6.8%
5	Not High	388	15	403	3.7%
(N = 551)	High	135	13	148	8.8%

*Criterion for High Risk: Greater than 4.9% (value for overall sample).

864

Table 2. Preformance of Final Set of Variables
on Overall Sample, by Deciles

Decile	N	Number Estimated Suicides	Number Observed Suicides	Observed Percent Suicides
1	275	1.17	0	0.0%
2	275	2.23	3	1.1%
3	275	3.28	4	1.5
4	275	4.68	7	2.5
5	276	6.43	7	2.2
6	276	8.72	10	4.0
7	276	11.71	9	3.3
8	275	16.52	17	6.5
9	275	25.33	22	7.6
10	275	55.92	57	20.7
TOTAL	2,753		136	

Comparison of observed vs estimated suicides. Chi-square = 4.1962
9 DF p = 0.8980

The final set of 15 predictors, when applied to the overall
sample, shows a close relationship between estimated and observed
suicide in every decile of estimated risk. (Table 2) Since this
is not an independent sample, we are only assured that the final
predictors do discriminate levels of suicide risk in the entire set
of subjects. The large size and diverse composition of this set
encourages our view that the predictors may have broader applicability.

The 15 final predictor variables were translated into a
paper-and-pencil scale that provides the user with an estimate of
relative risk of suicide within two years (low, moderate, high),
an approximate suicide rate (in percent), and the corresponding
decile of risk for persons in the population from which our subjects
were drawn. (Appendix A)

APPENDIX A

THE SUICIDE RISK ASSESSMENT SCALE

Instructions

1. The Suicide Risk Assessment Scale is designed to estimate the risk of suicide in adults aged 18-70, during a two year period following the time of assessment.

2. The Scale is primarily applicable to persons known to be at some risk, such as those in a serious depressive state, having suicidal thoughts or impulses, or having made a recent suicide attempt.

3'. The Scale is to be administered by a clinician, not self-administered. Responses to the items in the first column are best determined in the course of a clinical interview. The information need not be obtained in the listed order.

4. The subjective judgement of the interviewer is to be used throughout in categorizing the response, as data provided in the clinical situation may be incomplete, ambiguous or conflicting.

5. For the one most appropriate response category in the second column, the indicated "assigned score" in the third column should be entered into the last column as the "actual score." If any data are missing or unobtainable, score that item zero.

6. Total the fifteen actual scores and determine from the Table of Risk what category of risk is scored. This is expressed in three ways: 1) numerically, on a scale of one to ten, representing the decile of risk, 2) descriptively, from "Very Low" to "Very High," and 3) an estimated percentage of risk during the two years following assessment.

    The Suicide Risk Assessment Scale is intended as a supplement to, not a substitute for, clinical judgement. A thorough evaluation is indicated in any serious emotional disturbance. Individual uniqueness suggests that when the Scale is not consistent with clinical judgement, clinical judgement should be given precedence.

Date:_____	Total Score: . . . . . . _____
Subject:_____	Risk category, Table of Risk:_____
Interviewer:_____	Risk category, Clinical Estimate:____
Time needed to administer:____	Comment:_____
Ease of administration: 1 2 3 4 5 (circle number) Easy Difficult	_____

Suicide Risk Assessment Scale Appendix A (cont)

Item	Response Category	Assigned Score	Actual Score
1. Age at last birthday	Find age in table and enter corresponding score.	See table (page 4)	
2. Type of occupation	Executive Administrator Professional Owner of business Semiskilled worker Other	48 48 48 48 48 0	
3. Sexual orientation	Bisexual and sexually active Homosexual, not sexually active Other	65 65 0	
4. Financial resources	Negative (debts exceed resources) None 0 to $100 Over $100	0 0 35 70	
5. Threat of significant financial loss	Yes No	63 0	
6. Stress unique to subjects circumstances, other than loss of finances or relationship, threat of prosecution, illigitimate pregnancy, substance abuse or poor health.	Severe Other	63 0	
7. Hours of sleep per night (approximate nearest whole hour)	0-2 3-5 6 or more	0 37 74	
8. Change of weight during present episode of stress (approximate)	No change 10% or more weight loss Less than 10% loss Weight gain	0 0 60 60	

867

Item	Response Category	Assigned Score	Actual Score
9. Ideas of persecution or reference	Moderate or severe Other	45 0	
10. Intensity of present suicidal impulses	Questionable, moderate or severe Other	100 0	
11. If current suicide attempt made, seriousness of intent to die.	Unequivocal Ambivalent, weighted toward suicide Other or not applicable	88 88 0	
12. Number of prior psychiatric hospitalizations	None 1 2 3 or more	0 21 43 64	
13. Result of prior efforts to obtain help	No prior efforts Some degree of help Poor, unsatisfactory, or variable outcome	0 0 55	
14. Emotional disorder in family history	Depression Alcoholism Other	45 45 0	
15. Interviewer's reaction to the person	Highly positive Moderately or slightly positive Neutral or negative	0 42 85	
		TOTAL SCORE_____	

Total Score	Decile of Risk	Relative Risk	Approximate Suicide Rate
0-271	1	Very low	Less than 1%
272-311	2	Low	1-2.5%
312-344	3		
345-377	4	Moderate	2.5-5%
378-407	5		
408-435	6		
436-465	7		
466-502	8	High	5-10%
503-553	9		
over 553	10	Very high	over 10%

Age-Score Table

Age	Score	Age	Score	Age	Score
18	0	36	45	54	80
19	3	37	47	55	81
20	6	38	49	56	83
21	9	39	51	57	85
22	12	40	53	58	86
23	14	41	55	59	88
24	17	42	57	60	90
25	20	43	59	61	91
26	22	44	61	62	93
27	25	45	63	63	95
28	27	46	65	64	96
29	29	47	67	65	98
30	32	48	69	66	99
31	34	49	71	67	101
32	36	50	72	68	102
33	39	51	74	69	104
34	41	52	76	70	106
35	43	53	78		

DEPRESSIVE DISORDERS AND THE

PREVENTION OF SUICIDE

Peter Sainsbury

Lately Director Medical Research Council
Clinical Psychiatry Unit
Graylingwell Hospital
Chichester Sussex England

Recent research has not only established that the majority of suicides suffered from an unequivocal and treatable depressive illness, but that most of them also contacted their doctors in the period immediately preceding their death. Since this statement has important implications for suicide prevention, I propose discussing the sources of evidence for it.

First, regarding the incidence of suicide in depressives, many follow-up studies (Miles, 1977) consistently show that about one in six primary depressives will ultimately kill themselves. Table 1, for example, shows that about 15% of deaths in six cohorts of endogenous depressives followed through many years died by suicide. Longitudinal surveys of a whole populations' mortality are of particular interest (Helgason, 1964; Hagnell and Rorsman, 1978). Helgason, for instance followed over 5,000 Icelanders through 60 years; national records revealed that 103 (or 2%) developed a manic-depressive illness, 17% of whom died by suicide - the suicides accounting for more than half the deaths.

That this figure of about 15% is probably a valid estimate can be inferred by using it to calculate the expected number of suicides with a primary depression, when the life span of depressives is assumed to be 66 years (Oltman and Friedman, 1962) and the prevalence of severe depression to be about 2% of the population (Wing, 1976). The calculation in Table 2 deduces that England can expect about half of its suicides to be depressives (I.C.D. 296); a proportion that corresponds very closely to the 60% actually observed in clinical post-mortems of

Table 1. Death by Suicide in Affective Disorder
(adapted from Robins et al., 1959)

Reference	Cases n	Follow-up Years	Dead n	Suicide n	Death due to suicide %
Langelüddecke (1941)	341	40	268	41	15.3
Slater (1938)	138	30	59	9	15.3
Lundquist (1945)	319	20	119	17	14.3
Schulz (1949)	2,004	5	492	66	13.4
Stenstedt (1952)	216	10	42	6	14.3
Pitts and Winokur (1964)	56	death	56	9	16.0

Table 2.

1 The suicide rate of depressives can be estimated as:

$$\frac{\text{Fraction dying by suicide (0.15)}}{\text{Average life-span of depressives (66 years)}} \times 10^5 = 230/100,000\text{pa}$$

2 If 2 ± 0.62 of the population are depressives then England
and Wales (pop. about 50 million) can expect between 3,000
and 1,600 depressed suicides per annum

$$(\text{eg} \quad \frac{2.62 \times 50 \text{ million}}{100} \times \frac{230}{10^5} = 3,013)$$

3 As there are about 5,000 suicides per annum, we can expect
between 30 and 60% to have a depressive illness

4 This expected proportion agrees closely with the 65%
observed to have been depressed when 100 suicides were
assessed clinically

a consecutive sample of suicides (Barraclough et al., 1974).

The second source of evidence for supposing that a high
proportion of those who commit suicide already suffered from a
primary depressive illness originates from the work of Robbins
et al. (1959) in St Louis. Their method was to undertake diagnostic
interviews with suicides' relatives. From accounts given by the
families of 134 suicides they concluded that 94% had a definite

mental illness. We also obtained social and clinical data by
interviewing the relatives, friends and general practitioners of
100 consecutive suicides and 150 matched controls from the
population of Sussex and the City of Portsmouth (Barraclough et al.
1974). The sample was a representative one in so far as the
demographic characteristics of the suicides did not differ from the
national figures.

Whether each suicide was mentally ill and what the diagnosis
was, was decided by an independent panel of three psychiatrists
using our protocols. The panel agreed that 93% had an identifiable
mental disorder and that 64% had an uncomplicated primary depressive
illness; this increases to 77% if suicides diagnosed as alcoholics,
but who also had a severe depressive illness, are included (Table 3).

Most of the 64 depressives were of the endogenous type, but
17% had experienced manic episodes as well. But in order to see
in what respects the suicidal depressives differed from living
ones they were compared with a random sample of 128 endogenous
depressives drawn from the same population as the suicides
(Barraclough and Pallis, 1975). The rank order of 15 depressive
symptoms was the same for both groups; though the severity ratings
of the suicides were often higher. They differed significantly
on only three clinical items; the suicides manifested more
persistent insomnia, more self-neglect and more impairment of
memory. Insomnia has been shown by other workers to be
characteristic of the suicidal depressive (Rosen, 1970); but
its importance also lies in the further finding that many of our
suicides who had been prescribed barbiturates used this hypnotic
to kill themselves (Barraclough et al. 1971). As impaired memory
and self-neglect were not associated with organic cerebral
disease, they were probably effects of a severe depression on
cognitive function and morale.

As regards the history and course of illness in the two
groups, Barraclough and Pallis found that the depressed suicides
had made a previous suicide attempt ten times more often than the
living depressives; and that the suicide's illness had had a
longer course.

The social and demographic features which distinguished the
depressed suicides from other depressives were that they were
more often male, elderly, separated, recently bereaved (Bunch
et al. 1971) and socially isolated. For example, 42% of the
suicides lived alone, whereas only 7% of the living depressives
did.

The two groups did not differ however, on number of
previous episodes of illness, family history of affective illness

Table 3. Diagnostic Classification of 100 Suicides

	n
Depressive illness	77
Mixed affective state	2
Alcoholism[1]	15
Other disorders[2]	7
Schizophrenia	3
Diagnosis not possible[3]	2
Not mentally ill	7
Total	113

1 10 had alcoholism and depressive illness
2   2 had some other disorder with a depressive illness
3   1 had depressive illness with another but undiagnosable
    condition

and suicide in first degree relatives. In both groups, however, the incidence of these factors was similar to that reported in genetic studies of depressive psychoses, thereby further confirming the validity of the diagnosis given to the suicides retrospectively by the panel of psychiatrists.

The two groups were therefore clinically very similar; but the salient observations are that more than half of the suicides have been shown to have a treatable depressive illness and that their depression has some distinctive features denoting a suicide risk. The corollary of this is that the scope for preventive action is considerable.

A third source of data intimating that suicides are largely recruited from overt depressives, and should therefore be preventable, derives from studies on attempted suicides. These have been of two kinds: first, are those in which the statistical techniques of principal components and cluster analysis are used to identify categories of attempted suicides (Bagley, 1973; Henderson at al. 1977; and Kiev, 1976) and, they are consistent in differentiating a psychotically or severely depressed group of patients who make a serious attempt at suicide. Secondly, are studies in which the clinical characteristics of samples of attempted suicides are related to various measures of the medical seriousness of the attempt or of their 'intent to die'. The consensus of 10 such projects was that the variables most positively associated with seriousness of intent to die are a diagnosis of manic-depressive or primary depressive illness and a high score on a depression scale (Table 4).

Pallis, (1977), for example, scored 151 consecutive attempted suicides admitted to the Emergency Department of our District Hospital on Beck's Intent Scale and on a Suicide Risk Scale; he also obtained an independent rating of the medical seriousness of the attempt. Intent to die not only correlated significantly with the Suicide-risk Scores and medical seriousness, but also with the number and severity of depressive symptoms (Pallis and Sainsbury, 1976).

The depressive symptoms that distinguished the high from the low intent cases are shown in Table 5. The two groups also differed significantly on those socio-demographic variables which we have already seen to be strongly associated with suicide.

The depressive features of serious suicide attemptors are therefore very similar to those we found by interviewing the relatives of completed suicides.

So far we have established that:

1) both the seriously suicidal and completed suicides commonly suffer from a primary depression; and

2) attempted suicides in whom intent to die is serious are not only more likely to have an endogenous type of depression than those with low intent, but they also resemble completed suicides more closely. It therefore follows that recognising those cases with a depressive disorder is a priority in the assessment of the risk of suicide and hence its prevention.

However, the clinical differences between depressives who die by suicide and those who do not are few, so in order to identify those likely to commit suicide other factors need to be taken into account, our epidemiological studies (Sainsbury, 1973) have provided some clues.

First, the risk of suicide is strongly dependent on socio-cultural factors such as religious denomination, social class and occupation, as clearly emerged when our suicides and controls were compared on these items; and secondly, we also found suicide related significantly to psycho-social stresses - notably to bereavement and to moving house in the previous two years; unemployment was another predisposing event (Shepherd and Barraclough, 1980).

Table 4. Significant differences Between High and Low Intent
Groups for Symptoms Experienced in the Last Month (A)
and for Behaviour at Interview (B)

Variable	High Intent (n=75) %	Low Intent (n=75) %	x^2	p
(A) Insomnia	87	53	18.29	0.01
Pessimism	60	32	10.73	0.01
Impaired concentration	21	4	8.68	0.01
Loss of interest	32	13	6.43	0.02
Social withdrawal	29	12	5.85	0.02
Feeling useless or worthless	28	13	4.07	0.05
Weight loss	36	20	4.00	0.05
(B) Slow speech	19	4	6.63	0.02
Discouraged posture	47	25	6.22	0.02

No significant difference between groups: (A) depressive mood;
worrying; anger/irritability; weeping; anxiety/tension; agitation;
appetite; tiredness; self-blame; loss of confidence; depersonalization; (B) depressed; anxious/agitated; crying; histrionic;
hostile

Table 5. Period Between Most Recent Medical Contact and Death
for 64 Suicides Diagnosed Depression

	Family doctor %	Psychiatrist[1] %	Most recent contact of either %
0-7 days	34	9	42
8-30 days	19	8	20
31-90 days	16	3	17
91-365 days	13	2	11
366+ days	17	-	9
Total	99	22	99

1 Total under psychiatric care, 22; not under psychiatric care, 78.

In order to examine both the interdependence of risk factors and the hypothesis that more closely the individual attempting suicide resembles the completed suicide, the greater the risk of his dying by suicide. Pallis (1982) compared 75 suicides whose relatives were interviewed with the 150 attempted suicides he examined. He compared them on 55 clinical and social items from the standardised interview completed on both groups. Then using a step-wise discriminant function analysis he identified the best discriminators from which he correctly allocated 92% of the combined samples of attemptors and suicides to their respective groups. Once again the suicides were characterized by social features such as isolation and by depressive items. These findings next enabled him to construct long and short suicide risk scales. The scales were then validated by following up 1250 attempted suicides and significantly more of those that subsequently committed suicide had high-risk scores on both scales. The long scale, for example, predicted all subsequent suicides with only 17% false positives (Pallis, 1983).

The practical implications of this work are that risk (and intent) scales not only point to the severely depressed as being highly vulnerable, but that they can efficiently predict the short-term risk of suicide; hence they have potential value in assessing the preventive management of attempted suicides.

Indeed, the feasibility of prevention largely depends on the primary care services being able to: (1) recognise the depressive illness and those characteristics which denote a risk of suicide; (2) provide effective anti-depressant treatment, and, (3) organise efficient after-care. Support for those claims was obtained by evaluating how the depressive suicides were, in fact, managed.

Barraclough et al. (1974) found that over half of the suicidal depressives contacted their general practitioner in the month before death (Table 5). Moreover Pallis (1977), reported that most depressed suicide attemptors also did. It is evident that there are ample opportunities for therapeutic intervention. But were their doctors able to take advantage of them?

Our suicides' doctors clearly recognised their patients' distress because over 80% of depressives were prescribed tranquillisers and hypnotics (Table 6) but only a third of the depressives were given anti-depressants and in only one case was the dose or type appropriate (Barraclough et al. 1971).

Clearly in 1966 when we visited the suicides, G.P.'s lacked expertise in the diagnosis and care of the suicidal; but we have reasons to suppose that these skills have improved

Table 6. Prescribed Medical Treatment at Time of Death for
64 Suicides Diagnosed Depression

	%
Prescribed psychotropic drugs	81
Barbiturates	53
Antidepressants	30
Phenothiazines	20
Minor tranquillizers	23
ECT	5
Haloperidol	2
Hypnotics	70

since then.

The evidence derives from a comparison Mr Jenkins made of the consultation and diagnostic rates recorded in two large scale surveys of General Practice undertaken in England first in 1955 and again in 1970 (Logan and Cushion, 1958; OPCS, 1974). He found that whereas consultation rates for all illnesses fell in the later period, those for psychiatric disorders increased; secondly, the G.P.'s diagnoses in 1970 were more in accordance with the conventional psychiatric classification; and thirdly, the number of patients recognised as having a high suicide-risk disorder, especially depression, had increased greatly (Table 7). We tentatively inferred that G.P.'s attitudes to and management of, the depressive is changing in a way that could contribute to the recent decrease in suicide observed in England.

The management of depressives by psychiatric services is equally in need of appraisal. Time only allows me to refer to the disturbing increase in the suicide rate of resident patients in England and elsewhere (Sainsbury et al. 1978) a change which coincides with the introduction of more liberal regimes in our mental hospitals. Whether the current preference for early discharge and community care places the suicidal patient at greater risk has yet to be determined.

Walk (1967), however, has given grounds for supposing a well organised community service might reduce the incidence of suicide. He compared the suicide rate of all patients in contact with a psychiatrist during the 5 years before and after the introduction of the Chichester Community Psychiatric Service, in which 86% of all referrals were treated extra murally. He

878

Table 7. General Practitioners' Morbidity Study
(Logan & Cushion 1958; Office of Population
Censuses and Surveys, 1974)

		1956	1971	% change
A.	GP consulting rates per 1,000			
	All diseases or conditions	3,751.0	3,009.6	-19.8
	Mental disorders	187.4	297.6	+58.8
	Patients' consulting rate per 1,000			
	All diseases or conditions	670	671.1	+1
	Mental disorders	50	109.9	+119.8

	ICD No.	1956	1971	% change
B. Patient consulting rates (per 1,000) for various selected diagnoses: all ages, total male and female				
Anxiety neurosis	300.0	23.1	34.0	+47.2
Depressive neurosis	300.4	1.4	31.4	+2,142.9
Neurasthenia	300.5	5.7	2.3	-59.6
Other and unspecified	300.6- 300.9	7.0	0.7	-90

found a significant decrease in suicide among elderly patients.
Since it was the older, depressed patients who had benefited most
and whose referral had increased most after starting community
care, it is likely that it was an effect of the new service.

To sum up: The available facts on the relation of suicide
to depression, on the risk characteristics of the suicidal
depressive, and on the new opportunities we have for providing
effective treatment are such that most suicides must now be
considered preventable and services should be organised to promote
this goal. Were our present knowledge adequately conveyed to
doctors in training and to those medical and paramedical personnel
in the primary care services (and to whom the suicidal are known
to turn), and were emergency and psychiatric after-care services

better planned to profit from what is known about the affectively
disordered, a reduction in the incidence of suicide is feasible.

References

Bagley, C., 1973. Social policy and the prevention of suicidal
behaviour. Br.J.Soc.Work., 3: 473-495.

Barraclough, B., Bunch, J., Nelson, B., Sainsbury, P., 1974.
A hundred cases of suicide: clinical aspects. Br.J.Psychiat.
125: 355-373.

Barraclough, B., Nelson, B., Bunch, J., Sainsbury, P. , 1971.
Suicide and barbiturate prescribing. J.Roy.Coll. Gen. Pract.
21: 645-653.

Barraclough, B., Pallis, D.J., 1975. Depression followed by
suicide: a comparison of depressed suicides with living
depressives. Psychol. Med. 5: 55-61.

Bunch, J., Barraclough, B., Nelson, B., Sainsbury, P. 1971.
Suicide following bereavement of parents. Soc. Psychiat.
6: 193-199.

Hagnell, O., Rorsman, B. 1978. Suicide and endogenous depression
with somatic symptoms in the Lundby study. Neuropsychobiology,
4: 180-187.

Helgason, T. 1964. The epidemiology of mental disorder in Iceland.
Acta psychiat. scand. 40: suppl. 173.

Henderson, A.S., Hartigan, J., Davidson, J., Lance, G.N., Duncan-
Jones, P., Koller, K.M., Ritchie, K., McAuley, H., Williams,
C.L. Slaghuis, W. 1977. A typology of parasuicide. Brit. J.
Psychiat., 131: 631-641.

Kiev, A. 1976. Cluster analysis profiles of suicide attempters.
Am.J.Psychiat. 133: 150-153.

Langelüddecke, A. 1941. Über Lebenserwartung und Rückfallshaufig-
keit bei Manisch-depressiven. A. Psychiat. Hyg. 13: 1-14.

Logan,W.P.D., Cushion, A.A. 1958. Studies on medical and population subjects. Morbidity statistics from general practice.
General Register Office, HMSO, London.

Lundquist, G. 1945. Prognosis and course in manic-depressive
psychoses. Acta psychiat. neurol. scand. 35: suppl.,
pp 1-96.

Miles, C.P. 1977. Conditions predisposing to suicide: a review.
J. nerv. ment. Dis. 164: 231-246.

Office of Population Censuses and Surveys: Studies on medical
and population subjects, 1974. Morbidity Statistics from
General Practice. Second National Study 1970-71. HMSO,
London.

Oltman J.E., Friedman, S. 1962. Life cycles in patients with
manic-depressive psychosis. Am.J.Psychiat. 119: 174-177.

Pallis, D.J. 1977. The psychiatric assessment of attempted
suicide: personality, intent and suicide risk. Thesis,
Aberdeen.

Pallis, D.J., Barraclough, B., Levey, A.B., Jenkins, J.S., Sainsbury, P.,1982. Estimating suicide risk among attempted suicides. I Brit. J. Psychiat., 141: 37-44.

Pallis, D.J. ibid II. Brit. J. Psychiat. (in press), 1983.

Pallis, D.J., Sainsbury, P. 1976. The value of assessing intent in attempted suicide. Psychol. Med. 6: 487-492.

Pitts, F.N., Winokur, G. 1964. Affective Disorder. III. Diagnostic correlates and incidence of suicide. J.nerv.ment.Dis. 139: 176-181.

Robins,E., Murphy, G.E., Wilkinson, R.H., Gassner, S., Kayes, J. 1959. Some clinical considerations in the prevention of suicide based on a study of 134 successful suicides. Am. J. publ. Hlth. 49: 888-898.

Rosen, D.H., 1970. The serious suicide attempt: epidemiological and follow-up study of 886 patients. Am. J. Psychiat. 127: 764-770.

Sainsbury, P. 1973. Suicide: opinions and facts. Proc. R. Soc. Med. 66: 579-587.

Sainsbury, P., Baert, A., Jenkins, J., 1978. Suicide trends in Europe: a study of the decline in suicide in England and Wales and of the increase elsewhere. A report to the World Health Organisation Regional Office for Europe, Copenhagen.

Schulz, B. 1949. Sterblichkeit endogen Geisteskranker und Ihrer Eltern. Z.Menschl. Vereb. Konstitut, Lehre. 29: 338-367.

Shepherd, D. M., Barraclough, B., 1980. Work and Suicide: an empirical investigation. Brit. J. Psychiat., 136: 469-478.

Slater. E. 1938. Zur Erbpathologie des manisch-depressiven Irreseins: Die Eltern und Kinder von Manisch-Depressiven. Z. ges. Neurol. Psychiat. 163: 1-47.

Stenstedt, A. 1952. A study in manic-depressive psychosis, clinical, social and genetic investigations. Acta psychiat. neurol. scand. 79: suppl. pp 1-111.

Walk, D. 1967. Suicide and community care. Brit. J. Psychiat., 113: 1381-1391.

Wing, J.K. 1976. A technique for studying psychiatric morbidity in in-patient and out-patient series and in general population samples. Psychol. Med. 6: 665-671.

THE SELF-DESTRUCTIVE BEHAVIOUR OF EVERYDAY LIFE

Ahmed Okasha

Prof. & Head of Dept. of Psychiatry
Ain Shams University
Cairo - EGYPT

KEY WORDS

S.D.B - I.S.D.B. - Life "pleasures" - Rich food - Alcohol - Smoking - Risky sports - self sacrifice - patriotism - Martyrdom- Death instinct - Impulsive behaviour - Masochism - Noradrenergic reward system - Arousal.

It is rather hard to formulate a clear cut definition on concept regarding human behaviour and disorders of mental health. The study of self destructive behaviour has been hampered by semantic confusion, protean concepts and contradictory toxonomies. In a very broad sense self destructive behaviour can be defined to consist either in taking or in considering to take a life threatening risk, that need not necessarily aim at or lead to self destruction. Thus, it has nowadays become increasingly common to speak separately of indirect self-destruction and on the other hand direct self-destruction in a narrower sense, the latter includes three phenomena:suicidal thoughts, suicidal attempts and suicides. Indirect self-destructive behaviour may be defined as a behaviour characterized by taking a life threatening risk without the intention of dying, mostly repeatedly and often unconsciously, in such a way that the consequences are likely to be destructive to the individual before long (Lounqvist, 1978).

Indirect self-destruction comprises a wide variety of phenomena of great health importance. It is intriguing that all "Pleasures" in life lead to indirect self- destructive behaviour, rich food, alcoholic beverages, smoking, indulgence in coffee, gambling, risky sports, overindulgence in physical leisures, moreover, self-sacrifice for patriotic or religious causes, altruism for the sake

of the family and children, all the above phenomena are directed
towards social, physical and psychological decline. Even the search
for power and political disputes and aggression may lead ultimately
to a rebound effect with gradual loss of strength. Difficulty in
accepting one's own chronic illness, neglet of one's own health and
stress-seeking behaviour are also very frequently met forms of indirect self-destruction.

A person may damage himself by self-mutilation, by swallowing
foreign bodies or by repeatedly seeking surgical operations. Damage
may be caused by hunger strikes, ascetism or martyrdom.

Self-destructive risk may also manifest itself as a recurrent
breaking of social codes e.g. criminality or deviant traffic behaviour. A different type of risk taking is connected with dangerous
occupations and pursuits.

An inclination toward taking remarkable risks may be associated with any human activity e.g. in business life risk taking may
lead to public appreciation and reward, but on the other hand,
a failure may ruin not only the risk taker himself but other people as well.

The intentions underlying various forms of indirect self-
destruction are always individual in nature. What is usually involved is an individual's striving for a goal he regards as important for some reason or other without becoming consious of, or
without giving considerations to the other consequences of his
behaviour. The pursuit of a goal is often important to the individual for the maintenance of his-self- esteem and his inner integrity. However, the individual's motives are very often quite
different aiming to get rid of his inner sense of helplessness,
unworthiness and hopelessness.

A precondition of giving up self-destructive behaviour is
the coming about of a new inner balance with the help of therapeutic means or otherwise (Lonnqvist, 1978).

Freud (1927) implied the existence of indirect self-destructive behaviour (ISDB) in his hypothesis that among the characteristics of death instinct was a variable valence expressing itself
in fluctuating strength as time an situations changed. It was Karl
Menninger (1938) who developed the concept of the death instinct
to its fullest including ISDB, by postulating a change in the state
of balance between the opposing forces of the life and death instinct which under the influence of patterns containing guilt, aggression and eroticsm might produce a number of self-injuriours
or self-limiting behaviours. Menninger's classification included:
Focal suicide with self mutilation, Malingering, Chronic suicide

including asceticism or martyrdom, Neutrotic invalidism, Alcoholic addiction, Drug addiction, Antisocial behaviour, Psychosis with organic suicide, Meerlo (1968) called ISDB "hidden suicide", Schneidman (1968) used the term "subintentioned death" to describe the death which results from an individual's behaviour, which was not consciously intended.

Stress seeking behaviour with its negative and positive elements seems to play an important role in ISDB especially when the search for excitment and the degree of risk taking begins to exceed the boundaries of safety, survival and self- preservation. This area of stress seeking in relation to ISDB may have special significance for risk taking in its positive qualities which may have played a prominent role in the development of man in the form of mastering fear provoking situations, facilitating resolutions of developmental conflicts and fostering the drives for exploration and ambitious achievements.

Results of three studies of uncooperative diabetics, Buerger's patients and elderly chronically ill, comparing ISDB with direct self-destructive behaviour (DSDB) showed many differences in dynamics, cognitive and affective symptoms, relationships... etc. (Farberow, 1978).

Society attitude towards DSDB and ISDB is another variable. It may be condemned as in violent crime, assassinations or self-murder. However, it may be admired and glorified and somtimes national heroes are made through engaging in high risk taking and stress seeking climbers and explorers.

ISDB is not infrequently connected with impulsive behaviour : the person concerned thinks merely only of his momentary pleasure and satisfaction, being unable to take the longer term consequences of his behaviour into account e.g. smoking and drinking provide such an example. Again ISDB may manifest itself as a masochistic personality trait, where masochism becomes the only way be can express his disturbed aggression economy (Achte, 1978). Masochism may be seen as a character defence against anxiety.

There are many researchers dealing with the personalities of those behaving in an ISDB. If we take smoking as a model, which is ridiculed, condemned and known to represent a serious health risk and yet usually half the population does it. Why ? Is there something different about the personality of smokers ? Are they victims of a hereditary predisposition ? Studies by Eysenck (1960, 1980) and Hainus et al. (1980) showed that smokers are significantly more extravert, have early sexual experiences, risk taking, impulsivity, internal sensation seeking and drink more coffee and alcohol and are less likely to wear car seat belts. They are more frequently divorced, more subject to traffic accidents and more likely than non-smokers to change their jobs. Current smokers scored higher on the free floating and phobic anxiety scales of the Middlesex Hospital Questionnaire with some evidence of hysterical personality traits. There are a variety of explanations for smoking i.e. ISDB, which do not consider the substance e.g. nicotine is central to the behaviour. That it is a means of obtaining sensory gratification utilizing (Stepney, 1983).

a. sensory areas : e.g. smell, taste and appearance of smoke,oral and manual manipulation.

b. social areas : use of cigarettes to regulate and initiate social contact, exchange of cigarettes and social cohesion, image of smoker as adult, tough, and venturous and values as a displacement activity.

c. psychodynamic area : that smoking is a reflection of primitive sexuality, a reexperiencing of the pleasure of suckling. In children who had "constitutional" intensification of the erotogenic significance of the mouth region are expected to have a powerful motivation to drink and smoke would develop in later life. Also significance is attached to the phallic shape of cigarettes, pipes and especially cigars and to the symbolism of fire.

d. pharmacological areas : there is evidence that nicotine has intrinsically rewarding effect. Rats will lever press to obtain a dilute solution of the drug and prefer this to inadulterraded water. In rhesus monkeys some animals require primary shots of nicotine before they will self-inject the drug. These phenomena are presumably behavioural correlates of something equivalent to the "pleasure" reported by human smokers.

Jarvick (1970) suggested that nicotine facilitates the released noradrenaline and thus activates reward pathways in the limbic system. Again both nicotine and cigarette smoke release noradrenaline in the brains of cats, rats and monkeys.

Nicotine can be used in the manipulation of the psychological state i'e' arousal. Smoking can be either stimulant or depressant, depending on the smoker's environment. The contingent negative variation (CNV) is an EEG measure and like the proportion of alpha activity can be used as an index of arousal. When subjects smoked in their natural manner, some obtained consistent increase in CNV magnitude, indicative of stimulant effect, others under the same condition showed a consistant decrease. The direction of effect depended on dosage. Smokers with a low rate of nicotine intake tended to have stimulant effect e.g. extraverts, and those with a higher rate to have depressant ones e.g. introvert.

It seems that all types of ISDB stimulate the reward system in the limbic system through release of noradrenaline, whether the stimulus is a drug, food, sports, ascetism or martyrdom. It acts like the placebo effect and its release of opiate-like substances in the brain.

Because the immediate reward is physiological and the remote consequences and complications are psychological concepts for the mind of the individual undertaking ISDB, this sort of behaviour repeats and reinforces itself in spite of the fact that those people know the hazard of such a behaviour.

Has nature created those "pleasures" and "rewards" to instigate humans and animals in their self-elimination. Suppose one abstained from those pleasures for the sake of longevity and persistence, would this make for a happier life ??

REFERENCES

Achte, K. (1978): Some forms of indirect self destruction and their psychopathology. In proceedings of symposium on psychopathology of direct and indirect self-destruction. Edited by Achte, A and Lonnqvist? I. Psychiatrica Fennica supplementum.

Eysenck, H.J.; Tavant, M.; England, L. (1960): Smoking and personality. Br. Med. J., 1:1456-1460

Eysenck, H.J.; Eaves, L.J. (1980) The causes and effects of smoking. London: Maurice Temple Smith.

Farberow, N.L. (1978): Research in indirect self-destructive behaviour. In proceedings of the symposium on psychopathology of direct and indirect self destruction. Edited by Achte, Lonnqvist, I. Psychiat. Fennica supplementum.

Freud, S. (1927) Beyond the pleasure principle. London: Boul and Liveright.

Hainus, A.P. Jemeson, J.D.; Meade, T.W. (1980) Psychoneurotic profiles of smokers and non-smokers. Br. Med. J., 1:1422.

Jarvik, M.E. (1970) The role of nicotine in the smoking habit. In Hunt, W.A. (ed.) Learning mechanism in smoking.

Lonnqvist, J. (1978) Introduction: Self-destructive Behaviour. Proceedings of the symposium on psychopathology of direct and indirect self-destruction. Edited by: Achte, K and Lonnqvist, J Psychiat. Fennica Supplementum.

Meerlo, J.A.M. (1968) Hidden suicide. In Resnick, H.L.P.(ed.) Suicidal behaviour and management. Boston: Little Brown and Co.

Menninger, K.A. (1938) Man aginst himself. New York: Harcourt, Brace and Co.

Shneidman, E.S. (1968) Orientations towards death. A vital aspect of the study of lives. In Resnick, H.L.P. (ed.) Suicidal Behaviour and Management. Boston. Little Brown and Co.

Steppney, R. (1983) The psychology of smoking. Smith Kline and French publications.

OUTCOME OF ATTEMPTED SUICIDE

Jouko Lönnqvist and Esa-Matti Tolppanen

Department of Psychiatry
Helsinki Universtity Central Hospital
Tukholmankatu 8 C, 00290 Helsinki 29, Finland

INTRODUCTION

The purpose of this study is to determine the prognosis of attempted suicide in a long-term follow-up and to study whether a clinical interview can yield practical variables clinical significance to predict suicide.

MATERIAL AND METHODS

The series comprises all the 3,265 consecutive cases of attempted suicide treated at the emergency departments of Helsinki University Central Hospital in 1973-1979 and for whom a psychiatric consultation was arranged. Over 90 % of attempted suicides come for psychiatric consultation, in which a structured patient record form is used. The somatic severity, i.e. lethality, of the attempt was determined, together with the degree of intent to die according to the consulting psychiatrist, and the intensity of the psychiatric treatment arranged. A check was also made on all cases to establish whether they were alive or dead at the end of 1980.

RESULTS

By the end of the follow-up period a total of 305 patients had died, 217 of them male and 88 female (Table 1). In half of the cases (49.8 %) the cause of death was suicide. A quarter (25.9 %) had died from natural causes. The proportion of accidental deaths was higher among men, whereas in females the proportion of undetermined deaths was higher.

Table 1. Mortality During the Follow-up Period

Mode of Death	Males, % (N=217)	Females, % (N=88)	All, % (N=305)
Natural	24.4	29.5	25.9
Accident	18.0	6.8	14.8
Homicide	2.8	1.1	2.3
Suicide	49.8	50.0	49.8
Undetermined	5.1	12.5	7.2

The suicide rate among males was much higher than among females (Table 2). Those who committed suicide later on had received psychiatric treatment significantly more often and had also attempted suicide before the attempt related to this study. This attempt was significantly more severe both somatically and in regard to intent

Table 2. Characteristics of Suicides (N=152)

	Suicides, %	All, %
Male	71.1	42.7
Psychiatric patients	44.4	31.5
Previous suicide attempts	59.9	46.4
Lethality: mild	27.2	39.2
moderate	48.5	42.7
severe	24.3	11.7
Intent: mild	23.3	31.8
moderate	49.6	46.7
severe	27.1	14.2
Psychiatric after-care:		
no treatment	2.0	4.5
advice	32.9	39.4
referral	13.4	12.6
appointment	13.4	17.0
voluntary hospitalization	27.5	19.0
involuntary hospitalization	10.7	6.4
Age: under 20	5.9	9.5
20 - 29	41.4	39.3
30 - 39	24.3	25.0
over 40	28.3	25.2

Table 3. Annual Cohorts and Percentage of Suicides
During the Follow-up Period

Cohort		Percentage of Suicides in Population at Risk									
Year	Size	1.	2.	3.	4.	5.	6.	7.	8. year	Suicides	%
1973	333	1.5	0.6	0.0	0.6	1.3	0.3	0.7	0.0	16	4.8
1974	511	2.2	1.0	0.2	1.0	0.2	0.4	1.6		32	6.3
1975	489	2.9	2.4	0.7	0.4	0.9	0.9			38	7.8
1976	463	1.9	0.4	0.7	0.9	0.0				18	3.9
1977	481	2.1	1.3	0.9	0.0					20	4.2
1978	520	2.7	0.6	0.0						17	3.3
1979	469	2.1	0.0							10	2.1

in the survivor-victims who committed suicide. They had also been referred for psychiatric hosp ital treatment immediately after the attempt significantly more often than the others. Patients under 20 were underrepresented among the survivor-victims who committed suicide.

In all annual cohorts, the risk of suicide is greatest (1.5 - 2.9 %) during the first year of follow-up (Table 3). Even during the second year the risk is greater than normal. The rate of suicide subsequently falls, with cases divided unevenly throughout the follow-up period.

Among males the suicide rate was more than three times that among females (Table 4). The number of suicides among survivor-males increased immediately after the suicide attempt. 1.7 % (vs. 0.3 %) commited suicide within three months and 2.1 % (vs. 0.6 %) within six months. The suicide rate among males is high for several years after the suicide attempt. During the eight-year follow-up the risk of suicide among females is lower than that among males during the first follow-up year.

Among those who attempted suicide and who were receiving psychiatric treatment at the time of the attempt, the suicide rate during the first year of follow-up was over twice as high as the others (3.4 % vs. 1.6 %). The difference later decreases but nevertheless remains.

The suicide rate among those who had attempted suicide earlier

Table 4. Survival Analysis:
Cumulative Suicides by Sex

Follow-up Year	Males			Females		
	Suicides	At risk	%	Suicides	At risk	%
1st	49	1393	3.6	24	1869	1.3
2nd	71	1300	5.4	31	1833	1.7
3rd	77	1051	6.0	36	1573	2.0
4th	89	818	7.5	37	1283	2.1
5th	94	635	8.4	41	998	2.6
6th	100	468	9.6	42	717	2.7
7th	108	294	12.8	43	444	3.2
8th	108	109		43	174	

on was higher troughout the entire follow-up period (Table 5); these
cases were distributed more evenly throughout the follow-up period
(p<0.01). An earlier suicide attempt thus suggests a more long-term
risk of suicide.

The somatic severity, i.e. lethality, clearly distinguishes
between attempts in terms of the risk of suicide (p<0.001). When
lethality was rated as mild 2.9 % commited suicide during the follow-
up period; in cases of moderate lethality the figure was 4.7 % and
in cases of severe lethality 8.4 %. In females the prognosis after
severe attempts was clearly poorer (6.0 %) than after moderate
(2.3 %) or mild (1.3 %) attempts. The risk of suicide in males is
always high but increases along with the degree of lethality (5.4 %,

Table 5. Survival Analysis: Lethality of Attempts
and Suicides During the Follow-up Period

Follow-up Year	Degree of Lethality:					
	Mild		Moderate		Severe	
	At risk	%	At risk	%	At risk	%
1st	1282	1.1	1396	2.6	382	5.0
2nd	1247	0.7	1339	0.8	359	1.4
3rd	1065	0.2	1112	0.6	288	0.4
4th	876	0.6	864	0.6	219	0.9
5th	723	0.4	619	0.3	156	1.9
6th	547	0.2	416	0.7	92	1.1
7th	374	0.8	238	1.3	47	2.1
8th	150	0.0	75	0.0	18	0.0

Table 6. Survival Analysis: Predictive Value
of Intention to Die

Follow-up Year	Mild At risk	%	Moderate At risk	%	Severe At risk	%
1st	1039	1.2	1524	2.1	462	5.0
2nd	1007	0.8	1471	0.8	434	0.9
3rd	867	0.2	1204	0.4	364	0.8
4th	708	0.3	931	0.9	288	0.4
5th	588	0.3	669	0.4	209	1.4
6th	443	0.4	450	0.4	136	0.7
7th	299	0.7	258	1.2	88	1.1
8th	112	0.0	94	0.0	31	0.0

8.0 % and 10.6 %).

The predictive value of lethality is highly signigicant during
the first year of follow-up (Table 5). In cases of mild lethality,
the suicide rate during the subsequent year was 1.1 %, in cases of
moderate lethality 2.6 % and in cases of severe lethality 5.0 %.
Even later on, the degree of lethality correlated with the suicide
rate, but its predictive value was smaller.

The clinical global assessment of the psychiatrist in connection
with the suicide attempt on the intention to die correlated clearly
with the prognosis. In cases of mild intent, the suicide rate during
the subsequent follow-up period was 3.0 %, in cases of moderate intent
4.3 % and in cases of severe intent 7.8 %. In females the prognosis
was significantly better after attempted suicide but the degree of
intent classifies the females into different risk groups, too. In
cases of moderate intent the risk of suicide was twice as high as
for mild intent (2.2 % vs. 1.0 %) and in cases of severe intent six
times as high (6.0 % vs. 1.0 %). The risk of suicide among males in
cases of mild intent (6.1 %) is as great as that in severe intent
among females. In cases of moderate intent the risk is higher
(7.1 %) and in cases of severe intent it is signigicantly high
(9.9 %).

In cases of severe intent to commit suicide, the risk of
suicide during the first year of follow-up (Table 6) is over four
times greater than for mild intent (5.0 % vs. 1.2 %) and over
twice as high as for moderate intent (5.0 % vs. 2.1 %). Later on
during the follow-up period there were still differences in the risk
of suicide between the groups, though these were clearly smaller.

Both the lethality and intent clearly predict a higher risk of

Table 7. Psychiatric After-care and Suicides (%)
During the Follow-up Period

After-care	3 mo.	6 mo.	1 yr.	The end of follow-up
No treatment	0.0	0.7	1.4	2.0
Advice	0.7	0.9	1.6	3.8
Referral	1.0	1.5	2.2	4.6
Appointment	1.1	1.8	2.2	3.6
Voluntary hospitalization	1.1	1.3	2.9	6.6
Involuntary hospitalization	1.4	2.4	4.8	7.7

suicide in both long-term and short-term follow-ups. Within three months after the attempted suicide a 6-fold number of the survivor-victims with severe intent (2.4 %) and a 2-fold number of those with moderate intent (0.8 %) committed suicide compared to those with mild intent (0.4 %). During a 6-month follow-up, the differences in the risk are still more pronounced. In cases of severe intent, 3.5 % committed suicide within six months. The figures for moderate and mild intent were 1.6 % and 0.5 % respectively.

The intensity of further psychiatric treatment correlates with the suicide rate during the follow-up period (Table 7). The proportion of survivor-victims referred for hospital treatment against their will was clearly highest (7.7 %) during the follow-up. Likewise, voluntary hospital treatment is associated with an increase in the suicide rate (6.6 %). Ambulatory care (advice, referral, appointment) does not seem to significantly affect the prognosis. The prognosis for those who had not received treatment (2.2 %) was clearly better than for the others.

The intensity of further treatment correlates with an increase in the risk of suicide, even in a three-month follow-up.

PHYSICAL ILLNESS PRECEDING SUICIDE

Brian Barraclough

Faculty of Medicine
University of Southampton
Southampton, Hants, U.K

INTRODUCTION

Physical illness is believed to play a part in the chain of events preceding suicide. Many writers on suicide have made that observation with a notable exception in Durkheim. But why physical illness should be a precursor of suicide is not as obvious as why mental illness, which causes suicidal thinking as one of its symptoms, should be.

Terminal disease, particularly terminal cancer could induce suicide as a way of pre-empting a more horrible end. Some physical disease may be especially difficult to bear because of disfigurement, disability, pain or discomfort and cause death to be preferred to life. The metabolic effects of physical disorder or their pharmacological treatment may cause depression. The neuropathology of some disease may cause mood disorders, or alter behaviour, producing social stresses or inter-personal problems which themselves then become important factors in causing suicide. Physical disease and its treatment, surgery for example, might act as a stressful event predisposing to depression. Disease interfering with sight, hearing, speech or mobility might increase isolation and loneliness, factors considered important in the causes of suicide. The chance conjunction of physical disease and a depressive illness might result in a suicide which would not have occurred in an uncomplicated depression.

There are, therefore, grounds for hypothesising a link between physical disease and suicide.

The evidence linking physical disease and suicide is not as

convincing as that which has established the link between mental
disease and suicide. The evidence derives from long term follow up
studies to establish suicide rates of physical diseases and from case
studies of consecutive series of suicides describing prevalence of
physical disease.

METHOD

I searched the literature to find suicide rates of physical
illness and reports describing the occurrence of physical illness in
case studies of suicides. Physical illness excluded functional mental
illness, alcoholism and other addictions but included organic mental
illness, epilepsy and anorexia nervosa. Papers in English, French
and German were examined.

I used the following sources: a MEDLARS search under the term
suicide; a MEDLARS search for long term mortality studies under the
terms anorexia nervosa, amyotrophic lateral sclerosis, epilepsy,
multiple sclerosis, Parkinsonism, presenile and senile psychoses; a
MEDLARS search for long term mortality studies of conditions which
appeared in the suicide search - cardiac pacemakers, cardiac valve
replacement, diabetes, epilepsy, haemodialysis, head injury,
hepatitis, ileostomy, laryngectomy, lupus erythematosis, renal trans-
plant, rheumatoid arthritis, spinal cord injury, ulcerative colitis;
the bibliographies of Mayer Gross, Slater and Roth, the Handbook of
Clinical Neurology; standard medical and neurological texts; the
Statistical Bulletin of the Metropolitan Life Insurance Company of
New York and the Impairment Study, 1951. Likely references in the
bibliographies of relevant papers located were also examined.

I included a report if I was able to reach a decision about the
suicide rate. Few of the hundreds of papers I have read produced the
information to reach any conclusion about mortality. I decided the
disease had a raised suicide rate if the paper concluded so and,
failing that, if the suicide rate which I calculated from the data
given was higher than that for the general population or if the
percentage of deaths caused by suicide was much higher than expected.

I will summarise the results under four headings, medical,
neurological, surgical conditions and case studies.

Medical

Peptic or gastric ulcer is, in five studies (Krause, 1963;
Hirohata, 1968; Ihre et al., 1964; Viskum 1975; Lindskov, 1975),
reported to have a high suicide rate and the suggested link is
alcohol addiction.

Ulcerative colitis is reported in five studies (Jalan et al., 1970; Morowitz and Kirsner, 1969; Willard et al., 1938; Truelove and Witts, 1955; Spencer at al., 1962) as carrying an increased risk of suicide and in three (Lennard-Jones et al., 1974; Banks et al., 1957; Lioner et al., 1960) as not. Harrison's textbook of medicine asserts it does have a high rate and I believe that is correct. Furthermore the evidence suggests that systemic steroids may be the cause; the raised suicide rate has been observed since the introduction of corticosteroids and the related condition, recto-sigmoiditis (Farmer and Brown, 1971), treated with topical steroids has an average suicide rate.

Lupus in three studies (Dubois et al., 1974; Cheatum et al., 1973; Kellum and Haserick, 1964) has a raised rate and three not (Estes, 1971; Comerford and Cohen, 1967; Carpenter and Sturgill, 1966). The internal evidence is consistent with cerebral lupus, which can cause psychoses, being responsible and not other forms.

Haemodialysis in six studies (Tapia et al., 1973; Henari et al., 1977; Siddiqui et al., 1970; Popowuiak et al., 1975; Roguska et al., 1974; Heal et al., 1973) is reported as having a high suicide rate and in seven as not (Roguska et al., 1974; Stenzel et al., 1974; Palmer, 1971; King et al., 1975; Shapiro et al., 1974; Mathen et al., 1975; Foster et al., 1973). This variation probably results from differences in selection, for mental and behavioural abnormalities can exclude patients from dialysis, and differences in quality of psychosocial management. Suicide, I understand, can be concealed in dialysis deaths so may be understated.

In contrast to dialysis I found only one (Nielubowicz et al., 1971) of eight papers (Sellers et al., 1976; Simmons et al., 1977; Tersigni et al., 1976; Diethelm et al., 1976; Finkelstein et al., 1975; Ellis et al., 1972; Woods et al., 1973) on the outcome of renal transplantation even suggesting suicide was increased.

Seven (Theander, 1970; Morgan and Russell, 1975; Seidensticker and Tzagournis, 1968; Dally, 1969; Kay, 1953; Crisp, 1965, 1978) of nine papers (Nemiah, 1950; Ryle, 1936) on anorexia nervosa outcome report an increased incidence of suicide. That, I think, is accepted in psychiatry but may be an artefact of the selection of intractable cases for treatment by the psychiatrist after the physician or nature has failed.

One paper (MacGregor, 1977) reports suicide and attempted suicide to be increased in juvenile diabetes. In contrast there is excellent evidence for adult diabetics having an average rate (Armstrong et al., 1976).

Neurological

Of 11 studies on epilepsy, 10 report suicide to be increased; the association is stronger with temporal lobe epilepsy (cited in Barraclough, 1981).

Traumatic brain injury is, in two papers (Heiskanen and Sipponen, 1970; Society of Actuaries, 1954) of five (Wilkinson, 1969; Miller and Stern 1965; Fahy et al., 1967) reported as having a high suicide rate. The evidence is inconclusive in my view although most psychiatrists seem to believe the rate is increased.

A raised suicide rate is reported in one (Leibowitz et al., 1972) of four (Hutchinson, 1976; Gudmundsson, 1971; Kurtzke et al., 1970) papers on multiple sclerosis, the association being for cerebral disease.

Parkinson's disease may have a raised rate but the evidence of three papers is inconclusive (Cote et al., 1970; Slome, 1977; Zumstein and Siegfried, 1976). All patients were treated with modern drugs which can influence mental state.

The evidence for Huntington's chorea having a raised suicide rate rests on a single (Reed and Chandler, 1958) but convincing paper reporting a high rate for patients outside institutions and their relatives.

Four papers show spinal cord injury resulting in paraplegia or quadraplegia having a raised suicide rate (Hackler, 1977; Geisler et al., 1977; Nyquist and Bors, 1967; Price, 1973), and others have been published since this review was concluded.

Surgical

Total laryngectomy for carcinoma is reported in two studies (Barton, 1965; Shaw, 1965) as having a raised incidence of suicide. Alcohol excess is mentioned as being related to laryngeal cancer.

Ileostomy for colitis has two studies reporting a raised suicide rate (Ritchie, 1971, 1972). Steroids may be implicated since most cases were of ulcerative colitis. I have not found convincing evidence that colostomy has a raised suicide rate.

Limb amputations of the Finnish wars of the 1940's were associated with a high suicide rate (Bakalim, 1969) but I have not located satisfactory reports of a contemporary series.

Case Studies

With one exception the conclusions of published case studies are invalid because age, sex-matched controls were not used to evaluate the significance of physical disease found in suicides (Dorpat and Ripley, 1960; Seager and Flood, 1965) or, if controls were used, the method of comparison was faulty (Flood and Seager, 1968; McDowall et al., 1968; Farberow et al., 1966).

The exception is an English study of 17 male and 13 female suicides compared with 170 and 130 age matched controls (Jones, 1965). The male suicides but not the female had significantly more out-patient and in-patient hospital treatment for serious physical disease unlikely to be explained by depressed mood and hypochondriasis. 17 cases is insufficient for a conclusion in this type of work.

I will now summarise an unpublished enquiry of my own which compared the physical health of 75 consecutive suicides with 150 randomly selected living controls matched for age, sex, whether married and place of residence, two for each suicide. The result was more striking for similarities than differences. 40% in each group were physically healthy, 3% terminally ill and the same proportion had cancers.

But more suicides had serious illness, 33% compared with 25%, digestive system disorders 8% and 0%, epilepsy 4% and 2%, and deaf 4% and 1%. In the same study 93% of suicides were mentally ill (Barraclough et al., 1974).

CONCLUSIONS

Some physical diseases in my opinion precede suicide and contribute to it. The association is complex but involves at least four types of effect:

Cerebral pathology, for instance, in multiple sclerosis and lupus causes psychoses which have high suicide rates.

Addictive substance, alcohol for example, which are associated with an increased suicide risk, causes body changes, for instance peptic ulceration.

The disorder leads to breakdown of social bonds, for instance changed behaviour of Huntington's chorea or limitations of the paraplegic.

Treatment, for instance, with steroids affects mood.

However the independent contribution of physical disease to suicide is modest in comparison to that of mental disease and the contribution that it does make is, in my opinion, mediated through an adverse influence on mood.

The diseases mentioned in method but not results had an average suicide rate or only one report of a raised rate. Many reports included are of small numbers followed for short periods with few deaths, conditions which are well known to lead to the wrong statistical inference.

In the nature of things my literature search must have been incomplete so I would be pleased to hear of reports of suicide rates of diseases which I have left out.

REFERENCES

The references will be supplied on written application.

ACKNOWLEDGEMENTS

Mrs. Hazel Hills prepared this camera ready copy on an IBM Correcting Selectric III typewriter using Prestige Elite typeface.

FORENSIC PSYCHIATRIC ISSUES IN SUICIDAL BEHAVIOUR WITHIN AN EMERGENCY

PSYCHIATRIC SETTING

Jean-Pierre Soubrier, Jacques Feillard,
and Nicole Quemada
Infirmerie Psychiatrique
3 rue Cabanis
75014 Paris, France

Psychiatric clinic evolution, modern life, new therapies, have
led specialists, and more particularly those dealing with suicide,
to consider suicidal behaviours within a wide field, including mental
disorders which do not enter the nosologic frame, taking into account
any violence against oneself or against others, in an extended area
where border between normality and pathology is unstable, depending
on the acting out and on the position of the observer.

The question of suicide and the necessity of being helped in
case of suicidal ideas or attempted suicide and possibly get medical
care, arises in a general point of view as well as within the forensic
and legal system, with obligation of medical care in case of refusal.

What happens to attempted suicide when it is collected by the
police ? We will study, as an example, the Psychiatric Infirmary of
the Police Headquarters in Paris.

Briefly, an historical review. Created in 1872, the Department
depends on the Chief Commissioner of the Police, who asks a medical
team to give the first psychiatric aid to a given population including
all those who created a public disturbance, and determine who should
be sent to a mental hospital and not handed over to the Justice.
Psychiatric Infirmary was located in the Conciergerie, between the
Law-Courts and the Police Headquarters, on the banks of Seine river.

Some patients are also sent to the Psychiatric Infirmary by
the Penitenciary Administration, directly from prison or through
their medical and psychiatric departments.

In course of time, this department keeps its importance in

spite of the evolution of psychiatry and a better organization in orientating mental patients.

The special interest of this department lies in the fact that physicians have the administrative power to enforce the Law of June 30, 1838 concerning commitments. So patients are sent to the mental hospital where they get compulsory medical care if necessary, as per the law in force allowing to take action against those who are dangerous for themselves and for the others.

Therefore, according to P. Pichot, it is one of the first crisis center, in the most liberal sense of the word, and unique too from a historical point of view. It is the only medical psychiatric department where the patient, without a third party (family, friends ...) will not be allowed to refuse necessary medical cares and referral to a mental hospital.

Usually, in case of psychological crisis, the therapeutic attitude will be of the crisis intervention type. But when a severe pathological state, requiring a long psychiatric hospitalization, is evidenced or discovered, the orientation will be organized by our department.

Alcoholic pathology, psychopathies with or without associated delinquency, as well as the whole mental pathology, can be found at the Psychiatric Infirmary, with a high proportion of psychoses.

For today's meeting, we have set apart attempted suicide. Patients concerned are peculiar in the way that they do not need, or no longer need, intensive cares, but drew attention on themselves by attempting suicide in a usually spectacular, noisy, agitated way, using violent and dangerous means and (or) who did not accept to be kept in a general hospital. They can even require, during a short period of time, to be kept under observation in an inpatient milieu to give way from the acting out and make an estimate of the situation and of the residual lethal risk.

This department has carried out two successive epidemiological studies, each one of them considering a six months' period. The first one in 1964, centered on attempted suicides, which represented 3,36 % of a population including 63 % of males. The second one in 1978 in cooperation with I.N.S.E.R.M., dealing with the reasons for referral to the Psychiatric Infirmary, found 6 % of attempted suicides out of a population of 79 % of males. In this second study, which remains valid after a verification in 1982, we have compared this population of patients with suicidal behaviours to the normal population and have made differential findings about the type of suicide, the time referral occurred, later orientation with or without enforcement of the law. We first selected a particular group, characterized by violences aimed either against their own self or against the others by mean of threats or acting out.

These two types of violence, self-aggressive or hetero-agressive, have been correlated with various criteria, personal, social, family (sex, age, nationality, occupation, matrimonial situation, way of life, place of abode), psychiatric (diagnosis), as well as with the course covered during the crisis, before and after the Psychiatric Infirmary.

Out of 1883 patients studied during six months, we noted 111 attempted suicides (79 % of males, 21 % of females), 300 violences against others (87 % of males, 13 % of females).

Paradoxically, a certain proportion of suicides end up at the Psychiatric Infirmary in spite of a first visit in a general hospital, with eventually consultation of a psychiatrist.

Therefore, we actually are in front of patients with suicide ideation and intention, refusing treatment, for which enforcement of the law allows paradoxically a better prevention of suicide.

We do not want to side with or against the two theories in opposition : suicide as a "cry for help" or, as it is the case in some countries, enforcement of a law compelling to notify any suicide and to refer all those who attempted suicide to a psychiatric setting.

Difference between violent and agressive pathology and auto-agressive suicidal pathology is interesting. As a matter of fact, social characteristics (higher social level), age criteria (young people) and neuroses were prominent among attempted suicides. Violence against others was more typical of alcoholism and psychoses except manic-depressive psychosis which refers to attempted suicide.

Women do not have more suicidal tendencies than men. Suicide seems to concern more the city than the suburb. But the striking point of this study is the young age of the suicidal pathology (men and women).

Appealing to a third party seems to be connected to the "significant other" pathology, beyond the patient's environment. Most of the time, these patients have been dismissed from the general hospitals and it is very likely that a little more understanding and a better organization for receiving patients would appreciably reduce this percentage of attempted suicides which are taken over by the Police. In addition, this is not always well accepted or well understood by the policeman who expects a different attitude from the physicians and the general hospital.

In France, this law about commitments was supposed to be rescinded and replaced by a law making medical cares compulsory for any deviant pathological behaviour, not only those due to mental disorders but also those due to general diseases, epilepsy, renal diseases, alcoholism. Up to now, the Governmental Committee has not been able to come to a conclusion and move another law (hopefully).

As far as we are concerned, when we have to enforce this 1838 Law, we try to make the patient understand that we act in pursuance of the Legal power of the Chief Commissioner and not as a psychiatrist, in order to keep the dialogue between patient and therapist open.

As a matter of fact, compulsory medical cares could perfectly well be enforced without the assistance of the Police. Psychiatrists responsible for public mental health are legally responsible but not always dare to use this power.

A certain amount of carelessness seems to be of the psychiatrists' desinclination.

But when a suicide is committed in a nursing-home or a hospital, their responsability is involved, and the therapist can be reproached with not prescribing commitment. The usual "discharge against medical advice" will not release the therapist and the hospital from their responsability. In France, the Ministry of Health has been warned by the Insurance Companies of an increase of suicides within the General Hospitals. This question has also been raised in the United States in a recent article from R. Litman who suggests creation of Committees for prevention of suicide in the public hospitals.

As a conclusion, attempted suicide covers neither the whole of psychiatric emergency, nor the whole of psychological distress. It is now well-known that other behaviour abnormalities, including refusal of medical cares, are suicidal equivalents or indirect suicidal behaviours, according to Norman Farberow.

When dealing with suicidal acting out, with unquestionable purpose of dying, obligation to enforce the law is drastic and un-fortunate. This study showed the small percentage of genuine mental disorders for which the 1838 law was moved in the last century, at a time when biological and psychological therapies were not yet what they are nowadays.

When we compare 1982 to 1964 studies, we can see that the percentage of suicidal pathology was not so high in 1964 than in 1982, and therefore we can wonder whether attempted suicide is a mental health indicator, as Durkheim thought, a social health indi-cator or "social barometer" as per Hendin (1982).

We had rather come to the conclusion that attempted suicide is an indicator of social and moral pressure, that enforcing the law is a drastic measure which may have been therapeutically useful.

904

The legal psychiatric pathology reminds us daily of the frequency of post-homicidal suicides, melancholic or not, for which protection of the individual is necessary.

A temporary receiving structure inside the hospital would palliate the social reject from which suffers the one who attempted suicide.

This study has been carried out in collaboration with Unit 110 of the National Institute of Health and Medical Research (INSERM), and the Study and Research Centre of Forensic Psychiatry.

FAMILY AND SUICIDE

W. Poeldinger

Kantonale Psychiatrische Klinik Wil
Zürcherstr. 30
CH-9500 Wil/SG

Although it is a feature of modern psychiatry to include aspects
of motive forces within the family in the diagnosis and therapy,
connections between family and suicide can be traced back a long
way in literature. As far back as 1864 A. WAGNER,for example,
wrote on this subject in his book"Legitimacy in Apparently Arbitrary Acts from the Point of View of Statistics":
"According to observations made, we must also almost believe that
each year Nature seems to exact with equal certainty a fixed number
of suicides as it does other deaths, as it does abnormal marriag-
ges and immoral divorces. The annual number of suicides, broken
down by invididual provinces, sub-divisions of the state which in
themselves form a small organic whole, broken down by confession,
sex, age, civil state, occupation, means by which suicide was
committed, even by seasons, months and time of day, belongs in
some states to the most uniformly recurrent statistical facts
known.We have available much fine material and a wealth of observations on suicide; observations in the various countries show
some individual divergencies but great regularity within their
respective territories.

This indicates that primarily the general conditions of a people's civilazation have an influence on suicide, just as they do on so many other social factors."

In 1881 this line of thought was followed further by TH.-G. MASARYK in his book"Suicide as a Mass Social Phenomenon of Modern Civilization". These ideas were then taken up and elaborated by Emile DURKHEIM in his study of suicide,"Le Suicide",published in 1897.

In his theory DURKHEIM works out four basic types of suicidal behavior which can be attributed to different social causes. He divides these into two dimensions, namely that of social integration and that of social regulation. With regard to social integration he distinguishes between egoistic and altruistic suicide. He shows that cultures with high social integration also show a high rate of altruistic acts of suicide. He gives as an example the custom of suttee in India, the immolation of a widow upon the death of her husband, or martyrdom in early Christianity.

If, however, ties in a society have b-come loose, then the egoistic behavior of its members increases, whereas in an integrated society such behavior is neutralized by family, religious and political ties. As a result there ist also an increase in the number of egoistic suicides directes against society. The second dimension, social regulation, means that the society not only influences the thoughts and acts of the individual, but also has the power to regulate the motives and feelings of its members. From this point of view DURKHEIM distinguishes fatalistic suicides in highly regula-societies. His explanation is that in these highly regulated societies the individual can soon come to feel that he is entirely at the mery of such a society. In contrast, he describes the anomic suicide in a socially weak or not regulated situation and ascribes it to the prevailing lack of regulation, i.e.anomy. In addition to economic anomy as brought about by war or economic crises, he also examines the influence of anomy on familial relationships, for example on the frequency of divorce- and here, too, finds the expected connetion between the suicide rate and number of divorces. An empirically oriented sociologist, DURKHEIM naturally also examined the relationship to practice and verified his hypotheses with extensiv demographic material.Later works also confirmed the connections observed by DURKHEIM but sought, as for instance HALB-WACHS (1930) who revised DURKHEIM's works, to summarize the dimensions of social integration and social regulation in two types and thereby consider suicide under the general aspect of social integration or disintegration. In 1965 JONSON again revised the work begun by DURKHEIM and came to the conlusion that a society's suicide rate is always high when social integration is either low or high. If, however, a society's integration is within the average, the suicide rate is relatively low. JOHNSON thereby equated anomic and egoistic suicide. In both cases there is a striking lack of interaction between the members of a group as well as of generally binding norms or common goals. As, however, the term social integration is not at all exact, GIBBS and MARTIN then endeavoured through operationalzation to give a clearer definition of the term status-integration and to make it measurable on a scale basis.

It was thereby then possible to calculate quantitative differences between societies. These two authors reached the following five hypotheses:

1. The lower the suicide rate,the more stable and lasting the social relations.
2. The more stable and lasting the social relations, the more concordant the social expectations.
3. The more concordant the social expectations, the fewer the rôle-conflicts.
4. The fewer the rôle-conflicts,the fewer the individuals assuming

original, incompatible status positions.

5. The fewer individuals holding incompatible status positions,the higher the status integration.

Applying these perceptions to the family, as DURKHEIM already did, our own study of 440 patients hospitalized after attempted suicide showed that laver's grief,familial problems and isolation were amongst the most frequent triggering reasons and motives.

In all three motives we find the problem of the threatening loss of a partner. In the same study we could show that amongst patients hospitalized after attempted suicide, primarily divorced patients varied significantly from the normal distribution of the civil state of the population.It can be assumed that in the case of divorced persons,in addition to the loss,which has also been suffered by widowed persons, primarily feelings of guilt play a part.With regard to loss of a partner and on the basis of a number of statistics,BOJANOVSKY has been able to show that amongst widowed persons younger people are apparently in relatively greater danger of attempting suicide then older people.He explains this by the fact that the loss of a partner while still young is unexpected and therefore more difficult to accent and assimilate.He also points out that clinical experience has shown that a person can more easily overcome difficult situations if a majority of other people and not just that person alone has been similarly affected.This is also his explanation of the sinking suicide rate in older widowed persons and above all in women,as in these groups there are always many people suffering the same fate.In the case of divorced persons,however,his studies show no conspicuous differences in the separate age-groups.

Diagram 1 gives a graphic presentation of the absolute figures for divorces,suicides and deaths from traffic accidents in Switzerland compiled for the years 1970 to 1980 and shows the changes as percentages of the basic figures for the year 1970.These graphs also

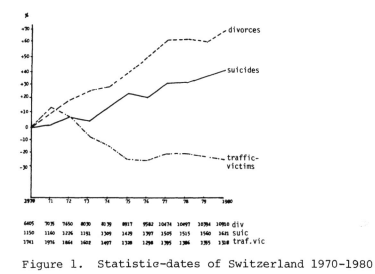

6405	7035	7650	8030	8139	8917	9582	10474	10497	10394	10910	div
1150	1160	1226	1191	1309	1429	1397	1505	1515	1560	1621	suic
1741	1976	1864	1602	1497	1320	1298	1395	1386	1355	1318	traf.vic

Figure 1. Statistic-dates of Switzerland 1970-1980

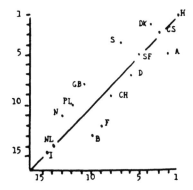

Figure 2. International comparison of rank orders in divorce
and suicide (average figures 1964-1965)

show that the developments in suicides and divorces show similar
trends,even if the increases in divorces(expressed as a percentage)
are higher than in suicides.In this connetion it is also of interest that in spite of increasing motorization the number of deaths
from traffic accidents has decreased in the same period of time.
In a macropsychological study of the family in Europe,FUCHS,GASPAR
and MILLENDORFER have also compared the relations between divorces
and suicides. They also found a strikingly close connection between the two socio-psychological indicators divorce and suicide.
Countries with a high suicide rate are at the same time those with
comparatively high divorce rate, with unstable marriges.These
authors say that in an international camparison of European countries this relation has remained constant since the 193o's,which
would indicate that this is a basic phenomenum. Diagram 2 shows an
international comparison of divorce and suicide,in order of frequency,under reference to GASPARI and taking account of the
average figures for 1964 to 1965. The solid line shows the legitimacy of these relations in the countries specified and indicated
by the appropriate international traffic signs.
A further connetion between family and suicide is shown by the
fact that suicide and attempted suicide run in some families. We
know that there are certain forms of depression,namely endogenous
depressions,which often run in families.Apart from heredity,it is
proble that suicides often run in families because acts of suicide
have a suggestive effect and people who are in mental distress and
who already know of cases of suicide within their families are more
inclined to take a similar course of action.I recall the case of a
young man of 23,who,after repeated failure in his studies,tried
to commit suicide by hanging himself. He said that memories of
stories about his grandfather were deciding factors.The grandfather had done much to contribute to the prosperity and reputation of the family and was much talked about long after his death.

912

He had,though,also blemished the family's name because he had ended his own life by hangig himself. His grandson,who was at a crisis point in his university studies suddenly felt that he understood his grandfather,whom he had silently always blamed for bringing shame to the family,although he had made it wealthy.Within himself he was in a way apologizing to his granfather,and amongst other thins wanted to make amends for the previous misunderstanding of his grandfather's act by hanging himself from the same tree as his grandfather had done. Fortunately so many years had gone by in the meantime that the tree had become rotten and the branch from which the patient wanted to hang himself broke.

In the medical treatment of persons with suicidal tendencies, familial relations are very important.We will,for example accept a risk of suicide and agree to out-patient treatment if the person concerned lives in a family unit where there is always someone to look after him and where he is not left alone at night.We will,however,not accept a similar risk of suicide if the person concerned is living alone in a bachelor flat and his no-one nearby to look after him.

In assessing suicidal tendencies,the pre-suicidal syndrome must be mentioned first and foremost(Diag.5).In this presuicidal syndrome we have the phenomenon of situational limitation,by which we mean primarily isolation.Such isolation is very often to be found in the family unit,namely when there is a situation of estrangement and growing apart.As GASTAGER says, it is unfortunately only too often the case that in such situations people do not direct their energies towards briding the gaps, but solely towards maintaining a facade towards the outside world. We are thus presented with the picture of a"facade family".In such a family,lonely persons have been shown to be especially prone to suicidal thoughts and impulses.Turning to the end of the question of how and to what extent an act of suicide is registered,the family should again be mentioned first,

as in most cases it is the family which is affected most, be it the
primary family from which one comes or the secondary family which
one has started oneself. Amongst other things this is also connected to the fact that every act of suicide is in some way at the
same time an appeal.In suicides this is often emphasized in a re-
proachful letter of farewell. It was STENGEL who first emphasized
that particular significance is thereby attached to an attempted
suicide.SHNEIDMAN and FARBEROW then talked about the"Cry for Help"
and it was KREITMAN and FEUERLEIN who introduced the term "parasuicide",or"parasuicidal act".

A further aspect of motive forces within the family has been registered by SPERLIN, taking as a starting-point Paul FEDERN's remark that"nobody kills himself,whom another does not wish dead".
He points out that in the families suicides there are incomparably
more early deaths in previous family history than in other families.
In this connection he speaks of a"trend towards death"predominating
in such families. Death as a solution to problems is the first
thing which occurs to members of such families. He also points
out that hostilities within the familiy,particularly on the part of
the mother, are more marked in the families of suicides. This makes
family-therapy,which would be the best form of therapy,in the sense
of tackling the problem together considerably more difficult.
Looking at several generations and on the basis of observing
casuistry and statistics, SPERLING comes to the following conclu-
sions:1. the familiy in which one is living at present has a protective effect as regards suicide. All statistics show that persons
living alone are in particular danger.2. There are several ways in
which the family of origin can affect a tendency to suicide:
1.if cases of suicide can be shown in the family history.2.if
threats of suicide by members of the family are used as blackmail.
3.An accumulation of more of less openly expressed wishes to die
made to the person who later commits suicide. These are expressed

914

relatively openly, for instance in the case of alcoholics and the chronically ill, but primarily also in the case of insubordinate children who have acted contrary to their parents'sense of values.

4.There have been premature,tragic deaths of respected persons in the family which have never been"mourned out".The premature death was understandably encapsulated as incomprehensible.

From the foregoing the following conclusions can be drawn:

1.More attention should be paid to the aspects of motive forces within the family,both for reasons of suicide prevention within the scope of medical care as well as with regard to diagnosis and therapy.

2.In a psycho-hygienic respect we must oppose all forces and powers which are destructive to the family and enure that in our society the family is again held in higher esteem.

Literature

Balint M.: Primärer Narzıssmus und primäre Liebe. Jb.
Psychoanal. *1,* 3–34, 1960. *Balint M.:* Die Urformen der
Liebe und die Technik der Psychoanalyse. S. Fischer,
Frankfurt 1969. *Battegay R., Haenel Th.:* Narzisstische
Störungen und Suizidalität. Sozial- und Präventivmedizin
24, 42–47, 1979. *Bojanovsky J.:* Partnerverlust als Auslö-
ser für Selbstmorde und Selbstmordversuche. Caritas *79,*
121–125, 1978. *Bojanovsky J.:* Ehepartnerverlust als Risi-
kofaktor für den Selbstmord. In: «Suizid-Ergebnisse und
Therapie.» Hrsg. C. Reimer. Springer, Berlin. Heidelberg, New York 1982. *Durkheim E.:* Le suicide. Etude de
sociologie. Alcano, Paris 1897. Deutsche Übersetzung:
Der Selbstmord. Luchterhand, Neuwied 1969. *Federn P.:*
Die Diskussion über Selbstmord. insbesondere den Schü-
lerselbstmord, im Wiener psychoanalytischen Verein. Z.
psychoanalyt. Päd. *3,* 334–379, 1929. *Feuerlein W.:*
Selbstmordversuch oder parasuizidale Handlung? Nervenarzt *42,* 127–130, 1971. *Freud S.:* Zur Einführung des
Narzissmus. Ges. W. Bd. *10,* 137–170, Imago Publish.
Co. Ltd., London 1946. *Fuchs A., Gaspari C., Millendor-
fer J.:* Makropsychologische Untersuchung der Familie in
Europa. STUDIA, Studiengruppe für internationale
Analyse, Wien 1977. *Gaspari C.:* Socio-ecological and
socio-hierarchical Aspects of societal systems; proceed-
ings on the 3rd European Meeting on Cybernetics and
Systems Research, 1976. *Gastager H. und S.:* Die Fassa-
denfamilie. Ehe und Familie in der Krise. Analyse und
Therapie.. Kindler, München 1973. *Gibbs J. B., Martin
W. T.:* Status integration and suicide. University of Ore-
gon Press, Eugene 1964. *Halbwachs M.:* Les causes de
suicide. Alcan, Paris 1930. *Hell D.:* Die Sozial- und
Familienbeziehungen Depressiver. Fortschr. Neurol.
Psychiat. *48,* 447–457, 1980. *Henseler H.:* Narzisstische
Krisen / Zur Psychodynamik des Selbstmordes. Rowohlt-
Taschenbuch-Verlag, Reinbek bei Hamburg 1974. *Hen-
seler H.:* Die Psychodynamik des suizidalen Erlebens und
Verhaltens. Nervenarzt *51,* 139–146, 1980. *Kreitman N.:*
Parasuizide. Brit.J. Psychiat. *115,* 746–747, 1969. *Masa-
ryk Th. G.:* Der Selbstmord als soziale Massenerschei-
nung der modernen Zivilisation. Konegen. Wien 1881.
Paykel E. S., Prusoff B. A., Myers J. K.: Suicide attemps
and recent life events. Arch. Gen. Psychiat. *32,* 327–333.
1975. *Perrez M. (Hrsg.):* Krise der Kleinfamilie? Hans-
Huber-Verlag. Bern. Stuttgart. Wien 1979. *Pöldinger W.:*
Die Abschätzung der Suizidalität. Hans-Huber-Verlag.
Bern, Stuttgart 1968. *Pöldinger W.:* Sozialpsychiatrische
Aspekte der Vereinsamung. Fortschr. der Medizin *88,*
1363–1366, 1970. *Pöldinger W.:* Suizidalität und Familie
Ars Medici *71,* 520–524, 1981. *Pöldinger W., Lange J.,*

Kirchmayr A. (Hrsg.): Psychosoziales Elend / Für ein menschliches Zusammenleben. Herder, Wien, Freiburg, Basel 1981. *Ringel E.:* Selbstmordverhütung. Hans-Huber-Verlag Bern, Stuttgart, Wien 1969. *Shneidman E. S., Farberow N. L.:* Clues to suicide. McGraw-Hill, New York 1961. *Sperling E.:* Suizid und Familie. Gruppenpsychother. Gruppendynamik *16,* 24–34, 1980. *Stengel E.:* Suicide and attempted suicide. Penguin, Harmondsworth 1964. *Wagner A.:* Die Gesetzmässigkeit in den scheinbar willkürlichen Handlungen vom Standpunkt der Statistik. Boyes & Geisler, Hamburg 1864. *Wellhoefer P. R.:* Selbstmord und Selbstmordversuch. Uni-Taschenbücher, 1078, G. Fischer, Stuttgart 1981. *Willi J.:* Die Zweierbeziehung. Rowohlt-Verlag, Reinbek bei Hamburg 1975. *Willi J.:* Therapie der Zweierbeziehung. Rowohlt-Verlag, Reinbek bei Hamburg 1978.

SUICIDE AND VOLUNTARY DEATH -

POSSIBILITIES OF HUMAN BEHAVIOR

Hermann Pohlmeier

Lehrstuhl für Medizinische Psychologie
West Germany D-3400 Göttingen, Humboldtallee 1d

On the occasion of the opening of the 12th German Hospital Day in Düsseldorf, the present President of the
Federal Republik of Germany, Karl CARSTENS, undoubtedly
a conservative and prudent statesman, claimed, "also we
must be allowed to ask the question how long we have to
painfully keep a human being alive by using every possible means...". The necessity of every medical help
may not be denied but we have to ask ourselves in which
way even dying can do justice to man and be humane.
(Süddeutsche Zeitung June 8, 1983). In these words we
have sketched the problem of suicide and voluntary death,
of suicide and euthanasia, of living and humane dying.
Due to the foundation of a Society for Humane Dying in
198o, this problem has become a topical item in the
German-speaking countries, but also worldwide the euthanasia problem has gained particular interest. In this
lecture, we will describe the present state of the
euthanasia discussion under the following three aspects:

1. Suicide and Voluntary Death
2. Suicide and Euthanasia
3. Human Dying and Living

Particular attention will be given to the relation of
suicide prevention, on the one hand, and the euthanasia
movement on the other. For this purpose, we have to
realize beforehand and especially demand from this VIIth
World Congress for Psychiatry that the discussion be unbiased and scientific and that any personal defamation
be rejected such as the suspicion that this discussion
were propaganda of a Communist ideology or a perversion
of the Hippocratic oath. Even now we may conclude that

the medico-psychiatrical prevention of suicide does not
exclude the discussion of voluntary death and euthanasia at all and that, were this happens nevertheless, it
is in danger of giving in to an ideology as well:
Suicide prevention as it has been established here in
Vienna for 30 years will have to theoretically and
practically ask new questions after such a long time
and face the possible rejection of unproved statements
presupposing that all sciences have two things in
common, namely freedom and truth.

1. Suicide and Voluntary Death

To grant people the right of suicide depends on the
norms and values that hold for the individual or whole
social groups. We may start out from the fact that in
the existing or desired pluralistic societies all over
the world people do claim this right of suicide. Phenomenologically there is no doubt about the possibility
of suicide commited as the practical consequence of
evaluating one's life which then occurs as an act of
one's own free will and as the result of consideration
and calculation (MEYER 1982, p. 65ff; HOCHE 1916).
Suicide is not necessarily and in every case "...the
end of a pathological psychic development..." as RINGEL
described it 30 years ago (RINGEL 1953, 3rd unchanged
edition 1983). There are even empirical studies which,
apart from the phenomenology of the individual case,
report on suicide in the non-medical field.

Apparently, we only have to reckon with a rate of
suicides of at most 70 per cent connected with (the
disease of) depression (SAINSBURY 1980). Whether the
rest of 30 per cent really consists of voluntary deaths
and suicides performed as a consequence of evaluating
one's life remains open. The voluntary deaths of several
artists and authors may here be mentioned (RAETHEL 1966,
DIETZE 1981). A good many artists put an end to their
lives with the final conclusion:
It is finished. We can furthermore point out some political suicides committed after serious thought of
either making oneself guilty of the betrayal of state
secrets in the case of espionage, or protesting against
political circumstances instead of tolerating them
(BRÜSEWITZ, PALLACH, WENNERSTRÖM, ROMMEL, REDL, POHL-
MEIER 1980). Following the ideas of the French Existen-
tialism, Jean AMÉRY, for the German-speaking countries,
has convincingly described suicide as a "...privilege
of the human being..." and showed that a person may
realize himself by means of committing .suicide, that

suicide creates freedom in certain situations of life
and that it is a basic right of man (AMÉRY 1976). The
latter is thus recognized in the legal codes of almost
all nations (WAGNER 1975, p. 84 ff, DEUTSCH 1983). By
describing attempted suicide chiefly as an attempt to
solve one's problems the Social Sciences and Humani-
ties, beyond that, confirm this anthropological and
philosophical interpretation empirically. Especially,
the French sociologist BAECHLER, to whom AMÉRY clearly
refers, has repeatedly tried to explain the individual
act of suicide beyond all theories and, in particular,
the medical theory from biography and concrete situations (BAECHLER 1975/1981). Years ago it seemed to me
sensible and well-motivated to make a distinction between suicide and voluntary death in order to differentiate situations of illness and disease from those
of human crisis (POHLMEIER 1980). The fact that the
group of suicides and attempted suicides constitutes a
minority deviating considerably from the statistical
norm does not establish a counter-argument to the
point of view that suicide is a possible choice of
the normal human being - almost all people are supposed
to think of suicide once in their life. The minority
proceeding to action leaves this possibility of human
behavior in the realm of human freedom outsice disease.
Suicidal behavior is not always psychopathological.

2. Suicide and Euthanasia

Prima facie suicide and euthanasia constitute two
different phenomena. Often no connection is established
between the two at all. Or they are not discussed in
any connection. A closer look, however, reveals common
characteristics and overlappings which have been
studied more carefully and have become clearer to us in
the past few years. It is the unnatural way of dying
that suicide and euthanasia have in common. In both
cases, death is not caused by external accidents but
brought about voluntarily. They differ as to the fact
that suicide is death by one's own hand and euthanasia
death by some other person's hand. What is the relation
of both phenomena with common characteristics and
distinctions mentioned above to each other and what
does it tell us about the meaning of human behavior?
If we recognize the right of suicide, we must equally
grant the right of euthanasia. This is a direct consequence of man's freedom. Of course, it is debatable
and may even be doubted whether the human will is not,
anyway, entirely determined and if the human being
does not, at least under certains circumstances, act

under compulsion. But on condition that the human being is able to decide independently, he is also able to decide on his life and death. This possibility of the human being is well-known to medicine and it is respected when the doctor asks the patient's consent before an operation. Whether a person really makes use of his right of self-determination where life and death are concerned in every situation is a different matter: consideration for one's neighbors, God or other ethical norms might restrict this right. It is a matter of conscience whether he makes use of it or not. This freedom of conscience must be maintained unless, owing to a mental disease, the ability to make a decision has been lost as, for example, in the case of a serious depression caused by a feeling of guilt due to forbidden aggressions, by the desire for self-punishment, by disappointment at unrealized wishes, or by total helplessness and hopelessness. Also, this freedom of choice must remain possible without being enforced externally. Finally, choice must be possible for the person that wants to decide on his life and death as well as for the one who is asked for help in such a case. Helping a person to end his life, a special form of euthanasia, becomes relevant when death by one's own hand is no longer possible. Euthanasia may then be a substitute for suicide. This is the reason why euthanasia societies publish guides to voluntary death. They are even ready to perform it, or at least assist a person in committing suicide. How are we to judge these endeavors towards decent death and humane dying for the purpose of which suicide is performed.

3. Humane Dying and Living

Humane dying and living appear to be natural human needs but are, at present, permanently disregarded and neglected all over the world. It is an old problem of politics that people talk about peace but actually plan and make war. To medicine, this problem is a new one as technical progress in the field of Intensive Medicine has brought about the possibility of lengthening life which is not necessarily compatible with human dignity and value of life. The mere possibility of lengthening physiological functions does not guarantee emotion, pleasure and communication, those essentials of human life. Endeavors towards a gentle death therefore date back to the beginning of our century.

Euthanasia societies are not a new phenomenon. Such a society was founded in England in 1935 and in the United

States in 1939. Even if at that time certain developments
in medicine influenced them we must, in addition to
that, take social changes into consideration.

As early as 1895,JOST published a study on the right
of one's own death (JOST 1895). And we have already
mentioned the work of the jurist BINDING and the psychiatrist HOCHE on the annihilation of unworthy life
(BINDING and HOCHE 1920). For a better understanding
of these developments the Göttingen psychiatrist MEYER
points to the revival of the so-called Social Darwinism
which, in quite a free and broad interpretation, strives
for an efficient human race via social selection. In
the sense of Social Darwinism, pain and infirmity are
unknown to such an efficent human race. HITLER's decree
of September 1, 1939 mentioned already which decided
"to extend the competence of physicians to be appointed
by name in such a way as to grant - as far as is humanly
possible to decide - incurable patients a mercy killing
after having critically evaluated their state of
disease..." thus coincides with the foundation of
Anglo-American euthanasia societies. This coincidence
at least indicates that the murder of patients by the
HITLER government has a historical background. This
hint may facilitate the present euthanasia discussion
without minimizing it. For it has worldwide entered a
new stage since 1975 in so far as it is since then no
more natural that just passive euthanasia or humane
dying are conderned but also the killing without the
consent of the person affected, either by way of judi-
cial decisions or a committee's resolutions. Particulary the publication of the Canadian psychologist Rut
RUSSEL, "Freedom to Die", of 1975 and that of KOHL of
the same year demand of physicians the active killing
in clearly determined situations (RUSSEL 1975, KOHL
1975). They are supposed to kill heavily defective
children on the parents' demand and people suffering
from dementia senilis or chronically insane persons
as far as they are legally incompetent on demand of
their (legal) guardians. Nobody should suffer just because he is not able to express his wishes, and ob-
stinate insistance on the patient's consent should
not prolong misery. In evaluating euthanasia societies
we should thus pay careful attention to their articles
of constitution and their objectives. In this connection it should be emphasized that the British Euthanasia
Society EXIT (MAIR 1980), which in 1980 published a
guide to suicide, and also the Australian Euthanasia
Society definitely reject active euthanasia.

Finally, the German translation of Jo ROMAN's book does not represent an instigation to active euthanasia even if, owing to her biography and extraordinary fate, she demands the "exit house" (ROMAN 1981). Up to the present day these attempts have in common the effort towards a decent death as well as a better life. They follow an excellent Western humanist tradition. The problem with euthanasia is that the person affected must be free to choose, i.e. he must not be forced into it. Any attempts to assess the value of a patient's life externally and thus end his life against his explicit wish do not agree with the Western humanist tradition mentioned. Hence, we must combat these attempts with all our strength. But medicine cannot resist efforts that want to make it possible for a person to die decently. Indeed, medicine with a human face has never acted that way (MITSCHERLICH 1947, 1960). Every physician is familiar with the situation where he stops medication so that his patient may die in peace and quiet (passive euthanasia). Compared with active euthanasia the basic difference certainly does not lie so much in the act as in terminology: death caused by failing to help and death caused by active intervention may easily be confused. Both manners of death would only have to rely on the patient's declared will. The declared and free will of a patient constitutes the connecting link between euthanasia and suicide, or, to be more precise, voluntary death. Voluntas aegroti suprema lex once was the motto of medical ethics which does not contradict the Hippocratic oath. Hippocrates had committed himself, in a broader interpretation, to do everything possible for the patient's benefit but not to stick to this principle of lengthening life at all costs. Why, then, should we prevent suicide? Does this not mean an attack on man's freedom and a prevention of a humane death, and does it not absolutely contradict the euthanasia movement? Not at all. Suicide prevention is hovering between arrogance and obligation (POHLMEIER 1978) and is allowed just in case we can definitely exclude a person's free will, or free will cannot decide ambivalently between life and death. Due to the widespread existence of both phenomena a large field of activity is open to suicide prevention. But in humility it must bow to the patient's free will and stop its work, like medicine, if the patient's free will demands euthanasie. It is obvious that we cannot apply laws in this case but have to respect a human being's freedom of conscience. Thus, suicide and euthanasia do not represent opposites, and efforts towards a humane death do not contradict efforts towards suicide prevention.

It was our aim to show that man is free and that
it is medicine and particulary psychiatry where man's
freedom demands our absolute respect. Hence it follows
that suicide is a matter of a "narrowing of mind" and
voluntary death a different kind of possible human
behavior. Suicidal behavior is not just psychopathology.

Literature

AMÉRY, J.: Hand an sich legen - Diskurs über den Freitod
       Klett, Stuttgart, 1976[3]
BAECHLER, J. Tod durch eigene Hand (1975)
       Ullstein, Frankfurt, 1981
BINDING, K. u. A. HOCHE: Die Freigabe der Vernichtung
       lebensunwerten Lebens
       Meiner, Leipzig, 1920
DEUTSCH, E.: Arztrecht - Arzneimittelrecht
       Springer, Berlin-Heidelberg-New York-Tokio, 1983
DIETZE, Gabriele: Todeszeichen- Freitod in Selbstzeug-
       nissen
       Luchterhand, Darmstadt, 1981
GUILLON, C. u. Y. le BONNIEC: Gebrauchsanleitung zum
       Selbstmord
       Robinson, Frankfurt, 1982
JOST, A.: Das Recht auf den Tod
       Dietrichsche Verlagsbuchhandlung, Göttingen, 1895
KOHL, M.: Veneficient Euthanasia
       Buffalo, Prometheus, 1975
MAIR, B.G.: How to die with dignity
       Exit - Euthanasie-Ges., Schottland, 1980
MEYER, J.E.: Anleitung zum Freitod
       Dtsch. Ärztebl. 78, (1982), 22-23
MEYER, J.E.: Todesangst und das Todesbewußtsein der
       Gegenwart
       Springer, Berlin-Heidelberg-New York, 1982[2]
MITSCHERLICH, A. u. F. MIELKE: Das Diktat der Menschen-
       verachtung
       Lambert & Schneider, Freiburg, 1947
MITSCHERLICH, A. u. F. MIELKE: Medizin ohne Menschlichkeit
       Fischer, Frankfurt, 1960
POHLMEIER, H. (Hrsg): Selbstmordverhütung - Anmaßung oder
       Verpflichtung
       Keil, Bonn, 1978
POHLMEIER, H.: Suicide as a Psychodynamic Problem of
       Depression
       Crisis - Int. J. Suicidol. 1, (1980), 27-34
POHLMEIER, H.: Social Background of Depressive Illness
       and Suicide
       Crisis - Int. J. Suicidol. 2, (1980), 134-141

POHLMEIER, H.: Der politische Selbstmord
Münch. med. Wschr. 122, (1980), 667-670
POHLMEIER, H.: Selbstmordverhütung und humanes Sterben
Münch. med. Wschr. 124, (1982), 1121-1123
POHLMEIER, H.: Selbstmordverhütung - Verhinderung humanen
Sterbens?
Nieders. Ärztebl. 55, (1982), 186-188
RAEITHEL, G.: Selbstmord und Selbstmordversuche ameri-
kamnischer Schriftsteller
Inaug. Diss. München, 1966
ROMAN, Jo: Freiwillig aus dem Leben (Exit House)
dtsch. Übers., Kindler, München, 1981
RUSSEL, R.: Freedom zu die
Human Press, New York, 1975
SAINSBURY, P.: Suicide and Depression
Psychiatria Fennica, Suppl. Helsinki, 1980, 259-267
WAGNER, J.: Selbstmord und Selbstmordverhinderung
Müller, Jur. Verlag, Karlsruhe, 1975

CHANGING PATTERNS IN SUICIDE BEHAVIOUR

John H. Henderson

Regional Officer for Mental Health
World Health Organization
Regional Office for Europe, Copenhagen, Denmark

Introduction

Suicide is one of the most common causes of death and among young people it ranks among the first in many countries of the European Region. The World Health Organization (WHO) considers suicide and attempted suicide as serious public health problems.

In 1968 WHO gave consideration to preventive measures, the organization of services, statistics and research, in the publication Prevention of Suicide, Public Health Papers No. 35, published by WHO Geneva, 1968.

In 1973 the WHO Regional Office for Europe convened a Working Group in Zagreb, Yugoslavia to review current knowledge in various aspects of suicide and attempted suicide, to consider international collaborative studies and to advise on national suicide statistic recording and reporting. The report of this group was included in Suicide and attempted Suicide, Public Health Papers No. 58, published by WHO Geneva, 1974.

In 1981 the WHO Regional Office for Europe convened a Working Group in Athens, Greece, to review changing patterns of suicide and attempted suicide, the validity and reliability of suicide statistics and to explore possibilities and strategies in suicide prevention.

Trends in suicide

This working group had available statistics on deaths by suicide from 23 of 33 Member States in the European Region and 18 of

927

these could be studied from 1961 to 1977 while all 23 provided data for 1979 or 1980. Appendix 1 gives the latest available information for those countries of the WHO European Region that provided data.

Throughout all European countries suicide is more common in the older age groups and more common in males than in females. There are large national differences which have persisted over the years with few changes in the rank order from the highest to the lowest.

The suicide rate for young adults has increased in both sexes in more countries than it has decreased and among the elderly, male rates have now started to rise along with the continuing rise in female rates.

Striking trends in suicide rates worthy of mention include the decline in rates for England and Wales where a reported 34% decline (2000 lives per year) occurred between 1961 and 1974. The countries in which the rates have increased in comparison to the decrease in England and Wales are Hungary (49%), Ireland (38%), Denmark (34%), Netherlands (34%) and Poland (34%).

Norway has for many years recorded rates half as high as in neighbouring countries - Denmark, Finland and Sweden. Studies are currently being carried out among the Nordic countries to investigate possible explanations.

Validity and Reliability of suicide statistics

The working group expressed confidence in the use of official suicide statistics from European countries for trend analysis. Consistent differences in rates between national, demographic and social groups have been recorded over long periods, differences which persist despite political changes that in many countries have altered the ascertainment procedures. To ignore the implications of such conspicuous regularities as the higher suicide rates of males, of the elderly the divorced and so on, and to diagnosis these as errors is surely an error of judgment.

Trends in Attempted Suicide

Variations in the rates of attempted suicide across major demographic and social groups show remarkably consistent patterns, changing little over the years from one country to another. Females outnumber males in all age groups. It is among teenagers and young adults that the rise in rates has been most marked, reaching levels that are now many times higher than among the middle-aged and elderly. There is a step gradient of increasing rates with lower social class. The unskilled lowest social class male group has more than eight times the rate of attempted suicide as the professional highest social class male group. Divorcees have substantially higher rates than the single, married or widowed. A large

928

proportion of patients in most series have alcohol problems, criminal, unemployment and debt records, and a history of family violence. Half of those who attempt suicide have done so before, and one fifth will attempt it again within 12 months. Again the figures are remarkably consistent from year to year and in different centres, as is the frequency with which suicide follows attempted suicide - 1% per annum according to many follow-up studies.

Validity and reliability of attempted suicide statistics

Underestimation of suicide attempts is likely to be much greater than for suicides. Surveys in general practice in Scotland and the Netherlands showed that hospital admissions underestimated the number of cases known to general practitioners by 30%. Field studies, in which everyone in a population sample was screened, suggested that 50%-60% of those who admitted to suicide attempts during the previous year had not reported the fact to a doctor. In countries where primary medical care and hospital provision is less available for these cases, the errors will be even greater. However the data gained from hospital studies should not be dismissed as valueless. A study in Edinburgh, Scotland, showed that hospital cases were representative of all those known to general practitioners. At least their demographic, social and clinical characteristics were the same, except that admitted cases were more medically serious than the non-admitted cases. The little we know about those who do not declare their attempted suicide to a doctor suggests that they contain relatively more self-injurers, more men, and more middle aged and older people.

Whilst sampling errors are always likely to be large, the main conclusion drawn from hospital data - that there has been a massive rise in rates all over Europe, particularly affecting the young - seems valid and reliable enough. That those who never report to a doctor may include many persons with characteristics close to those of successful suicides may be important for suicide prevention.

Possibilities and stategies for suicide prevention

The working group identified the following four groups as meriting particular attention for the improvement or development of methods of care to prevent suicide.

1. Persons known to be subject to depressive illness. Follow-up studies suggest that about one in six will kill themselves. There are effective treatments well within the capacity of general practitioners.

2. Psychiatric hospital inpatients. The number of suicide deaths is increasing where knowledge and skills to prevent this behaviour are most available.

3. Attempted suicides. Of those discharged from general hospitals 1% will kill themselves within the year, and up to 10% will die eventually.

4. Alcoholic and drug dependents. Both are at least as high for suicide risk as those who attempt suicide.

Conclusions

1. Suicide and attempted suicide should be considered separately. Although they are related, there are important demographic, social and clinical differences.

2. No change in the International Classification of Diseases (ICD) definition of suicide is proposed, nor any alteration in the traditional ascertainment procedures of European countries.

3. The term "attempted suicide" should include all non-fatal, intentional, self-inflicted injuries or poisonings

Suicide

4. The working group expressed confidence in using official suicide statistics from European countries for trend analysis. The errors are not such as to invalidate their use.

5. The following trends were studied and considered worthy of further investigation:

>   (a) the rising rates of suicide in most European countries, which have now reached particularly high levels in Hungary and the northern parts of Yugoslavia;
>
>   (b) the exceptional decline in rates in England and Wales and in Greece during the last two decades;
>
>   (c) the relatively low rate in Norway compared with other Scandinavian countries;
>
>   (d) the marked increases in rates for elderly women in most European countries, and
>
>   (e) the marked increase in rates for young adults in most European countries.

6. The working group related changes in social and economic conditions to changes in reported suicide rates. Changes in societies that are likely to lead to social isolation of more individuals may increases the suicide rate.

7.   The following were considered important high-risk groups for experiments in suicide prevention:

(a)   persons known to be subject to depressive illness;

(b)   psychiatric hospital inpatients;

(c)   those who have attempted suicide; and

(d)   alcoholics.

Attempted suicide

8.   Underestimation of attempted suicide is likely to be much greater than for suicide. Community field surveys suggest that as many as a third to a half of persons who attempted suicide never disclosed the fact to a doctor.

9.   Nevertheless, the following trends for hospital-referred attempted suicides have been identified in nearly all European countries where cases were related to the population at risk:

(a)   the overall rate of attempted suicide has been steadily increasing during the last twenty years;   and

(b)   teenagers and young adults have shown the greatest increase and have the highest rates.

10.   Attempted suicide rates are highest in poor city areas where other indices of social disorganization are high. Socioeconomic changes which put families under increased stress may lead to increased rates of attempted suicide.

11.   It was of the greatest concern to the working group that health care professionals in and out of hospitals so often have no training, and no coherent policy for managing attempted suicide.

12.   Just as the reduction in availability of coal gas does not seem to affect the suicide rate, so also the massive increase in medical drug prescribing does not seem to explain the rise in rates of intentional self-poisoning.

Acknowledgments

The author wishes to acknowledge the valuable contributions and work of the participants in the WHO Working Group on Changing patterns in suicide behaviour held in Athens from 29 September to 2 October 1981.

The report of the Working Group is published in Changing patterns in suicide behaviour, EURO Reports and Studies No. 74, Regional Office for Europe, World Health Organization, Copenhagen, 1982.

Appendix 1

Deaths from suicide in the European Region of the World Health Organization (latest year available)

Country	Year	Males		Females		Total	
		No.	Rate per 100 000 population	No.	Rate per 100 000 population	No.	Rate per 100 000 population
Austria	1980	1 342	37 8	590	14 9	1 932	25 7
Belgium	1977	1 201	25.0	673	13.4	1 874	19 1
Bulgaria	1980	842	19 1	364	8 2	1 206	13 6
Czechoslovakia	1975	2 345	32.5	896	11.8	3 241	21 9
Denmark	1980	1 039	41 1	579	22 3	1 618	31.6
Finland	1978	963	41.9	237	9.7	1 200	25 2
France	1978	6 447	24.7	2 711	10 0	9 158	17.2
Germany, Fed. Rep. of	1980	8 332	28.3	4 536	14 1	12 868	20 9
Greece	1979	186	4.0	91	1 9	277	2 9
Hungary	1980	3 344	64 5	1 465	26 5	4 809	44 9
Iceland	1980	14	12.2	10	8 8	24	10.5
Ireland	1978	106	6.4	57	3 5	163	4.9
Italy	1978	2 563	9 3	1 092	3 8	3 657	6.4
Luxembourg	1980	35	19.7	12	6.5	47	12 9
Malta	1977	0	—	—	—	0	—
Netherlands	1980	901	12 8	529	7 4	1 430	10.1
Norway	1980	370	18.3	137	6.6	507	12 4
Poland	1979	3 766	21.8	732	4 0	4 498	12.7
Portugal	1979	701	15.0	251	4.8	952	9 7
Spain	1978	1 094	6.1	413	2 2	1 507	4.1
Sweden	1980	1 137	27 6	473	11 3	1 610	19.4
Switzerland	1980	1 128	36 7	493	15 2	1 621	25 7
United Kingdom							
England & Wales	1980	2 629	11.0	1 692	6.7	4 321	8.8
Northern Ireland	1978	38	5.0	32	4 1	70	4.5
Scotland	1981	339	13 6	177	6.6	516	10.0

Source: WHO data bank.

ATTEMPTED SUICIDE IN BAVARIAN MENTAL HOSPITALS

Klaus-Dieter Gorenc

National Institute of Penal Sciences
Magisterio Nacional 113
14000 Mexico City

INTRODUCTION

The vast majority of the inquiries on suicide behavior have studied, primarily, the phenomenon of attempted suicide and completed suicide which occur in the general population. Only a reduced number of investigations have tried to determine the factors that could have triggering influence on suicide, and/or suicide attempt in mental hospitals, despite the fact that suicide rate is higher in the mental hospital population(1,2,3). The occurrence in mental hospitals is 3 to 4.5 times greater than in the general popualtion (3,4,5).

The few studies, which investigated the attempted suicide in the mental hospitals, show that the suicide is 3 to 4 times higher than attempted suicide (6,7,8). In contrast, Alsen (9) found that for each suicide occured 4 attempted suicides. This discrepancy is probably due to determinated methodological difficulties, which are evident in retrospective inquiries, such as incomplete data and uncontrollable data registration (10).

SAMPLE AND PROCEDURE

This retrospective inquiry proceed from a limited field of study of suicidology: the epidemiology, and tries to answer infrequent questions put formal such as a) which factors could unleash attempted suicides in mental hospitals, b) to establish whether the number of suicide attempts have increased in ten Bavarian mental hospitals which were analysed over a period of 2 decades, the first one from 1950 to 1959 and the second one from 1967 to 1976 and; c) to determine if this increase is relative or absolute and which

933

factors are connected with such an increase. The research is engaged in the area of general factors (size and prominence of the hospital, patient turn-over rate, physician and nursing personnel relationship with the patient and forced admission) which possible had a connection with the attempted suicide.

The data derived from the investigated variables: number of beds, physician- and nursing personnel relationship with patients will be denominated as "institution-related-variables"; patient's turn-over rate and forced admission will be named "event-related-variables". These data were obtained from the Statistical Annual Reports of the ten investigated mental hospitals. It was not possible to distinguish between a single or a repeated attempted suicide, because it was registrated as a numeric size. By taking each decade independently, it was possible to determine, if the occured changes in the mental hospital evolution have an influence on the suicidal behavior variation. The first decade was a transition period: from the somatic treatment to the psychopharmacological epoch, which began around 1954 (11). The second decade stood under the influence of the liberal treatment movement.

The statistics: since attempted suicide is, in principle, an independent event, it was used the Spearman-rank-correlation test to determine whether or not changes in institution- and event-related-variables were related to changes in suicidal attempts. The chi-square-significant test was used to determine whether or not there were significant differences in attempts of suicide between the two decades under study.

RESULTS

The number of attempted suicides which were registrated in the ten mental hospitals in both decades was 1639 and for the first decade the amount was 595 attempted suicides (2.8 suicide attempts for 1000 admissions) and 1044 (3.4 attempted suicides for 1000 admissions) for the second ten-years-period. From the first to the second decade the attempted suicide almost duplicated, while the number of all admissions increased only in the proportion of 1.5. For each year and hospital the average for the first decade was 5 attempted suicides and in the second one was ten suicide attempts ($p= \leq 0.01$), while in the first decade the admission average was 2094 patients and in the second 3066 patients.

In spite of the observed general significant increase in attempted suicide, it was necessary to investigate the differences among all hospitals that were studied. An absolute increase of attempted suicide was found in 7 of the ten hospitals. When the number of suicidal attempts is related to the number of admissions, there was found only a significant increase in four of ten investigated hospitals; therefore, this indicates that the increase in

934

attempted suicides was higher than the increase in admissons. In the other 3 hospitals there was found a significant decrease in attempted suicide, in spite of an increase in patient's admission.

The remaindering three hospitals did not show changes on the attempted suicide rate in relation to admissions.

From the investigated institution-related-variables a significant positive correlation resulted between the prominence of the hospital -measured with the indicator variable "number of beds"- and the attempted suicide in the second decade, but not in the first decade. The relation between number of physicians and beds meliorated in the second decade in all investigated mental hospitals. In 3 hospitals it was observed, that the physician to-bed ratio was near to the optimum of the ratio dictaminated by the German Psychiatry-Enquete (1:40 beds)(12); in spite of this, more frequent, attempts of suicide appear in the second decade. In two hospitals the ratio physician-beds meliorated above the optimun ratio, but there was also observed a significant increase of attempted suicide. In both decades a great defficiency in the amount of nursing personnel was not observed and as time elapsed the number improved, but a significant increase in attempted suicide was observed in 4 hospitals. In neither of these 2 decades a correlation between the amount of nursing personnel and the frequency of attempted suicide was observed (Table 1).

Table 1 Rank-correlation coefficients between attempted suicide and institution-related-variables

Institution-related-variables	1950 - 1959	1967 - 1976
	Correlation coefficients	
Number of beds	0.47	0.70
Physician-patient-ratio	0.20	0.45
Nursing-personnel-patient-ratio	0.09	0.43

Summarizing these results, it is possible to conclude, that with the increment of physician and nursing personnel the probability of occurrence of attempted suicide increases.

Of the 2 event-related-variables, a relation between the frequency of forced admission and attempted suicide was observed.

Table 2 Rank-correlation coefficients between the event-related-variables and attempted suicide

Event-related-variables	1950 - 1959	1967 - 1976
	Correlation coefficients	
Patient's admission	0.42	0.23
Forced admission	0.81	0.74

With this result (Table 2) it is possible to suppose, that with the increase of the number of forced admissions, the attempted suicide rate in the mental hospitals also increases.

DISCUSION

Apart from the numbers of forced admissions which correlates higher with attempted suicide, the analysis of the event- and institution-related-variables do not have a strong explanatory capacity. In spite of these results, a surprising tendency was observed; that with the quantitative ameloration of the clinical care of patients the probability of occurrence of suicide attempt grows. After these observations, it was necessary to try to explain the suicide attempt in relation to the inward situation of the institution "hospital" on the one side and on the other side with the social- and enviromental changes of the mental hospitals (3,7,13,14,15). These authors could not verify statistically the constructed thesis, because these events do not appear frequently enough, but these are not only conjectures.

The relation physician- as well as nursing personnel-patient has even a lower explanation capacity. In accordance with these results the number of attempted suicides increase as the relation of personnel-patient number increases. In our supposition these variables, attempted suicide and personnel, must show an opposite tendency, that is, increased attempted suicide frequency should produce a decrease in this ratio.

The quantity of physicians in mental hospitals does not allow to evaluate the quality of medical care. The German Psychiatry-Enquete (12) does not ignore the deficient qualification of physicians and nursing personnel. It is possible to suppose that the increase in attempted suicide frequency correlates with the deficiency of quality care, but at the present time there are no parameters which allow one to measure this factor objective.

Of the institution- and event-related-variables only the variable forced admission frequency shows a significant relationship with the attempted suicide frequency in the two investigated periods. This result would speak in favor of the notion that a high suicide risk is evident during the acute stage of mental disorders (16,17).

Other authors (1,18,19,20) demostrated that the increase of suicide behavior has relation with the implantation of the open-door-system in the mental hospitals, but the present investigation was not able to confirm this finding to its full extent.

Collective data are evidently not suitable for explaining the individual suicide behavior and these results show that it is necessary to explore general variables together with particular variables in relation to comparative data. It was not possible to obtain the personal data of each attempter, because these data are collected in the annuals only as numbers and it was also impossible to know what percentage of hospitals stations were opened during this period, but we presume that in the second decade the majority of stations stood open.

To study the phenomenon exhaustively, it is necessary to introduce a case register in mental hospitals and in accord once with these results find appropiate prevention measures, i.e. crisis intervention sections in mental hospitals.

REFERENCES

1. R. Hessö, Suicide in Norwegian, Finnish and Swedish psychiatric hospitals, Arch. Psychiatr. Nervenkr. 224:119 (1977).
2. B. Rorsman, Suicide among swedish psychiatric patients, Soc. Psychiatr. 8:140 (1973).
3. L.F: Saugstad, O. Ødegard, Mortality in psychiatric hospitals in Norway 1950-1974, Acta Psychiatr. Scand. 59:431 (1979).
4. S. Levy, R.H. Southcombe, Suicide in a state hospital for mentally ill, J. Nerv. Ment. Dis. 117:504 (1953).
5. J.W. Sletten, M.L. Brown, R.C. Evenson, H. Altman, Suicide in mental hospital patients, Dis. Nerv. Syst. 33:328 (1972).
6. H. Koester, Möglichkeiten und Grezen der Freizügigkeit in der Stationären Behandlung psychisch Kranker. Nervenarzt 37:421 (1969).
7. P. Mehne, Ursachen und Häufigkeit von Suiziden und Suizidversuchen über 65jähriger Patienten im psychiatrischen Krankenhaus, Acta Geronto 7:105 (1977).
8. J. Schwarz, Suizid im Krankenhaus, Beitr. Gerichtl. Med. 26:100 (1969).
9. V. Alsen, Selbstmord und Selbstmordversuch in der Klinik, Zbl. Gesamt. Neurol. Psychiatr. 196:3 (1969).
10. K. Boehme, Problematik der retrospektiven Auswertung von Suizidkrankenblättern. Zbl. Gesamt. Neurol. Psychiatr. 196:2 (1969)
11. E.H. Ackerknecht, "Kurze Geschichte der Psychiatrie," Enke Verlag, Stuttgart (1967).
12. Bericht über der Lage der Psychiatrie in der Bundesrepublik Deutschland, Deutscher Bundestag, Wahlperiode 7/4200 (1978).
13. E. Baecklin, Selbstmord im staatlichen Irrenhaus von Schweden in den Jahren 1901-1933. Zbl. Gesamt. Neurol. Psychiat. 92:274 (1939).
14. J.L. Kroll, Self-destructive behavior on an inpatient ward. J. Nerv. Ment. Dis. 166:429 (1978).
15. M. Rotov, Death by suicide in the hospital: An analysis of 20 therapeutic failures, Am. J. Psychother. 25:216 (1970).
16. K.A. Achté, A. Stenbäck, H. Teräväinen, On suicides comitted during treatment in psychiatric hospitals, Acta Psychiatr. Scand. 42:272 (1966).

17. J.B. Copas, D.L. Freeman-Brown, A.A. Robin, Danger periods for suicide in patients under treatment, Psychol. Med. 5:400 (1971).
18. K. Ernst, R. Kern, Suizidstatistik und freiheitliche Klinikbehandlung 1900-1972, Arch. Psychiatr. Nervenkr. 219:255 (1974).
19. K. Ernst, Die Zunahme der Suizide in den psychiatrischen Kliniken, Soz. Praeventivmed. 24:34 (1979).
20. J. Lønnqvist, P. Niskanen, R. Rinta-Mänty, K. Achté, Suicides in psychiatric hospitals in different therapeuthic eras: A review of literature and own study. Psychiatr. Fennica. 265 (1974).

TO THE PROBLEM OF AN INSTITUTIONAL SUICIDE

Jiri Modestin, Hans Brenner, and Urs Koch

Psychiatric University Clinic
Bolligenstrasse 111
3072 Berne, Switzerland

In spite of their relative constancy over time, there are long-term shifts in the suicide rates like drops during wars and increases during periods of economic instability. Switzerland has traditionally a high total suicide rate, and during the last years there has even been a distinct tendency for it to rise: 1959-62: 18.8, 1969-72: 18.3, 1979-80: 25.2. The suicide rates of Canton of Berne exceed those of the whole country and a comparable increase has been registered. At the same time a considerable increase of clinical suicides also has been observed at the Psychiatric University Clinic of Berne.

FREQUENCY OF CLINICAL SUICIDES

The systematic identification - the method has been described previously[1] - of all suicides committed by our patients while being on the hospital rolls revealed: in the years 1960-70 (Period I) 24 suicides, in the years 1971-1981 (Period II) 49 clinical suicides. Similar findings were reported by others[2-4]. Since parallel to this increase an increase of the general suicide rate in Canton of Berne has also been noted, it was necessary to compare both, the clinical and the general suicide rates with each other, taking the different composition of both populations into account. The actual suicide rates (per 100'000 admissions) were matched with the expected ones, i.e. with the general suicide rates adjusted with regard to the clinical population considering sex, seven age categories, and two categories of place of residency (communities with less or more than 30'000 inhabitants). The data for the reference population were obtained from the Swiss Federal Statistical Office; the data for the. clinical population are based on our investigation of a random sample of 1'100 patients (50 admissions per each of the 22 years), representing a clinical control group. Our data did not allow us to adjust for a marital status. The findings are summarized in Table 1. The

Table 1. General suicide rates of Canton of Berne,
expected clinical and actual clinical suicide rates by sex. Comparison of Period I
(1960-70) and Period II (1971-81)

	General Suicide Rates per 100'000 Population Canton Berne		Expected Clinical Suicide Rates		Clinical Suicide Rates per 100'000 Admissions (PUC Berne)	
	♂	♀	♂	♀	♂	♀
Period I 1960-1970	28.6	10.1	42.4	16.4	245.4	167.0
Period II 1971-1981	34.9	13.2	45.7	18.5	632.4	240.1
Increase	22.0 %	30.7 %	7.8 %	12.8 %	157.7 %	43.8 %

expected clinical suicide rates are higher than those of the general population. This is first of all due to the overrepresentation of older age groups, to some extent also due to the underrepresentation of the rural population among our inpatients. The actual clinical suicide rates do by far exceed the expected ones, being about 13 times as high for both sexes in the Period II. Comparing both periods, the increase (in %) of the actual clinical suicide rates also by far exceeds the expected one; for women it is about 3.5, and for men about 20 times higher.

COMPARISON OF CLINICAL SUICIDES WITH CLINICAL POPULATION

The total of 73 clinical suicides were compared with the control group of 1'100 inpatients. As can be seen in Table 2, in

Table 2. Clinical suicides and controls. Comparison of
Period I and II with regard to sex and age.

		Number of Patients		Sex Ratio	Statistical Significance	Average Age (years)		Statistical Significance
		♂	♀	♂ : ♀		♂	♀	
Period I 1960-1970	Suicides	15	9	1.7 : 1	n.s.	45.3 ± 16.8	44.8 ± 9.8	n.s.
	Controls	293	257	1.1 : 1		45.5 ± 17.9	46.0 ± 18.8	
Period II 1971-1981	Suicides	37	12	3.1 : 1	p < 0.01	39.5 ± 14.5	43.6 ± 21.0	p < 0.01
	Controls	299	251	1.2 : 1		38.5 ± 15.8	43.0 ± 17.0	

both periods there has been a predominance of men among suicides. In Period II this predominance becomes statistically significant. In Period I there is no difference in the average age between men and women, neither suicides nor controls; in Period II the age difference between both sexes becomes statistically significant, men being younger than women; however, there remains no difference between suicides and controls. In other words, the suicides, first of all male suicides, are younger on average in Period II, however, so are the controls.

There is a difference in the diagnostic distribution of suicides compared with controls ($p < 0.001$): among suicides there is an overrepresentation of schizophrenia and of manic depressive illness compared with other diagnostic categories (Table 3).

Table 3. Distribution (in %) of suicides and controls, specific for sex, by diagnosis.

		Schizophrenia	Manic-depressive Illness	Psychogenic Disorders	Organic Disorders	Alcoholism/ Addictions	Statistical Significance
♂+♀	Suicides	54.8	16.4	20.5	4.1	4.1	$p < 0.001$
	Controls	29.7	6.2	26.2	19.4	18.5	
♂	Suicides	55.8	15.4	19.2	3.8	5.8	$p < 0.001$
	Controls	23.2	4.0	28.2	19.7	24.9	
♀	Suicides	52.4	19.0	23.8	4.8	0.0	
	Controls	37.4	8.8	23.9	18.9	10.9	

There is also a difference between both sexes as to the diagnostic distribution within the control group ($p < 0.001$), a male predominance of alcoholism probably accounting for this difference in the first place. In the suicide group there is by contrast a distinct approximation in the diagnostic distribution between both sexes (the statistical evaluation being impossible because of the small number of women in our sample).

For male patients, Period I and II could be compared regarding the diagnostic distribution (Table 4). The observed increase in the male clinical suicides depends on the increase of suicides among schizophrenic patients as well as the patients with psychogenic disorders. Interestingly enough, there was no increase among the most suicide-prone group of manic depressive patients[5], in whom a morbogenic contribution, i.e. endogenous factors, play the major part. Thus, some exogenous factors like negative environmental influences might have led to the clinical suicide rate increase in the last years, influences possibly being generated by the clinical setting itself.

Table 4. Distribution (number and %) of male suicides and male controls by diagnosis. Comparison of Period I and Period II.

		Schizophrenia	Manic-depressive Illness	Psychogenic Disorders	Organic Disorders	Alcoholism/ Addictions
Suicides	Period I 1960-1970	7 (46.7%)	4 (26.7%)	2 (13.3%)	1 (6.7%)	1 (6.7%)
	Period II 1971-1981	22 (59.5%)	4 (10.8%)	8 (21.6%)	1 (2.7%)	2 (5.4%)
Controls	Period I 1960-1970	60 (20.8%)	11 (3.8%)	87 (30.2%)	70 (24.3%)	60 (20.8%)
	Period II 1971-1981	74 (25.5%)	12 (4.1%)	76 (26.2%)	44 (15.2%)	84 (29.0%)
Statistical Significance		p < 0.05		p < 0.05		

SUICIDE RATES: A COMPARISON OF TWO PSYCHIATRIC INSTITUTIONS

In the Psychiatric University Clinic of Berne in the Period II a lot of changes took place: important constructional innovations, retirement of a director, uncertainty about his successor, arrival of the new director, intensification of the treatment efforts with a consequent increase of the patients' turn-over, introduction of some of the principles of the therapeutic community, mixing of the sexes and open-doors on the majority of units - all conditions which have really been made responsible for the increase of the clinical suicides[3,4,6]. There is another state psychiatric hospital in Canton of Berne, the Psychiatric Clinic of Münsingen. In that institution, of course, some changes also took place in Period II, however, they were of a considerably smaller degree, they were not performed in a comparable incisive and comprehensive manner, and there was no change in the principal hospital policy, the director remaining the same. If the factors mentioned above were really responsible for the observed increase of clinical suicides, the suicide rates in Münsingen could be expected to increase to some extent, although not comparable to that in Berne. We have no complete data to calculate the expected suicide rates for the Clinic Münsingen, but we could compare small samples of the inpatients of both clinics. There was no significant difference with regard to the sex and the age composition, however, the patients of the Clinic Münsingen more frequently came from rural areas. Thus, we have no reason to suppose the expected suicide rates for this clinic to be higher than those for our institution. Table 5 compares the number of suicides and the suicide rates in both institutions, with regard to Period I and Period II. There are considerable differences as to the sex rates, however, in Münsingen a considerable increase of suicides also has been observed, even though

942

Table 5. Number of clinical suicides and
suicide rates per 100'000 admissions in PUC Berne and PC Münsingen. Comparison of Period I and II.

	PUC Berne			PC Münsingen		
	♂	♀	♂+♀	♂	♀	♂+♀
Period I 1960-1970	15 245.4	9 167.0	24 208.8	20 394.6	4 93.7	24 257.1
Period II 1971-1981	37 632.4	12 240.1	49 452.2	34 571.5	18 337.6	52 461.0
Suicide Rate Increase	157.7 %	43.8 %	116.6 %	44.8 %	260.3 %	79.3 %

totally it might be less pronounced than in our Clinic. This finding
points to the importance of extramural factors.

SUICIDE RATES AMONG PSYCHIATRIC EX-INPATIENTS

If the increase of clinical suicides depended on some general
factors even though effecting particularly psychiatric inpatients
as an especially vulnerable group, increased suicide rates also
should be observed among psychiatric ex-inpatients, who probably
remain an especially vulnerable group even after their discharge.
Table 6 presents the number of suicides among psychiatric ex-inpatients committed within one year after their discharge. Compared
with the increase of the expected clinical suicide rates of about

Table 6. Number of suicides among
psychiatric ex-inpatients committed within one year after
their discharge and corresponding suicide rates per 100'000
clinical discharges. Comparison
of two Clinics as well as
Period I and Period II.

	PUC Berne			PC Münsingen		
	♂	♀	♂+♀	♂	♀	♂+♀
Period I 1960-1970	33 537.6	15 277.1	48 415.5	30 583.9	22 503.4	52 546.9
Period II 1971-1981	34 562.8	19 367.9	53 473.0	59 970.9	27 497.2	86 747.4
Suicide Rate Increase	4.7 %	32.8 %	13.8 %	66.3 %	- 1.2 %	36.7 %

8 % for men and 13 % for women (the patients leaving the hospital are practically the same as those being admitted), the suicide rates among ex-inpatients also rose to some extent, however, this increase is by far not as pronounced as in the inpatients. This finding points to the importance of intramural factors.

CONCLUSIONS

The most important results can be summarized as follows: Clinical suicide rates are definitely higher than those of a general population. Moreover, in the period 1971-81 there was a considerable increase in clinical suicides as compared with the period 1960-70. This increase by far exceeds that observed in the general population. There has been a shift in the clinical suicides as well as in the whole clinical population towards the younger age. The diagnostic distribution of clinical suicides is different from that of general suicides. Schizophrenic patients account not only for the major proportion of clinical suicides but also for the major part of the increase observed. There are some factors operating at present in the society favoring the suicidal trend and effecting psychiatric inpatients in the first place. On the other hand it cannot be denied the increased clinical suicide rates also having to do with some intramural factors. We do not personally subscribe to the notion the increased suicide rates at this time observed in various institutions being a necessary price to be paid for the modern treatment methods, and thus for the benefit the majority of patients enjoys. Rather we would think this increase to be a temporary phenomenon due to the introduction of the new hospital and especially treatment policies; this being the case, a reduction of the clinical suicide rates is to be expected in our institution in the next future. Further follow-up will to be done may demonstrate this.

REFERENCES

1. J. Modestin, Suizid in der psychiatrischen Institution, Nervenarzt 53:254 (1982).
2. N. Retterstøl, Suicide in psychiatric hospitals in Norway, Psychiatria Fennica, Suppl.:89 (1978).
3. K. Ernst, U. Moser, and C. Ernst, Zunehmende Suicide psychiatrischer Klinikpatienten: Realität oder Artefakt?, Arch.Psychiatr. Nervenkr. 228:351 (1980).
4. O. Bjarnason, Association between changes in psychiatric services and increases in suicide rates, Arch.Psychiatr.Nervenkr. 232:15 (1982).
5. A. D. Pokorny, Suicide rates in various psychiatric disorders, J.Nerv.Ment.Dis. 139:499 (1964).
6. M. J. Kahne, Suicides in mental hospitals: a study of the effects of personnel and patient turnover, J.Health Soc.Beh. 9:255 (1968).

A TYPOLOGY OF ATTEMPTED SUICIDE

Heinz Katschnig and Geraldine Fuchs-Robetin

Ludwig Boltzmann Institut für Sozialpsychiatrie
Spitalgasse 11
A-1090 Wien, Austria

INTRODUCTION

One of the central issues of suicidology is the prediction of suicide following a suicidal attempt. There is no conclusive answer to this question yet available, as results of follow-up studies differ to a large extent. In an overview by Wilkins (1967) the percentage of suicide varied between 69 % within one year and 0,2 % within 9 years after the suicidal attempt.

The reasons for this discrepancy are probably manifold. Besides cultural and methodological differences the following explanation is possible: assuming that attempting suicide is not a homogenous phenomenon but may be regarded as consisting of different types of behaviour, each having a specific risk for subsequent suicide, a different composition of the populations studied could lead to very different suicide rates.

Although the prevention of suicide is by no means the only aim of caring for those who have attempted suicide, it is a legitimate wish of the practitioner, to get some guidelines as to which patients are at high risk of finally dying by suicide.

The topic of our presentation : "A typology of attempted suicide" is concerned with this aspect, and the question we try to answer is: Are there different types of attempted suicide with respect to the subsequent risk of a completed suicide?

STUDY DESIGN

In 1971, when all attempted suicides who had come to the knowledge of medical services were admitted to a central detoxification ward in Vienna, we selected a 1 in 4 sample of all 1104 patients admitted during the year. Of the 276 patients selected for this study, 14 had died within one week of admission, i.e. they finally had become suicides, and were therefore excluded from our follow-up, which was concerned with the remaining 262 patients.

We tried to establish the "fate" of these 262 patients as to whether they were still living or had died within a 5 and 10 years interval after admission. If a patient had died, we tried to establish the cause of death by checking all available administrative records, which means that our estimate of suicide risk is a rather conservative one.

RESULTS

After 5 and 10 years 94,7 and 93,5 % respectively of all patients could be traced. 35, i.e. 13,4 % had died in the first 5 years after admission, and a further 15 were found to be dead at the 10 year follow up giving a total of nearly 1 in 5 patients who had died within a 10 year follow up period. Of those who had died 11 (= 4,2 % of the original pupulation) had committed suicide within the first 5 years, a number which had risen at the end of the 10 year follow up period to a total of 14 (= 5,3 %).

Table 1. Fate of 262 patients who have attempted suicide, 5 years and 10 years after the attempt

	5 year follow-up	10 year follow up
traced	248 = 94,7 %	245 = 93,5 %
living	213 = 81,3 %	195 = 74,4 %
dead	35 = 13,4 %	50 = 19,1 %
suicides	11 = 4,2 %	14 = 5,3 %

The task we are confronted with in this paper is to find out whether this suicide risk of approximately 1 in 19 is differently distributed among possible subpopulations. In order to identify homogenous subpopulations in a given sample one of the many available cluster analytical methods is appropriate. The variables we selected for this cluster analysis were chosen on a priori grounds because of their theoretical interest and because of their accessibility. If a typology should be of any practical use then

variables have to be chosen which are easily accessible for all
staff involved in caring for suicidal patients.

In table 2 the basic frequencies of these variables in our
study population are presented showing the usual demographic
characteristics, such as low mean age, preponderance of women, an
overwhelming percentage of drugs having been used and a preponderance of patients with an interpersonal conflict as the only
motive (as opposed to what we have called "unhappiness motive",
i.e. basically a final loss, where no conflict is involved; see
Katschnig et al., 1979). Altogether 9 variables were used for
carrying out a cluster analysis.

Table 2. All patients (N = 262)

```
36,1 Mean age (years)
 64 % Female
 11 % Retired
 75 % First admission
 68 % Only conflict motive
 15 % Alcohol before attempted suicide
 10 % Unconscious on admission
 84 % Soft method
 96 % Only Psychogenic disorder
```

The cluster analysis yielded 7 clusters which cannot be
described in detail here. It was very astonishing that many
clusters had a high degree of homogeneity, i.e. many of the
variables showed a 100 % or a 0 % presence.

The largest cluster contained 92 patients, i.e. more than
one third of the total population, showing a much lower average
age than the total population, a higher percentage of women, all
92 patients were first admissions, all had admitted a conflict
motive only, and 99 % had used soft methods. This cluster
obviously represents the "typical" attempted suicide patient. We
called this the "cry for help" cluster.

Table 3. The "cry for help" cluster (II) (N = 92)

```
29,0 Mean age (years)
 77 % Female
  0 % Retired
100 % First admission
100 % Only conflict motive
  0 % Alcohol before attempted suicide
  0 % Unconscious on admission
 99 % Soft method
 99 % Only Psychogenic disorder
```

On the other hand, a small cluster, containing 28 persons, showed a very high average age, a high percentage of "unhappiness motives", and a higher percentage of cutting and hard methods; 100 % were retired. We called this the "failed suicide" cluster, as its demographic characteristics are close to those of a population of completed suicides.

Table 4. The "failed suicide" cluster (I) (N = 28)

62,9 Mean age (years)
64 % Female
100 % Retired
67 % First admission
25 % Only conflict motive
11 % Alcohol before attempted suicide
14 % Unconscious on admission
86 % Soft method
93 % Only Psychogenic disorder

Only one further cluster can be mentioned here, containing 36 persons all of whom were repeated attempted suicides at the time of entering the study. This cluster was, therefore, named the "chronic" cluster.

Table 5. The "chronic" cluster (V) (N = 36)

34,8 Mean age (years)
64 % Female
0 % Retired
0 % First admission
64 % Only conflict motive
0 % Alcohol before attempted suicide
0 % Unconscious on admission
92 % Soft method
92 % Only Psychogenic disorder

On clinical grounds one would expect a low suicide rate for the big cluster containing the "typical attempted suicide patient", and a rather high suicide rate for those who had predominantly unhappiness motives or who were already repeated attempted suicides when they entered the study. The next step of our analysis was, therefore, to calculate the suicide risk for each of the clusters separately. The results are only presented for the 3 of the 7 clusters described in more detail above.

No single suicide has occurred in the 10 years following the attempted suicide in the "cry for help" cluster. On the other hand the "failed suicide cluster" and the cluster of "chronic" suicidal patients had suicide rates of over 10 percent.

Table 6. 10 year suicide rates in three selected
         clusters of patients who have attempted
         suicide

                                    10 year suicide rate

"Cry for help" cluster (II)   0/92 = 0,0 %
"Failed suicide" cluster (I)   3/28 = 10,7 %
"Chronic" cluster (V)   5/36 = 13,9 %

II vs. I p <.01   II vs. V p <.001   I vs. V n.s.

A particular characteristic of the cluster analytic method
is that the originally resulting clusters, 7 in our study, are consecutively fused to form larger but less homogenous clusters. In
our case cluster II, III, and IV are fused to a large cluster in
two consecutive fusion steps, consisting of 142 patients. We have
contrasted the suicide rate in this cluster with that of the rest
of the population and found that there was a highly significant
difference between the two groups.

Table 7. 10 year suicide rates in two large clusters
         of patients who have attempted suicide

                                    10 year suicide rate

Low risk group
(fused cluster II, III, IV)   2/142 = 1,4 %

High risk group
(clusters I, V, VI, VII)   10/120 = 8,3 %

                  p <.01

Helpful as these results may be - we were able to allocate
each of the original 276 to one of the seven clusters with their
specific suicide risk (see Katschnig et al., 1979) - it is of
interest to know, whether the different suicide rates and the
clusters depicted are just a reflection of the different demographic
composition of these groups. The precise answer to this question
can only be given, when the suicide risk for a sex-age matched
general population sample is calculated for each of the clusters.
In table 8 we have presented the expected*) values in the small
clusters of persons who would have died by suicide in the respective
matched general population samples and contrasted them with the
observed values. It is evident that, apart from demographic influences, the cluster as such has a decisive influence on the

*) We are indebted to Dr. Richard Gisser and Dr. Peter Findl of
   the Austrian Central Statistical Office for calculation of the
   expected values from the Austrian mortality table 1975/77.

suicide rate. In cluster I, the "failed suicide" cluster, the observed value for suicide is thirty times as high as the expected value, in cluster V, containing the "chronic suicidal patients", this factor is even bigger (46). In cluster II, where no single suicide has occurred, the expected frequency would have been 0,19 persons. Similar results were obtained for the two large groups (table 9).

Table 8. Expected and observed numbers of suicides in three selected clusters of patients who have attempted suicide (10 year follow-up)

	expected	observed	factor
"Cry for help" cluster (II)	0,19	0	0 x
"Failed suicide" cluster (I)	0,10	3	30 x
"Chronic" cluster (V)	0,11	5	46 x

Table 9. Expected and observed numbers of suicides in two large clusters of patients who have attempted suicide (10 year follow-up)

	expected	observed	factor
Low risk group (fused cluster II, III, IV)	0,30	2	6,7x
High risk group (clusters I, V, VI, VII)	0,37	12	32,4x
All patients	0,67	14	20,9x

CONCLUSION

Attempted suicides have a more than 20fold risk of suicide in the subsequent 10 years if compared with the general population. Our results, confirming those of an earlier 5 year follow-up study (Katschnig et al., 1979) show that clinically meaningful subgroups with a very high and a very low risk can be identified. Whether scarce resources should be concentrated on the high risk groups only must, however, remain a question of debate. Not committing suicide does not tell us anything about the quality of life of those who "carry on". This question has to be answered by an other type of study which is especially designed for that purpose.

REFERENCES

Katschnig, H.,Sint, P.,and Fuchs-Robetin,G.,1979, Suicide and Parasuicide: Identification of High- and Low Risk Groups by Cluster Analysis, in:"The Suicide Syndrome", R. Farmer and St.Hirsch,ed.,Croom Helm, London

Wilkins, J., 1967, Suicidal behaviour, Am. Soc. Rev.,32:286

EMPIRICAL EVALUATION OF THE PSYCHOTHERAPEUTIC AFTER-CARE FOR

PATIENTS WHO ATTEMPTED SUICIDE

H.J. Möller, F. Bürk, A. Kurz, A. Torhorst,
C. Wächtler, and H. Lauter
Psychiatric Hospital of the Technical University
Ismaninger Str. 22
D-8000 Munich 80, F.R.G

The results of the different approaches of evaluative research in the field of suicide prevention are in general rather controversial and inconclusive. However, in some of the controlled studies a reduction of suicidal behavior as well as an improvement of psychopathological disturbances and social maladjustment has been shown. Motivational work and a more directive psychotherapeutic approach, which avoids frustration of the patients, seems to be correlated to a better outcome result in this target population (Kurz and Möller, 1982a, b). An important problem especially in the after-care of patients who attempted suicide, is a high rate of non-compliance (Möller and Geiger, 1981).

Up to now there is a lack of empirically based information concerning different methods of prophylactic and after-care treatment for people who are in suicidal crises or who attempted suicide. That is especially true for the situation in the Federal Republic of Germany. But also in the international field there are only few studies concerning this topic. To increase the knowledge on the situation of after-care treatment for patients who attempted suicide, we performed a controlled study using standardized rating instruments to describe actual psychopathological symptoms, social adjustment and personality traits. Among other we applied: Inpatient Multidimensional Psychiatric Scale (Lorr, 1974), Psychischer und Sozial-Kommunikativer Befund (Rudolf, 1979), Freiburger Persönlichkeitsinventar (Fahrenberg et al., 1978), Klinische Selbstbeurteilungs-Skalen (von Zerssen, 1976), Social Adjustment Scale (Weissman and Bothwell, 1976), Global Assessment Scale (Spitzer et al., 1976). Besides these psychopathometrical data we collected detailed information on socio-demographic and biographical data as well as on history of psychiatric illness and treatment.

The patients were selected of a sample of about 500 patients who were treated because of attempted suicide by poisoning in the Toxicological Department of the Klinikum rechts der Isar in Munich. Doctors of our Psychiatric Clinic are concerned with the psychiatric care of this ward under the conditions of a psychiatric liaison--service (Lauter, 1982). 226 of these 500 patients were chosen for a psychotherapeutic after-care on outpatient basis. The research program consisted of two phases. In phase I the standard-care stiuation was studied.The standard-care situation (N = 85) can be characterized by the following items: short crisis intervention during the hospital stay, after-care by specialized psycho-social institutions (e.g. "Arche"), fixed arrangement of after-care date to improve compliance. In the second research-phase additionally to this after--care arrangement a more intensified work on motivation was tried. Furthermore the patients were randomly assigned to two groups: the patients of the experimental group (N = 68) were treated on an outpatient basis by the same doctor, who treated them in the hospital. The psychotherapeutic after-care followed the rules of short-term psychodynamically oriented therapy (Kurz and Möller, in press). The duration of this after-care program was limited to about 12 hours during the three months after the suicide attempt. The after-care of the control-group (N = 73) was performed by the specialized psychosocial institutions mentioned above. In the two phases of the study the patients were randomly assigned to the four doctors collaborating in this project.

Comparing some relevant predictive variables it can be concluded that the three groups are rather well balanced concerning these variables. However, a tendency can be seen that the experimental group has a higher proportion than the control-group in some unfavourable characteristics like being divorced, living alone, unemployment in the last 12 months, previous stay in psychiatric hospital, history of alcohol/drug addiction or misuse. Although this discrepancy becomes only statistically significant concerning the item unemployment in the last 12 months ($p < 0.01$), it should be considered. On the basis of psychopathological data there is no relevant discrepancy concerning the relevant scores (Torhorst et al., in prep.).

The hypothesis concerning after-care treatment was, that the patients of the second research phase, that means the control group (and the experimental group), would have a higher degree of compliance than the patients of the first research phase, because of the intensified motivation work. Furthermore the experimental group should have a better compliance because of the continuity of care, which means, that the same psychiatrist treated the patients during the hospital stay and afterwards. As to the first hypothesis the compliance of the control-group shows only a small increase in comparison to the compliance of the standard-care group: e.g. the rate of non--compliance is 50% in the standard-care group, 60% in the control--group. As more convincing are the results of the experimental group:

Only 28% of the patients did not accept the after-care treatment. The data show that the lower degree of non-compliance in the experimental group is not compensated by higher drop-out rates during after-care treatment. The opposite is true: whereas only 12% of the control-group went to after-care treatment longer than five hours, 38% of the experimental group did so (table I).

Table I:

hours of aftercare treatment	standard care group (N = 85)		control group (N = 73)		experimental group (N = 68)	
0	51	60%	37	50%	19	28%
1 - 2	13	15%	14	19%	11	16%
3 - 5	7	8%	13	18%	12	18%
6 - 10	5	6%	4	6%	15	22%
> 10	6	7%	5	7%	11	16%
missing data	3	4%	0	0%	0	0%

$p < 0.005$

Thus it can be concluded, that the continuity of care is a very important factor to guarantee a high compliance in the after--care treatment of suicide attempters. The additional motivation work however seems not to be very successful under the tested conditions: That means, that the arrangement of a fixed after-care date, which proved as a very important factor of compliance in our former investigations (Möller and Geider, 1982), cannot be exceeded much concerning the increase of compliance rate by additional motivation work.

The patients were followed up one year after the index-hospitalization, using the same standardized instruments as before. We were able to collect at least some important data on 92% of the 226 patients. Six patients committed suicide. 23 attempted one or more suicides. The number of suicide attempts was 43, the number of recidives of suicidal behavior (suicide and suicide attempts) was 49.

To test the efficacy of the different after-care strategies, we compared the frequency of suicides, suicide attempters, suicide attempts and recidives of suicidal behavior between the three groups mentioned above. We had to notice the disappointing result, that the experimental group was worse than the control-group concerning some of these outcome-criteria (table I): The number of suicide attempters, the number of suicide attempts, and the number of recidives of suicidal behavior were significantly higher than in the control-group.

Table II:

	standard care group (N = 85)	control group (N = 73)	experimental group (N = 68)	significance control vs. experim. group
patients who attempted suicide	11	3	9	p = 0.052
patients who committed suicide	1	2	3	n.s.
patients with suicide or suicide attempt(s)	12	5	12	n.s.
number of suicide attempts	24	4	15	p<0.05
number of suicide attempts and suicides	25	6	18	p<0.05
no follow-up	3	3	2	n.s.
no recidive of suicidal behavior	70	65	54	n.s.

The experimental group is also a little worse than the control-group in two other outcome variables (stay in psychiatric hospital, inability to work), whereas the other outcome criteria (Global Assessment Scale, depression factor of the IMPS, Self-Rating Factor of Depression) show no discrepancy between the groups (table III).

In summarizing the latter data we have to conclude that the special after-care strategies in the experimental group were not able to prevent recidives of suicidal behavior more successfully than the usual after-care by specialized institutions of psychosocial care. The worse results concerning hospital stay and inability to work in the experimental group can possibly be explained by structural unequality between the experimental group and control-group concerning some relevant predictors.

Table III:

	standard care group (N = 80)	control group (N = 65)	experimental group (N = 62)
Global Assessment Scale (GAS)	66,9 (14,3)	66,9 (15,3)	65,5 (16,8)
Anxious Depression (IMPS)	12,7 (5,7)	12,9 (5,4)	12,9 (7,0)
Retardation and Apathy (IMPS)	3,1 (5,6)	2,9 (4,8)	2,8 (5,1)
Impaired Functioning (IMPS)	0,9 (1,3)	0,9 (1,4)	1,0 (1,5)
Depression Factor (selfrating)	7,1 (7,1)	6,2 (6,9)	7,6 (9,2)

Literature

Fahrenberg, J., Selg, H., Hampel, R., 1978, Freiburger Persönlich-
      keitsinventar, FPI, Hogrefe, Göttingen
Kurz, A., Möller, H.J., 1982a, Ergebnisse der epidemiologischen Eva-
      luation von suizidprophylaktischen Versorgungsprogrammen.
      Psychiat. Prax., 9:12-19
Kurz, A., Möller, H.J., 1982b, Ergebnisse der klinisch-experimentel-
      len Evaluation von suizidprophylaktischen Versorgungsprogram-
      men, Arch. Psychiat. Nervenkr. 232:97-118
Kurz, A., Möller, H.J., in press, Merkmale der psychotherapeutischen
      Kurzzeitbetreuung bei Patienten nach Suizidversuch, in: Aspekte
      der Suizidalität, Wolfersdorf, M., Faust, eds., Beltz, Weinheim
Lauter, H., 1982, Die psychiatrische Versorgung von Suizidenten auf
      internistischen Stationen, in: Herausforderung und Grenzen
      der klinischen Psychologie, Fiedler,P.A., Franke, A., Howe,
      J., Kury, H., Möller, H.J., eds. Deutsche Gesellschaft für
      Verhaltenstherapie, Tübingen
Lorr, M., 1974, Assessing psychotic behavior by the IMPS, in: Psycho-
      logical measurements in psychopharmacology. Mod. Prob. Pharma-
      copsychiat. Vol. 7, Pichot, P., ed., Karger, Paris

Möller, H.J., Geiger, V., 1981, Möglichkeiten zur "Compliance"-Ver-
        besserung bei Parasuizidenten. Crisis. Intern. J. of Suicide
        and Crisis Studies
Möller, H.J., Geiger, V., 1982, Inanspruchnahme von Nachbetreuungs-
        maßnahmen durch Parasuizidenten: Probleme und Verbesserungs-
        möglichkeiten, in: Psychotherapie in der Psychiatrie, Helm-
        chen, H., Linden, M., Rüger, U., eds., Springer, Berlin -
        Heidelberg - New York
Rudolf, G., 1979, Psychischer und Sozial-Kommunikativer Befund.
        Z. Psychosom. Med. Psychoanalyse 25:1-15
Spitzer, J., Endicott, R.L., Fleiss, L., 1976, The Global Assessment
        Scale. A procedure for measuring overall severity of psy-
        chiatric disturbances. Arch. Gen. Psychiat. 33:766-771
Torhorst, A., Möller, H.J., Bürk, F., Kurz, A., Wächtler, C., Lauter,
        H., in prep., Description of 247 patients with attempted
        suicide using standardized rating scales.
Weissman, M.M., Bothwell, S., 1976, Assessment of social adjustment
        by patient self report. Arch. Gen. Psychiat. 33:1101-1115
Zerssen, D. von, 1976, Klinische Selbstbeurteilungs-Skalen (KSb-S)
        aus dem Münchner Psychiatrischen Informationssystem (PSYCHIS
        München), Manuale. a) allgemeiner Teil, b) Paranoid-Depres-
        sivitäts-Skala, c) Befindlichkeits-Skala, d) Beschwerden-
        Liste. Beltz, Weinheim

CAN SUICIDE PREVENTION BE EFFECTIVE ?

Alexander Kurz and Hans-Jürgen Möller

Psychiatric Hospital of the Technical University
Ismaninger Straße 22
D-8000 Munich 80 F. R. G

In the field of suicide prevention, evaluative research faces special methodological problems. Insufficient consideration of these questions may result in unwarranted optimism or scepticism regarding the effectiveness of suicide prevention. In the present paper the available data will be briefly reviewed and discussed under methodological aspects.

WHAT DOES " EFFECTIVENESS " MEAN ?

The effectiveness of suicide prevention can be operationalized by different criteria of outcome. Each of them has its advantages and shortcomings. The suicide rate, being the " hardest " criterion, is appropriate only in large patient populations because suicide is a rare phenomenon. The suicide attempt rate can be applied to smaller patient samples but it is associated with problems of case recognition. " Soft " criteria such as psychopathology and social adjustment can be easily assessed but they do not exactly give the required information. Apparently, there is no optimal criterion of outcome and therefore the definition of effectiveness must be chosen in accordance with the question to be answered.

HOW CAN EFFECTIVENESS BE DETERMINED ?

Three major approaches have been developed to evaluate suicide prevention programs. In the first approach, which may be called epidemiological, the influence of a suicide prevention activity on the suicide rate in a defined geographical area is examined. In the second approach the evaluation of a preventive program is based upon its effect on treated patients, i. e. on individual outcome measures. This method will be referred to as the clinical approach. The third paradigm starts from the assumption that the utilization of a suicide prevention service by the target population is a crucial prerequisite of its effectiveness. In this approach epidemiological as well as clinical methods can be employed.

EMPIRICAL EVIDENCE

The Epidemiological Approach

Under this heading two different types of investigations can be subsumed. Type I compares the suicide rate in a town (or part of a town) where a suicide prevention service is available with the suicide rate in an ecologically similar town without such a service. The comparability of towns and the limitation of the catchment area of preventive services present the major problems in these investigations. The results are summarized in Table 1. Only in one study the effectiveness of the preventive service in question could be demonstrated using the suicide rate as a criterion of outcome. It is important to note that the investigation of Barraclough and associates (1977) is essentially an attempt to reproduce the positive result of Bagley (1968) with a refined method, particularly with more appropriate criteria of ecological similarity. Epidemiological investigations of type II compare the suicide rates in a town before and after a suicide prevention service is established. If a reduction

Table 1. Epidemiological Approach Type I: Results

Study	Bagley 1968	Lester 1973	Barra- clough et al. 1977	Bridge et al. 1977	Kreitman 1977
Insti- tution	Sama- ritans	Suicide Prevent. Centre	Samari- tans	Suicide Prevent. Centre	Mental Health Centre
Cri- terion	suicide rate	suicide rate	suicide rate	suicide rate	suicide attempt rate
Effec- tive- ness	yes *	no	no	no	yes

*p<.05

958

of suicides is to be regarded as an effect of the preventive activity the background variables must be constant which are known to influence the suicide rate of a town, e. g. population characteristics, structure of medical services and availability of important suicide means. The results are shown in Table 2. In two out of six studies the effectiveness of the preventive service in question could be confirmed.

The Clinical Approach

All clinical studies included in the review were designed as controlled trials. This type of investigation presents special problems when it is applied to suicide prevention. For ethical reasons, the control patients cannot be left without therapy and they cannot be put on a waiting list. They must receive some kind of treatment which may be expected to have a preventive effect and which is sufficiently different from the experimental treatment program. If the control group is recruited at some temporal distance from the experimental group, e. g. before the experimental treatment program is in operation, the problem is again encountered that the relevant background variables must be constant. The results of the clinical studies are summarized in Table 3. When all categories of outcome criteria are equally considered all but one investigations were able to demonstrate the effectiveness of the experimental program. It ist more informative, however, to examine the results with respect to the different outcome measures. Apparently, the suicide rate ist associated with a disappointing outcome whereas the softer criteria yield more positive results.

Table 2. Epidemiological Approach Type II : Results

Study	Sains-bury et al. 1966	Ringel 1968	Weiner 1969	Sawyer et al. 1972	Fox 1976	Cullberg 1978
Insti-tution	Commun. Mental Health Service	Lebens-müden-für-sorge	Suicide Prevent. Centre	Suicide Prevent. Centre	Sama-ritans	Community Mental Health Service
Cri-terion	suicide rate					
Effec-tive-ness	no	yes	no	no	yes	yes

The clinical studies differ from each other in a number of important methodological features, such as patients' characteristics,
nature and duration of treatment, and follow-up period. Generali-
zing conclusions are therefore only tentative. Interesting results
are gained when the investigations are compared with respect to
the following techniques of therapeutic management: keeping up contact with the patients, avoiding a therapist change and improving
patient compliance (all referring to the transition from hospital
to outpatient care). Experimental treatment programs which included one or more of these techniques were superior to the control
management in about half of the pertaining studies. Other treatment
variables, e. g. duration and professionality, had no comparable
influence on effectiveness.

The Utilization Approach

From the third approach of evaluative research only one aspect
will be considered. The readiness of patients who were hospitalized
after suicide attempts to avail themselves of subsequent outpatient
care has been examined in several clinical studies. The results are
shown in Table 4. Two special features of referral management were
associated with referral success: avoidance of a therapist change
and encouragement of utilization. Maximum compliance was achieved
by a combination of these two features.

Table 3. Clinical Approach : Results

Study	Chowd-hury et al. 1973	Welu et al. 1974	Ett-lin-ger 1975	Lit-man & Wold 1976	Motto 1978	Gib-bons et al. 1978	Wullie-mier et al. 1979	Liber-man & Eckman 1981
Effec-tiveness by sui-cide rate	-	-	no	no	yes*	-	no	-
by attempt rate	no	yes*	no	no	-	no	yes	both groups impro-ved*
by psycho-pathology or social adjustm.	yes*	no	no	yes	-	yes	-	

* P < .05

960

COMMENT

The efforts to determine the effectiveness of suicide prevention by epidemiological methods yielded controversial results which
are diffidult to interpret. More conclusive evidence was provided
by controlled clinical investigations. With some reservations due
to the methodological diversity of the studies it may be inferred
that suicide prevention programs can be effective. Three aspects of
therapeutic management seem to be intimately connected with effectiveness: avoiding a change of therapist, keeping up contact to the
patients and improving compliance. Obviously these techniques are
aimed at the pathology of interpersonal relationships which is
found in suicidal patients.

In reviewing the literature it becomes apparent that the potentialities of suicide prevention have not yet been fully developed.
Improvement my particularly be expected from further efforts to
adjust the therapeutic management to the requirements of the target
population.

Table 4. Compliance of Suicide Attempters

Study	Möller et al. 1982	Möller & Geiger 1981	Han-koff 1979		Bogard 1970	Paykel et al. 1974	Oast &Zit-rin 1974	Morgan et al. 1976	Möller 1982
Therapist change avoided	no	no	no	no	yes	yes	yes	yes	yes
Utilization encouraged	no	yes	no	yes	no	no	no	?	yes
Positive compliance per cent	31	62	34	45	11	45	26	70	72

REFERENCES

Bagley, C., 1968, The evaluation of a suicide prevention scheme by an ecological method, Soc. Sci. Med., 2: 1-14

Barraclough, B. M., Jennings, C., Moss, J. R., 1977, Suicide prevention by the Samaritans. A controlled study of effectiveness, Lancet, 2: 237-238

Bogard, M., 1970, Follow-up study of suicidal patients seen in emergenca room consultation, Am. J. Psychiatry, 126: 1017-1020

Bridge, T. P., Potkin S. G., Zung, W., Soldo B. J., 1977, Suicide prevention centers - ecological study of effectiveness, J. Nerv. Ment. Dis., 164: 18-24

Chowdhury,N., Hicks,R. C., Kreitman, N., 1973, Evaluation of an after-care service for parasuicide (attempted suicide) patients, Soc. Psychiatry, 8: 67-81

Cullberg, J., 1978, The Nacka project - an experiment in community psychiatry, in: " Proceed. 9th int. congr. on suicide prevention ", V. Aalberg, ed., The Finnish Association for Mental Health, Oy Länsi-Savo

Ettlinger, R., 1975, Evaluation of suicide prevention after attempted suicide, Acta Psychiat. Scand. Suppl. 260

Fox, R., 1976, The recent decline of suicide in Britain: the role of the Samaritan suicide prevention movement, in: " Suicidology ", E. S. Shneidman, ed., Grune and Stratton, San Francisco, London

Gibbons, J. S., Butler J., Urwin, P., Gibbons J. L., 1978, Evaluation of a social work service for self-poisoning patients, Brit. J. Psychiatry, 133: 111-118

Hankoff L. D., 1979, Situational categories, in: " Suicide ", L. D. Hankoff, B. Einsidler, eds., PSG Publishing Company Inc., Littleton, Mass.

Kreitman, N., 1977,"Parasuicide",Wiley, New York, Sydney, Toronto

Lester D., 1973, Suicide-prevention centers and prevention of suicide, New Engl. J. Med., 289: 380

Liberman R. P., Eckman T., 1981, Behavior therapy vs insight-oriented therapy for repeated suicide attempters, Arch. Gen. Psychiatry, 38: 1126-1130

Litman, R. E., Wold, C. I., 1976, Beyond crisis intervention, in: " Suicidology ", E. S. Shneidman, ed., Grune and Stratton, San Francisco, London

Möller H. J., 1982, Inanspruchnahmeprobleme bei der Betreuung suizidgefährdeter Patienten. Ergebnisse neuerer Untersuchungen, in: " Herausforderung und Grenzen der klinischen Psychologie" P. A. Fiedler, A. Franke, J. Howe, H. Kury, H. J. Möller, eds., Deutsche Gesellschaft für Verhaltenstherapie, Tübingen

Möller, H. J., Geiger, V., 1981, Möglichkeiten zur " Compliance "-Verbesserung bei Parasuizidenten, Crisis 2: 122-129

Möller, H. J., Torhorst, A., Wächtler. C., 1982, Versorgung von Patienten nach Selbstmordversuch - Aufgaben, Probleme und Verbesserungsmöglichkeiten, Psychiat. Prax., 9: 106-112

Morgan, H. G., Barton, J., Pottle, S., Pocock, H., Burns-Cox, C. J., 1976, Deliberate self-harm: a follow-up study of 279 patients, Brit. J. Psychiatry, 128: 361-368

Motto, J. A., 1978, Suicidal persons who decline treatment: a long-term program, in: " Proceed. 9th int. congr. for suicide prevention ", V. Aalberg, ed., The Finnish Association for Mental Health, Oy Länsi-Savo

Oast,S. P., Zitrin, A., 1975, A public health approach to suicide prevention, Am. J. Publ. Health, 65: 144-147

Paykel, E. S., Hallowell. C., Dressler, D. M., Shapiro, D. L., Weissman, M. M., 1974, Treatment of suicide attempters, Arch. Gen. Psychiatry, 31: 487-491

Ringel, E., 1968, Suicide prevention in Vienna, in: " Suicidal Behaviors ", H. L. P. Resnik, ed., Little, Brown and company, Boston

Sainsbury, P., Walk, D., Grad, J., 1966, Evaluating the Graylingwell hospital community psychiatric service in Chichester: suicide and community care, Milbank Memorial Fund Quart., 44:243-245

Sawyer, J. B., Sudak, H. S., Hall, S. R., 1972, A follow-up study of 53 suicides known to a suicide prevention center, Life-Threat.Behav., 2:227-238

Weiner, I. W., 1969, The effectiveness of a suicide prevention program, Ment. Hyg., 53: 357 - 363

Welu,T. C., Picard, K. M., 1974, Evaluating the effectiveness of a special follow-up program for suicide attempters: a two-year study, in: " Proceed. 7th int. congr. for suicide prevention " N. Speyer, R. F. W. Diekstra, K. J. M. van de Loo, eds., Swets and Zeitlinger, Amsterdam

Wulliemier, F., Bovet, J., Meylan, D., 1979, Le devenir des suicidants admis à l'hôpital général. Etude comparative de deux formes de prévention des récidives et des suicides, Sozial u.Präventivmed. Méd. soc. et prévent., 24: 73-88

THE PROBLEM OF SUICIDE IN PSYCHIATRIC PATIENTS

James S. Jenkins

Department of Sociology, University of Surrey
Gilford, Surrey,
West Sussex Institute of Higher Education
Bishop Otter College

INTRODUCTION

Perhaps the most important finding of both epidemiological and case studies of suicide has been the repeated observation of the association between mental illness and self-destruction. The findings are remarkably consistent; Barraclough and his colleagues (1974) report that 93 of the 100 completed suicides they studied were suffering from a mental illness at the time of their deaths, while Robins et al (1959) reported a figure of 94 per cent and Paerregaard (1963) found that 96 per cent of 1470 suicides in her study in the Copenhagen area had a psychiatric diagnosis. The most commonly diagnosed condition among suicides is depression, but alcoholism and schizophrenia are also, apparently, important conditions in the etiology of suicide. This strong relationship between mental illness and self-destruction can also be observed by examining patterns of mortality in various groups of psychiatric patients; for example, several authors, among them Hegalson (1964) and Sainsbury (1967), have reviewed studies of causes of death among manic depressives. There is substantial agreement in the studies, with a consensus that about 15 per cent of all those with this diagnosis die by suicide.

Similar high rates for suicide are to be found among groups of alcoholics and schizophrenics and indeed it appears that the majority of psychiatric conditions increase the propensity for suicide.

Since a large proportion of those who commit suicide are suffering from conditions that reputedly are treatable, it is not surprising that psychiatrists have argued that medical intervention

represents the most hopeful method of preventing suicide.
Barraclough, in a paper entitled "A Medical Approach to Suicide
Prevention" (1972), contrasting medical services with lay intervention, cites studies carried out in both Sussex and Scotland which
demonstrate a reduction in the suicide rate following improvements
in the psychiatric services of the area. Recognition is also given
to the improvements in the psychiatric care offered by general
practitioners; Sainsbury and Jenkins (1979) have suggested that some
of the decline in the suicide rate in England and Wales from 1963
onwards has been due to general practitioners, who are the most
likely professional group to have contact with the suicidal
immediately before their deaths, becoming more willing to diagnose
psychiatric illness in their patients, to use more appropriate
diagnostic categories and to see their mentally ill patients more
frequently than others.

     But the picture is not entirely favourable. In the case of
psychiatric in-patients, there is evidence from a number of countries
that suicide rates are increasing rapidly.

     Such trends have been observed in England and Wales, in the
Netherlands and in the Scandinavian countries. The reasons are not
clear: it may be that the psychiatric hospitals are now attracting
a population which is inherently more at risk for suicide than in
the past. But several authors have expressed concern that the
increased rate may reflect changed in-patient management away from
custodial care to the more liberal 'open-door' policies, which in
so many ways are desirable, but which may carry the cost of more
suicides occurring, which in less casual regimes may have been
prevented. Dismissing the deeper philosophical questions about the
right to kill oneself, suicides in patients can be seen, and are not
infrequently described by coroners as such, as failures of the
services. If this is so, then the evidence suggests that these
failures are increasing, despite the ever-expanding armamentarium
of psychiatric therapeutics.

The Present Study

     With this background it seemed important to a group of us at
the Medical Research Council Clinical Psychiatric Unit at
Graylingwell Hospital in Chichester (Director Dr. Peter Sainsbury),
to examine further the social and clinical characteristics of a
group of psychiatric patients who ended their lives by suicide and
to analyse their psychiatric care in the hope of being able to
suggest ways of preventing suicide in this extremely vulnerable
group. It was decided to examine all the suicides which took place
in a six-year period in an urban area of southern England. This
area, with a population of approximately a quarter of a million, is
covered by a psychiatric case register which contains computerised
records of all individuals living in a delimited catchment area who

come into contact with specialist psychiatric services. As well as
information about each patient's social and demographic characteristics, the register routinely collects data relating to diagnosis
and 'care events', for instance, admissions and discharges, commence-
ment and termination of some specialist forms of treatment and
attendance at out-patient and day hospital facilities. At the time
we carried out our study, about 13,000 people were known to the
register.

The investigation was carried out in three distinct phases.
Firstly, the coroner's notes of all inquests carried out in the
delimited area for the period of 1974-79 inclusive were examined.
These revealed a total of 110 suicides. Secondly, we searched the
register for known suicides: there were 56. Lastly, a control
group of patients who had not committed suicide was selected from
the register. They were matched with the "register" suicides on
age, sex, diagnosis (using wherever possible the ICD fourth digit
classification) and approximate date of inception to the register.

We thus had three groups. First, there were 54 suicides who
were not known to the register; the information we had about these
was limited to that which we had been able to obtain from the
coroner's notes. Secondly, we had 56 suicides known to the register
and, lastly, 56 controls who were known to the register but who had
not died by suicide. In order to obtain more information about
both groups of register cases their psychiatric case notes and,
where appropriate and available, their general hospital notes and
casualty records were examined.

Results

I should like to start by comparing the register suicides with
the non-register suicides.

There were identical numbers of men and women in the suicides
known to the case register, but in the non-register cases there was
a preponderance of men. As far as age is concerned, the mean ages
of all groups were similar except in the case of non-register
females who were considerably older. Thus the apparent tendencies
for those who commit suicide having not been in touch with the
psychiatric services are that they are more likely to be male and,
if female, older.

The two groups showed slight and non-significant differences in
the methods of suicide chosen, with the non-register cases favouring
overdoses and being more likely to use car exhaust fumes. The
register group used drugs less frequently but this was still the
commonest method. A quarter of them used unusual methods.

967

Non-register suicides were more likely to be single or widowed, while the register suicides were more likely to be married, divorced or separated (this finding is significant at the 5 per cent level). Similarly, the non-register cases are more likely to be living alone, but the difference between them and the non-register suicides is non-significant. However, overall one can detect a tendency for the non-register cases to be socially isolated, which is perhaps a reflection of the fact it is often the spouse or other family member who encourages a patient to seek help from the services. The register suicides were more likely to be unemployed (a frequent concomitant of long-termed psychiatric illness) while the non-register cases were more likely to be retired.

I should now like to turn to the more important comparisons, that is those between suicidal patients and the matched controls who had not killed themselves.

Although differences in the marital statuses of the two groups are small and non-significant the protective effect of living with others is shown by household composition, the suicides being much more likely to live alone than with others. But very similar proportions of both groups were employed; this gives some support for our belief that the severity of illness in the two groups was roughly similar.

Table 1

Depressives n = 35

	ECT	Current/3m Treatment	Apparently appropriate
Subjects	8	20	23
Controls	9	15	27
	n.s.	$x^2 = 1.4$ n.s.	n.s.

Other diagnoses n = 21

	ECT	Current/3m Treatment	Apparently appropriate
Subjects	1	11	15
Controls	1	3	13
	n.s.	$x^2 = 6.86$ $p < .01$	n.s.

N.B. Current/3m = was subject currently in treatment or was he within 3m of D.E.D.

When we come to consider treatment patterns and contact with the services, it must be remembered that since the two groups were matched on diagnosis it is expected that there will be great similarities between the two groups. This is borne out by the findings. The majority of cases, 35 out of 56 or 63 per cent, were diagnosed as suggering from depression. It can be seen from the table that very similar proportions of depressed subjects and controls received ECT, were receiving apparently appropriate drugs, etc. in the correct dosages, and were currently in treatment or had been in contact with the services within three months of the date of death. (Incidentally, for the controls the 'death equivalent' day is defined as the date following the same number of days the patient was known to the services as his matched suicide was.)

A similar pattern is observed with other diagnoses, of whom there were 21 cases. In this heading is included schizophrenics, of whom there were six, and a variety of other diagnoses including personality disorders, alcoholism, marital difficulties and so on. In this group, it can be seen that the suicides were more likely to be currently in treatment than the controls, but in effect this probably only means that, as would be expected, their condition was more active at the time immediately preceeding their deaths. For the controls the 'death equivalent' day is rather an arbituary time in this context.

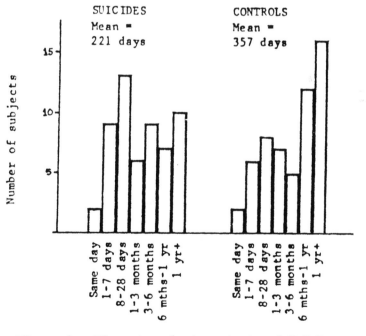

Figure 1. Time since last contact and D.E.D.

The mean length of time known to the service was similar for both groups, 2340 days for the suicides, and 2013 days for the controls. But there were significant differences between the suicides and non-suicides in the length of time since last contact with the service before death or 'death equivalent' day. The suicides were rather more likely to have been in recent contact with the service than the controls. But what is disturbing is that in both cases the mean number of days since last contact was so long. Indeed, nearly half the suicides had not been in contact with the service for more than three months.

It is well recognised that an important indicator of subsequent suicide risk is a history of previous suicide attempts. By careful examination of casualty notes as well as psychiatric notes it was possible to establish mean numbers of previous suicide attempts for our two groups.

Table 2

COMPARISON OF PREVIOUS SUICIDE ATTEMPTS

P.S.A.	Suicides	Controls
One	19 (34%)	8 (14%)
Two or more	23 (41%)	9 (16%)
Total	42 (75%)	17 (30%)

The suicide group was characterised by frequent suicide attempts; a total of 42 (75 per cent) had made previous attempts. More than half of them (23 cases) on more than one occasion compared with 17 (30 per cent) of the controls. This is significant at the .001 level. Interestingly, the suicides and controls had similar numbers of attempts in the month before the last contact with the services, 12 in the suicides and 9 in the controls; the suicides, however, were more likely to have had a history of attempts over the mid-term (1-12 months) and long-term (over 12 months) period.

Discussion

For medical intervention to be an effective means of preventing suicide, it is necessary for two criteria to be met. The first is that those at risk must be in contact with the services and secondly, once that contact has been established, effective care must be provided and continue to be provided while the individual is at risk.

As to the first requirement, it will be recalled that about
half the present sample was in contact with specialist psychiatric
care. But that is not to say that the remainder were not psychiatrically ill and in need of care. Psychiatric illness was mentioned
in the coroner's notes in 33 of the 54 cases. The commonest diagnosis was depression, which occurred in 31 cases, with alcoholism
also being frequently mentioned. In slightly more than a third the
subjects were receiving some form of psychiatric treatment, but as
Barraclough et al (1974) observed in their sample, this treatment
was often inappropriate for the condition or the dosage too small
to be therapeutically active. It appeared from the albeit meagre
coroner's notes that often if depression was seen as an appropriate
reaction to bereavement, physical pain or increasing disability, the
general practitioners paid little attention to it.

Turning now to suicides in patients known to the psychiatric
services, some of the findings of the present study are not new,
but serve to reinforce previous knowledge about the factors which
are associated with increased risk of suicide. Thus, we found that
social isolation, especially when it took the form of living alone,
was significantly related to subsequent suicide. Similarly, a
history of previous suicide attempt was far more likely to be found
in the suicide group; perhaps the interesting aspect of this finding
is the fact that previous attempts occurring longer ago were the
pertinent indicators of current high risk.

But possibly the most important finding of this investigation
is that risk for suicide in vulnerable patients extends long after
contact with the services had ceased; as has already been described,
46 per cent of the deaths occurred more than three months after the
last contact with the services. Unfortunately, we could find no
simple indicators of which patients need to be more carefully
followed up than others. When we compared the patients whose
suicides had occurred within three months of the last contact with
the services with those whose suicides had occurred after that, we
found that their sex, age and diagnostic characteristics were very
similar.

The implication of this finding is that, for prevention of
suicide by the psychiatric services to be effective in as many of
half of the vulnerable patients who had been in touch with the
services, follow-up monitoring and support needs to be offered for
a considerable length of time. It is perhaps necessary for psychiatry to perceive its responsibility in this function in much the
same way as those involved in general medicine follow up patients
with neoplastic or cardiac disease.

However, many of the patients most at risk may well not be
highly motivated to attend for out-patient appointments or at a
day hospital. We noticed that the records of our suicide patients

frequently revealed non-attendance at the last arranged appointment prior to their deaths. It would seem that the community-based services are more likely to be able to maintain effective contact with such patients.

In the British context such services would include the general practitioner, social workers based either in the psychiatric hospital or in community-based social services teams, and lay organisations such as the Samaritans. Mention also should be made of the community psychiatric nurse. But the efficiency and effectiveness of any of these groups depend on good quality of referral by the specialist services in the first place, continuing contact after referral, and a willingness by the agency to maintain the follow-up of patients over a long period. Unfortunately it appeared that referral back to general practitioners by the hospital-based psychiatrists was either non-existent or limited to a perfunctory discharge letter which frequently made no reference to the risk of suicide. Social work agencies, under the pressure of increasing workloads and an increasing tendency to use time-limited, task-centred methods, frequently see themselves as being unable to offer long-term supportive or monitoring care. Contact between specialist psychiatric services and some lay organisations is frustrated by different perceptions of confidentiality and the efficacy of each others' approaches. But the need for greater co-ordination between these different caring groups is clearly established and it is hoped that such co-operation will develop and improve.

In conclusion, it is important to say that the design of this study was such as to concentrate on failures rather than successes. It is difficult to identify patients who have been successfully saved from self-destruction by effective psychiatric care, but they are undoubtedly many. It is hoped that by recognition of the importance of social isolation, the warning signs of previous suicide attempts, and by improvement of follow up care their number can increase.

ACKNOWLEDGEMENTS

I am grateful to Dr. Peter Sainsbury, Jackie Kewell and Christopher Jennings for considerable help in the carrying out of this research.

REFERENCES

Barraclough, B., 1972, "A medical approach to suicide prevention."
    Soc. Sci. and Med. Vol. 6. pp. 661-671.
Barraclough, B., Bunch, J., Nelson, B., and Sainsbury, P., 1974,
    "A hundred cases of suicide: Clinical Aspects." (Brit. J.
    Psychiat.) Vol. 125. pp. 355-373.
Helgason, T., 1964, "The Epidemiology of Mental Disorder in Iceland."
    Acta Psychiatrica Scandinavica. Supp. 173.
Paerregaard, G., 1963, "Suicide and Attempted Suicide in Copenhagen."
    Vols. I, II, III. Kob: Akad au handling.
Robins, E., Murphy, G.E., Wilkinson, R.H., Gassner, S., Kayes, J.,
    1959, "Some clinical considerations in the prevention of
    suicide based on a study of 134 successful suicides."
    Amer. J. of Pub. Health, Vol. 49. pp. 888-898.
Sainsbury, P., 1968, "Suicide and Depression." Ed. Coppen. A and
    Walk, A., London.
Sainsbury, P. and Jenkins, J., 1979, "Suicide in Europe." Report
    to W.H.O. (European Office).

SUICIDE AND PARTNERSHIP: A BASIC EVALUATION

Christian Reimer and Friedrich Balck

Medizinische Hochschule, Lübeck

I. Introduction

Although Freud in 'Trauer und Melancholie' (1917), pointed out the
importance of the surrounding people for an act of apparent
self-aggression, his observations were sparsely reflected in
research. Paykel et al. (1975) found that a serious disagreement
with the partner was the most often mentioned life event preceeding a suicide attempt. Stengel (1969), remarking on the note of
appeal in attempted suicide, initiated studies on the communi-
cational aspect of suicide.

II. Questions and method

Using a post-suicide-attempt interview, we aimed to determine:
1) the emotional climate in the partnership, 2) the climate of
conflict and 3) the feelings towards the partner preceeding and
following the attempt. Our criteria were: a patient, at last 20 years

old, living in a steady, heterosexual realationship of not less than one year's duration, with no history of psychosis. The suicide attempt had to be at least partially motivated by partnership conflicts. Our random sample included 50 suicide partients and 47 partners (3 partners withheld co-operation) questioned as soon after the attempt as possible, since patients are most candid as to their motives in this period. Partners were interviewed separately.

III. Results

The emotional condition of those involved was measured by a free-answer open question and pre-conceived items with a five-stage scale, '1' being complete agreement, '5' being complete disagreement. The majority questioned described themselves as mostly sad and somewhat helpless. Male suicides agree least to item 3 (aggressive fighting mood) and to item 6 (estrangement from partner).Item 5 was rejected by all groups, expressing great concern about the suicide and its circumstances. The suicides differ from the partner group in the open question in that they express feelings of trust and affection for the partner. Women tend to depressively-tinged feelings, guilt feelings and emotional indifference. Aggressive feelings are rarer. Men also tend to depressive feelings.

Table 1: the emotional situation after suicide attempt; calculated group average of the amount of agreement to the items presented

	groups			
items	s/m	p/f	s/f	p/m
1. I'm sad at the moment	2.07	2.33	1.97	2.29
2. I greatly blame myself	2.50	3.25	2.72	3.11
3. I'd like to give him/her a piece of my mind	3.86	3.50	3.53	3.57
4. I've no idea how to behave now	2.36	3.00	2.61	2.94
5. I don't feel especially troubled	4.36	4.58	4.39	4.40
6. He/she isn't close to me at the moment	4.50	2.83	3.08	3.78

Partners, in contrast, feel concern and pity, but even more accusation, estrangement and being put under pressure. Guilt feelings are mentioned by 4 male partners, but by no female partners. The open-question evaluators rated the answers on 3 additional scales: ambivalence, climate of conflict and emotional climate. The evaluators rated all groups as low on ambivalence (female partners lowest) and all partner groups as clearly feeling a climate of conflict. Partners were more unemotional, suicides more engaged emotionally.

Table 2: the naming of emotional contents in the open question after suicide attempt:

emotional categories	groups			
	s/m (N=14)	p/f (N=2)	s/f (N=36)	p/m (N=35)
trust, love, affection	12	2	17	1
troubled, worry about partner	–	5	3	13
blaming towards partner	–	4	5	11
pity	3	4	3	6
uncomprehending, estrangement	–	–	1	13
disappointment, insulted	2	–	8	2
guilt feelings	4	–	3	4
feel being put under pressure	–	4	–	7
fear of oneself	1	1	–	7
helplessness, uncertainty	–	1	2	5
anger/rage	–	2	–	4
surprise	–	1	–	3
abandonment	–	–	4	–
afraid of partner	–	–	3	–
hatred	–	–	3	–
worthlessness	–	–	2	–
disliking	–	–	2	–
contempt	–	–	1	–
indifference	1	–	8	–

In estimations of the emotional situation before the suicide attempt, item 6 is accepted by all groups, by suicides somewhat more, and item 5 is widely rejected. In the open question the suicides express more depression and aggression, the partners more aggression and indifference. 'Blaming towards the partner' is frequently named, but never by female partners, who, to 20%, feel 'love, trust and affection' for the partner. Evaluations of answer forms show a low ambivalence for all groups (lowest for male suicides and their partners). Climate of conflict was tense, female suicides having the highest admitted conflict tension. On 'emotional climate', suicides were more involved than their partners. The partners of male suicides were least emotionally involved.

IV. Discussion

Male suicides are emotionally bound to their partners and the partnership. They feel disappointment and rage before the suicide attempt, mixed with helplessness. They are more emotionally in-volved than their partners. The suicide attempt reduces conflict tensions, increases involvement, but doesn't affect feeling of trust. Their female partners feel indifference and pity. They are emotionally involved in the situation, yet estranged from their partner. The suicide attempt doesn't reduce tension for them. They feel pity, but reject the attempt at manipulation. The emotional distance remains.

Female suicides feel aggression (rage and hatred) for their

partners before the suicide, but also disappointment and insult. They have a high 'climate of conflict'. The attempt reduces aggression and disappointment and increases trust (as among men), but also indifference. The estrangement remains to their partners. 1/3 of the male partners feel rage before the attempt, 1/3 indifference and 1/3 trust and affection. After the attempt, they feel pity and incomprehension. As among female partners, tension is not reduced, but the male partners are not so emotionally distant. Male suicides hold fast to their relationships even when their partners have internally left them. The attempt perhaps follows their recognition of the true situation. Female partners tend to mention their partners' involvement, but not their own, thus perhaps reducing their guilt feelings.

Our results demonstrate the importance of partnership interactions in suicide causation, and the need to involve partners in therapy.

LITERATURE:

1. Freud, S.,   1946, Trauer und Melancholie, in:
                  Ges. W. X, Imago Publ. Co., London.

2. Paykel, E., Prusoff, B. and Myers, J.,   1975, Suicide attempts
                  and recent life events,
                  Arch. Gen. Psychiat., 32: 327.

3. Stengel, E.,   1969, "Selbstmord und Selbstmordversuch",
                  Fischer, Frankfurt a. M.

SUICIDE AND PARTNERSHIP: THE CONFLICT BEHAVIOUR

Friedrich B. Balck and Christian C. Reimer

Medical College Lübeck, Clinic for Psychiatry
Lübeck, Federal Republic of Germany

I. Introduction:

Suicidality and partnership were seen as close connected
long time ago already.
Conflicts in a partnership played often a role in the
causation of a suicide attempt (BANCROFT et al., 1977)and
like KATSCHNIG and STEINERT (1975) mentioned, the suicide
attempt itself becomes a strategy of nonverbal influence.
Other authors classified the suicide attempt as a pattern
of transaction- and communication (GOLDBERG & MUDD,
1968).

Some ideas can be found by STENGEL & COOK (1958) who
viewed the suicide attempt not as a "demonstration", but
as an unconscious expectation for help. For this reason
it is possible, that there follows either a reinforcement of the partnership or a definite break in it.

These specific social-effective aspects of suicide attempt
are short-ranged, don't cause profound changes and have
only an effect by a certain percentage of the patients.
We found no detailed investigation of the conflict behaviour in the partnership of a suicidal person.
The partnership of the suicide is the central concern of
the present study, and especially the conflict behaviour
in conflict situations. It will be characterised by means
of the emotional climate, the feelings between the partners, and their behaviour during conflict. If one takes
the suicide attempt to be a non-verbal form of communication with the partner, then one may ask whether any chan-

ges appear in the partnership as a result of this communication.
We have examined this question with regard to the emotional climate, the behaviour during conflict, and the "density" of the relationship, i. e. whether the partners want to separate or to come together.

To investigate this range of variables, the following instruments were used:
- an instrument composed of 7 questions, to investigate feelings towards the partner,
- a questionnaire about behavior during conflict (BALCK, 1982) which derives from the conflict theory of COSER (1956) and DEUTSCH (1969),
- a questionnaire describing the outcome of fights (11 questions),
- a questionnaire with 8 questions measuring changes in the partnership after the suicide attempt, and
- social data about the suicides and their partners.

Suicides and their partners were included in the study who were older than twenty years old, whose partnerships had lasted at least one year and who had no history of psychosis. The procedure of the investigation was as follows: 50 suicides and 47 partners were interviewed immediately after the suicide attempt. All of these persons received a questionnaire sent to them after one week. 27 suicides and 22 partners responded to this questionnaire.

This random sample of suicidal persons and their partners in the second questioning was composed of 23 men und 26 women; almost three- fourth of the persons were married, where as the remaining pairs were composed of single, widowed or divorced persons. The average age of the suicidal pairs lay at approximately 35 years, the mean duration of the partnership was 11 years and two months. 84 % had a school certificate from the basic or middle school.

II. Results:

Our results from the double questioning are concerned with three aspects:
- the feelings towards the other and the tensions in the partnership in the time preceding the suicide attempt.
- the climate of conflict and the conflict behaviour immediately following the suicide attempt and after approximately one week.
- the short term changes in the partnership which resulted from the suicide attempt.

982

The feelings towards the other preceding the suicide
attempt:

The feelings of the suicide and his partner for each other
are determined by close agreement, good emotional contact
and a more or less developed uncertainty. This uncertainty ist greater in the suicide than in the partner following the suicide attempt. Both persons feel only minimum
rage and do not greatly blame themselves. Their feelings,
however, sway back and forth between tension and harmony.
The feelings of having pity for the other differentiates
between the suicides and their partners. The partner pi-
ties the suicide to a much greater degree than it is
conversely the case.

This evaluation of the feelings towards each other in the
time preceeding the suicide attempt doesn't even change
in the retrospective evaluation farded in one week later,
outside of one exception. This change in evaluation concerned the question: "I simply had no idea how to behave
towards him". This question indicates some confusion in
the communicative situation in the marriage of the
suicide.

Immediately following the suicide attempt, the partner
and to much greater degree the suicide had spoken of just
such an uncertainty in communication preceding the suicide. This uncertainty was seen by both to be of small
degree in the retrospective after one week. This perceptual correction, which possibly is activated as a
defense against a situation which calls forth a feeling
of hopelessness, is especially apparent in the suicide's
partner.

This period before the suicide attempt is on the one hand
characterised by uncertainty in the couple's relationship,
but not by increased tension. Only 38 % of the suicides
and 45 % of the partners in the period immediately after
the suicide attempt spoke of increased tensions in the
time before the suicide attempt. These statements change
amazingly after one week. Now, 100 % of the suicides and
86 % of the partners speak of increased tension in the
period before the suicide attempt.

The climate of conflict and the conflict behaviour in
the period after the suicide attempt

The period after the suicide attempt is characterized by
fights and discussions. Both, suicide and partner, achieve
significantly higher values than the normal population

on a scale of the conflict questionnaire, on which the degree of conflict is measured. The suicide attempt appears as a non-verbal act, possibly giving the opening signal to this incipient verbal battleing. This behaviour does not change for either of those involved in the following week.

If the suicide and the partner are requested to evaluate whether more the conflicts or more the understanding and enjoyment dominate in their partnership, both answer on the average "neither". The answer strongly deviates from the answer found in the average population: this group says, the 'understanding and enjoyment' dominate. It appears to us, however, that with this question, an indication of the emotional climate in the partnership is made on the one hand, while on the other hand a reduction in the socially acceptable response behaviour takes place. The couples, so it would seem, are able to view the tensions in their partnership more honestly after the attempted suicide.

Just, how do persons in these partnerships manage conflicts? The scores of the suicides and their partners are increased on the scale "destructive conflict behaviour" ($p \leqslant 0,05$) and strongly reduced among the suicides, somewhat reduced among the partners on the scale "constructive conflict behaviour" ($p \leqslant 0,05$) compared to a normal population. These partnerships may be characterized by a non-open form of communication: for example, an attempt may be made to manipulate the other by tricks, and to avoid a talk about the problems and the future of the partnership. The scores of both are high on the scale "avoidance of conflict by the partner" ($p \leqslant 0,01$). It is especially the suicide who accuses his partner of going out of the way of conflict. The partner expresses this opinion somewhat more weakly. This is not surprising in view of the recent suicide attempt.

These characteristics of a suicidal partnership do not change in the course of the week following the suicide attempt.

They may not seem to be very original for these partnerships at the first glance. A comparison with strongly dissatisfied couples from the normal population however shows that the values of the suicidal couples go far above their values.

A furhter insight into the conflict behaviour in these partnerships is given by a questionnaire which asks after

the results of disagreements. Suicides and their partners
say, in contrast to control groups, that they don't speak
to each other for a longer time after a fight, that one
of them frequently leaves the domicile after a fight and
each of them wants to be left alone.
A feeling arises among suicides during argumenting that
the other one could leave him in the end. This finding
is clearly connected with his low-self-esteem, and fits
into theoretical considerations about a basic narcisstic
disturbance in suicidal persons (e.g. Henseler, 1974).

Let us summarize the results about conflict behaviour in
partnerships with suicidal persons. Destructive and few
constructive manners of conflict behaviour dominate in
these partnerships. A discussion about problems is avoided as much as possible. Should this not succeed, an
agreement is reached more seldomly than in a normal couple.
Such conflict discussions end more probably in a breakdown in communication and usually in a flight from the
domicile. It is in our opinion conceivable, that these
useless behaviours for solving conflicts can reawaken
fears of separation and abandonment in a narcisstically
disturbed personality, and thus re-activate the basis
for their suicidal behaviour.

Changes in the partnership:

What changes result from the suicide attempt in these
partnerships?

We presented the suicides and their partners with eight
possible changes. These ranged from separation, a deterioration of the partnership, stability in the partnership to reconciliation in the relationship.
A reconciliation was caused by the suicide attempt among
a quarter (1/4) of those questioned. It came to a worsening of the partnership likewise among a quarter of the
persons. The suicide attempt led to a separation among
40 % of the persons, which was predominately initiated
by the partner of the suicide.

III. Summary and discussion:

Initially, we had characterised the suicide attempt as a
non-verbal act of communication, and referred to similar
approaches by KATSCHNIG and STEINERT (1975).

If we view the results from this angle, it is apparent
that the suicide attempt is indeed an impulse to resume
verbal communication, but that very few people succeed

in overcoming their destructive behaviour.

A basic tendency of destructive conflict behaviour is
the mutual manipulation and the tendency to make mountains out of molehills. At the end of any such disagreement there is then a tendency to run away from the
scene of battle as the only manner of behaviour which
leads to a reduction of tension. This scheme for solving
conflicts is especially activated by the suicide attempt,
so that it comes to a parting among many couples.

IV. Literature

1. F.B. Balck, Zufriedenheit in der Zweierbeziehung.
    Eine empirische Untersuchung zu Konfliktstra-
    tegien und zum Konfliktverhalten zufriedener
    und unzufriedener Freundes- und Ehepaare.
    Diss. Hamburg 1982.
2. J. Bancroft, A. Skrimshire, J. Casson, O. Haryard-
    watts and F. Reynolds, People who deliberately
    poison or injure themselves: their problems
    and their contacts with helping agencies.
    Psychol. Med. 7: 289-303 (1977).
3. L. A. Coser, The functions of social conflict.
    Glencoe Ill., Free Press 1956.
4. M. Deutsch, Conflicts: productive and destructive.
    J. of Social Issues 25: 7 - 41 (1969).
5. M. Goldberg and E. Mudd, The effects of suicidal
    behavior upon marriage and the family, in:
    Resnik, H.L.P. (ED.), Suicidal behaviours,
    Boston, Little, Brown and Co. 1968.
6. H. Henseler, Narzißtische Krisen. Zur Psychodyna-
    mik des Selbstmordes. Rowohlt, Reinbeck 1974.
7. H. Katschnig and H. Steinert, The strategie func-
    tion of attempted suicide. Mental Health Soc. 2:
    288 - 293 (1975).
8. E. Stengel and N.G. Cook, Attempted suicide. Its
    social significance and effects. Oxford Uni-
    versity Press 1958.

LOOKING-GLASS-SELF AS A SUICIDE-PREDICTOR

Armin Schmidtke and Sylvia Schaller

Zentralinstitut für   Otto-Selz-Institut
Seelische Gesundheit   für Psychologie und
Mannheim, FRG   Erziehungswissen-
                             schaft, Mannheim

INTRODUCTION

In recent theories the development and changes of the self-concept are considered in functional rela- tionship to metaperspectives and through this to the cognitive socialization of individuals (Laing, Phillipson & Lee, 1966; Epstein, 1973; Wylie, 1974; Orlik 1979). It is thought that self-assessment gradually approaches the "Looking-Glass-self" (how a person thinks he is seen by others) particularly by people to whom he relates (Laing et al., 1966). The recording of metaperspectives and their changes, therefore, could gradually offer possible opportu- nities to record changes in self-worth early and con- sequently to assess the suicidal risk.

Defining the reference groups more precisely could possibly even allow a more differentiated judge- ment of the suicidal risk. The hypothesis could be derived in this way from the temporal covariation of the changes in metaperspectives and self-image, that metaperspectives of suicidal patients with intended lethal suicide attempts are generally more negative than those of patients with more manipulative-type suicide attempts. With the latter, it should not, of course, be assumed that they feel misunderstood by all groups and people in their environment, if the part- icular purposes (of the attempt) are only directed towards specific people or groups, for example, the family.

It is likely that this differentiation is even possible with such groups to which a more negative self-image is a priori ascribed. Above all, because the ideal self-image is relatively similar and stable interindividually (according to the literature) a comparison of the "looking-glass-self" and the former could lead to a differentiation.

A purpose of this study was to examine part of these hypotheses.

METHOD

The subjects were 33 male (average age 16.8 years) and 84 female adolescents (average age 16.2 years) after a suicide attempt. They were examined in the years 1973-1978. Until 1982 a follow-up was carried out to record further suicide attempts. There was a minimum catamnestic time span of 4 years. 5 male and 10 female juveniles made another suicide attempt after the testing. The average interval between the testing and the second suicide attempt was 14.2 months (δ) and 14.4 months ($\female$). The control groups were 44 male and 34 female juveniles in psychiatric treatment and 131 male and 150 female adolescents without psychic abnormalities. The average age of the comparative groups did not differ significantly from that of the suicidal groups.

The following groups were also examined: 34 male prisoners with attempted suicide during imprisonment (average age 23.2 years); 22 male prisoners with self-mutilation during imprisonment (average age 24.11 years); 72 male prisoners without suicide attempt or self-mutilation (average age 23.9 years)

The self-concept (S), the ideal self-concept (I-S) and the metaperspectives of the self-concept were assessed. As reference groups 2 groups were chosen: a narrowly defined group closely related to the patients "LGS-Family, (LGS-F)" (how I believe I am regarded by the family) and a more broadly defined group, LGS-environment (LGS-E; how I believe I am seen by the people in my environment).

As a scale a semantic differential of 7 grades with 25 word-pairs was used. Based on the concept/-

scale interaction the SD consisted of two essential
factors which in pre-examinations were identified as
"Emotionalism" and "Assertiveness/Self-Confidence" as
specifications of the potency and evaluation factor.

The similarities of the concepts, after centring
on the mean value (in order to exclude the effects of
social desirability and therewith heightened coefficients of correlation), were calculated pro S with the
coefficient r_c of Cohen (1969). This correlation-
coefficient takes into consideration the haphazard
arrangement of the word pairs. With the z-transformed
similarity coefficients 3 (group) x 2 (sex), analyses
of variance for the juveniles and single-factor
analyses of variance for the prisoners, respectively,
were carried out. The factor scores for the single
concepts were assessed besides.

RESULTS

Up to the analysis of variance for the similarity S/LGS-E, all analyses of variance of the other
similarities of concept yielded significant main
effects for the factor "group": S/LGS-F: $F = 10.46$; $p <$
.01; η^2 (x 100) = 5.7, ω^2 (x 100) = 5.2; I-S/LGS-F: F
= 24.53, $p < .01$, $\eta^2 = 12.1$, $\omega^2 = 11.6$; I-S/LGS-E: F =
7.37, $p < .01$, $\eta^2 = 4.0$, $\omega^2 = 3.5$; LGS-E/LGS-F: F =
6.58, $p < .01$, $\eta^2 = 3.6$, $\omega^2 = 3.1$. The LGS-F turned out
to be the most negative in both suicidal groups.
While, for example, the self-concept correlated with
the LGS-E at .27 in the male suicidal juveniles and at
.87 in the female, the LGS-F's do not correlate more
significantly or only negatively (-.37, -.09) with the
self-concepts. These differences are also significant
mostly in the comparisons "suicidal" vs. the psychiatric groups.

The results also allow the hypothesis of differentiated metaperspectives of persons with different lethal intention of the suicide attempt, if one
supposes for the groups of male and female juveniles a
different lethal intention in the sense of a statistical hypothesis sensu Bunge. As the analyses of
variance of the similarities S/LGS-E and the corresponding comparisons of the group profile show, the
male and female juveniles differ significantly, particularly in reference to this assumed judgement.
(Comparisons of the correlation S/LGS-E: $t = 3.58$, $p <$
.01; I-S/LGS-F ♂: $r_c = .82$, ♀: $r_c = .56$, $t = 1.69$, $p <$
.10; I-S/LGS-E ♂: $r_c = -.14$, ♀: $r_c = .70$, $t = 3.35$,

p < .01; LGS-F/LGS-E ♂: r_c = .44, ♀: r_c = -.13, t = 1.99, p < .05.)

The differences in the factor-scores show this very clearly also. While among the male juveniles both assumed judgements deviate towards the negative, among the females only the assumed judgement of the family is negative. Only this judgement contains negative opinions generally for both factors in this group.

Each of the suicidal subjects with further suicide attempts after testing also have a correspondingly lower S/LGS-E similarity. The comparisons S/LGS-F and S/LGS-E of the male and female juveniles with further suicide attempts after testing also differ significantly. The similarities of judgement I-S/LGS-F differ as well.

The metaperspectives of all prisoners deviate also towards the negative. Because of the low self-concept of prisoners, no significant differentiation between the groups (main effect "group": F = 2.91, p< .10) was shown in the analysis of variance of the self concept/LGS similarities. The analyses of variance for the similarities of metaperspectives with the ideal-self judgements however resulted in significant main effects for the factor "group" (I-S/LGS-F: F = 2.52, p <.10; I-S/LGS-E: F = 6.22, p < .01). The groups of prisoners with self-mutilation or suicide attempts, each possess significant lower similarities in comparison to the control group.

DISCUSSION

The results show relatively unanimously in all groups, that the assessment of metaperspectives can differentiate suicidal groups from control groups. The metaperspectives in suicidal groups prove to be more negative in general than the self-concept and deviate from the ideal-concept also in corresponding negation. Above all the comparisons of similarities of the meta-perspectives with a relatively unchanged standard of ideal judgement (average similarity of ideal judgements .90) also allow therefore a differentiation of suicidal groups with different types of suicide attempts from each other. As the results of the groups of prisoners show, this also holds true for groups whose self-image proves to be more negative in general and where for that reason the similarity self-con-cept/LGS does not differentiate. The results also permit the hypothesis that with greater lethality of the suicide attempt the metaperspectives prove to be generally negative and also more negative than in groups with less lethal attempts. Based on the available results, it could therefore be assumed, that in a comparison of differentiated metaperspectives, not only with the self-concept (as a changeable variable) but also with a relatively less changeable standard, the simultaneous recording of the concept judgement, its similarities and their change over time could provide a contribution to the assessment of the suicidal risk.

REFERENCES

Cohen, J., 1969, r_c : a profile similarity coefficient invariant over variable reflection, Psych. Bull., 71: 281 - 284.
Epstein, S., 1973, The self-concept revisited. Or a theory on a theory, Am. Psychol., 28: 404 - 415.
Laing, R. D., Phillipson, H. & Lee, A. R., 1966, "Interpersonal Perception," Tavistock, London.
Orlik, P., 1979, Das Selbstkonzept als Bezugssystem sozialer Kognitionen, Zeitschrift für Sozialpsychologie, 10: 167 - 182.
Wylie, R., 1974, "The Self-concept," Univ. of Nebraska Press, Lincoln.

ATTEMPTED SUICIDE: A REPORT ON GENERAL

HOSPITAL PSYCHIATRIC UNIT PATIENTS

Montejo-Iglesias,M.L., Crespo- Hervás, M.D.
and   Ramos-Brieva,J.A.

Hospital Clínico de "San Carlos". Madrid
Instituto de la Salud Mental, Madrid (SPAIN)

INTRODUCTION

Suicide and attempted suicide have been recognised as one the most important public health problems which exist in all countries. The incidence has been on the increase. This fact has been observed since the beginning of the seventies in Spain. However, in our country, there have only been a few investigations about this problem.

This paper tries to reflect the social and demographic conditions, the ecological aspects and the clinic characteristics of a limited sample: parasuicides in general hospital urgencies of Madrid.

MATERIAL AND METHODS

The sample is composed of 104 inpatients (71 females and 33 males) of a general hospital psychiatric unit (San Carlos' Hospital) for parasuicide. The patients came from the hospital Emergency Unit and they were admitted for evaluation and treatment. The patients who denied suicidal intentions are excluded.

The data had been collected during nine consecutiv months using a questionnaire of 65 items which looked for information about social and demografic aspects, clinical characteristics and facts about the attempts (method used, day and hour, etc). Where also applied the followinf tests: Raven-test, Bricklin, Piotrowsky and Wagner's agressivity test (1962) and Beck's Depression Scale (1961) when patient's physical and psychological conditions permited it.

This paper only considers a part of that variables.

The criteria for socioeconomic levels are Hollingshead and Redlich's criterion (1958). For the clinical diagnosis we used the I.C.D.-9ª (W.H.O., 1977). To value the social adaptation we followed the DSM-III classification (1980). The "upper", "very good" and "good" levels are our GOOD group; "fair" is our FAIR and "poor", "very poor" and "grossly impaired" levels are our BAD group. None of the impatients were in the "grossly impaired" group.

Statistical comparisons were carried out using non parametric chi-squared test (Siegel, 1956)

RESULTS AND CONCLUSIONS

The sample was composed of 104 inpatients: 71 females (68%) and 33 males (33%)(see Table 1). This distirbution is different to the general population: 48% males and 52% females (I.N.E., 1977)(df=1; x^2 Yates'= 14.53; p<.o5). Other spanish samples have found similar distributions to ours (Santo Domingo, 1968; Salon-Serra, 1971).

The most outstanding age group is between 21-30 yr. The number of attempts decreases after 50 yr.

If we compare the results with the general population distribution we find differences with statistical significance, as much for the totals as for the sexes (totals: df= 8; x^2 = 86.11; p<.05; males: df= 7; x^2 = 23.82; p .05; females: df= 8; x^2 = 59.77; p<.05). In our sample, children under 15 yr. and women between 61-70 yr. are underrepresented with respect to the general population. The cases accumulated between 21-30 yr., was shown by Pöldinger (1969) and Hawton et al. (1982). The decrease after 50 yrs. was shown by Kennedy and Kreitman (1973).

The majority of our patients were single. This does not coincide with other authors (Jacobson and Tribe, 1972; Kreitman and Chowdhury,1973; Santo Domingo, 1968). Salon Serra (1971) has also found a majority of single people (55%) in Spain. As far as the general population is concerned significant differences are found too, but there are fewer widowers, more divorced (or separated) people and more single people.

The more overrepresented socioeconomic levels are number IV and V, which relate to the socioeconomic profile of the population attending that hospital (Ayuso y Calvé, 1975).

With regard to their occupation, we have found more housewives (24%), unskilled workers (19%) and unemployed people (14%). There are statistically significant differences related to sex, but they are

994

mainly influenced by the housewives group. The other variables do not yield statistically significant differences (df= 6; x^2= 7.07; p<.50).

According to their neighbourhood, 58% of the sample dwelt in Madrid downtown (men as well as women, and no statistical significance can be inferred form this distribution), 35% lived in the outskirts of the city and 8% of the sample lived in the country. Kennedy et al. (1974) report having found high figures in downtown slums, average figures in the outskirts of the city (working class) and lower figures in the suburbs (middle class). Weltz (1979) reports for Manheim is as follows: figures oscillate form 5% in residential areas up to 21% in the center of the city and low figures in the villages.

A 76% of the sample lived with their own family or with their parents, a fact that can also be found in the general Spanish population. There is a greater tendency among men than among women towards living alone (27% vs 10%) though we have found no statistically significant differences. This data has also beeen reported by Kreitman and Chowdbury (1973).

Though as a rule, there is a leaning towards GOOD social adaptation (45%) (without statistically significant differences depending sex) there seems to be worse social adaptation among men than among women (39% vs 18%). Nevertheless, Paykel et al (1974) report the opposite figures with a majority (72%) of BAD social adaptation (data are not fully comparable since they worked a sample of general population with suicidal ideas).

Most of the parasuicides happen in the evening. Females seem to prefer the period form 19 to 24 hours (37% vs 24%), while males tend to concentrate their attempts in the period from 14 to 19 hours (30% vs 30%). Differences without statistical significance. Jacobson and Tribe (1972) found out that most of the attempts place in the first half of the night, followed by the first half of the day which agrees with our own results.

There seems to be no special day of the week to attempt suicide. However Jacobson and Tribe (1972) report that women tned to favour Twesdays and men Mondays.

A 61% of the total sample asked for medical aid before attempting suicide. Women ask for more help than men (not statistically significante differences). Of the people who asked for help, 43% asked psychiatrists and 38% asked general practitioners.Kleitman and Chowdhury (1973) found that 15% asked for help but to general practitioners (74%) and, in second place, to social services.

The 41% of our sample had two or more precipitator factors (Ta-

Table 1 Sociodemographic Characteristics

		FEMALES		MALES		TOTAL		level signific.
		N	%	N	%	N	%	
SEX		71	68	33	32	104	100	
AGE	15 yr	6	8	1	3	7	7	
	16–20	14	20	5	15	19	18	
	21–30	26	37	13	39	39	38	
	31–40	6	8	5	15	12	12	p<.30
	41–50	15	21	5	15	20	19	
	51–60	4	6	1	3	5	5	
	61–70	––	—	2	6	2	2	
	71–80	––	––	1	3	1	1	
MARITAL SATUS								
single		38	54	17	51	55	53	
married		30	42	13	39	43	41	p<.90
widowed		1	1	1	3	2	2	
sep/divorced	2		3	2	6	4	4	
SOCIAL CLASS								
II		1	1	3	9	4	4	
III		13	18	7	21	20	19	p<.30
IV		43	61	16	48	59	57	
V		13	18	8	24	21	20	
EMPLOYMENT								
unemployed		10	14	5	15	15	14	
unskilled		11	15	9	27	20	19	
skilled		6	8	7	21	13	13	
administratv.	8		11	2	6	10	10	p<.01
housewife		25	35	—	—	25	24	
student		8	11	4	12	12	12	
cualified professional	3		4	4	12	7	7	
retired		––	—	2	6	2	2	

ble 2), similar figures to that found by Paykel et al. (1974). Men, usually, have one or no precipitator factor and women, usually, have two or more (p<.05). The premenstrual phase is a important factor in women (32%) and the alcohol in men (30%), similar data to that found by Corbett et al. (1974), Goldney (1981) and Hawton et al. (1981).

The clinical diagnosis of the majority of patients was NEUROSIS (63%) above all in women (70% vs 48%). Bagley and Greer (1971), in a psychiatric hospital sample, found 46% of neurosis. Salon Serra (1971), in a liaison psychiatry sample, found a different relation

Table 2 Precipitator Factors in Last Month and Diagnostic

		FEMALES		MALES		TOTAL		level
		N	%	N	%	N	%	signific
NUMBER	one	22	31	18	55	40	38	
	two	24	34	5	15	29	28	p<.05
	three(⟩)	11	15	2	6	13	13	
	none	14	20	8	24	22	21	
PATTERN								
premenstrual phase		23	32	—	—	23	22	
physical disease		13	18	4	12	17	16	
alcohol		14	20	10	30	24	23	
near suicidal exampl.		11	15	8	24	19	18	
puerpery		6	8	—	—	6	6	(*)
struggle of couple		16	23	5	15	21	20	
loss of object		15	21	9	27	24	23	
disputes		7	10	1	3	8	8	
none		14	20	8	24	22	21	
DIAGNOSTIC								
Schizophrenics and paranoid states		1	1	—	—	1	1	
Affective disorders		10	14	6	18	16	15	
Neurotic disorders		50	70	16	48	66	63	
Dementias and other organic conditions		3	4	3	9	6	6	p<.30
Sociopathic personality disorder		3	4	4	12	7	7	
Alcohol dependence		4	6	4	12	8	8	

(*)various patterns for each patient are possible

between men and women as far as neurosis is concerned (6% vs 11%). In samples carried our in three general hospitals and a psychiatric hospital 15% neurosis is found (Jacobson and Tribe, 1972). Corbett et al. (1974) found 50% neurosis in a general hospital.

Our results suggest that in many suicidal attempts of this Spanish sample there is no real desire to die. It is nothing but a desire to overcome an emotional stress, it is a manipulation of environment.

REFERENCES

Ayuso Gutierrez,J.L., Calvé Perez,A., 1976, "La psiquiatría en el Hospital General". Paz Montalvo. Madrid.

Bagley,Ch.,Greer,S., 1971, Clinical and Social Predictors of Repeated Attempted Suicide: a multivariate Analysis". Brit. J. Psychiat., 119: 515.

Beck,A.,Ward,C.,Mendelson,M.,Erbangh,H.,1961, An Inventory for Measuring Depression. Arch. Gen. Psychiat.,4:561.

Bricklin,B.,Piotrowski,Z.,Wagner,E., 1962.,"The hand test".,Charles Thomas, Sprinfield

Corbett,J.,O'Flaherty,A.,Malone,J., 1974., Attempted suicide:a six month hospital., Irish. Med. J., 67:533.

Diagnostic and Statistical Manual of Mental Disorders .,1980.,American Psychiatric Association (3ª ed), Washington D.C.

Goldney,R.D., 1981., Attempted suicide in young women: correlates of lethality, Brit. J. Psychiat., 139:382.

Hollingshead,A.B., Redlich,F.C., 1958., "Social class and mental illness". Wiley. New York.

Instituto Nacional Estadistica.,1977.,"Caracteristicas de la población española deducida del padrón municipal de habitantes.Provincia de Madrid". Ministerio de Economía. Madrid.

Jacobson,S.,Tribe,P., 1972., Deliberate self-injury (attempted suicide) in patients admitted to hospital in Mid-Sussex. Brit. J. Psychiat., 121: 379.

Kennedy,P.,Kreitman,N., 1973.,An epidemiological survey of parasuicide ("attempted suicide") in general practice. Brit. J. Psychiat.,123: 23.

Kreitman,N.,Chowdhury,N.,1973., Distress behavior: a study of selected samaritan clients and parasuicides ("attempted suicides" patients). Part. I: general aspects., Brit. J. Psychiat., 123:1.

Manual of the International Statistical Classification of Diseases ., 1977.,World Health Organitation., Geneva.

Mawton,K.,Fagg,J.,Marsack,P.,Wells,P., 1982., Deliberate self-poissoning and self-injury in the Oxford Area:1972-1980., Soc. Psychiat. 17: 175.

Paykel,J.K.,Myers,J.,Lindenthal,J.J.,Tanner,J., 1974., Suicidal feelings in the general population: a prevalence study., Brit. J. Psychiat., 124: 460.

Pöldinger,W., 1969.,"La tendencia al suicidio". Morata. Madrid.

Salon Sierra,R., 1971., Problemática psiquiátrica de las tentativas suicidas. Estudio en un hospital general. Med. Esp., 65: 85.

Santo Domingo,J.,Carrasco,J.J.,León,G., 1969., Contribución al estudio epidemiológico de las tentativas suicidas en España., Rev. Esp. Anest. y Rean., 191: 208.

Siegel,S., 1956.,"Nonparametric statistic for the behaviorial sciences". McGraw-Hill. New York.

Welz,R., 1979., Social and ecologicla background of attempted suicides in Mannheim. in "Estimating needs for mental health care: a contribution of epidemiology". Häfner,H.H. ed.,Springel-Verlag, Heidelberg.

INTRODUCTORY ADDRESS TO THE 7th WORLD CONGRESS OF PSYCHIATRY

Robert Volmat

Clinique de Neurologie et Psychiatrie
C.H.U. St Jacques
25000 Besançon (France)

My dear colleagues,
Ladies and gentlemen,

Please permit me as your President to make a brief historical
sketch concerning the evolution of our society, in examining principally its connections with the World Association of Psychiatry and
the World Congress.

As a member of the secretarial organization at the First World
Congress in 1950, I was very interested in the first complete
exposition of psychopathological art. This display, however, was
accompanied neither by work-sessions nor individual commentary.

At the second World Congress in Zurich in 1957, with the aid
of Christian MULLER, a more modest exposition was organized, this
time accompanied by work-sessions which were extremely animated.
Two years later, I had the opportunity, during the lombrosian
celebrations in Verone, of promoting, with the help of Cherubino
TRABUCCHI, the first International Congress of Art and Psychopathology. A constituent assembly formed the International Society
of Art and Psychopathology (S.I.P.E.). This was in 1959.

In 1961 at the Third World Congress in Montreal, the Society
was asked to organize a symposium. Similar demands were renewed in
1966 at the Fourth World Congress in Madrid, and in 1971 at the
Fifth World Congress in Mexico where the remarkable exposition
was staged with the aid of models from Basle, thanks to the kind
cooperation of SANDOZ International. Our last participation was
in Honolulu in 1977 at the Sixth World Congress.

The S.I.P.E. organizes, concurrently, its proper International Congresses which take place actually once every three years, the 10th being held in Munich in October 1982. We also organize International Symposia with the aid of different member organizations ; the 16th is slated for Barcelona in 1984.

We are deeply grateful to the successive dirigeants of the W.P.A. for having regularly given us the possibility of organizing symposia of our own. We are also grateful to the President of the W.P.A., the general secretary, and members of the executive committee for, upon your proposition at the Regional Symposium in Hong Kong in 1980, a Section of Art and Psychopathology was created. This step is clearly in line with the natural evolution, both of the International Society of Art and Psychopathology and of the World Psychiatric Association. A Board was thus formed and the relevant statutes proposed.

This Section has just, in fact, been approved here in Vienna last night during the General Assembly meeting.

The actual organization of our scientific sphere of action comprises two structures : The International Society of Art and Psychopathology (S.I.P.E.) which is a member of the W.P.A., its national and affiliated Societies, and the Section of Art and Psychopathology of the W.P.A., a more independant body.

These two structures, however distinct, remain closely coordinated as the same members comprise the two boards of direction (executive boards). It is therefore to this administrative ensemble that we owe the organization of the present Symposium. The links between the S.I.P.E. and the W.P.A. are now firmly established.

We would like to salute Professor Irene JAKAB of Pittsburg who has constantly been by our side since the Society's incipiency at Verone, as well as Professor Leo NAVRATIL, our Austrian colleague, responsible for the admirable exposition at the Museum of Modern Arts.

I would like to thank the orators who have come to Vienna to expose their works. Equal thanks go to all the participants who come the observe and perhaps discover a field of research hitherto unsuspected.

1000

Finally, on behalf of all my colleagues, I extend felicitations to the different committees as well as their presidents who have participated in the minute and perfect organization of this 7th World Congress of Psychiatry, warm wishes to our President, Pierre PICHOT, our General Secretary, Peter BERNER, members of the Executive Committee, as well as the Committee of the World Congress of Psychiatry.

Thank you.

WRITTEN EXPRESSION IN DEPRESSION

C. Ballús and J. Obiols

Department of Psychiatry
Facultat de Medicina
Universitat de Barcelona

INTRODUCTION

Speech, as a primal form of expression, constitutes a valuable indicator of the psychopathological state of depressive patients. It is well known that the verbal expression's course and content shows shades of its own in depression.

These shades have been described by many authors (Ey et al., 1978; Freedman et al., 1980) and confirmed more recently by others (Weintraub, 1967; Pope et al., 1970; Castilla del Pino, 1978; Andreasen, 1979). They all point at the poverty and the low pressure of speech found in depression. These descriptions tend to be more accurate with the help of accoustic analyzers which allow us to decode emotional and affective aspects of speech (Alpert 1982).

We have less information concerning the written expression of depressive patients. However, certain particular aspects have deserved special attention. For example, related topics like analysis of depressive characters in novels or the meaning of the notion of spleen in poetry have been deeply studied by literary critics. We could even go back to Aristotle when he ruled that the adequate emotional state for Philosophy was melancholia.

Another aspect which deserves particular interest is the analysis of suicidal messages. These documents -full of pathetic meaning- are, notwithstanding, a partial aspect of the globality of written expression in depression.

We might as well mention a field of undoubted value: the graphological analysis of the documents of depressed people. For obvious reasons we will not discuss it here.

Leaving aside the three mentioned aspects, we have tried to deepen in the written expression of these patients beyond mere sub-jective impressions derived from the analysis of speech. In that sense we agree with what Leroi-Gourhan (1965) stated: "Graphism is independent of voice" and what Hecaen (1972) more recently reaffirm-ed: "The graphic code cannot be considered as a simple transcrip-tion of the oral code: The graphic activity constitutes a model of specific accomplishment".

EXPERIMENTAL STUDY RESULTS

We have done a diachronic analysis of the written expression of nine depressive patients enroled in a weekly therapy group. This group only accepts patients diagnosed as depressive: Three of them with major depression and the other six with a minor depressive dis-order.

Before the beginning of each session they were invited to fill the Beck's self administered rating scale for depression (13 items, rated from 0-to-3, 0-to-4 or 0-to-5) and to write a text with the heading "Today I feel..." without any specific limitation.

The study brings together the data of nine consecutive sessions. We must point out the fact that most of the patients did not attend the totality of the sessions.

We were interested in analysing the possible correlations to be found between the clinical state of depression (according to the Beck rating scale scoring) and the written texts. Psycho-linguistic indexes deductable from a text are, of course, almost limitless. An adequate index -a simple and important one at the same time- is the length of the text (scored by the total number of words).

So, words were counted in each of the texts and the scores obtained in this way were compared to the Beck's scores. In a total of 48 observations, the independence test was made through the Sperman rs coefficient and a value of 0.2658 was obtained (significant for $p < 0.05$). Consequently, we can state that a correlation between the clinical degree of depression (as measured by the Beck scale) and the length of the written text exists. We must also state that the intensity of this relationship is moderate. This finding seems interesting because it shows —at least in our 48 texts— a reversed tendency to the one described in the speech of depressed patients. The poverty of speech classically described by psychopathologists and experimentally confirmed by Andreasen (1979) seems to be diluted. The opposite tendency appears in the written expression: The more depressed the patient feels, the longer and more detailed texts he writes.

We may assume there are some explanations to this effect. It is possible that the depressed patient, feeling inhibited in his/her social communication, would tend to express him/herself more easily by writing than by speaking. Furthermore, we can assume that these patients might find a relief through writing their thoughts and emotions. Indeed, we frequently find that depressed patients keep a diary, make poems and seem to benefit from this.

We have looked over other psycholinguistic indexes like (i) the percentage of verbs and (ii) the percentage of negative particles (no, never, nothing, etc.) in each text. We expected to find a lower percentage of verbs —as elements indicating activity— in patients with higher ratings of depression. In the second case, we expected —following Weintraub's (1967) assumptions— a positive correlation between the score of depression and the percentage of negative particles. Nevertheless, none of these correlations proved to be significant.

Another approach comes from the thematic analysis as shown in Table 1. The simple phenomenological systematization of each text allows us to observe the tendency towards the repetition of the topics in each patient. From the diachronic analysis, week per week, of each patient separately, we get the impression of a cyclic closed discourse. In that sense, what has been described by

Table 1. Thematic Analysis of the Texts

1.1 Feeling –/getting better at session/job problems
1.2 Feeling –/getting better at session/job problems
1.3 Job and family problems/guilt/suicidal thoughts
1.4 Feeling –/getting better at session
1.5 Feeling +/possible job
1.6 Feeling 0/possible job/family problem
1.7 Feeling +/possible job/family problem
1.8 Feeling 0/possible job/family problem
1.9 Feeling 0/possible job/family problem

2.1 Inability for self autonomy/pride
2.2 Atheism/agnosticism/pride
2.3 Pride/interdependency

3.1 Feeling 0
3.2 Feeling +/comments about group
3.3 Feeling +/medication
3.4 Feeling +/future perspectives
3.5 Feeling –/daughter illness
3.6 Feeling –
3.7 Feeling +
3.8 Feeling +

4.1 Feeling +
4.2 Feeling –/general problems/struggle
4.3 Feeling –/struggle/withdrawal/alcohol/fear
4.4 Feeling –/anxiety/struggle
4.5 Feeling –/insomnia/struggle/withdrawal
4.6 Feeling –/struggle/withdrawal
4.7 Feeling +/seeing the doctor
4.8 Feeling –/anxiety
4.9 Feeling +/seeing the doctor

5.1 Feeling +/comparing passed and future feelings
5.2 Feeling 0/comparing passed feelings/suicide/fear of illness
5.3 Feeling 0/comparing passed feelings/children problems
5.4 Feeling +/comparing passed feelings/repetition/no solution
5.5 Feeling 0/comparing passed feelings/repetition/no solution
5.6 Feeling 0/comparing passed feelings/doubts about medication

Table 1 (Cont.)

5.7 Feeling –/comparing passed feelings/repetition/no solution
5.8 Feeling –/comparing passed feelings/stolen purse/repetition/no solution
5.9 Feeling 0/comparing passed feelings/repetition/no solution

6.1 Feeling –/symptoms description/social phobia/obsessions
6.2 Feeling –/symptoms description/social phobia/obsessions
6.3 Feeling 0/symptoms description/drawing/violence
6.4 Feeling +/symptoms description/drawing/future perspectives
6.5 Feeling +/future perspectives/alcohol
6.6 Feeling +/future perspectives/obsessions

7.1 Feeling +/social relations problem/body
7.2 Insomnia/thoughts/social relations problem
7.3 Feeling +/tiredness
7.4 Tiredness/aggressivity

8.1 Feeling –/fear/insecurity
8.2 Feeling –/tiredness/solution in sleep
8.3 Feeling –/tiredness/solution in sleep/problems
8.4 Feeling +
8.5 Feeling +/problems solution
8.6 Feeling –/loss of thoughts

9.1 Feeling –/problems/perspectives
9.2 Feeling 0/perspectives/withdrawal

Note: "–" stands for negative feelings
       "+" stands for positive feelings
       "0" stands for in-between

Fernandez-Zoila (1981) as the lack of productive differentiations in the psychopathological discourse is ratified.

FINAL COMMENT

We are conscious about the relative value of the data here stated. On one side, the limited number of cases does not allow us to draw final conclusions. On the other, the technique employed –writing a text beginning with "Today I feel"– may cause loss of interest and tiredness by being presented to the patients week per week and may condition a tendency to shorten writings at the same time that depression improves. We think that further developments of this methodology will allow us to reach more valid conclusions. Anyway, the study of the written expression of the depressed patient can bring quantitative and qualitative data useful for the diagnosis and the knowledge of the evolutive process.

REFERENCES

Alpert, M., 1982, Encoding of Feelings in Voice, in: "Treatment of Depression: Old Controversies and New Approaches", Clayton, P.J. and Barret, J.E., eds., Raven Press, New York.

Andreasen, N., 1979, Thought, Language and Communication Disorders. II Diagnostic Significance, Arch Gen Psychiatry, 36:1325.

Castilla del Pino, C., 1978, Lenguaje y Depresión, in: "Vieja y Nueva Psiquiatría", Castilla del Pino, C., ed. Alianza, Madrid.

Ey, H., Bernard, P. and Brisset, C., 1978, "Tratado de Psiquiatría", Toray-Masson, Barcelona.

Fernández-Zoila, A., 1981, L'écriture dans la tête. Du processus psychopathologique envisagé comme un récit écrit, Confrontations Psychiatriques, 19:259.

Freedman, A., Kaplan, H. and Sadock, B., 1980, "Comprehensive Textbook of Psychiatry", Williams and Wilkins, Baltimore.

Hecaen, H., 1972, "Introduction à la Neuropsychologie", Larousse, Paris.

Leroi-Gourhan, A., 1965, "Le geste de la parole", A. Michel, Paris.

Pope B., Blass, T., Siegman, A. and Raher, S., 1970, Anxiety and Depression in Speech, J Consult Psychol, 35:128.

Weintraub, W. and Aronson, H., 1967, The Application of verbal behaviour analysis to the study of psychological defense mechanisms. IV Speech pattern associated with depressive behaviour, 3 Nerv Men Dis, 144:22.

JOCHEN SEIDEL: WORD DRAWINGS

Harry Rand

National Museum of American Art
Smithsonian Institution
Washington, D.C

When written language was new, when it represented the very
furthest advance of technology (and what is technology but the amelioration of the environment by knowledge) writing and drawing were
the same thing. Today we often forget that the acquisition of
writing by children involves acquiring two separate skills. First we
must learn to scan a page just above its surface. If we look too
closely we see the texture of the paper and the ink, ragged at the
letters' edges. The second skill, the one that is easier to observe
in practice, is the physical dexterity that needs to be acquired to
form the letters. A difficult and demanding job to teach a child, it
is almost impossible to teach an illiterate adult to form letters
precisely because the muscular dexterity involved is so great; the
hand-eye coordination for writing is so imperiously insistent to
very strict tolerances that, like a musical instrument, it is best
learned in childhood. Thus, during the dawn of the age of writing,
the craft of the scribe was a closed guild, and a mysterious and
exhalted one. The professional scribe drew sounds on a page or
tablet or scroll that shaped the breath of those who saw his work,
however far away or even after the scribe's death.

Those first symbols still survive within our letters, the
distant offspring of hieroglyphs. In the letter 'A' is the upside
down picture of a bull; in 'B' a house; and so forth. To some
degree even the original sounds have been retained--and why not?
There has never been a need to improve on the alphabet once it
emerged from the chrysalis of hierogpyphics. The primordial function
of letters as abbreviated words, and hence sound radicals, is mostly
forgotten in our everyday usage. Yet, glimmers of the substrate of
written language color our choice of words, effect the connotational

network by which we labor from the urge to expression toward more-or-less satisfying communication.

But if the process were willfully reversed, if by sheer force of concentrated attention the whole history of western art could be reversed and made to avalanche backwards in headlong flight toward its most basic assumptions, what would such a superhuman effort resemble? In short, could there be a conceptual Cézanne, an artist forcing us to see--with the clarity of Chinese/Japanese calligraphy-- the quidity of our utterances written out shamelessly as billboards? (Other modern artists have used writing as part of the content of their work. The early Cubism of Picasso/Braque solicited the page as a virtual surface, precisely because the page possessed such special properties as a plane--it disintegrates when the letters are read: that first skill of childhood reading, focusing the eyes just above the inscription for symbol isolation. De Kooning also used letters to start works but, if initiated by writing, de Kooning's works did not maintain the integrity of the inscription. Torres-Garcia and many others could be cited in this way as well.) Only Seidel, with a stubborness as breathtaking as Morandi's and an obstinancy as fatal as DeStaël's made of letters, of utterances, a landscape he wandered, alone. Sometimes his statements were howled (Fig. 1) and lept up before us as the walls of glaciers. The sentences themselves are bits of wisdom, fragments, of which adult articulation are made; but here, solitary: "I Did Not Know" is a nightmare of guilt, of gone opportunity, of missed paths untraceable. The writing, whatever its literary worth as *subject matter*, is secondary to the works as drawings. Calligraphy, scale, use of material, composition-within-the-page, and all the other canonical virtues by which we judge an artwork a

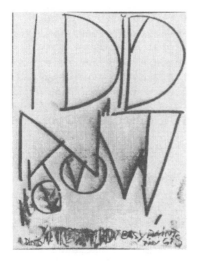

Fig. 1

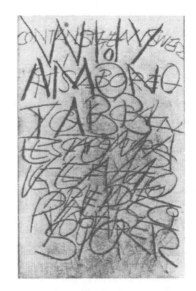

Fig. 2

success, all these operate upon us before we read Seidel's words. Becuase of this--whatever their diaristic component, their autobiographical or poetic effect upon us - -his drawings stand among the pantheon of occidental draftsmanship, distinguished for their purely linear accomplishments.

Another drawing (Fig. 2) densely packs the surface, choking off the work from the center to the edges. Penetration into the space behind the letters is halted; this is a "field composition" in which the field ceaselessly mumbles to us that it is composed of letters, of a human statement. This subject matter can be arranged more "classically" (Fig. 3), and tell us "Got the Bad Girl Treatment..." as news, incidentally reminding us that Ezra Pound called Art "news that stays news." *Montevideo Para Noja* (Fig. 4) loosens the field a bit more, but includes the complex pun on "paranoia." In that state of mind a network of assumptions is thought to reside behind the appearance of the world and to generate a causality parallel to the apparent, i.e., the rational, relationships between effects. In this drawing the letters mediate between shapes. A hazy field rests within the picture plane: blurred letters create a deep space aerially and implied sculptural volumes vie with the immaterial existence of 'words,' as breath. The very condition of paranoia is thus reified, but in a work of astonishing calligraphic beauty arising from the urgency, the willfulness and necessity of its creation.

Other works possess an aura of assimilated knowledge that bespeaks Seidel's exquisite grasp of art history. In one drawing (Fig. 5) J. M. W. Turner's swirling storms and centripetal compositions are recalled. Giacometti's portraiture--itself laden with the

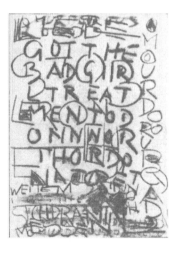

Fig. 3

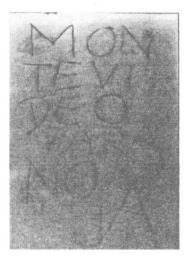

Fig. 4

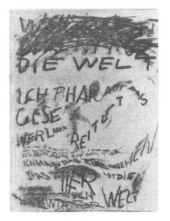

Fig. 5

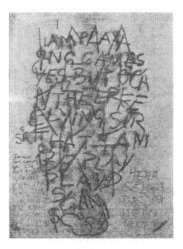

Fig. 6

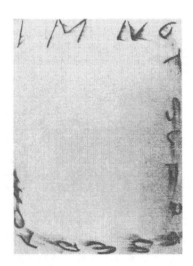

Fig. 7

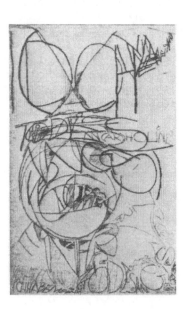

Fig. 8

incense of ancient culture--is suggested by another work (Fig. 6),
while Sam Francis' evacuation of the center of the composition is
employed, with a self-contained warning about the 'rules' of
composition in *I'm Not Supposed To* (Fig. 7). Seidel's clusters of
letters loom up before us, at times like fantastic formations of
clouds (Fig. 8), and we apprehend such works as being in indefinite
scale, both intimate and gigantic. In one drawing (Fig. 8), the
scale of the heaped up forms is such that we seem to be the Lilli-
putian *Monk* (By the Sea) whom Caspar David Friedrich painted, gazing
out for portents of the universal condition. Friedrich's world,
however charged, was mute. But Seidel's shreiks: Seidel's is a
truly psychotic world in which every branch, rivulet, rock, cloud and
breeze murmurs. No Romantic invitation to devine the common nature
of the world and man, Seidel's landscapes are composed of
letter-middens, great barrows, tumuli of implements--words.

Art historically Seidel is a challenge for he re-covers ground
covered by others, but examines assumptions left fallow by a previous
generation. He was dauntless and obsessive, and a marvelous artist.
Psychologically Seidel poses the enigma of a man of very real disorientation, genuine mental ill-health, who was not incapacitated by
his illness. Yet it would be macabre to suggest that his self-destructive madness--an illness that led to suicide--fostered his art,
although it did inform his subject matter and propel him to a wholly
uncompromising authenticity.

NOTE:

This essay was previously published in:
    Jochen Seidel "Word Drawings", Galerie Heike Curtze, Vienna &
                                    Düsseldorf, 1983

PICTORIAL ART AND THE MEDICAL THEME

Joseph Fusswerk-Fursay

13, boulevard des Batignolles - 75008 PARIS

The artist and the scientist are very often sharply contrasted one
with the other, and the average man gets the impression that art
and science are contradictory disciplines, to such an extent that
the rare artists who have carried out scientific research, such as
Leonardo da Vinci are considered to be two-headed geniuses, exceptional beings. Nevertheless all artistic as well as scientific
creative work has been imbued with its author's philosophy of man
and reflects the changing patterns of thought and customs then prevailing.

Psychiatry cannot remain indifferent to this eminently human occupation: art which above and beyond its efforts to represent the
world for us in an aesthetic fashion, is in itself an outstanding
form of expression of the human mind.

The oldest prehistoric drawing that we know of, is one depicting a
sorceror working his magic, and if this can be taken as symptomatic, equally the fact that medical themes are relatively rare in
artistic productions, including modern painting is no less so, and
this in spite of the fact that Psychiatry, has for decades been
trying to get a better understanding of the many questions studied
in the very wide firld of the relationships between art and psychopathology.

Although doctors, have for various reasons, studied some of the
most remarkable painters of the 19th and 20th centuries, and
although following the studies done by Prinzhorn, Morgenthaler,
and Minkowska, psychiatry has done research on the "world of Forms"
that is to say the relationship between mental illness and its sufferings, his struggles and their pictorial reflection, they have

developed the idea of the creative act as having a therapeutic role. Painters, on the other hand, have only accorded an insignificant place to the medical side of things when compared with the immense progress that medicine has made, and when compared with the importance that the doctor and the healing arts hold for us all during our lives. When then does painting which mirrors our everyday preoccupations and anxieties, reflect our aspirations and why do painters despise to so great an extent medical science, which is an ingredient of our everyday lives?

Far be it from me, in the course of this simple expose, to give a deep analysis of the many relationships that can be shown to exist between pictorial art and psychiatry. I would simply like to point out that there are extremely few paintings dealing with illness and its cure, and this is by no means accidental but springs from man's prevailing opinion of himself.

Charcot, to whom psychiatry owes so much, was one of the first to have studied the relationship between painting and medicine (and we find this sponsorship an encouragement in our research work), a study from which he thought there was much to be learned, and not one of minor importance; and so, in collaboration with Richer he published two works "The Diabolical in Art" in 1887, "The Deformed and the Sick in Art" in 1889. Charcot recounts how struck he was to find portrayed on a grotesque mask in the Church of Santa Maria Formosa in Venice, and clearly represented, all of the morbid facial distortions on which he had been lecturing his students in the Salpêtrière a few days previously, while showing them some remarkable specimen. Thus he could point out as he wrote that hysteria which up to recently has not been studied as a neurosis is nevertheless a very ancient disease ... and to show the place that external symptons of hysterical neurosis took in paintings, at a time when it was considered not as an illness, but as a perversion of the soul, due to the power and influence of the devil.

By proclaiming loudly that this "Demonology" was a false science, since the patients suffering from "diabolical possesion" were in his opinion, showing characteristic signs of hysteria, Charcot replaced these explanations based on religioustheories alone, by conclusions drawn from scientific investigation, and more radically still, laicized the medical thinking of his day. He underscored how true to life many paintings were, while also reflecting as they did the religious beliefs of the artist (miraculous cures, diabolical possession,...) they at the same time faithfully reproduced the objective symptoms of the disease, and hence could be the subject of scientific study, and thus he inaugurated a kind of retrospective medicine, full of interest for its adepts. Thus he diagnosed, on the grotesque mask in Venice, the hysterial spasm portrayed, on it, which it is quite impossible to confuse with any other, such as a nerve spasm.

If Charcot expressed astonishment by implication at the rarity of paintings dealing with medical themes he had his own opinion of Taine, "The relationship applicable between Art and Science honors both one and the other". Almost a century later Leon Binet in collaboration with Charles Maillant, wondered at the decreasing number of contemporary paintings dealing with medical themes, in spite of the fact that never before had medicine made such great strides forward.

Let us now consider paintings and the medical theme before the close of the 19th century. Witnesses to the religious beliefs of their times, the painters up to 17th century, had always bracketed therapeutics and religion together. Raphaël, Poussin and Rübens always pictured healing as taking on a miraculous form, or as taking place on the steps of a Church or Temple, thus implicitly bringing out God's role in man's biological destiny.

In the 17th century, with the Flemish masters, the medical theme made its appearance in their works. Many of their paintings have it as their subject matter; we know that Brueghel spent long hours at the Gate of Brussels, observing there the epileptics and the sick. Also numerous other painters such as A. Brouwer, Gerard Dow, Franz Hals and Gabriel Metzer looked on medical subjects in a new light.

The 17th century was the decisive period and at this time painters reflected after their fashion the struggle between ideas based on religious faith, and the incipient efforts now being made to interpret reality by reason alone ane the experimental sciences a decisive century as we have said during which Rembrandt, this great master of the Chiaroscuro (about which psychiatry would have much to say), showed himself to be at one and the same time an observer along scientific lines, with his remarkable "anatomy lesson" while painting with equal conviction "The 100 guilders", a work in which he represents Christ curing the sick and the little children, and thus picturing for us a scene, details of which we do not find in any of the Gospels.

Elie Faure, like many other commentators on the History of Art, like H. Focillon and R. Hamann, cannot help thinking that this evolution in pictorial themes has some connection with the ongoing scientific revolution, and that while Harvey was discovering the circulation of the blood, and Newton was studying the motions of the heavenly bodies, the painters felt like starting a veritable aesthetic revolutionary movement. And as Pastor Valery-Radot remarks, "Finally people realized that beauty could be found in other places besides Mount Olympus or the Christian firmament. Not alone the ill, the degenerate and the mad but also corpses and more generally all the aspects of the medical and surgical world could be shown by the artist to have beauty hidden in them."

During the 19th century, both medicine and painting took parallel paths in the sense that both took giant steps forward, became revolutionized even. Thus in the first quarter of the century, corresponding to the discoveries of Pasteur, to the theories of Lamark, the research done by Laennec and Esquirol, the painters of the Romantic period sought out subjects they could treat in a style both dramatic and tormented and became interested in medicine, hospital scenes, asylums, in epidemics which were decimating whole populations both in France and throughout the world. This fact (which seems praiseworthy to us) led the psychiatrist Georget to ask the great painter Gericault (1791-1824) to do some paintings of some of his most representative patients, and thus add to clinical observations.

Although during the second half of the 19th century, great medical events took place, with the discovery by Jackson of the anaesthetic properties of ether, the introductions of antiseptics into surgery by Semmelweiss, and with Claude Bernard publishing his "Introduction to experimental medicine", painting also progressed in a comparable fashion, with the springing up of the Realist School of painters, amongst whom were to be numbered painters such as Courbet, Millet, Manet, Degas.

At the close of the 19th century and on into the 20th century there were an abundance of schools of painting like Impressionism, neo-Impressionism, Pointillism, Divisionism, some of these movements were sometimes opposed to one another, but nevertheless they had one feature in common, namely their independance of their subject matter.

According to Leon Binet this change, confirmed by modern day paintings, reflected the beginning of the adoption of a new view of man's nature or rather of his place in the physical and intellectual scheme of things. He tries to show that the bonds between art and medicine in the 20th century are more intimate, deeper and more meaningful then ever before.

What the scientist is trying to bring out while rejecting scientifically unfounded theories about man and the world, the artist is expressing out of a visceral reaction with the consequent rehabilitation of all art forms - from naive art to art in the rough! Henceforth the artist does not tend to study the subject outside of himself, objectively, but rather will project himself outwards, and use his works as a means of self-study, to study his mental universe, and thus we can say that different painters project their pathological troubles onto their works of art.

For some this movement, in which the artist tries to express himself in a surrealist way, making the appearance of the things he paints dependent on his own subjectivity, is a corollary of the doubts raised by science in modern times. The law of relativity, wave mechanics, the general evolution of modern physics have as their counterparts as a matter of fact the birth of abstract painting, cubism, geometric paintings, together with surrealism, as if science and art in unison, each in its own fashion were throwing doubts on the validity of ideas inherited from far off times. In this respect the profusion of works done by Picasso bear witness to the great changes taking place in scientific thought. This theory is an interesting one, but seems to tie the progress of science up too much with the movements in the schools of painting. The theory of relativity, wave mechanics, and the discovery of DNA, or the endorphines, even if they are fairly well known, still have not modified the mental universe of all and sundry.

Lastly, it would lead mainly to only wanting to consider form, aesthetics, the plastic side, and to forgetting the setting of the work of art. René Huyghe denounced such restrictive rules of art appreciation and heavily underlined the fact that is as much a mode of self-expression as the solution to a plastic problem. We agree with Huyghe and André Malraux that the work of art is at one and the same time an artistic interpretation on canvas and also a reflection of the period during which the painter lived, as well as of the ambient philosophy of man. Thus for the author of the "Metamorphosis of the Gods", the change from the neo-Gothic to the Renaissance, from van Eyck to Botticelli is to be explained above all by a profound change in the philosophy of man, and Botticelli introduces a new kind of art where Venus appears as the rival of the Virgin, the nymph of the Angel, and the unreal of the Divine.

Of course if painters are witnesses to their times, it is generally held that in art theme is less important than form. But if there is no gainsaying this face, if it is true that the painter paints with his blood, and that theme is secondary, it remains nevertheless true that the latter reflects the artist's impression of his times, and what appears to him to be of exemplary value. And there is a striking contradiction between the importance man attaches to health and illness, to medical treatment and therapeutic effectiveness, and how little these things are reflected in art. If we had to judge nowadays the importance of medicine in our society from the number of works of art devoted to it, we would quickly become convinced of how insignificant a role it has.

For our part, we believe that this absence of theme so crucial to human life, pinpoints a phenomenon we have tried to analyze elsewhere in a more specifically psychiatric setting. In our age when science and psychiatry have apparently become so much a part of life, the human mind persists in entertaining irrational ideas without realizing it, and where the mind is concerned, cure is thought to have necessarily come, in every case, wholly or partially from phenomena outside the ordinary scope of nature, as well as rationally unintelligible phenomena. Truly, works of art force us to face up to this unpleasant fact but one that is still with us, that science is fighting a losing battle against the convictions of our patients.

In this never ending struggle between health and sickness with people taking the view that consulting the doctor is just one way of getting cured, along with others, like magical practices, or going to healers, simply because superstitious ideas still have a strong grip on the human mind. The progress of medicine has succeeded in changing people's mentalities, and making them recognize everyday cures as a biological phenomenon, and consequently as a possible subject of a work of art. Besides the mentality which admits the possibility for medical science to bring about a cure, there is another based on irrational notions which pictures health as coming from irrational methods of healing.

This incursion into a sphere which interests me a great deal, namely the one about people's beliefs, may seem foreign to this expose. Still I remain persuaded that as long as man has not come to realize his capacity to understand illness and believe it biologically curable, cures will continue to seem to belong to the non-medical field, and illness continue to be practically absent from works of art. Let us not make any mistake about this and certain films prove my point, that the public at large is more ready to believe in "diabolical possession" of certain patients, rather than admitting that they were suffering from hysteria, as the scientific analysis by Charcot of their cases makes clear.

THE BASIC PRINCIPLES OF

DYNAMIC EXAMINATION OF DRAWING

Istváns Hardi

Pest County Council
Semmelweis Hospital,Psychiatric Center
1085 Budapest, Stáhly u.7

The research work of dynamic examination of drawing started in the 1950-eth. Is was an individual initiation and so it continued (Hárdi 1-7). Especially the developmental psychology of the children's drawing impressed the work. Meanwhile the author got acquainted with Machover's draw-a-man test and the Goodenough-test. The results didn't only converge with the traditions of the field but with Volmat's and Jakab's statements, with the observations of Marinow, Navratil, Bader and Navratil, Suchenwirth dealing with "drawing of a man", and with the recently published results of Kraft.

The dynamic examination of drawing is a serial comparative method of drawing of a man. Its basis is the consequent practical and theoretical follow-up of the serial-comparative principle of clinical and graphical changes, processes, dynamisms.

What are the basic principles of dynamic examination of drawing ?
1/ The formal changes of the drawing.
2/ The temporal aspects of the drawing.
3/ The personality levels.
4/ The observations of contents.

1/ The formal changes in drawing can be followed

e.g. at therapies with psychotropic drugs. As the result
of the favourable therapeutic effect the quality of line
gets better, the drawings become more perfect, esthetic,
harmonic, rich.(When the patient is getting worse all
these take the opposite direction, Hárdi 1-3.)

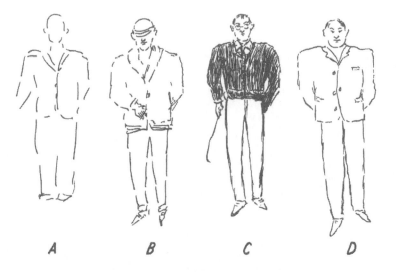

Fig.1. A 40-year-old schizophrenic man had been staying
in bed for years secluded from the world. He was taken
care by his widow mother. He was hospitalised after an
examination. After the hospital treatment we began a
combined psychotropic cure at the inhibited, withdrawn
patient. His first drawing /A/-coming back to our Out-
patient Clinic -drawn with dotted lines is a figure
with an empty face, his limbs are deficient. He got better as the result of the cure. This goes to show on his
drawing /B/ the figure is richer in details, though he
covers the face with the edge of his cap. Later he draws
a more plastic - informal figure though wearing glasses
/C/ with more coherent lines as the result of further
therapy. His last drawing /D/ - a walking figure, with
his hands behind him, his expressive face reflecting vitality - shows the period of rehabilitation (he works 4
hours daily). The patient feels today still good, he works.

        2/ The serials of drawing give a temporal informa-
tion as well. Most of the people make a drawing of a certain style on a certain level. The average man inclines

to draw a simply learned pattern. Some of them make a
cliché-like drawing with a little change. This pattern
bursts in acute psychoses or in intense emotional shocks,
e.g. at a schizophrenic exacerbation, and something new,
mostly a more primitive one is produced. If a drawing,
especially in acute state differs essentially from others, we can compare so to say <u>confront</u> them (Hárdi 4).
This comparison gives useful conclusions e.g. of the
cases of acute alcoholic intoxications, acute schizophrenia etc.

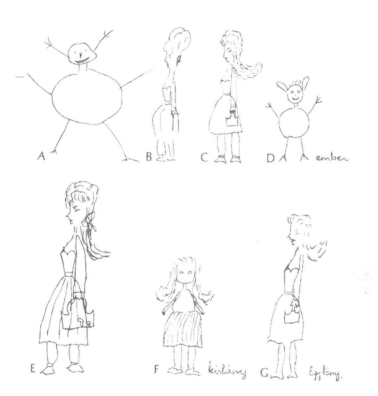

Fig.2. P.J. - a 20 year-old woman with schizoaffective
psychoses had been staying in hospital for 3 month with
her newborn baby as it had a pylorus stenosis. When the
problem was solved and they left the hospital, she got
ill: she couldn't eat, spoke incohaerently, could have
run. Her parents have died recently, they committed suicide. She had been suffering from suicide thoughts, she

couldn't sleep. She was hospitalised because of uncertain psychogenic depressive complaints drawing a primitive laughing, clinging figure with opened, clinging arms and spread legs. There are some lines coming out of the head paralel with the arms instead of the ears /A/. Returning from the hospital she is "too calm", "she can't be glad of anything" /B/. She draws a more differentiated woman with the arms straight at her body. She was also given antidepressants to the previous psychotropic cure. Some years later paranoid delusions, experiences of depersonalisation are observed beside the depressive complaints. Her drawing /C/ is a differentiated one having a conspicuous hair with a part of it in the air. An extreme perplexity occurs after repeated cures, she can't do anything especially take of her baby. She is afraid of everything and in this severe state there appear suicide intentions: she feels, she must die, this is her last day. Now - she is hospitalised again - she draws again a primitive figure /D/ similarly to the first one, the difference is only the hair, standing upwards and the enormous ears. Her later drawings of a balanced state are better than the previous ones, she draws a mature, differentiated woman-figure /E/. She gets a Valium-Lithium cure in her new anxious,perplexed period drawing a little girl with a queer, empty face and eyes, without a mouth /F/. Her last drawing after a repeated hospital treatment delineates a tilting girl, her skirt is opened underneath. It is similar to the previous ones though of a minimally weaker output /G/.

Besides acute states we can follow chronic ones too (Hárdi 4,7), e.g. personality changes at alcoholics, schizophrenics.

3/Through the temporal aspects we get to the question of regression. Considering it closer we arrived to the field of the personality - levels of adults (Hardi 7). The patients fullfill under their usual, developed personalitiy-levels at the dissolution of patterns or in acute states when the changing, mature individualised drawings regress. When the acute state is over, it returns on its own characteristic original level. On the basis of these I devided the adult personality-levels into six basic levels, similar to the childrens' /see Fig.3/.The simple level drawing realistically is d;

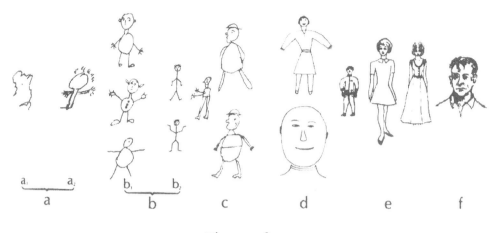

Figure 3

e means a higher level, a plastic way of designing, rich
in details, following reality flexibly; level f may express individual experiences, or may even artistic effect.
The primitive categories from a till c are similar to the
well-known child-scheme, head and leg or circle-line
scheme. Here we can distinguish the circle and line from
the stick-figure as a special scheme drawn by adults
(Hárdi and Saághy 6). A special change is level c, when
the cicle-scheme appears in double-lines. These observations were collected at 2.600 patients in serial examinations and this classification helped a lot at the various problems and changes in the expression of personality.

The formal categories and personality levels together allow a special quantitative evaluation. On a certain personality-level, in a balanced state, a characteristic achievement is observed. In better states it may
result in richer drawings, in worse states in poorer, incomplete ones, so to say it may lead to achievement-de-
crease. This also give a useful information about the condition of our patients.

4/Drawing a man - seems at first - not to give any
information about the content. In practice it is very important in positive and in negative respects as well. The
mimics, the posture, etc. can be regarded as adjacent to
expressive movements, but the action, the possible delin-

eation of the surroundings, the style of clothing, etc. can also be valued as positive content-elements. On the negative side there are insufficiency, neglect and impoverishment of the figures of lower levels. On the other hand the <u>omitted parts</u>, e.g. the mouth at alcoholics, the genitals at sexual conflicts, etc. as a result of the defence mechanisms.

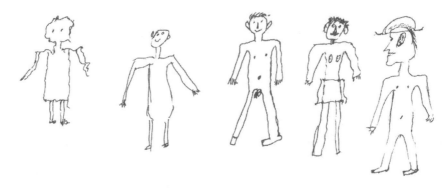

A   B   C   D

Fig.4. A 56-year-old diabetic and hypertoniac man was an alcoholic. He was very restless: he wanted to cut his leg, he threatened his wife with murdering her and he had a suicide intention as well. Sometimes he spoke incohaerently. At the first examination the strong tremor of the hands and the mental deterioration were remarkable. His state got worse in some days: he saw "more eyes", "a policeman", his tension, anxiety, depression increased and he was hospitalised in a delirous state. He drew an uncertain atactic, tremorous, deformed,"ragged" figure without a mouth /A/. After the hospital care he carried on relatively still with medicines drawing with quick lines a schematic figure smiling deformed /B/. It is interesting because of it's <u>opened underneath</u>. Meanwhile he persecuted his wife with jealousy.The patient interprets it, that he "wasn't enough good" to his wife because of his sexual potency troubles. He doesn't take his medicines, he drinks. Now he delineates a naked man with **genitals** /C/. The patient was drinking on and in his worse state he draws an uncertain woman-figure with a skirt and bosoms /D/. We succeeded in treating the isolated man diminishing the drinking, taking medicine regularly. He tries to do his best, he goes to work now. His last drawing reflects a relatively calm, self-controlled state /E/: it is a naked man wearing a transparent hat on his head, having a relatively big,detailed chin, big mouth - in profile. He adds, that he had omitted the genitals, though he wanted to draw a naked child.

The delineated four trends are the basis of evaluation and interpretation in the dynamic examination of drawing. We mustn't forget, that these <u>aren't static, descriptive categories but can be serially followed in alterations, changes: they are dynamisms, processes.</u>

REFERENCES

1. I. Hárdi: Elektroshock hatása a kézirásra.
Ideggyógyászati Szemle,Suppl.: 247 (1956).
2. "   "   : Psychologische Beobachtungen der Schrift
und Zeichnung nach vorangegangener Elektro-
schok-Therapie.
Arch.Psych.Neur.203:610 (1962)
3. "   "   : Dynamische Zeichnungsuntersuchungen im Laufe
von Behandlungen mit psychotropen Mitteln.
Arch.Psych.Neur.205:49 (1964).
4. "   "   : Confrontation in Dynamic Drawing Tests. In:
Jakab, I. ed."Art Interpretation and Art Therapy"
Karger, Basel (1969).
5. "   "   : Alcoholic Diseases in the light of dynamic
drawing tests. Psychiatria Fennica, 47.(1977).
6. "   "   : The problem of the stick-figure. In:Andreoli,V.
ed.:"The Pathology of Non-Verbal Communications".
Masson, Milano (1982).
7. "   "   : A dinamikus rajzvizsgálat. Medicina,Budapest
(1983).

NONVERBAL EXPRESSION AND CONGENITAL APHASIA

Irene Jakab

Univeristy of Pittsburgh, School of Medicine

3811 O'Hara St., Pittsburgh, PA 15213 USA

The review of the literature reveals that the classical early publications on aphasias deal essentially with problems of localization. They rarely mention the gesture communication of the aphasic as a diagnostic criteria of their language disturbance. The correlations of language function and the brain are still of interest to researchers (Segalowitz, 1983). Detailed studies deal also with the neural models of language processes (Arbib et al, 1973). The role of the right hemisphere in language disorders is studied by Millar and Whitaker,(1983);Netley and Rovet,(1983);Dennis and Whitaker,(1977);and Gazzaniga,(1970). Naeser et al,(1982),and Damasio et al,(1982),deal with atypical aphasic processes due to subcortical lesions. An analysis of the correlation of the neuropathological substratum and the clinical symptoms of transcortical aphasia is given by Környey, (1975).

Lately several papers correlate the aphasic verbal language deficit with the deficits of nonverbal expression in spontaneous gestures and pantomime (Kadish, 1978; Feyereisen and Seron, 1982; Daniloff et al, 1982; Duffy and Duffy, 1981; Varney and Benton, 1982; Snyder, 1978; Varney, 1978). While other authors relate sign language proficiency to aphasias (Metellus et al, 1981; Peterson and Kirshner, 1981; Moody, 1982; Meckler et al, 1979; Guilford et al, 1982), the aphasia cases in which the lesion has been in the dominant hemisphere, and extended to the parietal lobe and angular gyrus, show the most extensive disturbance of the gesture language (Chiarello et al, 1982). In subcortical Broca type aphasia, with intact internal speech, the nonverbal expression of gesture, writing and drawing may remain intact. Cicone et al, (1979), found that Broca aphasics equaled, or surpassed, the normal controls in the clarity of their gesture communication, which has parallelled their speech

1029

output. The studies of graphic expression of aphasic patients have been restricted essentially to the study of writing and less frequently to the study of their drawings.

The early childhood communication disorders are described in a developmental context of brain-language function (Rapin and Allen, 1982; Dennis, 1982; Kirk, 1982), and the term Developmental dysphasia, used by Wyke,(1979),does cover also the congenital aphasias.

In early childhood, the communication disorder is a common symptom of several psychiatric disorders. In these cases the proficiency in nonverbal communication is one of the most reliable differential diagnostic signs. This applies not only to spontaneous gestures and pantomime, but also to the drawings of nonverbal children. Of the 105 mentally retarded-emotionally disturbed children (3-12 years old), treated 1975 to 1981 at the John Merck Program (Dept. of Psychiatry, University of Pittsburgh) 43 were nonverbal. Their graphic expressions corresponded generally to their mental age, especially on the "Draw a person" test. However those patients who exhibited autistic features showed pathological distortions and discrepancies in the level of maturity within the details of any given drawing.

The children diagnosed as aphasics, in addition to the global mental retardation, exhibited a higher level of performance in their drawings than their overall mental age level and specifically in contrast with their failure on subtests requiring to produce verbal speech. Slides presented at the Congress are not reproduced here due to restricted space in this publication.

The following case will illustrate the complexity of the diagnosis and the need for multimodality treatment in congenital aphasia. This case of a mentally retarded child suffering from congenital aphasia and severe, secondary, emotional-behavioral disturbance is published more extensively by Jakab (1982, pages 93-95).

Peter is a 10 year old Caucasian boy. Before admission, at the age of 9.5, Peter obtained an MA of 1:9 (IQ 25) on the Bayley Scales of Infant Development. At admission, the clinical neurological evaluation revealed several minor anomalies: metatarsus varus; height in the 20th percentile; Peter's teeth were discolored and ground down by bruxism. He had no gag reflex. Muscle hypotonia and hyperreflexia were also found. Psychiatric evaluation showed withdrawal, anxiety, negativism, almost continuous screaming in extremely shrill, high-pitched voice; self-abuse and aggression and total lack of verbal or gestural communication.

Peter suffered from expressive, Broca aphasia, with essentially intact internal speech and adequate receptive language. His screaming and most other symptoms developed secondary to the frustration of being unable to communicate.

A dramatic turning point in the differential diagnosis came about when Peter wrote spontaneously a word on the blackboard, as an answer to the teacher's question, addressed to another child. After this episode intensive educational efforts were instituted in order to teach Peter to communicate through reading and writing. Furthermore, a behavioral therapy program has decreased his screaming and made him more accessible to a multimodality treatment, which included speech therapy and sign language communication, physical therapy and art therapy. In art therapy Peter used finger painting, at first, and amidst colored streaks spontaneously wrote letters and numbers. Art therapy, as a nonverbal modality of expression, enhanced both Peter's willingness to communicate, and his concept formation, by drawing objects and naming them in writing with correct spelling. At the time of his discharge Peter achieved a MA of 3-4 years on the Stanford Binet L.M. and a social age of 6.0 years on the Vineland Scale.

DISCUSSION

The three major pathological conditions of early childhood which constitute differential diagnostic problems are the following: mental retardation, early infantile autism and congenital aphasia.

The question of differential diagnosis is most likely to be asked around the age of 3 years. (At this time even the late speaking normal child would have acquired both receptive and expressive verbal language). Hearing loss should be excluded.

In the mentally retarded child there is a global delay in the acquisition of verbal language or a ceiling at a low preverbal level, with prolonged babbling, perseveration and syntactic errors. The retarded child's delayed motor development and delayed intellectual functions are usually parallel to the language delay, although Mahoney et al,(1981),found that children with Down syndrome are more delayed in their rate of language acquisition than might be predicted from general indices of their level of intellectual functioning. These findings substantiate the need for the careful review of the psychological profile gained from evaluating the subtest performances on a given test in addition to establishing the overall mental age. The intelligence profile will document specific deficits as well as the strengths (assets) which should be utilized in the treatment design of aphasic retarded children (Jakab: 1982 pages 270-332; Reynolds, 1983). In the differential diagnostic evaluation we should take into consideration Eisenberg's (1957) concept of the interdependence of the basic pathology with the resulting reorganization of the personality in face of the functional deficit, as well as the influence of the environment.

In early infantile autism, the language delay shows an inconsistent pattern. There are discrepancies between the receptive and
expressive language proficiency. The examination may reveal a pattern of language disorder in which the receptive language appears
to be less developed than the expressive language: the child appears not to understand the words, which he occasionally uses correctly in spontaneous speech. At repeated testing it becomes evident, that it is a lack of being 'tuned-in,' or a refusal to listen
and follow instructions, rather than an inability to understand the
verbal instructions used in language testing. Autistic children
often reject the interaction with people and they use language
mostly to express their own needs and to communicate only on their
terms, while disregarding the demands of others. They may also use
idiosyncratic, distorted language, with well pronounced sounds (not
real words), but with specific "coded" meaning. The echolalic tendency (immediate or delayed variety) may show a more basic pathology
in communication.

The gesture language of the nonverbal retarded child is generally at the same level as his mental age, while the gesture
language of the autistic child, if he is willing to use gestures,
may show a more sophisticated level than his verbal production, although it may be bizarre. Similar discrepancy can be observed in
the graphic products of retarded children with autistic features,
especially in their drawings of human figures. For example head-leg
figures may score low on mental age scale, while they include details
which are only drawn at higher mental age, such as teeth, eyebrows
and hair. Frequently their human figure drawings are also distorted.

In congenital aphasia, specifically if this aphasia is not a
global one, (extending both to receptive and expressive language),
but rather a case in which the receptive language is essentially
intact and the expressive language is delayed, or nonfunctional, the
child would use spontaneously similar gestures and pantomime for
communication as a verbal child of the same age (Snyder, 1978).
This happens, however, only in the early stages at which time the
child still attempts to communicate. If the child's communication
efforts are met by lack of understanding, on the part of the adults
in his/her environment, he/she will give up the use of spontaneous
gestures and pantomime, and may develop behavioral problems due to
the frustration caused by the inability to communicate (Agranowitz
and McKeown, 1964; Jakab, 1972). Following this stage it is very
difficult to determine if the lack of communication is due to true
aphasia or if it is at least partially caused by emotional disturbance. It is well known that even among non-aphasic children of
immigrant families, severe emotional disturbance such as school
failure, depression, suicide, aggressive unsocialized behavior,
and substance abuse may develop, before they learn the language of
their new home country. Some of their deficiencies in adaptation
may become permanent (Cantwell et al, 1980; Laxenaire et al, 1982;

Skhiri et al, 1982; Moussaoui and Sayeh, 1982; Marcos, 1982). A very detailed history (if it can be elicited from the parents) about the child's early communication skills, at the time of language development, between age 1 and 3, could help to clarify the diagnosis. Children with congenital aphasia and additional broader language pathology may have difficulties in understanding gesture language and imitating it. Lesions of the parietal lobe and angular gyrus causing asymbolia prevent the understanding of the written word and of the sign language.

The evaluation of the total communication potential of a very young child is hindered by the time lag of the sequences of the normal early developmental stages (Rapin and Allen, 1982). It is at age 6-7 years of normal maturity that the child, is ready to understand written symbols, such as letters and numbers, and their meaning in various combinations of forming the words or multidigit numbers. If an aphasic child has reached a mental age of 6-7 years on testing on all other items except verbal language, he may be ready to learn written communication as a substitute for the expressive verbal language.

The most promising cases for rehabilitation (or habilitation in cases of congenital aphasia) are those in which the expressive language deficit is caused by subcortical lesion. These patients are unable to produce meaningful speech sounds, inspite of an intact Broca area. Based on the assumption of the plasticity of the young brain, the early global communication skill training with gesture language, pantomime and later reading-writing training may lead to the development of verbal communication skill. It is known that an important factor in recovery after brain damage, even in adults, is the plasticity of the brain (Finger and Stein, 1982). An example from the literature is the case of a quadriplegic boy with global aphasia, who was introduced to sign language at age 6 yrs. 9 months. Subsequently he was able to read, write, converse and produce imaginary stories (Fuller et al, 1983). In some cases of atypical caudate/putamen aphasias the correct diagnostic localization resulted in the successful use of 'melodic intonation therapy' (Albert et al, 1973; Sparks et al, 1974). In the rehabilitation of adults Glozman et al,(1980), have found that speech activity has increased by using drawings of objects. Art therapy with aphasic children can increase their vocabulary of concepts by representing action pictures. It can also help them express feelings through nonverbal media. Art therapy can be a useful tool in addition to early and vigorous communication skill training in preventing the secondary emotional disturbance due to the frustration of being unable to communicate.

CONCLUSIONS

Complete neuropsychological evaluation and the best possible localization of the lesion, may help designing the best intervention method for the habilitation of children suffering from congenital aphasia. The neuropsychological and anatomical diagnosis may also help in predicting the long range potential for rehabilitation.

In the treatment of congenital aphasias, or broader categories of developmental dysphasias, multidisciplinary diagnosis and intensive multimodality treatment is most useful, including nonverbal communication training through art therapy by using graphic expression as a tool for concept formation. Psychiatric treatment may be required in cases with secondary emotional disturbance caused by the inability to communicate.

It is suggested that training with total communication method be instituted with all children who are diagnosed as suffering from congenital aphasia, knowing well that some may have difficulties even with simple sign language, while others may acquire sign language rapidly and develop verbal expressive language and written language. They may acquire verbal language gradually, most likely by using untapped cortical reservoirs for developing specific language skills, based on the plasticity of the young brain.

It is strongly recommended to attempt to teach reading and writing to nonverbal, retarded, children whose mental age has reached the 6- to 7-year level, on test items other than the spoken language.

Through correct differential diagnosis and therapeutic trial, the practitioner may save a retarded aphasic youngster from a life-long frustration due to the inability to communicate.

References

Agranowitz, A., and McKeown, W.R., 1964, "Aphasia Handbook," Thomas, Springfield, Illinois.
Arbib, M.A., Caplan, C., and Marshall, J.C., 1982, "Neural Models of Language Processes," Academic Press, Inc., New York, N.Y.
Cantwell, D.P., Baker, L., and Mattison, R.E., 1980, Psychiatric disorders in children with speech and language retardation, Arch. Gen. Psychiatry 37:423-426.
Chiarello, O., Knight, R., and Mandel, M., 1982, A Left Parietal Infarct in a Prelingually Deaf Person Resulted in an Aphasia for Both American Sign Language (ASL) and Written and Finger-Spelled English, Brain 105(Pt.1):29-51.

Cicone, M., Wapner, W., Foldi, N., Zurif, E., and Gardner, H.,
    1979, The Relation Between Gesture and Language in Aphasic
    Communication, Brain & Language 8(30):324-349.
Damasio, A.R., Damasio, H., Rizzo, M., Varney, N., and Gersh, F.,
    1982, Aphasia with Nonhemorrhagic Lesions in the Basal Ganglia
    and Internal Capsule, Arch. Neurol. 39:15-20.
Daniloff, J.F., Noii, J.D., Fistoe, M., and Lloyd, L.L., 1982,
    Gesture Recognition in Patients with Aphasia, J. Speech-Hear.-
    Disorder 47(10)43-49.
Dennis, M., and Whitaker, H.A., 1977, Hemispheric Equipotentiality
    and Language Acquisition, in: "Language Development and
    Neurological Theory," S. Segalowitz and F.A. Gruber, eds.,
    Academic Press, Inc., New York, N.Y.
Dennis, M., 1982, The Developmentally Dyslexic Brain and the
    Written Language Skills of Children with One Hemisphere, in:
    "Neuropsychology of Language, Reading and Spelling," U. Kirk,
    ed., Academic Press, Inc., New York, N.Y.
Duffy, R.J., and Duffy, J.R., 1981, Three Studies of Deficits in
    Pantomimic Expression and Pantomimic Recognition in Aphasia,
    J. Speech-Hear. Res. 24(1):70-84.
Eisenberg, L., 1957, Psychiatric Implications of Brain Damage in
    Children, Psychiatric Quarterly 31:72-97.
Feyereisen, P., and Seron, X., 1982, Nonverbal Communication and
    Aphasia: A Review. II. Expression, Brain & Language 16(2):
    213-236.
Finger, S., and Stein, D.G., 1982, "Brain Damage and Recovery,"
    Academic Press, Inc., New York, N.Y.
Fuller, P., Newcombe, F., and Ounsted, C., 1983, Late Language
    Development in a Child Unable to Recognize or Produce Speech
    Sounds, Arch. Neurol. 40(3):165-168.
Gazzaniga, M.S., 1970, "Le cerveau dédoublé," Bruxelles-Dessart et
    Mardaga, eds., in: Une observation d'aphasie chez une illettrée
    (analphabète) Réflexions critiques sur les fonctions cérébrales
    concourant au langage, J. Mettelus, H.P. Cathala, Mme. Aubrey-
    Issartier, and A. Bodak, Annales Médico-Psychologiques 139(9):
    992-1001.
Glozman, J.M., Kalita, N.G., Tsyganok, A.A., 1980, On One System
    of Methods of Aphasics Group Rehabilitation, Int. J. Rehabilit.
    Res. 3(4)519-526.
Guilford, A.M., Scheuerie, J., and Shirek, P.G., 1982, Manual Com-
    munication Skills in Aphasia, Arch. Phys. Med. Rehabil. 63(12):
    601-604.
Jakab, I., 1972, The Patient, The Mother, The Therapist: An Inter-
    actional Triangle in the Treatment of the Autistic Child,
    J. of Communication Disorders 5:154-182.

Jakab, I., 1982, Diagnosis and Differential Diagnosis of Mental
    Retardation, in: "Mental Retardation," I. Jakab, ed.,
    S. Karger, Basel/New York.
Jakab, I., 1982, Psychiatric Disorders in Mental Retardation, in:
    "Mental Retardation," I. Jakab, ed., S. Karger, Basel, New
    York.
Kadish, J., 1978, A Neuropsychological Approach to the Study of
    Gesture and Pantomime in Aphasia, S. Afr. J. Comm. Disorders
    24:102-117.
Kirk, U., 1982, Introduction: Toward an Understanding of the
    Neuropsychology of Language, Reading, and Spelling, in:
    "Neuropsychology of Language, Reading and Spelling," U. Kirk,
    ed., Academic Press, Inc., New York, N.Y.
Környey, E., 1975, Aphasie Transcorticale et Écholalie: Le Problème
    de L'Initiative de la Parole, Rev. Neurol. 131.(5): 347-363.
Laxenaire, M., Ganne-Devonec, M.O., and Streiff, O., 1982, Les
    problèmes d'identité chez les enfants des migrants, Annales
    Médico-Psychologiques 40(6):602-606.
Mahoney, G., Glover, A., and Finger, I., 1981, Relationship between
    Language and Sensorimotor Development of Down Syndrome and
    Nonretarded Children, American Journal of Mental Deficiency
    86(1):21-27.
Marcos, L.R., 1982, Adults' Recollection of Their Language Depri-
    vation as Immigrant Children, Am. J. Psychiatry 139(5):607-610.
Meckler, R.J., Mack, J.I., and Bennett, R., 1979, Sign Language
    Aphasia in a Non-Deaf-Mute, Neurology (Minneap.) 29(7):1037-40.
Metellus, J., Cathala, H.P., Aubrey-Issartier, Mme., Bodak, A.,
    1981, Une observation d'aphasie chez une illettrée (analphabète)
    Réflexions critiques sur les fonctions cérébrales concourant
    au langage, Annales Médico-Psychologiques 139(9):992-1001.
Millar, J.M., and Whitaker, H.A., 1983, The Right Hemisphere's
    Contribution to Language: A Review of the Evidence from Brain-
    Damaged Subjects, in: "Language Functions and Brain Organiza-
    tion," S. Segalowitz, ed., Academic Press, Inc., New York, N.Y.
Moody, E.J., 1982, Sign Language Acquisition by a Global Aphasic,
    J. Nerv. Ment. Dis. 170(2)113-116.
Moussaoui, D., and Sayeh, H., 1982, Les enfants de migrants ou
    l'impossible identité, Annales Médico-Psychologiques 149(6):
    588-592.
Naeser, M.A., Alexander, M.P., Helm-Estabrooks. N., Levine, H.L.,
    Laughlin, S.A., and Geschwind, N., 1982, Aphasia with Predomi-
    nantly Subcortical Lesion Sites, Arch. Neurol. 39:2-14.
Netley, C., and Rovet, J., 1983, Relationships among Brain Organi-
    zation, Maturation Rate, and the Development of Verbal and
    Nonverbal Ability, in: "Language Functions and Brain Organi-
    zation," S. Segalowitz, ed., Academic Press, Inc., New York,
    N.Y.

Peterson, L.N., and Kirshner, H.S., 1981, Gestural Impairment and Gestural Ability in Aphasia: A Review, Brain & Language 14(2): 333-348.

Rapin, I. and Allen, D.A., 1982, Developmental Language Disorders: Nosologic Considerations, in: "Neuropsychology of Language, Reading and Spelling," U. Kirk, ed., Academic Press, Inc., New York, N.Y.

Reynolds, C.R., 1983, Strength Models of Remediation in Neuropsychology and the Process of Ipsative Score Interpretation, Child Neurology 2(2):9-10.

Segalowitz, S., ed., 1983, "Language Functions and Brain Organization," Academic Press, Inc., New York, N.Y.

Skhiri, M.D., Annabi, M.D., and Allani, M.D., 1982, Enfants d'immigrés: facteurs de liens ou de rupture? Annales Médico-Psychologiques 40(6):597-602.

Snyder, L.S., 1978, Communicative and cognitive abilities and disabilities in the sensorimotor period, Merrill-Palmer Quarterly 24:161-180.

Sparks, R.W., Helm, N.A., and Albert, M.L., 1974, Aphasia rehabilitation resulting from melodic intonation therapy, Cortex 10: 303-316.

Varney, N.R., 1978, Linguistic Correlates of Pantomimes Recognition in Aphasic Patterns, Journal of Neurology, Neurosurgery & Psychiatry 41(6):564-568.

Varney, N.R., and Benton, A.L., 1982, Qualitative Aspects of Pantomime Recognition Defect in Aphasia, Brain & Cognition 1(1): 132-139.

Wyke, M.A., 1979, "Developmental Dysphasia," Academic Press, Inc., New York, N.Y.

SELF-HEALING TENDENCIES, ART AND THERAPY

Wolfgang K. Mueller-Thalheim

Rehabilitation Center BBRZ Linz
A-4600 Wels, Gross-Str. 8
Austria

Artistic actions as a therapeutical means have a long history, reaching back to times of the Holy Bible. Therefore it would be worth it to investigate, how the term art-therapy was established in the last years.

The term "art" is as difficult to define as the term "therapy". Both seem to be ambivalent, either in consideration of an ideal expectation, or even in doubtful distrust. Just at this moment even methods of psychotherapy have been inflated and depreciated, and "art" has a suspicious touch for many people. Now both terms are combined for a new one. This may be an unconscious demounting of the ideal model "art" (A.Reiter, 1981). From this corner too some aggression rises against the "art of the insane", which should not be estimated as an artistic achievement. But here we do not need justify the high esthetic value of some of these works.

Art and creativity deserve to get to the point of view, as symbols as well as criterion of the original abilities for development of personality and culture. What will be created and how it will be done, that decides about the estimation of the work. Of course, it shows a weak point of this art-therapy: it can grow up to work-centric tendencies, instead of client-centrics, as it would be its task by medical responsibility.

The self-demonstration of abilities, the expression of inner tensions, just so the impulse for movement and determined meaningful motion, taking aim at a certain result, these are the pure motivations and drives, efficient in art-

1039

therapy. It activates initiative, courage and joy in creativity. At the psychotic patient it is the healthy part of the personality, which gets stimulated.

If therapeutical aims should be reached, the creative process moves mainly in a pre-logical level. The symbolism of forms and colour has archaic roots and avades largely the hermeneutical grasp. Especially this explaining of symbols is not seldom tried, in each case with the risk of loss of the efficiency. Today we know that the way of realisation and interpretation has become less efficient, according to the worldwide knowledge of popular psychoanalytical facts.

What Reiter calls the "symbol-optimismus" is no more than a satisfied explanation of pictural fragments from deeper layers. They hardly are actualized any more, but gathered, collected, in naive hope of a broad result of this kind of art-therapy.

Now we are coming to the central question, to which extent the creative process, respectively the artistic expression does get a therapeutical quality ? The depth-psychological theory may be presumed as wellknown. We are interested if and how the creative process distinguishes between healthy and sick people. Supposing, that the dynamics are the same, as Bader and Navratil and others described it, then we can a priori neglect a precise psychiatric diagnosis at art-therapy. It can be applied in neuroses, psychoses and even organic cerebral diseases, as far as the general requirements are given.

The healthy artist lives aware, eager to produce, and ready to controlled regression too, in order to reach the creative base. He works out of an inner impulsion, whom he does not know for the most part. He is overcome, "statebound" (Navratil, 1975), even he had to seek and experiment for a long time to find his personal way and style. His life is not very different in its outward appearance from the others. Nearby see however we find rather in any case very strong tensions, which form his live events extraordinary and often tragically. Psychobiographics speak volumes about that.

The artist makes use of his production not only to earn his living, but particularly to maintain his psychic balance. The self-concept regulating function ("selbstwertregulierende Funktion") of artistic work has been described by Kohut 1966, and the self-healing tendencies by Müller-Thalheim 1975. One should not be reluctant to regard those self-defensive and self-healing mechanisms in a greater scope of natural science, as an achievement of human nature. Without this neither a wound can be cured, nor the work of mourning can be done, nor a psychosis gives way. If we finally do not know exactly how its dynamic, we should keep a watchful eye upon it, when therapeutical methods are to be examined. Errors can thus be avoided and also the hubris of thinking: "It's me, who has cured, with my methode !"

The artistic act grows out of the dissociation of high tensed patterns as the ideatoric component, and the psycho-motoric impulse of creation. Navratil, 1965, mentions a dis-integration of the compulsively emotional and the rational as the starting point of all creativity. There exists a "height of fall" in production: the mill runs as long as there will be water enough. This hypothesis may explain the character-istical ecstasy-like periods of work, which we know from many artists, just so from Aloyse (Bader, 1961), Hauser (Navratil, 1978), Schröder-Sonnenstern (Gorsen, 1969), Reischenböck(Mül-ler-Thalheim, 1972).

If we take ubiquitous "basic schizomorphic structures " for granted as a tension factor of creativity (Müller-Thal-heim, 1968), creative achievement could be encouraged and observed in every psychotic but also in neurotic cases. Following Navratil we regard this disposition as the precondi-tion of artistic work at sound and sick. It may be gradual-ly marked, but nevertheless efficient, whatever psychical diseases are present.

The schizomorphic structures are available as well as an artist consciously intends to step down to the sources, or a psychotic patient cannot avoid that.

Thus, self-healing tendencies act as a mere stabilisation and protection against losing reality. The patient is strug-gling to find a modality of expression, just so the artist is striving to achieve integration. The creative abilities of the individual provide a fascinating object for study. Not only the works of symbolical expression, created by the indi-vidual, but also apparently trivial psychiatric symptoms such as delusions and hallucinations do in no way lack originality and aim. Delusion may functionate as a defense and an imagi-native interpretation of a pathological situation, from the side of the patient. This reveals a certain teleological char-acter.

The confines of art-therapy and its limited influence on the course of a disease are avowedly well-known. The authen-tic clinical successes of art-therapy are more or less modest. Otherwise the artists know the way of stabilisation and self-confidence by symbolisation. Already the little child makes

himself symbols, small objects with features of idols, star-
ring at it, snuggling up to it, for abreaction, so far as
the child will not be inhibited by the presence of ready made
toy. It seems to be that the creative, whose essential factor is the playful, exists in human being as a constitutional
autoregulative function of self-defense.

Therefore the art-therapy, which supports these functions
would deserve a more important place, as it worldwide gets
conceded. Let us ask, why art-therapy does not succeed to a
greater extent.

The artistic production always is a delivery outward, in
relation with self-esteem, self-confidence, with symbolic accomplishment of desires, last not least with narcissistic experience. Who produces, delivers himself to the labile value
judgement of the world around us. Non-success may intensify
the discord between personality and work, and increase the
danger of secundary neurotic reactions. Therefore art-thera-
pie should never be executed without accompanying psychotherapy.

My own experience with long-term patients over nearly
three decades exemplifies that. This type of therapy was recommended to me by R.Volmat, when I visited him and his
"painters rooms" in Paris, 1956.

Meanwhile we learned, that lasting success and the necessary consent of the patients, their relatives and the medical colleagues can only be earned if the main accent is laid
on the state of health and on the course of the disease and
not on the production of pictures as interesting as possible.

Another source of fallacy may be the upgrading of products of the art-therapy by ideological concepts. If the artist is mentally sick, perhaps even hospitalized, his oeuvre can
be praised more than its artistic value. In spite of the real
often admirable accomplishment, these things will be mixed,
which better would be separated. It should be the fatal inclination of the society on the one hand, to pretend its tolerance, on the other hand to self-defend reckless against a
lot of anxieties, as it is fear of illness, decline and death,
fear of uncalculable, of the numinous.

By reason of those hitherto hardly discussed considerations it is necessary to ask, whether art-therapy has developed encouragingly. We believe, that much is going on. A permanent critical considering is indicated, to avoid that this
precious therapeutical method stagnates in self-complacency.

Reference

Bader, A., 1961, "Insania pingens"   DuMont,   Köln

Bader, A., and Navratil, L., "Zwischen Wahn und Wirklichkeit"
      Bucher,   Luzern / Frankfurt a.M. (1976).

Gorsen, P., Das Schizophrene als Kunst. Der Fall Friedrich
      Schröder-Sonnenstern,   in "Das Bildnis Pygmalions",
      Rowohlt,   Reinbek bei Hamburg. (1969).

Kohut, H., 1966, Formen und Umformungen des Narzissmus,   in
      Psyche,   20:513

Müller-Thalheim, W., 1968, Die bildende Kunst und der Begriff
      des Abnormen,   Österreich.Ärztezeitung, 23:1430.

Müller-Thalheim, W., 1972, Sexus und Religion,   Confin.psychi-
      at., 15:91.

Müller-Thalheim, W., 1975, Selfhealing Tendencies and Crea-
      tivity, in "Transcultural Aspects of Psychiatric Art",
      I.Jakab, ed.   Karger, Basel.

Navratil, L., 1965, "Schizophrenie und Kunst",   dtv, München.

Navratil, L., 1975, "Der Himmel Eleno. Zustandsgebundene Kunst"
      Kulturhaus,   Graz.

Navratil, L., 1978 "Johann Hauser. Kunst aus Manie und Depres-
      sion",   Rogner & Bernhard,   München.

Reiter, A.,   1983 Kunsttherapie - eine neue psychotherapeuti-
      sche Methode ?,   Kunst u.Therapie,   3:1.

Volmat, R.,   1956, "Expression plastique de la folie", M.C.F.
      Paris.

RELATION BETWEEN SPEECH, WRITING AND PAINTING

AT THE PSYCHIATRIC PATIENTS-PAINTERS

Drazen Neimarevic

Neuropsychiatric department
of the Medical Center
Karlovac-Yugoslavia

In this study we were investigating sixteen psychiatric patients from whose ten were treated in the Psychiatric Hospital Vrapce, two in the Psychiatric Clinic Rebro-Zagreb, two in the Psychiatric Department Medical Center Karlovac, one in the Psychiatric Hospital Rab and one in the General Hospital in Belgrade. By profession seven were academic painters (six were ill from schizophrenia and one from chronic alcoholism), two were self-educated painters (one ill from schizophrenia and the other from epilepsy, oligophreny and psychopathia), two were collaborators at Art Centers in Zagreb and in Berlin. The first was ill from chronic alcoholism and the second from schizophrenia. One was amateur-painter (psychosis epileptica), one finished the Art Academy (he is suffering from schizophrenia), and three were of other professions and began to paint spontaneously during their illness (schizophrenia, paranoia and depressive psychoneurosis.

Nine of previously mentioned patients died, five of them are still living but we don't have any data about two of them. Twelve of them are men and four are women. Marital status:eleven single, three married and of two of them we don't have any information. All the History records have been checked, we talked with eleven patients, the linguistic analysis of written text or poems have been made, and finally we analysed their paintings or plastic expressions.

We have been studying primarily the process of thinking from its formal aspect (excluding the delusions), then we scrutinized his oral product; furthermore we analysed syntaxis and its disturbances (excluding the context) and finally we studied the paintings in particular the plastic expressive mediums (line, colour simetry, proportion, rhytm and space).

This project was made by the collaboration of the Academy of Art Zagreb and by the Institute of Literature of the Yugoslav Academy of Science and Art, Zagreb.

The first patient was an academic painter-schizophrenia-paranoid. Her speech was permanently confused and later on, she became autistic. In her writing we saw the dissociation (the letter written just before her disease was from the linguistic aspect, entirely normal). The painting during the disease practically ceases but for some paintings (lockets) of changed thematic. Ductus in her paintings is completely normal.

Our second patient was a pianist-schizophrenia hallucinatoria. Her speech was completely coherent in spite of terrible auditive hallucinations from which she was suffering for over than 3o years. Written word like plastic expressions are also coherent. Yet the melancholy is dominating in her expressions. (Fig. 1).

The third case is an academic painter suffering from schizophrenia simplex. Ductus of his speech, at first slightly incoherent became gradually completely incoherent and lasted 37 years, while his writing was stereotype and infantile. His poems are without dissociation, with no literary quality. For example:
    "I created the master piece
    So this occasion
    That the painting immediately
    I could sell easy."
The painting is infantile academism, but quite coherent.

With the fourth case (signpainter-paranoia) the formal thinking was always preserved and his speech and the writing entirely coherent (but with plenty of paranoid delusions and the ideas of reference). The plastic expression is also preserved in the plastic expressive mediums (means) which are "petrified" and they are "showing" his abnormal ideas. (Fig. 2).

With the fifth case (academic painter-schizophrenia paranoid) the speech production with the illness is always incoherent (dissociated), but before death his ductus (stream of thought) was quite logical! The painting is at the highest artistic level especially the watercolourings as we can see on Fig. 3 from the year 1923. But on Fig. 4 which was painted much later during the disease, we see the darker colour as the reflection of his depression. At Fig. 5 we see his most famous painting representing the mountain Klek, without human beings. He painted the mere landscape in into which he himself escaped. The painting is always entirely coherent.

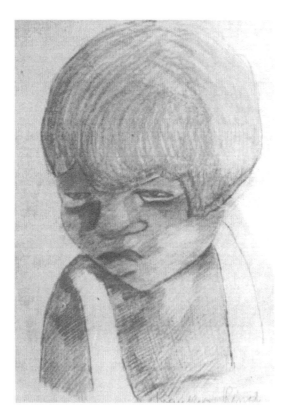

Fig. 1

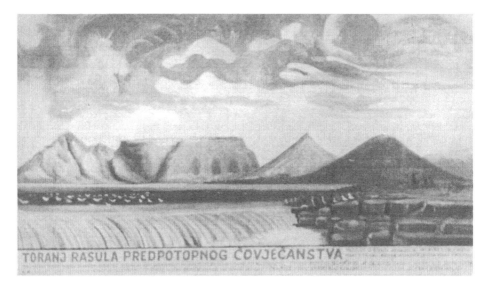

TORANJ RASULA PREDPOTOPNOG ČOVJEČANSTVA

Fig. 2

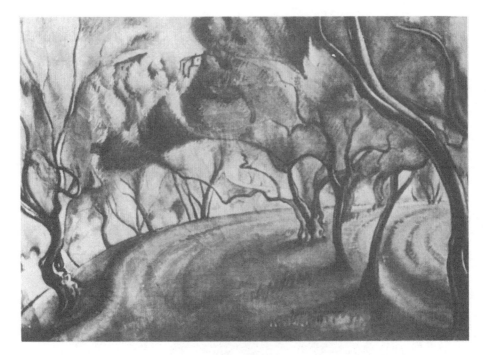

Fig. 3

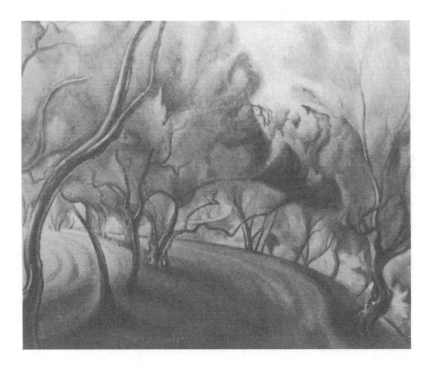

Fig. 4

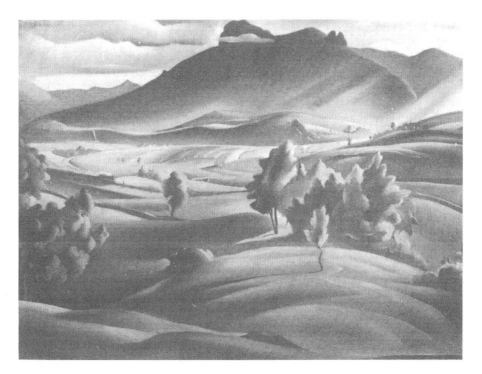

Fig. 5

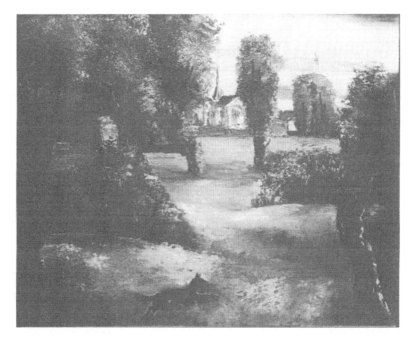

Fig. 6

With the next case (academic painter-schizophrenia paranoid) the illness began with ideas of persecution and with visual hallucinations. The painting (Fig. 6) from that period, he painted in Paris, represented the black dog which persecuted him (there are no human beings in the painting). The stream of thought was coherent during the illness except for a period of autism which lasted for 3 months.In the course of that time he neither spoke nor wrote, and didn't paint. (Fig. 7) is from the phase, when he was in the remission, and it has been painted quite coherently(like other paintings).

In our seventh case we studied a painter-collaborator of the painting atelier of Max Oppenheimer in Berlin who suffered from a catatonic form of schizophrenia. The stream of thought was incoherent during his whole disease. His writing was also dissociated. (Fig.8) he painted after the first year of his illness, but the next painting (Fig. 9) he made after 7 years from the beginning of his mental disease at the Psychiatric Hospital Vrapce, one year before his death. The painting is confused representing human bodies scattered all around in all directions. The figures of various dimensions are gathered in great number. The painting is entirely incoherent and the style is changed to surrealistic.

Further we have the example of the woman, an academic painter suffering from schizophrenia simplex with the constant normal stream of thoughts with the orderly association of writing and with the original coherent style (Fig.10). She is giving the diagrams of her subconsciousness with the curved lines.

The next patient has finished the Academy of Arts, suffered from schizophrenia inveterata. The thinking was coherent, but with the transition to the dissociation parallel to the writing. We present the part of one of his poems:
"The lunatic asylum is now the scene the place of dreaming,
where is the echo of my waving
like the flourished undersee source
in which the sun its hues interweaves."
The drawing is completely coherent, but entirely stereotype and without creativity.

The next is a self-educated painter ill from schizophrenia paranoid with the coherent till light faded away the stream of thoughts. The analogy to this is his writing, but the painting is completely coherent but schematic and without creative invention.

Further-on we present one self-educated painter, ill from epilepsy, oligophreny and sociopathia with the coherent oral, written and plastic speech. (Fig. 11) represents the author himself embracing vigorously Psychiatric Hospital Vrapce in which he was treated four times.

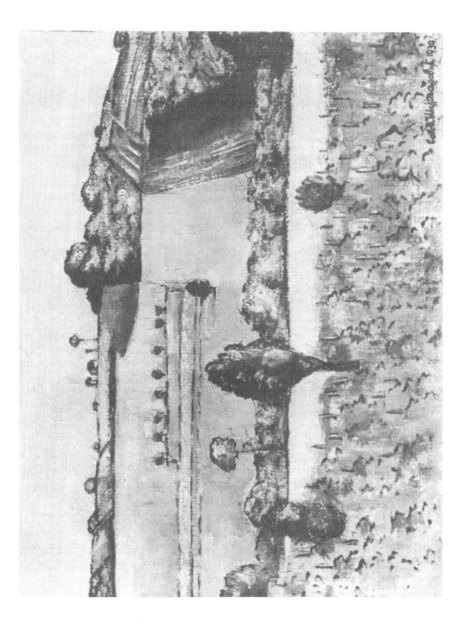

1051

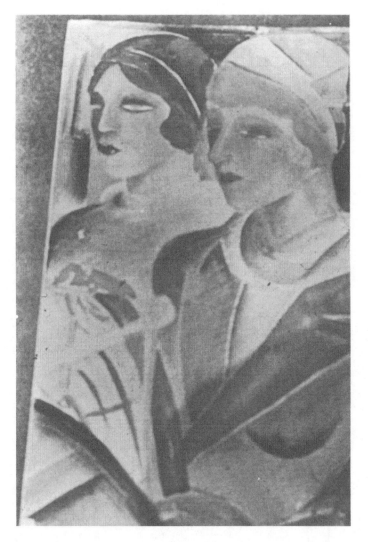

Fig. 8

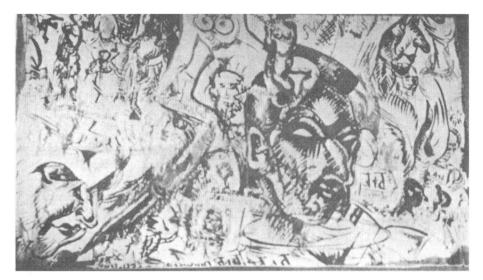

Fig. 9

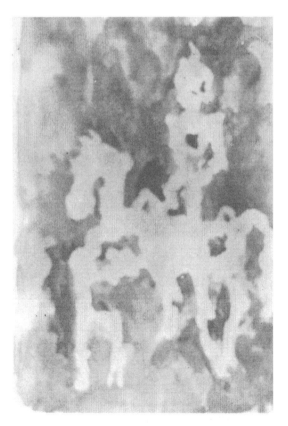

Fig. 10

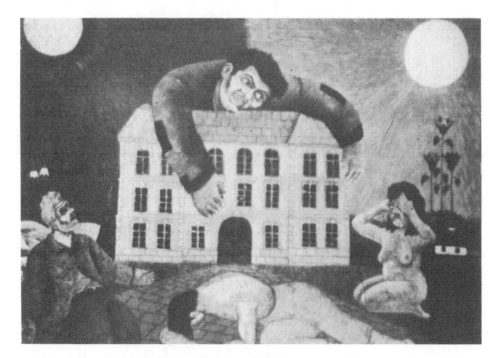

Fig. 11

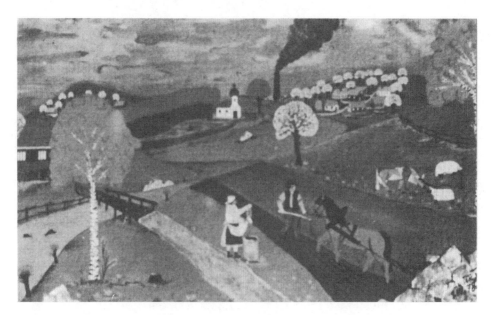

Fig. 12

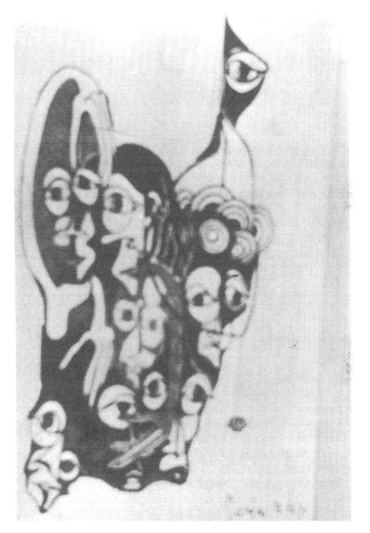

Fig. 13

The twelfth case is an academic painter who sufferes from chronic schizophrenia. His oral and written stream is dissociated as we can see in one of his poems:
    "that come these these known
    who make time horses,
    the painting is the excitement of the soul
    haloa wise there is no bread."
We cannot stop his schematical painting of female silhouettes.

The thirteenth case is the   amateur-painter who at first suffered from epilepsy with grand mal attacks, afterwards from epileptic psychosis with incoherent stream of speech and in the written composition, while the stream in the poems is less dissociated but becomes faded away. The painting is incredibly concentrated namely coherent in the colour nuance arranging creating special loveliness (Fig. 12). He died in the epileptic status.

The next is one woman patient treated under diagnosis depressive psychoneurosis who began to paint spontaneously at the hospital. Her speech and her poems are well linked and expressed in the miniature lyric form. The plastic works are manneristic in one exaggerative style. Her depression created dead figures like on (Fig. 13), but still in the coherent stream.

The fifteenth case was the collaborator of one of the painting ateliers, treated due to alcoholism and psychopatia. His stream of thoughts is quite normal and is reflecting in his speech a strange hallucinatory poetical prose, which is in the boundaries of literaty boldness. He paints coherently empty constructions and his "painting" is far from being art.

The last case is the academic painter- alcoholic whose stream is coherent in speech, writing and in painting.

THE CONCLUSION:
    It was found that there was accordance between the course of speech and writing, but there is no such accordance in certain cases between the stream of thoughts and the painting or artistic expression. Accordingly the thoughts may be incoherent, but the pictorial expression can be coherent.

SYMBOLIC EXPRESSION AS MESSAGES AND THEIR THERAPEUTIC SIGNIFICANCE

Y. Tokuda

Neuropsychiatric Research Institute
91, Benten-cho, Shinjuku-ku
Tokyo, 162, Japan

I. INTRODUCTION

The phenomena encompassed in the phrase "Symbolic Expression as Messages" are related to fields such as philology, information theory and symbolic theory, on which there has already been a great deal of research.

My objective here is to touch on the symbolic content and therapeutic significance to be found in cases that are familiar to us in the therapeutic processes of Art Therapy, where the client entrusts his inner images in symbolic expressions and goes through an auto-therapeutic process.

II. THE SIGNIFICANCE OF SYMBOLIC EXPRESSION

When psychological content is expressed in some form of image, it is very often merely a sign and sometimes a symbolic expression. It is necessary for the therapist to receive such expression as a message, and the way in which the message is interpreted is dependent on the therapist.

At the same time, such symbolic expression depicted by the client, either on a conscious level or an unconscious level, is also a factor in the process of self-insight. In other words, it is necessary to recognize anew the significance of symbolic expression as essential and gradual messages to the client himself for the attainment of integration.

III.   CASE STUDY - ANOREXIA NERVOSA

Let us take a case study as an interesting example of the way in which symbolic expression works.

Recently, anorexia nervosa has received attention as a major disorder creating problems that are pressingly relevant to our time and age. The case study is a 19-year-old and the younger of twin sisters. Her dietary habits became abnormal from high school age and she was prone to vomiting, which gradually became habitual. She was caught between the desire to eat and the emotional repression of that desire. This state was accompanied by constant feelings of regret and conflict, with a tendency to emotional instability.

After graduating from high school, she went through an unhappy love affair, as a result of which she experienced an identity crisis and became emotionally unstable. The eating disorder became more conspicuous and she fell into a state of self-hate. She attempted suicide by cutting her wrist and turning on the gas, but was found and saved, in time. She felt that her body had become obese and that her face was swollen and resembled a monster. Contrary to her low self-esteem, however, she was in fact adequately slender with quite a good figure.

There was an identity diffusion in the case's feelings, which can be described for example as "not wanting to grow up", "wishing to have a better understanding of society but not wanting to see the sordidness", "feeling shameful about her obscure image".

The programs for hospitalized treatment were planned on an individual basis and included not only immediate treatment for mal-nutrition, but more importantly, an individual art psychotherapy to facilitate non-verbal communication. During the month and a half of hospitalization, some 20 pencil drawings and water colors were produced spontaneously by the patient in therapeutic situations. The patient's graphic representations are characteristic in terms of symptomatology and also show the personal conflict underlying the disorder. But much more than that, some of the expressions in her graphic representations show unique expressions of self-image and self-esteem as well as unusual symbolic expressions such as the clown image and the clock image.

Groping for a Self-Image

Representations related to a search for self-identity can be seen throughout the series of drawings. One of the first depictions in the art therapy sessions was that of a very thin and stylish nude female. The female figure is an expression of self-image, depicting the patient standing in front of some males and what seems to be the figure of the sun. The drawing represents a symbol of her body image and her emotion.

Following this, there was a picture containing an upside-down, tear-streaked female face on the left side and the figure of an ancient warrior. The female image is a self-image. The longing for a strong male is depicted in the ancient warrior image. There was also a sequence of elegant female figures in pencil and water color, all showing narcistic self-images.

Some double images appeared in the patient's expressions, and one of her pictures showed a triple image. The case was one of a pair of twins and her own image overlaps with the image of her twin sister. A strong psychological conflict against her intelligent and beautiful sister could be recognized.

Another representation portrays a female hand apparently seeking a male. The hand is groping earnestly for the establishment of self. It is probably also a hand searching for someone to depend on.

The Clown Image

Midway in the sessions, there was a representation of a clown figure with an accompanying poem. The work projects the self-image as a clown. The clown has a personality that symbolizes one shadow aspect of man and is an ambivalent existence. The patient has written a poem underneath the clown image in which she gives vent to the sad emotions associated with the fun-loving, humorous, pleasure-giving clown on the one hand and his role on the other to be laughed at and despised. Bruch (1962) describes this as "the anorexic's desperate struggle for a self-respecting identity". The existence of the clown has also been indicated in the case reports made by Marianne A. Crowl of the U.S.A., and it is interesting to note this curious trans-cultural coincidence at a symbolic level.

The Clock Image

Another representation depicts time, self-image and a male figure. The lower figure is the male and the soaring figure above it is the female. In anorexia cases, it has been observed that there are many instances of fear of time passing, wishing to stop the clock or hide it, or hoping that the night would last forever. One interpretation is that the patient's fear for the future is projected to his daily life and that this symbolizes his refusal to mature. The present case wavered between the polarities of orientation towards and rejection of maturity, and it may be conjectured that her works represented the time dimensions related to a moratorium on maturity.

After this, the patient continued to grope for her self-image in the course of self-integration.

IV. DISCUSSION AND CONCLUSION

Symbolic expression appears in the psychotherapeutic relationship between client and therapist in Art Therapy. It is a message directed to the therapist who is an outsider. At the same time, it is directed towards the client himself and the image of such symbolic expression is a major factor in auto-therapeutics. Regardless of whether the client's symbolic image expression or drawing is an unconscious expression or not, it provides a meaningful impact on self-integration and works favorably in the process of self-insight.

Bruch (1973) has written on the significance of art therapy for anorexic patients that he has found "art work particularly useful, not so much for the unconscious symbolic content but as an aid in evoking a patient's self-awareness, as illustrating his own pattern of experience, and of his way of expressing his concepts of functioning and interaction with others." Also, Mitchell (1980) has written that "art therapy offers the patient new ways to discover herself. Through the creative process, greater opportunities for further self-expression are provided."

I have used a case of anorexia nervosa and have tried to provide examples showing very high levels of symbolic content. From a clinical iconographical viewpoint also, examples showing such high quality of symbolization are indicative of a direction towards good integration and, from our own experience, tend to follow a satisfactory recovery path. When symbolic expression in the form of image expression is complemented by verbal images, the messages thus expressed become qualitatively superior and more complete as information.

My presentation has been made with some reference to the comparative cultural aspect.

REFERENCES

Bruch, H., 1962, Perceptual and conceptual disturbances in anorexia nervosa, Psycho. Me. 24.
Bruch, H., 1973, "Eating Disorders", Basic Books, New York.
Crowl, M.A., 1980, Art therapy with patients suffering from anorexia nervosa, The Arts in Psychotherapy Vol.7, No.2, pp.141-151.
Mitchell, D., 1980, Anorexia nervosa, The Arts in Psychotherapy Vol.7, No.1, pp.53-60.

GRAPHIC EXPRESSION OF TWO NEUROSES : HYSTERIA AND OBSESSION

R. Volmat and Cl.J. Belin

Clinique de Neurologie et Psychiatrie
C.H.U. St Jacques
25000 Besançon (France)

Pathological handwriting like normal handwriting is worthy
of a double approach : psychopathological and somatic. These
different techniques complete each other and can play a role
in diagnosis.

The graphological analysis gives the possibility of
apprehending in a stable manner the major traits of the personality of the patient and is a test that is sensitive to the
variations in the clinical state with the changes in handwriting
being clearly visible according to the variability of the context.
Speech presents a host of connotations for those who know how to
listen. Writing evokes a deeper world for the graphologist :
that of symbolic thought and family and collective unconscious.

Graphological work taking into account cerebral functioning
began with POPHAL. The scale that he has provided enables the
research worker to consider the pathological or non-pathological
aspect of handwriting.

Research which has been sensitive to these methods has
continued in two directions : analytical and neurophysiological
with the organic and mental illness sometimes being confused.
Both in graphology and clinical psychiatry the concept of
structure reflects the way a mental state is constituted by the
fundamental elements of the personality forming a group of
coherent signs which correspond to a syndrome. This grouping
together of comparable signs corresponding to certain illnesses
forms the reference basis.

Both in clinical psychiatry and graphology one needs to maintain and distinguish the particular dynamics of the neurotic and psychotic structures as indicated by the psychoanalytical works.

The techniques used in graphology demonstrate the essential characteristics of the written signs in a structural perspective by taking into account the forms and their dynamic features to show the types of characteristic handwriting in different illnesses. The research is based on spatial symbolism and the objective criteria of shape, movement and arrangement and the different Freudian stages of personality maturation have been respected. Characteristic examples of the entire personality will be presented. The study of these characteristic examples can lead to a diagnosis.

To obtain samples of handwriting requires a non-directive attitude and in the clinical environment the graphologist is trained for the interviews where samples can easily be obtained once the patient is made aware of this approach.

So as to give some idea of the diversity of the graphical presentations two series of handwriting will be presented : one from a study of hysteria and the other from that of obsessional neurosis.

HANDWRITING OF HYSTERICS

The portrait of this woman illustrated by a post card with several lines of handwriting was sent by a patient suffering from hysteria. The picture seems to be a projection of herself as she would like to be : beautiful, ideal, sophisticated, impeccable. "Hysteria, this supreme means of expression" (ARAGON). The hysteric wears masks, adopts fashions of the moment with their excesses and artifices, but at the same time lacks a true identity. FREUD started his work with a study of hysteria (Dora, 1901) and according to FREUD "hysteria would be a deformed work of art" (Totem and Tabou, 1912).

Faced with somatic conversion there is the expression of a type of personality put forward by different authors :
    - emotional lability : the graphism is unstable in its strokes and it is affected ;
    - the poverty and facticity of the affects can be seen in the artificial shapes of the script, a slowing down, a cold pressure, multiple irregularities coming from awkwardness and the powerlessness to be able to project and ideal image of oneself ;

- egocentrism : the handwriting is narcissistic and self-centred ;
- the histrionism produces artificial shapes and extravagant capital letters ;
- the erotisation of the social relationships is revealed by a lack of warmth in the graphism ; she never expresses empathy. Only the need of others so that she can show herself off. The strokes lack depth ;
- immaturity is present in the childish items (E) on the GOBINEAU and PERRON scale. This scale sets out the childish and adult criteria which should be dominant in the handwriting of a person with a satisfactory maturity level.

Hysteria which is generally attributed to women is not limited solely to women. The male hysteric lacks virility and his handwriting is feminine. In our sample range which represents a yearly average of 30 hospitalised cases 6 were men.

The male or female hysteric has difficulty in putting up with the family and professional environment. He maintains a better relationship with the medical staff who knows how not to make him feel his deficiencies and who can lead him to more authentic self expression.

Each example of handwriting maintains its own characteristics. However, both the graphologist and layman can see that the deformations of the strokes do correspond to a state of morbidity. For the graphologist specialised in psychopathology all the cases presented show hysteria in the dramatisation of symptoms and situations.

HANDWRITING OF OBSESSIONAL NEUROTICS

Here the graphical presentation, semiology and dynamic is completely different. In hysteria, the oedipian conflict takes place at the oral and phallic libidinal levels and shows itself in the round upward shapes. In obsessional neurosis regression to the sadic-anal stage is characterised graphically by the black and smuggy strokes and the narrow rigid shapes. This is the pensive type with the all powerful invested in rituals, verifications and conspiracies. The stroke lacks vitality and evokes JANET's psychasthenia.

The movement, arrangement and lack of rhythm show power-lessness at the diversity of approaches to problems. The repetition of "I" would be the expression of an obsolute will not to lose the control of oneself and events. Sight is turned inwards towards oneself and the "I" is in the mirror. Whereas the "I" of the hysteric is aimed at seducing others.

In this second series of examples the handwriting is contracted and aged. The rigid super-ego can be seen in the rectilinear margin on the left. This super-ego exerts a ferocious pressure on the devitalised "ego".

This second series of examples includes a drawing of a patient of 45 years of age who is completely inhibited, rigid and anxious. In contrast to the drawing in bright colours of the hysteric this drawing is black. Here nothing is left to chance. The details are precise and meticulous : the eyes, around the ears and the freckles on the face. There is little imagination in this drawing. It is tight and difficult to see.

The difference in structure between these two neuroses is graphically evident.

Under no circumstances can a graphological investigation replace clinical observation. It is a para-clinical examination and perhaps even a privileged one in relation to the batteries of tests that are often given. There is no doubt that it should be an integral part of the examination. However, the information provided by the graphologist should not be considered as infallible. It requires interpretation in relation to the patient and the clinical context. It is under these conditions that the graphologist can add to the knowledge of the patient and undoubtedly help in the therapy.

PSYCHOPATHOLOGY IN A CRISIS? 10 BASIC TRUTHS

ABOUT THE CRISIS AND ITS POSSIBLE SOLUTION

B. Pauleikhoff

Psychiatrische und Nervenklinik
der Westfälischen Wilhelmsuniversität
4400 Münster

1) Soul and personality have been banished from
   psychiatry since the times of Griesinger, thus
   giving rise to a psychopathology without psyche,which
   was striving for pure empiricism only to miss it
   more thoroughly.

2) Since only the brain was considered the basis of
   psychic functions, there developed, despite many
   counter-currents and resistances, a materialistic
   view of inner life that took pattern from chemistry
   and physics.

3) This approach came to a dead stop in a mist of
   hypotheses (Dilthey) and led to a grave scientific
   crisis.

4) To overcome this crisis the reintroduction of soul
   and personality as the core and foundation of
   scientific experience and perception is indispensable and needed most urgently.

5) Soul means the biography of a temporal "Gestalt"
   reaching from birth to death, in which the personality is centered.

6) This biographic reality is no spatial object in
   the natural sciences, rather a reality with
   temporal limits that is lived through and experienced by the individual.

7) It is realised in recurrent cycles of daily life
    as a structure of meaning, influenced by present
    and past.

8) In the encounter between ego and non-ego an
    access to situation and biography of personality
    is opened. The interview gives the physician
    direct insight into situation and biography.

9) On the one hand psychology and psychopathology
    are no natural sciences in the usual sense ,on the
    other hand they are empiric sciences too, they
    have to look for their principles of experience
    and perception rather in time than in matter.

10) Within the framework of all psychic phenomena and
    disturbances the problem of time has to be cleared
    necessarily in order to secure a solid base for
    unadulterated experience in psychopathology and
    to make further genuine progress possible in both
    diagnosis and therapy.

IDENTITY AND DIFFERENCE AS MOMENTS OF SELF

Bin Kimura

Department of Psychiatry
Nagoya City University School of Medicine
1 Kawasumi, Mizuhocho, Mizuhoku, Nagoya 467 Japan

Being the self in the sense of relating-to-oneself constitutes
the fundamental determination of a human existence. In fact, there
are many psychiatric disturbances in which this determination seems
to be seriously affected. Most schizophrenics show their first symptoms in adolescence, when juveniles are facing toward an inevitable
work to enter into adulthood, that is to say, when the self has now
to relate to itself basically otherwise than in childhood. If one
fails in coping with this inward task, one must fall into a critical
distress of which the most conspicuous manifestations in clinical
psychopathology are such typically schizophrenic symptoms consisting
in a pathological conviction that the most intimate intention of
oneself be radically at disposal of others.
     Schizophrenic patients often say, "Others are coming into my
soul, so that I can never be myself", "They catch continuously my
thought and rob me of any secret. So I can keep no more my self",
"There are no more boundary, no more difference between myself and
others" and so on. Such assertions demonstrate unequivocally that
the issue of the self is inseparably connected with that of the
other, that the self is able to be self only remaining clearly
distinct from the other and securing its innermost against him.
It means however that it is for the self necessary to meet the other
every time and to get to itself only through this continuous encounter. It is only in an interpersonal situation between myself and
the other that I am in a position to identify myself as myself.
So the self is *per se* a modality of primordial difference that always differentiates itself from the non-self and so actualizes the
originality of the I distinct from the other.
     The self does not exist in any way as an object belonging to
oneself as everguaranteed property. In order to identify myself as
myself saying I am I, I have everytime to differentiate myself from

1067

the other and to join always anew the inner historicity of my own
identity. It is only after I have experienced myself as a difference from the other that I am enabled to say I am I. Before it
there can be neither myself nor the other. The difference itself
is thus always differentiating itself from the other and identifying itself as the self. This difference is not a symmetrical one
between two equally differenciated sides but constitutes a characteristic asymmetry. The self is not merely one of both sides. It
takes rather the whole difference on its hand alone, producing it
by itself. The other on the contrary does not behave as a proper
half of it , taking a role to evoke the self to its act of differentiation and being the medium through which the self comes to itself
as this difference *per se*. The difference proves itself thus as a
inner difference which is the self as such.

The other needs not always be a real human being. I can also
relate and behave to myself just when I am quite alone. The schizophrenics tend to become aware of deprivation and alienation of their
own self especially when they are withdrawing from any interpersonal
relationship. Certainly, a real encounter with actual other persons
may be necessary for an infant for whom the own inner existence and
the outer world are not yet differentiated. So he has to obtain the
first germ of his own self only through encounters with his mother
and other family members. His long life history thereafter represents nothing but the very process of symbolization and internali-
zation of those real encounters. This process makes him possible
little by little to realize himself as an inner difference, an inner
relationship to himself, even when he remains alone.

To be myself can be secured for me only when I succeed to integrate this inner difference into my own inner historicity in the
manner of the "consequence of natural experience" characterizing the
sane way of the being-in-the-world according to L. Binswanger(1).

Such an identity of the self does not rest upon itself like
sameness of things but refers always to its past, to its just accomplished act of differentiation as well as to its immediate future
in order to come to itself continuously. We see here exactly such
a difference which differentiates and at the same time is differentiated, a difference as a transcendence that can be nothing other
than the structure of the existence demonstrated by M. Heidegger (2)
as temporality of the being-in-the-world.

All these things go now basically wrong with the schizophrenics.
Our clinical observations as well as results of family studies of
schizophrenics show unanimously how the patients attracted the attention of their surroundings already in shildhood because of their
quite weak self-assertion and, on the other side, how little was
readiness to a true interpersonal encounter among the family members,
no matter whether we may conclude from these findings a hereditary
predetermination of schizophrenia or a specific family dynamics
called schizophrenogenic. In any case, the later schizophrenics
were destined long before manifestation of psychoses to have to

1968

relate to themselves as well as to the other in such a way that it was quite difficult for them to integrate the inner difference into the consequence of natural experience of their historical identity. In critical interpersonal situations which they must go through in adolescence it often occurs that they do not know how they can identify this inner difference with their own self. Then must the difference get to be to such an extent alienated and deprived that it appears still only as a agency of non-self. In other words, the asymmetry of difference cannot prove itself any longer. The patients come thus to experience all of their own intentions as influenced or perceived by the other. These characteristic symptoms of schizophrenia may not be understood in any way in terms of thought disturbances or pathological cognitions, for these represent essentially answers of patients to a critical inner situation of interpersonality.

All that we have seen imposes to us explicitly a question about basic structure of interpersonality. To other with whom I encounter each time and as difference from whom I have each time to appropriate myself to myself, such other appears here no more as an objective thing but as a personal self with his own subjectivity. How is it possible and how looks it phenomenologically that one self meets another intersubjectively.

As to the problem of constitution of *alter ego*, there are a number of philosophical theories. Nevertheless, all of these seem to have failed to solve the question what the other subjectivity really is, because they all simply believe that they can construct an alternative ego as copy of the original one into the other, that the subjectivity of the other can anyhow be approached from outside. However, does not the very subjectivity of the other consist in its absolute unapproachability or in the fact that the inside of it remains for me absolutely unknown? It must be only an objective other person who can be approachable from outside as an alternative ego.

This absolute unapproachability of the subjective other was conceptualized phenomenologically be J.-P. Sartre (3) as a "hole of my world", i.e., a deficit of my objectifiable world. However, his theory of the being-for-the-other (*l'être pour autrui*) seems in so far still inadequate as he remains to consider an absolute "either-or" without any compromise between myself and the other. Either the other looking at me objectifies me to a mere thing or I myself looking at him objectify him on my part. A true interaction between two equally subjective selves seems here shut off from the beginning.

It was now A. Schütz (4) who introduced in his theory of intersubjectivity the bergsonian concept of "duration" (*durée*). He says that I experience not only my own duration as an absolute reality as well as you experience yours as such. It is rather true that your duration is given to me just as my duration is given to you at the same time, both as an absolute reality. In this contemporality of two durations I am becoming older together with you.

His conception of becoming-older-together (*Zusammenaltern*) may serve further as a guideline for us. This duration does not mean something like a time span extending quasi spatially from now to now

but must be understood as a horizon of temporality in the sense of
a openness toward both directions of earlier and later, until now
and from now on, a horizon which I am continuously experiencing as
my own present and my own subjective self. Every object in my surroundings given in my duration including human beings appears for me
as something more or less known. I am always ready to categorize it
as this or that taking it in as a particle of my own world. The difference of my self-identity keeps thus its fundamental asymmetry.

It is not the case with the other I encounter intersubjectively.
I do not experience him simply in my own duration as something belonging to my identity but as someone who participates with his own
duration in mine and so becomes older together with me. My present
appears now to be splitted inwardly in two parts: the one belongs to
me but the other does not, being not idenfiable for me. The latter
must keep an asymmetrical difference in itself. Its center of grav-
ity exists on the side of the other, beyond of my own world. It is
what Sartre designates as a hole, as a deficit of my world, a hole
through which my world is flowing out incessantly. Here come across
two asymmetrical differences one another, differentiating and identifying themselves each for its part. But, far from being two win-
dowless monads without any interactional communication, there is
between them a true intersubjective encounter based on the contemporary becoming-older of both durations. Since the duration constitutes in its true sense nothing but the deepst foundation of the
inner difference, this contemporality means a common participation
of both subjectivities in the same intersubjective world. So we see
that the "between" (*Zwischen*) of the intersubjectivity between myself
and the other proves a real phenomenon of time, as B. Pauleikhoff(5)
has pointed out recently with full reason.

It will seem now quite obvious to us that such an act of contemporary becoming-older must be getting so precarious with schizophrenics. Not only in his psychotic state but already in his preceding life history it seems hardly possible for the patient to keep
his own inner difference and its asymmetry as well as to integrate
it into the inner historicity of his self-identity. The self as
inner difference or reality of duration is deprived of its natural
self-evidence (*natürliche Selbstverständlichkeit*) in the sense of
W. Blankenburg(6) and deeply alienated, sometimes in the way of a
schizophrenic depersonalization, sometimes in a form of delusion of
influence , sometimes of a cenesthopathic feeling of the body image.

Psychopathology as a branch of psychiatry looks today lower
estimated in its actuality. It is generally convinced that psychiatrists have to make more efforts to research neurobiological conditions of psychic disturbances. It seems actually true if subjects
of psychopathology remain restricted within merely symptomatological
issues. If psychopathology wants to keep itself as independent discipline, it must turn its attention much more to the transcendental
problems like intersubjectivity above discussed.

REFERENCES

1. L.Binswanger, "Schizophrenie", Neske, Pfullingen (1957).
2. M.Heidegger, "Sein und Zeit", 7. Aufl. Niemeyer, Tübingen (1953).
3. J.-P. Sartre, "L'être et le néant", Gallimard, Paris (1943).
4. A.Schütz, "Der sinnhafte Aufbau der sozialen Welt", Suhrkam, Frankfurt a.M. (1974).
5. B.Pauleikhoff, "Zeit zwischen Ich und Du", in:"Kriminologie-Psychiatrie-Strafrecht", Festschrift für H.Leferenz, publisher unknown (1983).
6. W.Blankenburg, "Der Verlust der natürlichen Selbstverständlich-keit", Enke, Stuttgart (1971).

THE CASE HISTORY AND THE "UNLIVED LIFE"

Albert Zacher

Institut für Psychotherapie
der Universität Würzburg
D - 8700 Würzburg

The term "case history" is being used in a different sense. The medical disciplines oriented organically are understanding by that term just the facts of symptomatology and etiology of a specific illness, the psychopathologists however are equating case history with the life history of a patient, especially since K. Jaspers performed his psychopathological theories (Jaspers, K., 1973).

Viktor von Weizsäcker has pointed out that both in the history of states and in the history of a single person the opportunities not realized are really more effectful than the realized ones. He initiated that surprising conception of the "unlived life" and made clinical and philosophical investigations in order to detect its importance for medicine (von Weizsäcker, 1950; Zacher, 1978).

THE RISE OF THE "UNLIVED LIFE"

By choosing and deciding between the possibilities of future man creates history in the present - thus he separates each moment "unlived life" from lived historical reality. Therefore "unlived life" is a consequence of man's temporal existence.

THE EFFICACY OF "UNLIVED LIFE"

Our daily experience obtained through the contact with patients shows that our omissions are just as able to disturb the state of health as our activities. Both, changes and events of life as well as monotony and ennui can shatter health - W. J. Revers (1949), Viktor von Weizsäcker (1956, S. 244 ff) and D. Wyss (1980, S. 442ff) have clearified this fact for psychology and medicine.

SUGGESTION TO STRUCTURE THE TERM OF "UNLIVED LIFE"

Consideration of inner and outer world enables us to subdivide the totality of the term "unlived life". Opportunities of the outer world for example can either be taken and developed or be failed. Omitted opportunities can disturb the state of emotions such as grief, sorrow and the feeling of being guilty. All those literary works telling of self-realization and discovery of one's own ego - all the philosophical works aiming at the same theme, are born by the knowledge that the "unlived life" of our inner world can cause many burdening effects concerning our well-being.

Other structures of "unlived life" can be deduced from the existentialistic planning (see Tellenbachs term of "Remanenz" (Tellenbach, 1976)) or from the modes and structures of communication as described by Wyss (see below).

RENOUNCING, REJECTING, MISSING AND LETTING SLIP

Rilke's poems include the idea of "unlived life". In his remarks upon missing of decisions Rilke was convinced that missed opportunities and decisions burden the present state and necessitate a subsequent mastering of those decisions in the past (Bollnow, 1962, S. 214 ff).

Contrary to noticed but missed opportunities - the opportunities which had been let slip have not been noticed. "Unlived life" originating in that way cannot be mastered when the inner situation is ready for decision but only if the circumstances of the outer world rereturned once again - because it is more related to outer than to inner causes. Letting slip is not as burdening as missing.

The effect of ascetism and its existence within all
religions is an important cultural and historical example
for the serious consequences of "unlived life". Renouncing and missing differ through the decision. Renouncing
means to step foreward, missing throws back behind the
moment of decision. But the uncertainty in renouncing and
missing will be existing for life: the opportunity to re-
value the past will not end as long as life is going on.
Men are permanently kept in the suspense wether the re-
liefing renounce of today might change to a burdening
sick-making missing of tomorrow. Tragedy as well as hope
of human life are captured in this dialectic relation.

PARALLELS TO THE COMMUNICATION THEORY OF DIETER WYSS

The communication-modi of the existence shown in
the structures of space, time, body and performance:
to reconnoitre, to discover, to open up, to argue with
oneself, to bind and to loosen, all that precede the
mastering (Wyss, 1976). Remaining behind one of these
steps means to fail mastering and thus, possible or
even challenged life remains unlived. Binding and loosening are joint to the decision, include renouncing and rejecting. Man who doesn't surpass discovering, opening
up and arguing with himself is missing the opportunity
to decide. Those people who only reconnoitre and thereby don't see their possibilities, lose the possible richness of life.

THE ANAMNESIS OF "UNLIVED LIFE"

Besides the direct questions for omissions and re-
nounces during the life the doctor can indirectly get
down to the "unlived life" of a patient by listening to
hints of resignation, dissatisfaction and so forth.
Revers (1978) has managed to use the TAT as an indicator
for this essential part of the past. Wyss (1982) has created the Würzburg-questionnaire as a systematically elaborated instrument for detecting unlived communication.

"Unlived life" causes undoubted effects on the present state and on judgement of the future; therefore case
history cannot exclude this widely overlooked element of
the past, should it represent the totality of a person's
life.

Reference

Bollnow, O. F., 1962, "Maß und Vermessenheit des Menschen" Vandenhoeck & Ruprecht, Göttingen.

Jaspers, K., 1973, "Allgemeine Psychopathologie", Springer, Berlin - Heidelberg - New-York.

Revers, W.J., 1949, "Die Psychologie der Langeweile", Meisenheim, Hain.

Revers, W. J., 1978, "Der thematische Apperzeptionstest", Huber, Bern - Stuttgart.

Tellenbach, H., 1976, "Melancholie", Springer, Berlin - Heidelberg - New-York.

Weizsäcker, Viktor von, 1950, "Diesseits und Jenseits der Medizin", Koehler, Stuttgart.

Weizsäcker, Viktor von, 1956, "Pathosophie", Vandenhoeck & Ruprecht, Göttingen.

Wyss, D., 1976, "Mitteilung und Antwort", Vandenhoeck & Ruprecht, Göttingen.

Wyss, D., 1980, "Zwischen Logos und Antilogos", Vandenhoeck & Ruprecht, Göttingen.

Wyss, D., 1982, "Der Kranke als Partner. Lehrbuch der anthropologisch-integrativen Psychotherapie", Vandenhoeck & Ruprecht, Göttingen.

Zacher, A., 1978, "Der Krankheitsbegriff bei Viktor von Weizsäcker", Medizinische Dissertation, Würzburg.

APROPOS OF CHANGING CONCEPTS OF CONSCIOUSNESS IN PSYCHOPATHOLOGY

Toshihiko Hamanaka and Hiroshi Ohashi

Department of Neuropsychiatry
Kyoto University School of Medicine
606 Kyoto Sakyo Shogoin, Japan

If we find in "Philosophy of symbolical forms"(Vol.3, 1929) a remark of E. Cassirer: "...The concept of consciousness seems to be a real Proteus of philosophy...", and if we again read in an introduction of C.-F. Graumann (1966) to the problems of consciousness in psychology: "...For too many discussions, sustained up to this day in order to clarify the notion of consciousness, carry the character of concept-exegesis", — then nobody would surely refuse to recognize that also in psychiatry the state of affairs in this respect is not much different; psychiatry borrowed indeed in her modern cradle the fundamental concept in question from nowhere else than the two older sciences mentioned above, thereby being compelled at the same time, however, to put up with the very same complications as theirs. These conceptual difficulties have not remained in fact without being mentioned in numerous textbooks and contributions of psychiatry, leading not a few authors, by reason of its alleged obscurities, to dismiss the notion of "disturbed consciousness" held to be of no clinical use, while others have found themselves entitled to consider every phenomenon of derangement in human psychical life in view of disordered consciousness.

If we are to begin further back in the historical change of the concept of consciousness, there is a basic fact attracting our attention in the history of medicine, namely that the psychopathology, and consequently the whole medicine with essentially "biological" tendency, in antiquity could do largely without a notion of consciousness. At first sight it may sound rather strange, especially since in those days there existed a well developed system of clinical symptomatology describing disorders of consciousness on the one hand, and the Cartesian concept "conscientia" (Latin) goes back etymologically, as widely known, to the classical "conscientia"

1077

and further to "syneidesis" (Greek) on the other. These antique notions however appear at no time in the medical literature of the Greco-Roman age. Galen, for example, attributed "caros" to abolition, "coma" and "lethargos" to weakening of "phantasia", which should have its organ in the anterior part of the cerebrum; patients afflicted with "caros" were described as those who "lost their intelligence, movement, and sensibility" resp. became simply "anaisthes" (insensible), whereas "phrenetic" (febrile-delirious) patients should get back their "nous" (reason) in the course of restoration.

The consequences of this Aristotelian-Galenic tradition were extraordinary far-reaching, so far as to remain further authoritative and influential not only till the end of the arabic-scholastic middle age, but beyond the Renaissance and the baroque period even down to the 18th century, that is, till one hundred years later than the establishment of the concept of consciousness in philosophy by Descartes as "cogitatio", by Locke as "tabula rasa", and by Leibniz as "miroir vivant" resp. "apperception/perception".

Still in the writings of Th. Willis (1664/72) "carus" as well as "coma" was interpreted as a consequence of hindered radiation of "spiritus animales" out of the corpus callosum, the site of "imaginatio" and "sensus communis", toward the cerebral cortex lodging the "somnus" and "memoria". Also in the clinical descriptions of epileptic seizures and apoplectic attacks by H. Boerhaave (1730/35) there appear only such terms as "functiones animales", "sensus internus" etc, but never the "conscientia".

It is very characteristic of the process introducing step by step the concept of consciousness into medical science, that it was destined to be accepted in the course of the 18th century by psychiatry as the first discipline, which was setting up on its own just at that time as one special branch of medicine, to be assimilated with considerable delay by the doctrine of nervous diseases. What illustrates paradigmatically this circumstance, is the doctrine of W. Cullen (1977), a Scottish nosologist, who conceived in his medical psychology, designed upon the model of Locke's empiricism, the "vesaniae" as disorders of "intellectual functions", especially of "judgement", that represents one form of the "sensations of consciousness" constrasted with the "sensations of impression", whereas not a single mention of "consciousness" is found in his teachings on "neuroses" otherwise, all kinds of "neuroses, inclusive of "vesaniae", being defined as "affections of the sensorium".

In the doctrines of German authors at the end of the 18th century, in contrast to the empiricist-sensualistic trend of British psychiatry, the concept of consciousness was largely coined by faculty psychology which is interpreted as "manifestation of the psychological theory of German idealism" with "das Ich und das Bewußtsein" in its "key position" (Leibbrand and Wettley 1961). The faculty psychology, in its original form scarcely concerned about physiological knowledge, started from "consciousness of himself" among other things, which was formulated by I. Kant in his "Anthropologie" (1798) as follows: "That the human being is able to have the I in his thought, raises him infinitely above all other creatures on the earth. Thereby he is a person and that one and the same person, by virtue of unity of consciousness maintained amongst all changes befalling him." It reminds us in the first place of corresponding psychiatric conceptions of J.C. Hoffbauer (1802/07) as well as of J.C. Reil (1799/1803). Hoffbauer, a Kantian, views the "self-consciousness or subjective consciousness" as that through which the "personality" "becomes possible", describing its "alienating phenomena." For Reil likewise the "consciousness" resp. "self-consciousness" along with "prudence and attention" constitutes the "triumvirate of closely related psychic forces", which integrates the human being with his various qualities toward a personal unity." The medical universalist Reil does not however remain without commenting upon the physiological aspect of the problem, writing further that "with this equipment (the cerebrum) raising the manifold-bodily toward one individuum, ... the cause of self-consciousness seems to be related." The notion of consciousness plays further a role of unequalled importance in the sin-doctrine of J.C. Heinroth (1818/31), re-interpreted recently in anthropological terms, in so far as, according to him, "a human-morbid state is ... that, in which the human being finds himself more or less restricted", i.e. "unfree" in consciousness, so that "every consciousness, not admitted in conscience or reason, ... should be a consciousness in a morbid state." For Heinroth therefore, consciousness is neither the consciousness referring to psychic quality nor some conscious part of psyche, but unmistakably a "psychic system", in the meaning of Bash (1955), that possibly is able to form the bodily too. A number of related conceptions of consciousness are further read in other psychiatric doctrines of varying origin out of the first half of the German 19th century. Among medical students orientating themselves in the current of romantic medicine, it is noteworthy to remark that C.G. Carus (1846) initiated the shifting of emphasis to the negative side of consciousness, anticipating the later depth psychology.

Confronted with the notion of consciousness, the French psychiatry in the corresponding period holds a peculiarly isolated position. It talks about consciousness almost exclusively in such cases as it is a matter of a patient's insight into his own disease resp. of related forensic notions: "folie avec conscience", "perte de conscience de ce desordre" etc. This attitude persisted through all the generations of French psychiatrists in the 19th century, beginning with Ph. Pinel (1801), and leaving some followers still at the dawn of our century. In contrast to the confined status of the concept of consciousness, the preponderance of the notion of "intelligence" resp. "understanding (entendement)" strikes our eye, illustrated by the definitions of mental disease given by a series of French authors (Esquirol 1938, Georget 1820, etc.).

Coming back to the German 19th century, we find it in the process of "dissoluting the concept of soul" (Leibbrand and Wettley, 1961), originally initiated already by Locke. Now there was merely a question of the "organ of consciousness" and of the "facts of consciousness" as starting-point of all the psychological thinking (Herbart 1823/25). What underlies this trend, is not so much the faculty psychology or natural-philosophic conception as rather the "psychology without soul" (F.A. Lange 1866), i.e. J.F. Herbart's "mechanics of representation", conceived after the mathematical model, with increasing propensity toward experimental-physiological psychology in the following generations (C.T. Fechner 1860, W. Wundt 1873/74). Thus, German psychology is now exhibiting at this time certain common features with empiricist sensualism in England and France. What illustrates the circumstance exemplarily, is the essentially intimate relationship between W. Griesinger's psychiatric conception (1943/67) on the one side and those of T. Laycock (1838/45) and J. Baillarger (1845/65) on the other. In the medical psychology of Griesinger, based on Herbart's representation psychology, consciousness is a "vacant space for representations", where develops eventually a "conflict" resp. "competition" among representations "in accrodance with the laws of association of ideas", producing "favoured" representations which find finally "passage to actions" instead of "unconscious" representations "repressed" under the "threshold of consciousness" (Herbart). The whole process was conceived as "psychical reflex actions", taking pattern from the physiological reflex theory as its model, which was being accomplished just in those days by M. Hall (1832/50) and J. Müller (1831/40) continuing the pioneering andeavours of R. Whytt (1751), F. Prochaska (1780/84) etc (Canguilhem 1977). Let us remark by the way, that the notion of consciousness in Herbart's and Griesinger's doctrines reminds us readily of the "stage theory" ("Theatrum internum") of D. Hume (1739/58), finding itself later in the conceptions of E. Hering, the physiologist (1870), as well as in K. Jaspers' psychopathology (1913) among others in hardly modified form. — Laycock's doctrine of "cerebral reflex action or automatic action" as well as W.B. Carpenter's theory of "unconscious cerebration" (1853) was likewise constructed on the basis of reflex theory combined with English association psychology, and found its application for instance in explanations of hysterical disorders of behaviour with somnambulism etc brought into focus at that time, whereas in Baillarger's conception of "automatism", interpreting such psychotic phenomena as hallucination etc in essentially the same manner, there is no mention of consciousness. Thus for Baillarger as well as other French psychiatrists who followed him, the concept of automatism was destined to play a much more important role than that of consciousness.

It is a noteworthy, yet unexpected turning in the history of psychiatry, that two opposite trends of neuropsychiatric thinking of our century came apart, growing out of this same root: association-ism since C. Wernicke (1874/1905) with the concept of consciousness as epiphenomenon of associative functions of the cerebral cortex on the one hand, and hierachic holism on the other since J.H. Jackson (1864/94) with the notion of consciousness as a phenomenon psychologically determined, that "concommits" with the sensori-motor activity of the nervous system on the highest level (Hamanaka 1982/83). One notion however was lacking in both cases: that of the Unconsciouss, being to be saved by S. Freud.

The Herbartian-Griesingerian conception of consciousness, besides, gave rise to probably the first comprehensive symptomatol-ogy of disorders of consciousness by R. Krafft-Ebing (1877/79) in neuro-psychiatry with the introduction of the notion of "twilight state", as well as to the elaboration of a psychophysical concept of "clouding of consciousness" by E. Kraepelin (1889) based on Fechners doctrine. Kraepelin's conception of consciousness with its attribute "clarity" referring no more to particular representations as in Griesinger's doctrine, but to consciousness as such, is to be considered as a basis of most of contemporary theories of disturbed consciousness in neuropsychiatry, which endeavour to estimate it as accessible to description or even measurement in the function of stimulus-reaction (e.g. a series of "coma-scales" proposed in recent years), as pointed to by U.H. Peters (1974).

Thus, we have arrived at the beginning decennia of our century, and would like now to get over its first three quarters in order immediately to proceed to our own age, because whatever change the concept of consciousness has undergone meanwhile, must surely be well known to you in every detail. At present the state of the problem of consciousness looks in such a way that we find ourselves called upon to subject it once more to a through examination no less than ever, — confronted with a scientific situation of neuro-psychiatry, which seems, so to say, to be flooded with "labels" of (disordered) consciousness. Nowadays "consciousness" is again indeed in everyone's mouth, thus for instance in the context of "altered states of consciousness" (Ludwig 1966), further with the "Institute of human consciousness" (R.E. Ornstein 1972), which is willing to achieve "expansion of consciousness", or also with the "prolonged coma" (since P. Wertheimer et al. 1953), in which case it is hard to determine, whether it is a question of disturbed consciousness or severest dementia, further more with the problem of "disorders of consciousness" pretended to have a higher incidence in cases with left- than right-hemispheric lesion (Albert et al. 1976 etc since Lewandowski 1910), or with the alleged "division of consciousness" and even of "soul" in split-brain patients (Sperry et al. 1966/79), as well as with the localization of "circuits of consciousness" in the corpus callosum (S.J. Dimond 1980), and last but not least with the "lateralization" of the Conscious in the left-dominant and of the Unconscious" (in the sense of depth psychology) in the right-nondominant hemisphere (Galin 1977). — We are sorry not to be able to proceed to closer examination of the notion of consciousness used by every author because of limitted time for presentation today. If we allow ourselves nerverthless to summarize in few words some striking features of their concept-applications, we should readily be able to confirm that there is to observe a certain reductionism or else arbitrariness in dealing with the notion of consciousness, common to all of them, even though in different conceptual dimensions: consciousness is simply equated now with contents of perception,now with attention, or again with vigility, not rarely are conceptual dimensions scarcely differenti-ated or kept apart.

All that is the actual motive of our modest attempt today to clarify the changing concept of consciousness to some extent. We think, that we find ourselves not so much in an age' of "crisis of psychopathology" as rather in an age of "crisis arising from lack of psychopathology" as a fundamental science in psychiatry, — psychiatry, which — in modifying a formulation of Boring (1933) a little — would never have come into being indeed just as psychology and philosophy, if it were not for the problem of consciousness, whatever objectivists, behaviourists—operationalists, and biolo-gists — might have said about it.

N.B.: The part in the original paper, treating the historical episode of introducing the European concept of consciousness into Japanese medicine, is omitted by reason of limitted space.

REFERENCES

Hamanaka, T., 1978, Disorders of consciousness, in: "Gendai Seishin-Igaku Taikei (Handbook of Contemporary Psychiatry)," Vol.3/A/1, ed. Y. Ushimura et al., Nakayamashoten Publ. Co., Tokyo (in Japanese).
Hamanaka, T., and Ohashi, H., 1983, Possibility of neuropsychologi-cally orientated psychiatry, in: "Proceedings of World Psychiatric Association Regional Symposium, Kyoto/Japan 1982", ed. H. Ohashi et al., the Japanese Society of Psychiatry and Neurology, Tokyo.

THE PROBLEM OF TIME IN PSYCHIC PHENOMENA:

AN APPROACH TO METHODOLOGICAL CRITICISM

W. J. Revers

Psycholog. Institut

Akademiestraße 22, A-5020 Salzburg

It was only the critical analysis of the tenets or
"Grundannahmen" as Kurt Huebner[1] calls them on which
we base scientific cognition and the "proposed solutions", as they are termed by Mario Bunge[2], that showed
their dependence on a historical context. This analysis
also showed the historical relativity of the theories
and methodologies based on these tenets. This insight,
however, should not lead to our rejecting the methodology hitherto employed in science. The epistemological
problem lies rather in the unchecked influence of our
premises on scientific planning and the interpretation
of scientific findings. In the history of science a
methodologically misinterpreted reality has enforced
the "correction" of these tenets over and over again.

All disciplines of empiric science established in
modern history at first followed the example of the
model science of "physics". Like the physicists themselves they were at first captivated by the "fascination of the universal"[3] that seemed to have been
attained in clascical Newtonian mechanics.

1) Kurt Huebner: Kritik der wissenschaftlichen Vernunft.
   Freiburg/München 2/1979.
2) Mario Bunge: Scientific Research I – The Surch for
   System. Berlin/Heidelberg/New York 1967.
3) Ilya Prigogine & Isabelle Stengers: Dialog mit der
   Natur. München 1981.

As a "classic science" it still remained an effective model when in physics themselves the study of nature had clearly shown the limitations of the universality of the dynamic laws. The laws of classical physics are independent of time: "Once the initial conditions are given, these eternal laws will determine the future forever, as they have determined the past."4) But the advances of physics in the field of thermodynamics showed that there are things like waste or irrecoverable loss, i. e. irreversible processes. Prigogine gives the following resume: "We find ourselves in a world governed by chance, a world in which the laws of reversibility and determinism can be applied only to simple borderline cases."5)

This confrontation of physics with the problem of "time as an indestructible ground weave"6) did not fail to leave its mark on the other empiric sciences like biology or psychology but also sociology. This will be illustrated by the exemplary case of psychology.

Wundt and the other pioneers of experimental psychology were striving for another Newtonian position, so to speak, for empiric psychology. From its very beginnings Wundt's construction—to characterize an early psychological tenet with his name—met with opposition from W. James, to name only one scientist who deemed individuality, the central "self" of the conscious subject indispensable. Again and again attempts were made to prove the universality (and reversibility) of emotions, performances of the memory and mental processes, and again and again the provocations of concepts like typology, characterology, psychology of personality or motivation research emerged— not to mention psychoanalysis and its consequences. When under the influence of psychoanalysis and psychosomatic medicine even psychology could no longer evade the epochal engagement for the distressed individual, when public demands necessitated the establishment of a clinical psychology it seemed as if psychology was undergoing a schism between "genuine" empirical science and more or less unscientific practice.

---

4) ibid., p. 11
5) ibid., p. 18 (The italics are mine)
6) ibid., p. 245 ff.

The hypothesis of a universal mental structure in any
test person, of any individual case as "a case of"
proved to be unsuitable for the recognition of problems posed by therapeutical practice. Here it became
clear how dubiuns even the intentions of personality
research were, since the personal reality of the individual could no longer be overlooked. If psychology
was to be "science" at all it had to develop a concept
of "person in time" i. e. of the irreversible development of personality and had to work out methods that
did not miss this same concept by their very definitions. Its fundamental problem lies - to overstate
the point - in the contradiction between the - ex
definitione - given uniqueness and singularity of the
person with its irreversible development on the one
hand and the scientific demand for generality of knowledge on the other hand.[7] Does not the "incomparabi-
lity" attached to the concept of person[8] exclude any
possibility of finding generally comparable features?
Persons who are the objects of psychological observation are not as timeless as the person as a concept.
But they are living persons, living beings whose
existence takes its course in time, for whom time is
both transience and duration; they are "persons in
time" as well as "persons with a body", they are
"materialized" and it is only thus that they can develop concretely and exist: as "persons incarnate " in
time. And this is precisely why there are features
suitable for comparisons and generalisations. Other
such features are given in the field of social background and biography, such as descent from parents,
dependence on the family, the fact that one is born
into a sociocultural community and culture, determining one's habits, rituals, language, traditions,
way of life, sociocultaral norms and religious world
wiews. But not only the sociocultaral rules governing
life are given facts for any individual, but also the
tides of his or her life, phases of continnous growth
on the one hand and of expansive development on the
other hand with every period of life posing new
problems. And it is also a given fact that no individual can undergo this development without learning,

---

7) A similar complex of problems in physics is described by Prigogine in his chapter:"Vom Sein zum
Werden" ibid., p 201 ff.
8) Revers: "Der Begriff 'Person' in der Psychologie",
in B. Gerner ed.:Personale Erziehung.Wege der Forschung,Vol. 29

without maturation, without independent decisions,and
that the development of personality does not take place "automatically" like a biological process of growth
and without the constant demand to realize one's self
through decisions. In these features-which have been
brought forward quite unsystematically- lies the
potential for a relative universality that enables us
to compare different developnents of personality: What
has happened to individuality at what time under what
kind of physical conditions and sociocultural circumstances? Everyone is, so to speak, the only "case of
himself". And yet the recordable "rules" of individual
development offer approaches to this problem of singularity, to observe general conditions for the development of these individualities and to understand
personal development as typical answers to these conditions. Just to understand the importance of such
single processes, given and limited in time, for the
overall project of personal development is the aim of
biographical analysis. Prompted by Erich Rothacker's
notion that one could best understand a fellow human
being if one had a life-film of him depicting him in
all public and private situations, Hans Thomae[9] chose
the method of "Lebenslaufanalyse" as the via regia of
longitudinal studies in developmental psychology. Where
psychology was "clinically" orientated from the outset,
as in psychonalysis, the principle of order and reference system of analytical hermeneutics has always been
the biographical chronology[10] of the patient - often
in striking contrast to psychoanalytical theory, whose
mythological basis was determined by the "Zeitgeist"
of physicism. The temporality of phenomena, the chronological order of personal development and maturation
urges one to find out in a biographical analysis what
has happend to the individual in certain fundamental
situations, lived through by any human being, and
particularly in critical situations (or threshold
situations) of transition from one period of life
to the next.

---

9) H. Thomae: Das Individuum und seine Welt, Göttingen
   1968.
10) Cf. my article: "Das Zeitproblem in Freuds Psycho-
    analyse." in: Zeitschr. f. klinische Psychol. u.
    Psychoth. 3 (23) 1975, S. 214 ff.

The failure in any phase seems to have its typical
symptoms, symptoms of the failure to deal with the
prevalent theme of a particular phase of life: themes
such as nutrition and growth, the integration into
the ritual of cleanliness, the confrontation of
one's own will with authorities, finding one's role
within a group of brothers and sisters and children
of the same age, the integration into the institution
"school" and the motivation of learning, the
enlargement of the field of one's activities, the
"flight from home" — the emotional transcendence
over egocentrisen, the detachment from the self, the
search for ideals (or idols) and discovery of the
non-ego in the Eros.

APPLICATION OF KLAGES' CHARACTEROLOGY TO PSYCHIATRY

Toyoji Akada

Tokyo Women's Medical College

10 Kawada-cho, Shinjuku-ku, Tokyo, Japan

The appeal of Prof. Pauleikhoff, that we must get back the soul which has been lost in psychiatry since Griesinger, is very significant especially concerning the fact, that his appeal is connected closely with a general trend of our time. Ludwig Klages was warning against destroying the nature and losing the human soul, which are both going on hand in hand. As his psychology including his characterology is based on his philosophy of the life and its connection with the ego (life or biocentric philosophy), it is quite useful to apply this psychology to psychopathology or psychiatry. Klages himself made a great contribution to psychopathology with his theory of hysteria and psychopathia, and some psychiatrists made use of his psychological findings for their psychopathological study. In Japan 25 years ago Chidani and his collaborators analysed and reported symptoms of fugue, obsession and hysteria which appeared on the basis of endogenous depression, and also symptoms of children depression. Then he made a unique diagramm of manic-depressive disease applying fundamental notions of Klages' characterology. In 1975 at the 1st meeting of the austrian-german-japanese society for psychiatry Shibata reported that in some cases of acute delusion of percecution a manic life process is the basis for this psychose. In 1980 at the 2nd meeting of that society I analysed a case in which such a delusion occured several times.

Now I present a tridimensional view of endogenous psychoses applying Klages' sketch of the personality architecture. According to him a person consists of life and ego. The life can be expressed as an ellipse polarized to the foci of the body and the soul. (Fig. 1) The ego as the centre of human activities is located above the ellipse, in equal distance from both foci, and communicates, while

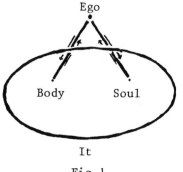

Ego

Body   Soul

It

Fig.1.

Table 1. Fundamental notions of characterolog,

1. Material (talents, quantative properties)
2. Structure (properties of relation, proportional attributes)
3. Nature (driving forces, properties of direction)
4. Framework or architecture
5. Pseudo-typical action of character upon communal life
6. Constant qualities of behaviour

Table 2. System of Driving forces

Spiritual driving forces	
Releases	Bonds
A. Spiritual self-devotion= Capacity for enthusiasm	A. Spiritual self-assertion=Reason
1.Thirst for truth	1.Theoretic reason
2.Formative impulse	2.Aesthetic reason
3.Love of justice	3.Ethical reason Sense of duty, Conscience (Sense of remorse)

Personal driving forces	
B. Personal self-devotion= Depth of feeling	B. Personal self-assertion=Egoism
1.Spontaneous trendencies towards devotion	1.Driving forces towards the extension of the ego (spontaneous egoism)
2.Passive tendencies towards devotion	2.Driving forces for preservation of the ego (passive egoism) Prudence, Watchfulness, Suspicion, Timidity
3.Reactive tendencies towards devotion	3.Driving forces for rehabilitation of the ego

(simplified)

awake, always with both poles of the life. The signs of this
communication are the feelings. The acts of will arise from the
ego, being accompanied by feelings. The ego is the spirit, which
has found its dwelling in a human being. The life and the ego work
together or struggle with each other, so that various relations
arise between life and ego. Both principles take part in each of
the six fundamental notions of Klages' characterology.[2,3] (table 1,
table 2).

For the psychopathology of endogenous psychoses two of them
are specially important: proportional attributes (Verhältniseigen-
schaften) and driving forces (Triebfedern). The former include
    a capacity for stimulation of feelings,
    a capacity for stimulation of will,
    and a personal capacity for expression.
These capacities consist of a driving factor and an inhibiting
factor which both stand in the same relation as dividend and divisor
in a fraction, for example

    capacity for stimulation of will=urge force (Triebkraft):
    inhibition (Widerstand).

Those three quotients are personal constants in one's usual life,
but undergo a change by manic-depressive psychoses.

While animals are driven to a target by a feeling of want
(urge-force), human being strive to attain a purpose which they
have set for themselves. The cause of an act of will is a driving
force, which at the same time is the disposition of a feeling.
The will gets its moving energy from the urge-force and steers it
to its own purpose so that a driving force possesses energy and
direction. Klages classifies the driving forces first into those
of releases (self-devotion) on the left hand and those of bonds
(self-assertion) on the right hand. Then each is divided into two
groups: spiritual driving forces above and personal driving forces
below. Thus we obtain the four main groups. The group right below,
that is that of personal self-assertion, is the most important one
for psychopathology. Klages divides it further into three subgroups:
driving forces for the extension of the ego (spontaneous egoisms),
those for its preservation (passive egoisms) and those for its
rehabilitation (reactive egoisms).

Now I try to applicate these notions to the symptomatology
of endogenous psychoses. In manic forms on the life level at the
body pole such symptoms as light, quick and excessive movements,
flushing of the skin etc. are dominant. At the soul pole bright
mood is found, which changes abruptly to irritation, being influenced
by the ego. Symptoms such as strong impression, short sleep and
awaking in the early morning are in the middle between body and soul.
The middle stage which mediates the life and the ego is governed by

symptoms, speaking in usual terminology, of hyperbulia and flight of ideas on the left hand and emotional lability on the right hand. We can explain these as results of an increase of the proportional attributes which is due to a growth of the driving factors as well as a reduction of the inhibiting factors in the fractions mentioned above. In this way the inhibiting factors are overcome by the growth of the driving factors. The symptoms of the middle stage as well as on the life level are characteristic rather for a disease than for a person. Above on the ego level, accentuated by a high-pitched self-feeling, a tendency of self-extension prevails in general. But a personal disposition of resistance to expression, connected with inhibiting driving forces, struggles with the manic energy and brakes the self-extending tendency. These inhibiting driving forces are driving forces of self-preservation and ethical reason (sence of duty, sence of remorse), which is one of the driving forces of spiritual self-assertion. On the right hand we see the symptoms in which the high-pitched self-feeling appears almost without inhibition: self-conceit, haughtiness, arrogance and megalomania. In the middle there are the symptoms of somewhat stronger inhibition, that means symptoms which are most common to manic states: impudent, shameless, too familiar, optimistic etc. On the left hand there are the symptoms, in which we find a strongest tendency of inhibition against self-extension: expressly, artificial, criticism, sarcastic, litigious. These symptoms on the ego level are personal attributes, which have been provoked to appear by the changes in the middle stage and in the life level. The variety of the symptoms on the ego level is due to the degree to which the ego is benumbed by manic energy like in a drunken state. When the struggle between manic energy and inhibition is or becomes very serious, schizophrenic forms appear.

The depressive forms are in almost all points contrary to the manic forms. The quotients of the proportional attributes become smaller and the self-feeling is low-pitched. Various symtoms on the ego level can be explained as depending upon the degree to which the ego is carried away by the low-pitched self-feeling (fugue, delusion of bilittlement) or the self-esteem struggling against this feeling (obsession, hysteria).

The schizophrenic forms appear, as mentioned, from a serious struggle between increase of the urge-forces deriving from a manic energy and resistance to expression plus inhibiting driving forces. A person of such a character cannot accept the least excess of energy, which could lead to self-extension, because it means a step over the limit, that is to say a delict in his eyes. According to Klages the resistance to expression consists of a tendency to hide some feeling and a sense of honour. The former can be traced back to the world of the animals and the latter is proper to the human society. The resistance to expression has a deep root in the human nature and shows fairly great variety for different races or persons. The increase of urge-forces derives from the manic life process, the resistance to expression belongs to the personality. Both have originally nothing to do with each other. But when an increase of the urge-forces occurs in a man of strong resistance to expression, an internal struggle begins between ego and life. So I have made the arrows of feelings (partially also those of willings) in the personality skech by Klages confront each other, particularly for schizophrenic forms. The energy, which would be used otherwise for hyperbulia, is exhausted by the inner struggle, so that in the middle stage we see incoherence and bloking of thinking, ambivalence, bewilderment on the left hand, anxious tension and delusional mood on the right hand.

The self-feeling is threatened with ruin, against which the self-esteem stands up. On the ego level the symptoms of watchfulness, self-relating and ideas of perception appear, which are often connected with auditory hallucinations. Also disturbance of activity-consciousness or obstruction of will arises often which are expressed by patients as "thought is made, understood, taken off, broadcast etc." Those belong according to K.Schneider to schizophrenic symptoms of the first rank. Concerning their essence, the theories of "permeability of the ego-circumstance-fence" by Schneider and "unhiddening(Entbergung)" by Zutt are very interesting, because these conceptions put in words what the patients fear most: to be exposed defenceless in public. There is reflected an internal process, in which the resistance to expression, though it is strong, cannot completely overcome the increase of urge-forces.

Below on the life level there are symptoms, which show the increase of urge-force, being modified by the ego in danger: impulsive or automatic movements, stiffness and catalepsy at the body pole, uncanny or extatic mood at the soul pole.

While in fairly many cases of catatonic and paranoid forms the symptoms disappear sooner or later like in the case of a simple mania, some cases recover after their symptoms have first changed into those of simple mania. But in other cases such symptoms as megalomania, delusion of perception and hallucinations on the state of abulia continue to exist even after the manic life-process has passed away. They result from the struggle of a person against the world, which is the struggle of the ego against the life from the viewpoint of personality architecture. In these cases, I suppose, that loosening or slit has occured between ego and life (chronic forms).

In hebephrenic forms the symptoms of watchfulness, anxiety, fractional ideas of perception and grandness appear on one hand and an optimistic, euphoric mood and childish, foolish behaviours on the other hand. The patient talks sometimes about his own doings or states, as if he were a looker-on. We notice here twofold egos: the one, which is driven by an increased urge-force, and the other, which remains still observing the former coolly. That is one of the facts which prove the loosening mentioned above. In hebephrenic forms it occurs probably from the beginning. Though it is provoked by an increased urge-force due to manic life-process, its disposition being provided in the personality architecture. Figure 2 shows that both factors, manic life-process and fall of character architecture, participate each differently, may be nearly in inverse ratio, in varions syndroms of endogenous psychoses.

Klages says, that the basis of schizophrenia is separation of an individual life from the universal life. I add to this that we must search for the premise for such a separation in the ego-life-loosening in one's character architecture.

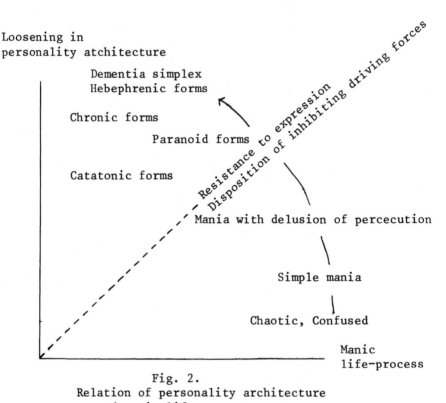

Fig. 2.
Relation of personality architecture
and manic life-process

REFERENCES

1. L.Klages, Vorschule der Charakterkunde, in:"Ludwig Klages Werke, Bd. 4," Bouvier, Bonn (1976).
2. ditto, Die Grundlagen der Charakterkunde. in:ditto.
3. ditto, translated by W.H.Johnson, The Science of Character, George Allen & Unwin, London (1929).

BORDERLINE SITUATIONS AND DELUSION

Hermann Lenz

Chiefdoctor

4020 Linz, Landstraße 32, Austria

Science is based on the laws of logic and causalation.
Life is a most complex event and so it will be understand only
partly by scientific research. Much more it is complicated to
make use of science in psychopathology. Psychopathology is in the
first time experience of the verbal and non verbal contact between Ego and Thou, it is a subjective experience. Thou are not
only humans thou is also the culture and the nature.
Psychopathology is based on a phenomenological description of
subjective experience of thou. By the method of comparisons of
psychopathology experiences with same meaning it is permitted
to come upon relative valid statements. But we have to examine
the relation of Ego and thou in all directions and we have also
to grasp psychopathology experiences in the space of time.

The borderline situations of human existence is a most interesting psychopathologic phänomenon. The humans will be aware
frequently of his own spiritual Ego in such situations. Borderline situations cannot be understood only on a logical way, here
it is also necessary on irrational way. Borderline situations are
always polar situations. The following different borderline
situations are in reality only the various facets of one and the
same borderline situation of humans. In such a situation it is
possible to see ever the border of our real existence, but our
insight into the Transcendency will be remain incomplete.

Following situations will be explained:
1.) The harm and suffer of ourselves and with other persons and
    the polar situation: the experience of love.
2.) The guilt and the acknowledgement of sin closly bound up
    with responsibility. The polar situation is the experience
    of salvation.
3.) The experience of loss of personal freedom closly bound up
    with existential anxiety. The polar situation is hope — as the
    Roman poet Cicero wrote.
4.) The loss of thou, the infinite loss of all. It would be the
    experience of eternity, if there is no process or becoming
    in such experiences but it means death, if something runs its
    course.
5.) The loss of his own Ego. The normal man cannot make it clear
    himself, we can it experience only in delusion. The polar
    situation is the regeneration (rebirth) of Ego.
6.) The loss of time, which the man experiences in the loss of
    thou and Ego. The polar situation would be the experience of
    eternity.
7.) The borderline situations of dying. It can be experienced only
    in rare and favourable situations and it was described in
    former times in the death—books. There are horrible events
    but also experiences of bliss.

New experiences of much situations are refered by Hampe,
Kübler-Ross, Moody, etc.
Delusion is also a borderline situation, it is the sacrifice of
man as a spiritual human (H.Ey.)
Delusions demonstrates us all the different facets of borderline
situations. Such situations can we also observe in the beginning
of creative acts (art, science, religions)

Now I intend to give you examples of borderline situations in
delusions and also opposite to it examples of borderline
situations in art. I shall select examples of modern literature.
I hope to make it evident, that there is no crisis of
psychopathology.Certainly, the presupposition is, that
psychopathology has no permission to exclude the human as a
spiritual being and have to realize the connection of Ego and
Thou and also the in-definiteness of his history. Examples of
modern literature will make all borderline situations more
understandable for anybody as borderline situations in delusions.

1.) The borderline situation of harm:
    A women with delusions has had the opinion to be Theresia von
    Lisieux,who was well known by her intercessions and so has
    healed many people. She told us she could heal another nun
    with a paralysis of the leg, because she have had two stars —
    belief and hope — in front of her and Christus in her mind.

Upon a time she had bad luck, she could not arrest the two
stars and now all was lost and harm was immeasurable. The
patient had two years later a similar delusion. In the opinion
to take over the harm of the people of Biafra by meditation
she experienced some time later the rupture of her meditation.
Harm and feeling of guilt remained in her mind.
A.Camus describes the borderline situations of harm in his
novel:"The pest". All doors of the city were closed and so
the inhabitants were excluded from what was happening in the
world. The only future of the inhabitants was to dy earlier or
later in their city. But that was no real future and A.Camus
describes how the heart of the inhabitants turned into stones.
All love disappeared more and more and harm becomes infinite.
The clergyman Paneloux says in the novel infront if his own
death:"Such borderline situations can only be tolerated by
self-sacrifice as it was realized by the medical doctors in
the city, or by faith in god".

2.) The borderline situations of guilt:
A wood-carver accused himself in his delusion to have sold his
masterworks (Christus or angels) and not have made a present
of it. He accused also his sister not have made a present of
her big inheritance for poor people. He have had a life of sin
and he heared the last trumpet to condemm him. In his opinion:
"He will be sent to the hell, because he was the origin of
all human death".
Max Frisch describes in the parabel: "In the time of the end
of the war", a woman, who could not bear for longer time her
guilt. In a German city she had to give a Russian officer
lodging. She hided in her cellar her husband, a German officer,
who has participated in the Jew massacre in Warschau.
The wife invited the Russian officer for a dinner and have gone
to bed with him. All that was done to take away any suspicion
somebody could be hided in her house. But the jealous husband
looked up to the room and was discovered as a German officer
participated in the massacre. The Russian officer went out to
take care for the woman. Now begins a discussion between the wife
and husband.He defends his behaviour with self preservation and
his wife would have acted in the same way. But the wife has
taken the guilt of adultery to save his life. Now she could
not bear guilt and commit suicide. Guilt remains always.

3.) The borderline situation of loss of freedom:
A psychotic woman has lost her speech and handwriting, but
also her own thinking, will and feeling. All was raped by a
medical doctor and she could speak, think, write only as the
doctor demanded. Laser-rays produced by a computer controlled
her behaviour, she was a "ray-model" for the science. Her
own did not exist, she was the instrument or the machine of
an other human.

1097

E.Canetti delineated the loss of freedom in the novel
"Delayed". The persons in his novel bear a capsule around the
neck, which contains the date of birth and death. The persons
didnt know their age and it was forbidden to open the
capsule. For the persons was the prohibition of opening a restriction of their freedom. Later the discussions of the
persons give as a result, that opening of capsules succeeded
in loss of freedom, because now all is determinded, everybody
lives in death-agony.

4.) The borderline situation of loss of thou:
In a melancholic delusion was the patient of the opinion,
that the houses of the city were only traps, the wire from
the head to her hands were dead. She had lost her feeling,
her heart was absorbed. In the place of heart was only ice.
All confidence was put away. The world stands still, nothing
becomes, darkness was dawned to all eternity. She wished
passionately to die, because dying is a process, which comes
to an end.
G.Benn has given an example for such a person in the figure
of Rönne in his novel "The brains".
Rönne told us he has no opposite, he could not be in relation
to anything, he has no influence on space or time. He rested
and didn't come in contact with anything. Benn declares such
a borderline situation as a life in crystal. Such a
constitution is labelled in psychiatry as petrification

5.) The borderline situation of Ego - loss.
The loss of Ego is frequently reported in delusion. One
patient informed us, that the former Ego was vanished, but
now she has got the real Ego. She had two father, one is the
material father, one-namely god - the spiritual father. Some
weeks later she had lost her real Ego, she called herself as
a dead person and later as a machine, which "lives
theoretical". Another psychotic man designated himself as
magic-puppet, he would not be a human. His eyes were put in or
are wood-eyes. He "Dies permanent", his situation would be
everlasting and he would be also on other planets.
V.Gesattel reports about a psychotic man: " I am the
nothingness and so I dont't exist. The death would be better,
but the death doesn't exist as death. I am dead and so I
don't need the idea of death, because I am the death".
The loss of Ego is scarcely described in poetry. Only
Hölderlin have experienced such a situation. He wrote:
"I feeling myself dead","I don't participate in the time" or
"I shout to myself the horror-word: You are a living dead man".
E. Jonescu have written upon the loss of identy of the persons
Smith and Martin in the novel "The bald-headed singer".

6.) The loss of time will be described by psychotic patients with
the words "Time is stopped" or I experience the eternity. In
her delusions expressed a patient "she are dying endless",
"she was, is and will be in anytime", "She originate in
nothingness", she speaks with dead people, etc. We can hear
also that they are "ghost".
In poetry S.H.Lawrence mentions the experience of "Time is
stopped" in his novel "The rainbow". The lovers Will and
Ann tell us, that there was "Eternity in their embrace", or
"all was a moment, all former events were extinguished".
"Will was with Ann entombed in darkness" or "The big cycle
in the centre was without any movement, here dominated
celibrated stillness with-drawn from time". In blessed moments
we can experience eternity as it is asserted in the great
religions.

7.) The borderline situation of dying is not observed in
delusion, only the death of the own Ego. In poetry dying is
narrated in so far as the death of closely connected person is
described. The closely connected person is a part of myself and
so I can experience - partly - my dying. Th.Bernhard has written
a book named "Breathing". A young patient sees continuous how
other patient die without to be disconcerted. But he can for
the first time experience dying, as he stands on the extreme
point of his own life. Such a situation makes up one mind in
order that we become not engulfed in worth-lessness.
Bernhard is of the opinion, that the borderline situation of
dying guide to the mind of ourself. Th.Wilder tells about
the meeting with death in his novel "We got off once more".
Here is the death represented as iceberg, with which everyone
is confronted. Iceberg is also a symbol of life without love.
The meeting with death is only possible if hope and love is
in our heart. (Th.Wilder)

The borderline situations of human namely harm and love, guilt and
salvations, loss of freedom and hope, Loss of Thou, loss of time
and eternity, loss of Ego and reincarnation, dying, and bliss are
all phenomenon of the human. In delusion we observe first of all
the negative part of borderline situations. The cause of it is,
that loss of freedom and existential anxiety is in the forefront of
delusions. In delusion we are often not able to hope.
Borderline situations are reported within the memory of man.
An example for it is the admixture of ochre in the tombs of ancient
China, which are dated in the old Stone age. Ochre was the sign of
ritual blood and probable the borderline situation of dying was
the oldest one. I think we can better unterstand delusions if we
have experienced borderline situations or have read about it in
novels or romances. To comprehend psychopathology, especially

delusion we cannot only make use of rational arguments, we have
also to take in account the subjective experience. The origin of
Such experiences belongs frequently to the irrational sphere.
Delusion is a model of behaviour restricted to humans. The
subjective and irrational experience in the borderline situation
of myself and also feeling with others in similar situations has
also a validity, although it has not the same validity as the
result of rational arguments. But delusion as borderline
situation can never be fully explained, it can at best be understood.

AUTHOR INDEX

SUBJECT INDEX

SUMMARY

CONTENTS OF

VOLUMES 1-8

VOLUME 1

CLINICAL PSYCHOPATHOLOGY

NOMENCLATURE AND CLASSIFICATION

VOLUME 2

BIOLOGICAL PSYCHIATRY

HIGHER NERVOUS ACTIVITY

VOLUME 3

PHARMACOPSYCHIATRY

VOLUME 6

DRUG DEPENDENCY AND ALCOHOLISM

FORENSIC PSYCHIATRY

MILITARY PSYCHIATRY

VOLUME 7

EPIDEMIOLOGY AND COMMUNITY PSYCHIATRY

VOLUME 8

HISTORY OF PSYCHIATRY

NATIONAL SCHOOLS

EDUCATION

TRANSCULTURAL PSYCHIATRY